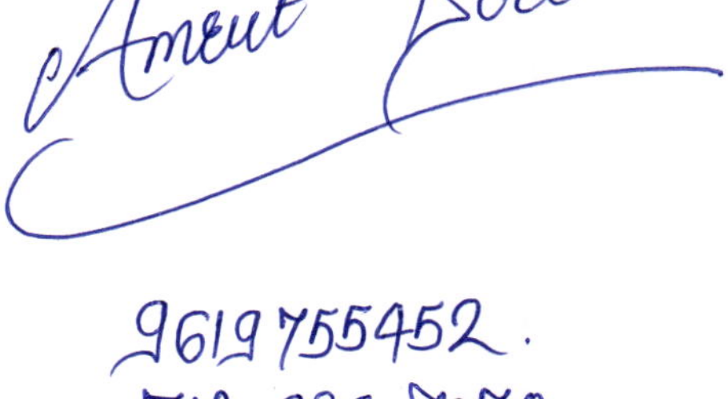

9619755452.
312-626-7030.

ARTHROSCOPIC SHOULDER SURGERY *and* RELATED PROCEDURES

HARVARD ELLMAN, M.D.

Associate Clinical Professor
Orthopaedic Surgery
University of California at Los Angeles
Center for the Health Sciences
Medical Director
The Shoulder Institute
Los Angeles, California

GARY M. GARTSMAN, M.D.

Clinical Associate Professor
Department of Orthopedics
Baylor College of Medicine
Fondren Orthopedic Group
Houston, Texas

TIMOTHY C. HENGST, FAMI

Medical Illustrator
Thousand Oaks, CA

ARTHROSCOPIC SHOULDER SURGERY *and* RELATED PROCEDURES

1 9 9 3

Lea & Febiger

PHILADELPHIA • BALTIMORE • HONG KONG
LONDON • MUNICH • SYDNEY • TOKYO

A WAVERLY COMPANY

Lea & Febiger
Box 3024
200 Chester Field Parkway
Malvern, Pennsylvania 19355-9725
U.S.A.
(215) 251-2230

Executive Editor–Darlene Barela Cooke
Development Editor–Sharon R. Zinner
Project Editor–Denise Wilson
Production Manager–Michael DeNardo

Library of Congress Cataloging-in-Publication Data

Ellman, Harvard.
Arthroscopic shoulder surgery and related procedures / Harvard Ellman, Gary M. Gartsman.
p. cm.
Includes index.
ISBN 0-8121-1492-2
1. Shoulder joint—Endoscopic surgery. 2. Shoulder joint—Surgery. I. Gartsman, Gary M. II. Title
[DNLM: 1. Arthroscopy. 2. Rotator Cuff—surgery. 3. Shoulder—surgery. 4. Shoulder joint—surgery. WE 810 E47a 1993]
RD557.5.E45 1993
617.5'72059—dc20
DNLM/DLC
for Library of Congress 92-48440
CIP

NOTE: Although the author(s) and the publisher have taken reasonable steps to ensure the accuracy of the drug information included in this text before publication, drug information may change without notice and readers are advised to consult the manufacturer's packaging inserts before prescribing medications.

Reprints of chapters may be purchased from Lea & Febiger in quantities of 100 or more. Contact Sally Grande in the Sales Department.

PRINTED IN THE UNITED STATES OF AMERICA

Print number: 5 4 3 2 1

DEDICATION

To the educators and innovators in shoulder surgery and arthroscopy who have guided us and inspired this text, and to Noël and Carol for their love and understanding throughout this endeavor.

FOREWORD

It is a privilege to write this foreword for "Arthroscopic Shoulder Surgery and Related Procedures" by Dr. Harvard Ellman and Dr. Gary M. Gartsman. Their objective in this work is to integrate arthroscopy into the diagnosis and treatment of shoulder disorders. Because both authors are experienced open shoulder surgeons as well as pioneers and leaders in the development of shoulder arthroscopy, they have been able to present the use of the arthroscope in the shoulder in a most authoritative and responsible manner.

With the greater understanding of shoulder pathology and the rapid improvements in operative technique and rehabilitation of the shoulder that have developed during recent years, shoulder surgery is now frequently performed all over the world. As expected, shoulder arthroscopy has become widely used. Unfortunately, arthroscopy is too frequently misused. The arthroscope is an instrument of great value when properly applied in the right situation. However, it does not alter the need for correct diagnosis and understanding of the pathology and it does not alter the objectives of surgery. At times, these objectives may be better achieved with the scope but at other times may be better achieved with open surgery. In each section of this book, the authors have defined the pathology under discussion as well as the uses and limitations of the scope. Wherever the scope may be of value, their preferred technique is expertly described.

This book is so well written and illustrated that it makes reading pleasant. The content is timely and important for all surgeons and residents who contemplate doing shoulder procedures. Undoubtedly, it will be widely quoted and of lasting value.

Charles S. Neer, II, M.D.
Professor Emeritus and Special Lecturer
Orthopaedic Surgery
Columbia University
New York, New York
Founding President
American Shoulder and Elbow Surgeons

PREFACE

The era of treating shoulder disorders without benefit of arthroscopy has ended. The arthroscope has established its value in many avenues of research, diagnosis, and treatment of this complex joint.

It is as implausible to consider that all future shoulder surgery will be done by arthroscopic techniques as it is inconceivable to believe that all such surgery will be done solely by open operative intervention in the future. It is equally implausible to consider that a surgeon who has been trained in the discipline of open surgical reconstruction can become a proficient arthroscopist without arduous instruction and practice in gaining these new techniques.

In a similar vein, the surgeon who has acquired great skill performing arthroscopy within the knee or other joints cannot expect to enter the shoulder and operate successfully without acquiring diagnostic acumen and the ability to perform open surgical procedures when indicated.

To the extent that orthopaedic subspecialization extends to include only a single joint, there should be no "shoulder arthroscopist"—only a shoulder surgeon who is skilled in both open and arthroscopic techniques and has the judgment to apply each appropriately.

The shoulder joint, all too neglected in the past, has enjoyed an explosion of interest in the recent decade. More original research, clinical studies, and textbooks have been published during this period than ever before. Lectures, seminars, and hands-on laboratory sessions are widely available and maximally attended. The resultant level of competence among the orthopaedic community is becoming comparable to that enjoyed by the hip and the knee in prior decades.

This book is designed to instruct surgeons and allied medical professionals in the skills and understanding necessary to perform and assist in shoulder arthroscopy. The constraints of space within this text require that we assume the reader has acquired a basic level of competency in the use of arthroscopic equipment. Many will have acquired these skills within the knee over years of practice. Recent residents and fellows have learned techniques in both the knee and shoulder simultaneously. We intend to guide both groups into the advanced techniques of arthroscopic shoulder surgery.

This text does not dwell extensively on the anatomy and function of the shoulder. Others have already done so admirably. We will, however, consider in detail the preoperative evaluation and arthroscopic findings in most of the frequently encountered shoulder disorders. The various sections include rotator cuff disease, instability, glenohumeral arthritis, and miscellaneous affections of the shoulder. When the established diagnosis is amenable to arthroscopic technique, the reader will find step-by-step guidance. When open surgical intervention is indicated, the authors will present their preferred technique or refer to the classic sources.

Operating room personnel will find a section describing in detail the equipment necessary for shoulder arthroscopy. Instrument placement on the back table and Mayo stands will be illustrated. Positioning of mechanical instruments, instrument drivers, and video equipment in relation to the patient will be outlined. Rehabilitation, both nonoperative and postoperative, will be described in detail.

The goal of this textbook is to integrate shoulder arthroscopy into the study and treatment of shoulder disorders. The arthroscope is a tool to be used by the skillful surgeon when appropriate, sometimes to supplant and at other times to supplement a previously established open technique. The proper application of arthroscopic techniques presented in this text depends on two skills: cognitive and mechanical. Each must be acquired. The practice of both authors is dedicated to shoulder surgery. At this writing, approximately 50% of shoulder procedures are arthroscopic and about 50% require open surgical intervention. Although we anticipate that this percentage will gradually favor the arthroscope, it is our basic premise that the surgeon who brings a patient into the operating room for shoulder intervention should be competent in the performance of both open and arthroscopic techniques.

Los Angeles, California — Harvard Ellman
Houston, Texas — Gary M. Gartsman

ACKNOWLEDGEMENTS

My interest in the shoulder originated from my ignorance of this joint when I began to practice orthopaedic surgery 40 years ago. While Ernest E. Codman and many pioneers who followed him contributed greatly to my lifelong endeavor to learn more about the shoulder, I feel a deep personal debt to Charles Neer II. His research, writings, and teachings have led me and many others to a greater understanding of shoulder disorders and their treatment. Credit also is due to those dedicated physicians (Rowe, Rockwood, Cofield, Post, Matsen, Hawkins, Neviaser and many others) who, along with Neer, created and nurtured the American Shoulder and Elbow Surgeons. This society is dedicated to shoulder research and education and provides a forum through which our knowledge of the shoulder will continue to advance.

There would be no textbook on shoulder arthroscopy without the arthroscopic instruments that were originally developed for use in the knee. The contributions of Takagi, Watanabe, O'Connor, and Johnson, among others in this area, are gratefully acknowledged.

Just as in the knee, shoulder arthroscopy was originally used for diagnostic purposes. I must confess that the idea to perform an acromioplasty using arthroscopic techniques occurred when I blundered into the subacromial space while attempting to enter the glenohumeral joint. The cadaver surgery that followed at UCLA in pursuit of this goal could not have occurred without the cooperation of Phil Mundy, who loaned the Dyonics mechanized shavers and burs, and Judy Lindstrom, who provided the Concept electrocautery system so essential to provide hemostasis when the procedure was moved from the anatomy lab to the operating room in 1983.

In 1985, a preliminary report on the first 10 cases of arthroscopic subacromial decompression was presented at the First Open Meeting of the American Shoulder and Elbow Surgeons. The one- to three-year follow-up results of the initial 50 cases were presented to the Arthroscopy Association of North America in March 1987. This study was awarded the Richard O'Connor Research Award and was published later that year in *Arthroscopy: The Journal of Arthroscopic and Related Surgery*. Ward Casscells, in his Editor's Comments, noted that "This paper appears to push the frontiers of arthroscopic surgery beyond anything that was dreamed of just a few years ago." Dr. Casscells' comments were prophetic of the explosion in surgical arthroscopy of the shoulder that has followed.

To make one small advance beyond the existing knowledge of medical science is the fulfillment of a childhood dream. This text is designed to stand as a way station in the inexorable journey toward better understanding and treatment of shoulder disease. The reader is encouraged to consider and challenge the existing dogma. Surely the techniques advocated here will be modified and improved, and just as surely, the passage of time will prove some of the principles espoused to be inaccurate.

I am most appreciative of the efforts of my co-author Gary Gartsman, whose many contributions and genial collaboration have allowed us to speak in one voice. It is hoped that the reader will recognize the outstanding talent of Timothy Hengst, who worked so diligently with us to produce the many original illustrations in this text. The intra-articular photographs that are such a prominent portion of this book are electronically generated images taken during actual surgery. Much credit is given to Ed and Jan Morgan of Professional Photo Laboratory, Marina Del Rey, California. Their wizardry with computer and film is apparent.

No acknowledgement would be complete without expressing appreciation to my associates over many years (Herman Epstein, Eugene Harris, Irwin Bliss, the late Stanley Katz, Scott Graham, Stephen Kay, and William Brien) for their encouragement and forbearance during this endeavor. Special kudos to Maureen McAdam and Julie Martina, who transcribed this text; to George Mundorff, Darlene Cooke, and the editorial and production staff of Lea and Febiger; and to brother Edgar Ellman, an author of merit, who said this could be done.

HE

Dr. Ellman has paid tribute to the pioneers in shoulder surgery and arthroscopy and I echo his thanks.

Drs. J. Cutler Roberts, Richard Felmus, Robert Replogle, and George Wantz stand out as men who were important in my career.

Dr. Allan Inglis shared with me his enthusiasm for learning and teaching and is really responsible for my interest in academic orthopedics and shoulder surgery. One man can make a difference. He did.

In 1983, Dr. James B. Bennett suggested to me that the arthroscope might be a useful tool in the shoulder. His encouragement continues to this day.

The cadaver work in the Orthopedic Research laboratory at the Baylor College of Medicine demonstrated that an acromioplasty was possible with arthroscopic techniques (later published in *American Journal of Sports Medicine*) and gave me the confidence to proceed in the clinical arena.

The support provided by Dusty Sullivan of Dyonics was invaluable. Pioneering a new field was wonderful yet frightening. Not everything went as smoothly as it does now.

My arthroscopic skills were underwhelming. Drs. G. William Woods and James R. Bocell were kind enough to share their considerable arthroscopic experience.

The Fondren Orthopedic Group, The Methodist Hospital staff, and the Houston and Texas Gulf Coast Orthopedic communities supported my practice of shoulder surgery and provided the patient referrals.

1985 was an exciting year because Harvard Ellman presented his preliminary report on arthroscopic subacromial decompression and suddenly I felt less lonely. Dr. Hugh S. Tullos helped guide my clinical investigations by restraining youthful impulses and encouraging me to publish my work only when I had sufficient numbers with adequate follow-up. The 1990 publication in the *Journal of Bone and Joint Surgery* was the first article in that journal devoted solely to shoulder arthroscopy.

The importance of professional accomplishments assumes some perspective with the passage of time. What will not diminish for me is the great and wonderful experience of collaborating with Harvard Ellman.

He was my orthopedic surgeon when I was injured as a child, a role model during my youth, a source of inspiration in shoulder arthroscopy, and forever a friend. Thanks, Harv.

GMG

CONTENTS

SECTION I THE BASICS

SECTION II ROTATOR CUFF DISORDERS

SECTION III INSTABILITY

SECTION IV THE ARTHRITIDES AND MISCELLANEOUS AFFECTIONS

SECTION V RELATED CONSIDERATIONS

SECTION VI REHABILITATION

I

SECTION

THE BASICS

EVALUATION AND DIAGNOSIS OF PRIMARY SHOULDER DISORDERS

1

This chapter presents a clinical approach to the evaluation and diagnosis of primary shoulder disorders. Shoulder pain may be provoked by a variety of *extrinsic* sources, such as cervical radiculopathy, thoracic outlet syndrome, angina, gallbladder disease, penetrating ulcer, or Pancoast's tumor. These and other less common disorders refer pain *to* the shoulder. The primary shoulder disorders that cause pain to originate *from* the joint are presented in four categories:

1. Rotator cuff disorders (from tendinitis to full-thickness tears).
2. Instability.
3. Arthritis.
4. Miscellaneous affections.

In each of the primary shoulder disorders, symptoms are provoked when the joint is moved. This characteristic is not common when shoulder pain is based on extrinsic sources.

A diagnostic evaluation of primary shoulder disorders begins with a comprehensive history. The "Comprehensive Shoulder Questionnaire" in Appendix I helps to gather pertinent historical data. Age, hand dominance, level of activity, duration of symptoms, trauma, and associated medical conditions can be important to both diagnosis and treatment. The history is followed by a sequential physical examination that includes inspection, palpation, range of motion, and strength determination. Joint stability and neurologic status are carefully assessed.

ROTATOR CUFF DISEASE (IMPINGEMENT SYNDROME)

The impingement syndrome, as delineated by Neer,[1] unifies a constellation of terms, such as bursitis, tendinitis, and partial or full-thickness rotator cuff tears, into a single clinical entity that describes the reactive and degenerative changes that occur within the rotator cuff. The classification further embraces both pathomechanical and therapeutic implications.

Stage I (edema and hemorrhage) is a relatively mild, reversible form of tendon involvement. Stage II (fibrosis and tendinitis) connotes more chronic involvement with fiber failure likely in the more advanced cases. Stage III is the designation used when the rotator cuff is torn. Arthroscopic inspection, which permits the identification of partial tears of the articular surface of the cuff, has led to the classification of rotator cuff tears into partial or full-thickness tears.

CLINICAL FINDINGS

IMPINGEMENT SIGN

The primary physical finding in impingement syndrome, regardless of the stage, is pain on forward elevation with the joint internally rotated (palm down). the scapula should be stabilized (Fig. 1–1). The occurrence of pain within an arc of 70 to 120° is considered a positive impingement sign. Pain occurring when the shoulder is flexed forward to 90° and then internally rotated and adducted may be referred to as the impingement II sign (Fig. 1-2). In this position, pain develops as the greater tuberosity and attached musculotendinous cuff tissue are rotated under the anteromedial aspect of the acromion and beneath the taut coracoacromial ligament.

TENDERNESS

Tenderness is elicited over the anterior margins of the acromion and the coracoacromial ligament. Direct palpation of the tendinous insertion of the supra or infraspinatus in the region of the greater tuberosity is painful. Tenderness of the long head of the biceps as it enters the intertubercular sulcus from above is commonly present.

RANGE OF MOTION

Antalgic restriction of motion in forward flexion, adduction, and internal rotation is frequently noted. Range of motion should be carefully measured in forward flexion, adduction, and internal and external rotation. External rotation is measured with the arm at the side, as well as at 90° of abduction. The degree of motion should be recorded as R/L, except for internal rotation. Internal rotation is described by the anatomic location reached by the thumb behind the back. The inferior tip of the scapula is roughly level with the spinous process of the seventh dorsal vertebra (D7). Mobility in internal rotation then can be expressed, for example, as right thumb touches right sacroiliac joint or lumbar 2 (L2) or dorsal 10 (D10) depending on the spinous process level achieved in the lumbar or dorsal spine. The range of internal rotation with the shoulder in 90° of adduction may be recorded in degrees. The examiner should be aware of the "paradox of the shoulder," i.e., the joint must be fully externally rotated (palm up) to achieve full overhead elevation in pure adduction. External rotation moves the tuberosity posteriorly to avoid impingement directly beneath the acromion. The shoulder capsule tightens as elevation increases, and when the arm is elevated fully overhead, neither internal nor external rotation is possible.

A goniometer should be used for accurate measurements of the angle achieved between the humerus and midline of the trunk in forward flexion and adduction. Measurements are most accurate when made with the patient seated to avoid lumbar hyperextension. When pertinent, both active and passive motion requires documentation. Except for younger individuals and those with

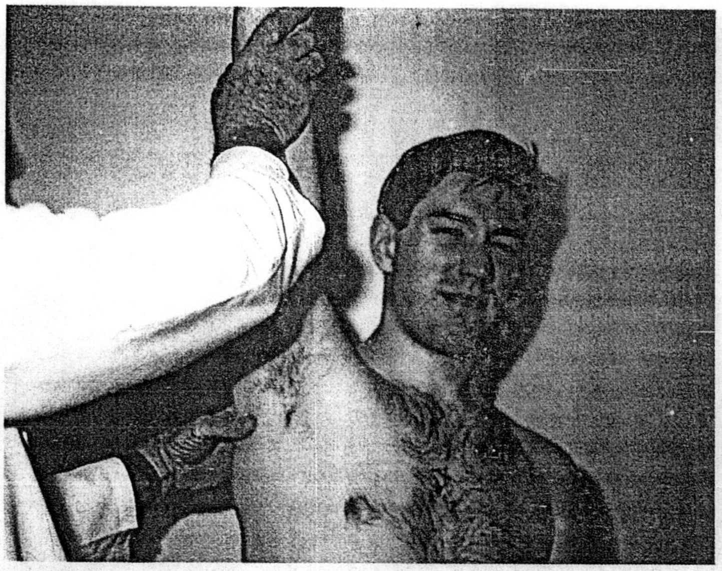

FIG. 1–1. Impingement sign I: Forward elevation with forearm pronated. Stabilize scapula.

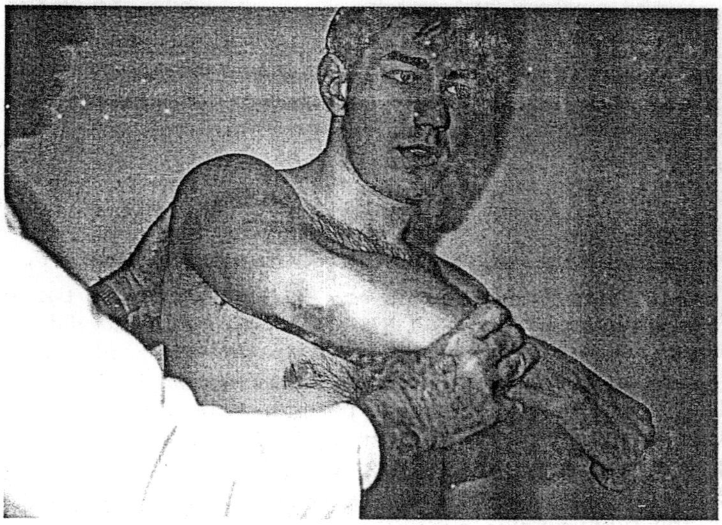

FIG. 1–2. Impingement sign II: Forward flexion to 90° in external rotation, followed by internal rotation and adduction.

increased capsular laxity, a measurement beyond 160 to 170° is unusual for either of these ranges. Elderly and more muscular individuals are usually 10 to 20° below these levels bilaterally. Scapulohumeral rhythm should be observed. The individual contributions of scapulothoracic and glenohumeral joint mobility in patients with stiff joints may be difficult to assess.

STRENGTH

Strength is evaluated in forward flexion, abduction, and external rotation. The result of strength testing is graded on a scale of 0 to 5. (0 = paralysis; 1 = trace;

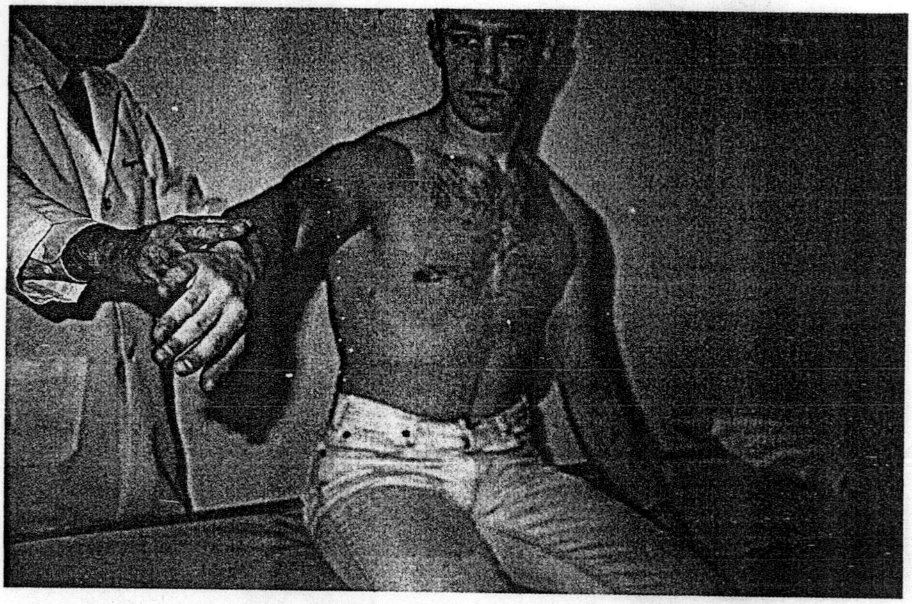

FIG. 1–3. Strength testing with the arm held at shoulder level in the scapular plane. The forearm is pronated.

2 = able to move with gravity eliminated; 3 = able to overcome gravity, but unable to sustain any resistance; 4 = can elevate against gravity and sustain moderate resistance; 5 = normal strength.) Pain inevitably inhibits performance when strength is tested in the area of impingement. Many patients who test clinically weak on the initial examination during elevation can demonstrate normal strength when tested in the subimpingement range of 40 to 60° of flexion or abduction. Ablation of pain by the subacromial injection of local anesthetic (impingement test) permits a more accurate evaluation of the patient's strength. The medication must be properly placed for the test to have validity.

Weakness is the cardinal sign of a full-thickness rotator cuff tear. When weakness is demonstrated in the absence of pain or neurologic disorder, a cuff tear is probable. A full-thickness tear of a portion of the supraspinatus still permits overhead elevation of the arm, but strength is impaired in comparison to that of the opposite extremity. Strength testing with the arm pronated while abducted in the plane of the scapula, midway between forward flexion and full abduction, isolates the supraspinatus directly superior to the joint. Weakness associated with relatively small tears can be determined in this position (Fig. 1–3). If the tear involves both the supra- and the infraspinatus, the patient may be unable to elevate the arm overhead, and the classic "shoulder shrug" may be seen. Weakness in both elevation and external rotation indicates a massive tear.

NEUROGENIC WEAKNESS

Although persistent weakness following pain ablation strongly suggests a cuff tear, other causes of weakness should be considered. Entrapment of the suprascapular nerve may seriously compromise shoulder strength. Other neurogenic factors include post-dislocation deltoid paralysis secondary to axillary injury (Fig 1–4), "winged scapula" secondary to injury to the long thoracic nerve (Fig. 1–5), or "pseudo-winging" secondary to involvement of the trapezius caused by

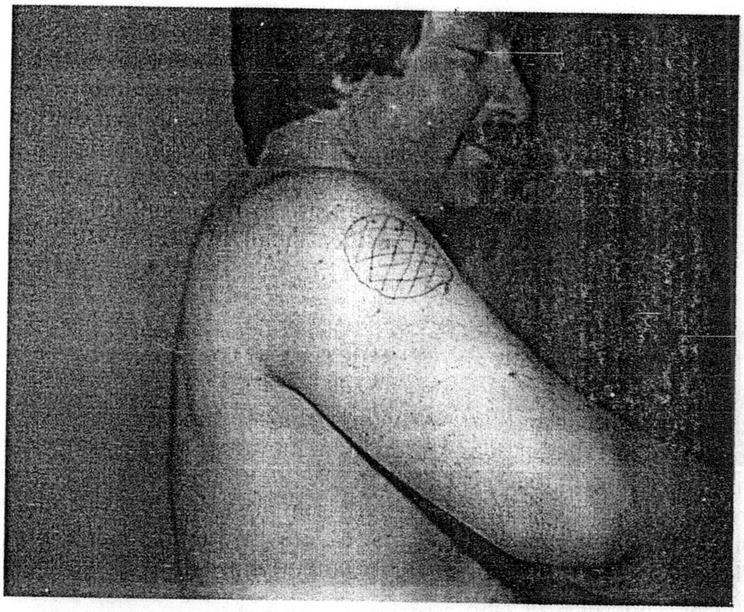

FIG. 1–4. Post-dislocation deltoid paralysis secondary to axillary nerve injury.

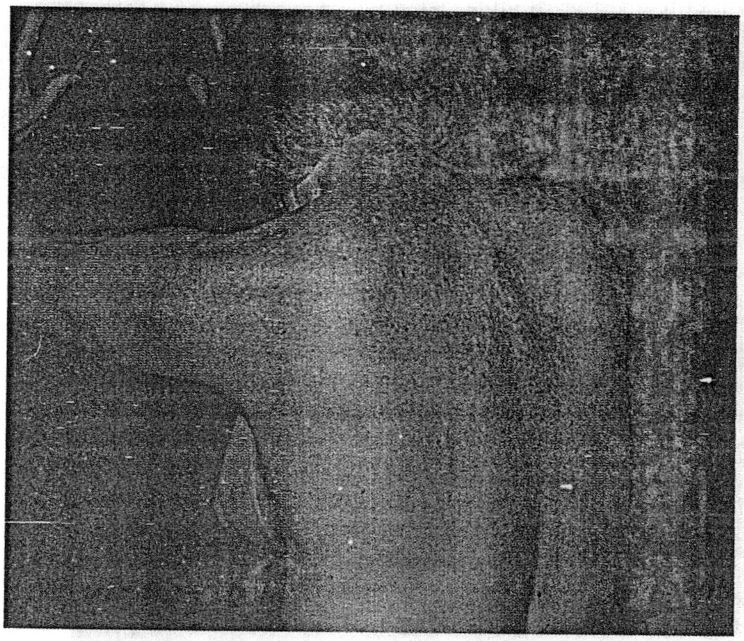

FIG. 1–5. Winged scapula, right, secondary to long thoracic nerve paresis.

injury to the spinal accessory nerve. This trapezius-induced pseudo-winging most commonly occurs when a lymph node biopsy or tumor excision has been performed in the posterior triangle of the neck. Pseudo-winging may also occur in patients with posterior instability. Brachial plexopathy, either viral or traumatic, produces a protean pattern of shoulder girdle and upper extremity weakness. Electrodiagnostic studies can help to sort out these neurogenic factors.

ATROPHY

Subtle atrophy may be discovered by comparison with the opposite shoulder. The scapula may appear skeletonized in long-standing cases of rupture of the supra- and infraspinatus (Fig. 1–6) or of suprascalpular nerve entrapment. Deltoid or trapezius paralysis may also produce profound muscular wasting and can cause the scapular spine and acromion to appear subcutaneous.

The pathomechanics and diagnosis of rotator cuff failure, including diagnostic imaging, are described in further detail in Section II, entitled Rotator Cuff Disorders.

ACROMIOCLAVICULAR JOINT EVALUATION

The acromioclavicular (AC) joint must be independently evaluated during a shoulder examination. A prominent joint may be caused by trauma or degenerative changes. The clavicle rotates with shoulder elevation, and pain originating within the AC joint must be differentiated from the discomfort associated with subacromial impingement. Indeed, downward protruding spurs from an arthritic AC joint may produce impingement independently from a hooked anterior acromion.

Localized tenderness or pain associated with palpation or elevation is the primary clue to AC involvement (Fig. 1–7). Pain occurring with adduction of the arm across the chest at shoulder level is a provocative sign for AC disease (Fig. 1–8). The selective injection of an anesthetic agent into either the AC joint or the subacromial space helps to determine the region from which pain is arising. Plain radiographic films differentiate AC arthritis from chronic second- or third-degree AC separation and demonstrate any spurs arising from the undersurface of the clavicle that might be associated with impingement. The less common condition of osteolysis of the AC joint, occasionally seen in weight-lifters, may

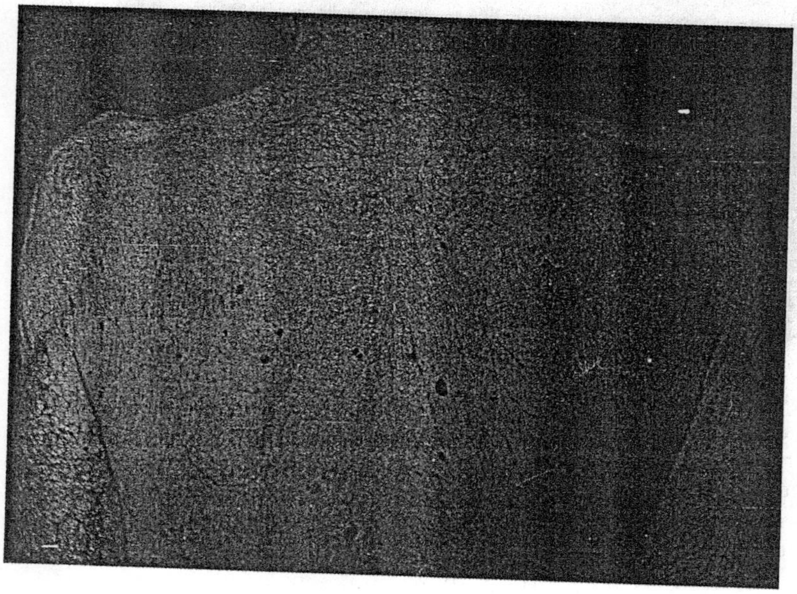

FIG. 1–6. Skeletonized appearance of scapulae following chronic rupture of supra- and infraspinatus.

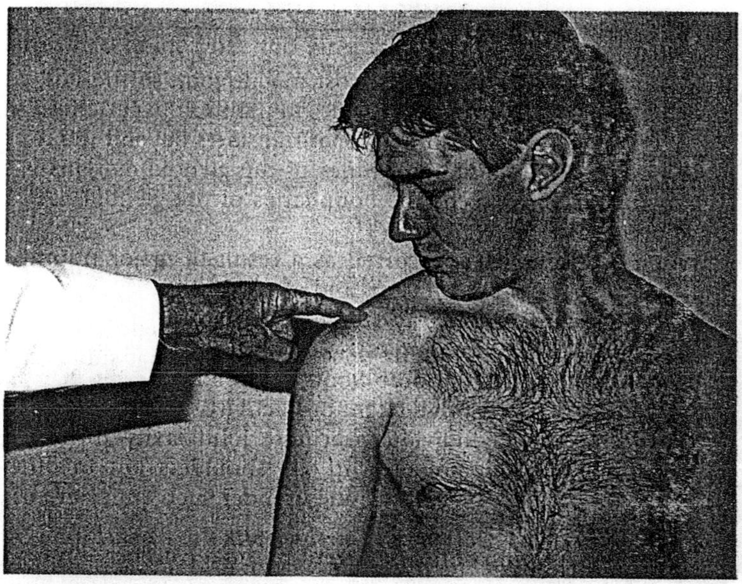

FIG. 1–7. Localized tenderness is a primary symptom of acromioclavicular joint involvement.

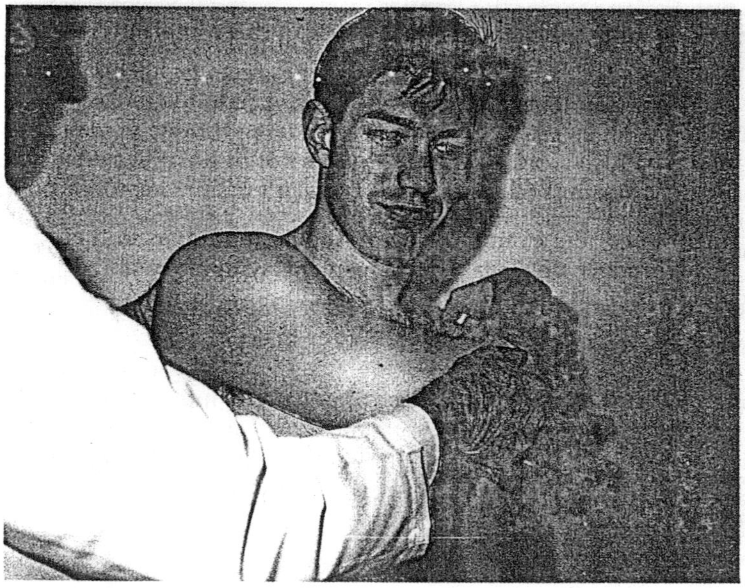

FIG. 1–8. Cross-chest adduction provokes pain in a pathologic acromioclavicular joint.

also be determined by a plain radiographic film. An anteroposterior radiograph of the AC joint taken with 15° cephalic tilt will enhance visualization of the joint.

The differential diagnosis between impingement syndrome and AC disorder can be difficult. A Mumford resection of the outer end of the clavicle does not cure impingement, nor does anterior acromioplasty eliminate the pain of AC derangement. The two disorders may arise concurrently and require a combined procedure.

INSTABILITY

The shoulder is inherently the most mobile joint in the body. The diagnosis of instability can be challenging at times to the most experienced shoulder surgeon. By definition, the humeral head that translates beyond the range of normal but does not totally escape the confines of the glenoid margins is said to *subluxate*. When translation exceeds the boundaries of the glenoid, a *dislocation* is said to have occurred.

When dislocation has occurred as a result of major trauma, the diagnosis is quite simple. The original event, and often subsequent recurrences, may be documented by numerous x-ray studies. Trauma of a less significant degree may stretch or tear the restraining capsule only to the extent that subluxation occurs from that time forward. Some joints are rendered unstable by the cumulative microtrauma of a repetitive strenuous activity, such as throwing, swimming, or weight-lifting. Other individuals acquire joint laxity from their forebears and demonstrate the trait not only in the shoulders but in other joints as well. Trauma, sometimes quite trivial, may render such an inherently lax joint symptomatic.

With the exception of the recurrent traumatic dislocation or of the congenitally lax joint in an individual who has discovered that the voluntary ability to dislocate the shoulder is entertaining to others, the patient with shoulder instability simply appears with a painful shoulder. The examiner must determine from a myriad of possible disorders the cause of this complaint.

HISTORY

The history of shoulder instability is often subtle. The patient may comment that the shoulder slips, slides, clicks, feels loose, or goes dead. If these terms are not mentioned, the examiner always should inquire as to their presence. Instability may produce secondary impingement symptoms, and the patient may erroneously be diagnosed with primary impingement unless instability is searched for and ruled out.

The role of trauma must be carefully considered in the history to determine whether the event was major enough to produce significant injury or something more trivial. The role of repetitive strain must also be analyzed. Finally, the examiner should determine whether the dislocation is *involuntary* or *voluntary*, and, if voluntary, whether it had been initially involuntary and then became voluntary.

PHYSICAL EXAMINATION

Most normal shoulders permit translation of the humeral head in the glenoid fossa. The range of normal varies from one individual to another. As many normal shoulders as possible should be examined to appreciate the degree of laxity that may be present without symptoms. Posterior translation of up to 50% of the head circumference may be normal in the relaxed or anesthetized individual. Anterior translation of from 25 to 33% of the head circumference may be possible in an otherwise asymptomatic shoulder.

DIRECTION, DEGREE, AND CONTROL

The examiner must determine both the direction and the degree of instability. The examiner should conclude whether the *primary direction* of instability is anterior, posterior, inferior, or a combination (multidirectional). The *degree of displacement,* whether subluxation or dislocation, must be determined. Finally, the determination of whether *control* is voluntary, involuntary, or combined should be made during the examination.

INSTABILITY TESTS

Instability testing requires a systematic method of stressing the musculoligamentous supports of the shoulder in an effort to confirm the degree and direction of instability. A description of the most valuable tests follows.

APPREHENSION TEST

This test may be performed with the patient seated (Fig. 1–9A) or preferably, supine (Fig. 1–9B). As the arm is gradually abducted and externally rotated, the examiner presses from behind to translate the humeral head gently forward. The patient's response should be noted at 45°, 90°, and 135° of abduction. The patient with anterior instability becomes increasingly apprehensive as the humeral head translates anteriorly across the labrum toward the position of potential dislocation. The subscapularis no longer exerts any restraining effect of anterior displacement as the arm approaches 90° of abduction. In a positive test, muscular guarding develops at this point. A "positive grab test" may occur as the patient suddenly reaches with the unaffected hand to forcibly restrain the examiner. The patient may complain of posterior and anterior pain caused by capsular stretching. As this

FIG. 1–9. A, Apprehension test, seated: As the arm is abducted and externally rotated, the examiner exerts pressure from behind to translate the humeral head anteriorly. The stability should be tested in 3, 45, 90, and 135° of abduction.
B, Apprehension test performed in a similar fashion while supine. Gentle pressure is applied to translate the shoulder anteriorly.

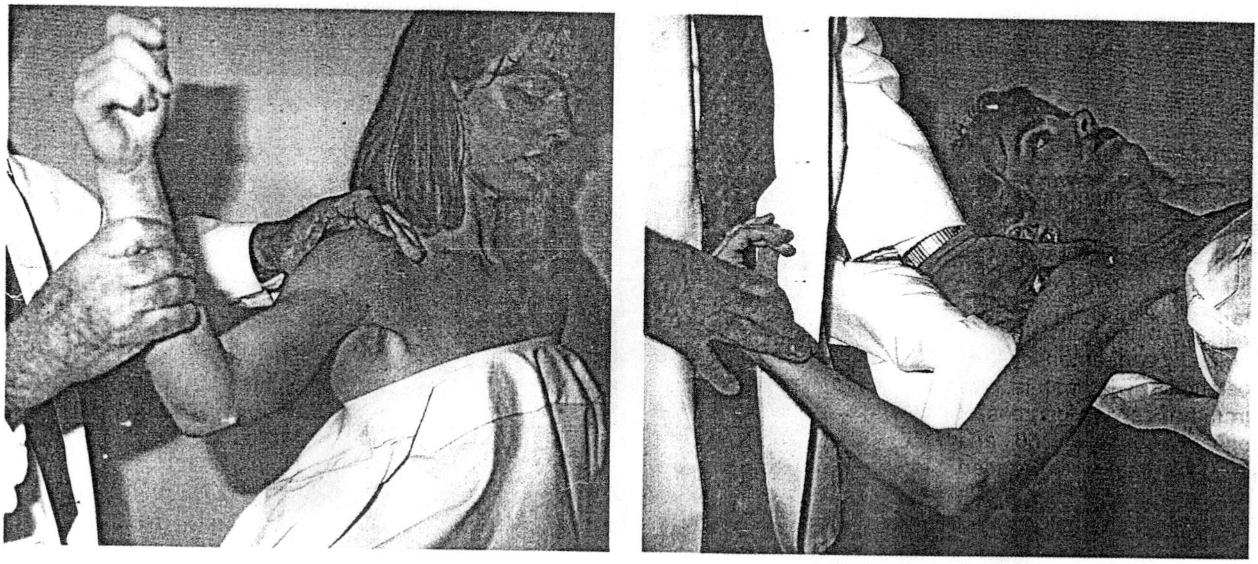

A B

test is performed, a flap of anteroinferior labrum may produce a clicking sound or sensation. This maneuver must be carried out cautiously in patients with recurrent dislocations and a sizable Hill-Sachs' lesion, because external rotation in such patients may produce an unpleasant anterior dislocation during the examination.

ANTERIOR-POSTERIOR DRAWER TESTS[2]

These tests are quite valuable in assessing both anterior and posterior laxity, expecially in the apprehensive patient who will not permit examination in abduction and external rotation. The test is most reliable when the patient is supine. The patient lies comfortably with the arm at the side. The goal is to stabilize the scapula and attempt to translate the humeral head anteriorly or posteriorly in relation to the glenoid without evoking apprehension and muscular guarding. The classic *anterior drawer test* is described with the examiner facing the affected shoulder. The right shoulder is examined by gently lifting the arm from the patient's side and placing the hand in the examiner's right axilla. The hand is held there by adduction of the examiner's humerus (Fig. 1–10). In this position, the humerus is flexed forward about 20° and slightly externally rotated. The scapula is stabilized with the examiner's right hand, which reaches over the top of the patient's shoulder to grasp the patient's scapular spine with the fingers while exerting pressure on the coracoid with the thumb. The examiner's left hand grasps the shaft of the humerus just below the axilla to compress the humeral head against the glenoid and then translates it anteriorly with significant force. The test begins at about 50° of abduction, and abduction continues to increase to as much as 120° as stability is tested.

The examiner must become familiar with normal laxity by examining many shoulders and invariably comparing the affected with the more normal side in each individual patient. If the scapula is not well stabilized, a sense of false anterior laxity may be elicited. Labral clicks may be reproduced, and the patient may volunteer that the shoulder is "about to slip out" when a disorder is present. A patient with anterior labral detachment may give the sensation of both anterior and posterior laxity. This sensation is a false posterior laxity in which posterior subluxation is actually permitted by the lax or torn anterior capsular attach-

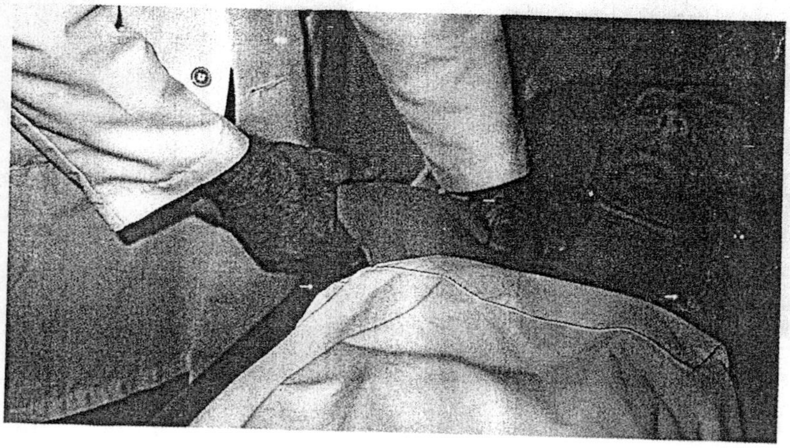

FIG. 1–10. Anterior-posterior drawer test, supine: The patient's arm is supported in the examiner's axilla. One hand stabilizes the scapula while the other translates the humeral head anteriorly and posteriorly. The test is performed at varying degrees of abduction between 50 and 120° while the joint is loaded by slight medial pressure.

ment. In a somewhat similar fasion, patients with marked posterior laxity may simply be subluxed when supine, and efforts to translate the head anteriorly merely move it from behind back into the fossa.

During the *posterior drawer test,* the patient's right elbow is flexed to 90° and lifted by the examiner's right hand to position the shoulder in 20 or 30° of forward flexion and 20 to 30° of abduction (Fig. 1–11). The left thumb of the examiner is placed just lateral to the coracoid process, directly overlying the humeral head anteriorly, the fingers stabilize the spine of the scapula. When downward pressure of the thumb on the humeral head produces abnormal posterior displacement, the effect can be both felt and observed. The patient may confirm that the shoulder feels as though it is slipping out.

A variation of the drawer tests may be performed with the patient seated (Fig. 1–12). The examiner stands behind the patient and, to examine the right shoulder, uses the left hand to hold the lateral clavicle with the fingers and the scapular spine with the thumb for stabilization. With the patient's right hand resting at the side, the examiner's right hand grasps the humeral head and attempts to

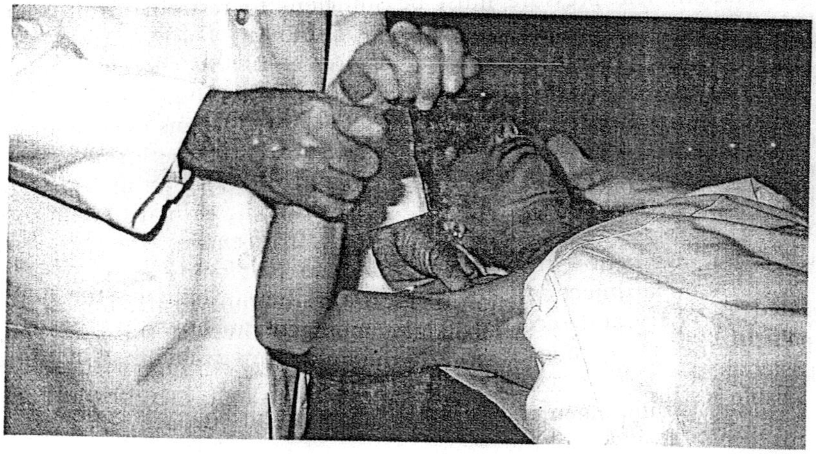

FIG. 1–11. Posterior drawer test: The fingers of the examiner's left hand stabilize the spine of the scapula while the thumb moves lateral to the coracoid and exerts posterior pressure on the humeral head. The patient's arm is held in a position of mild forward flexion and 20 to 30° of abduction.

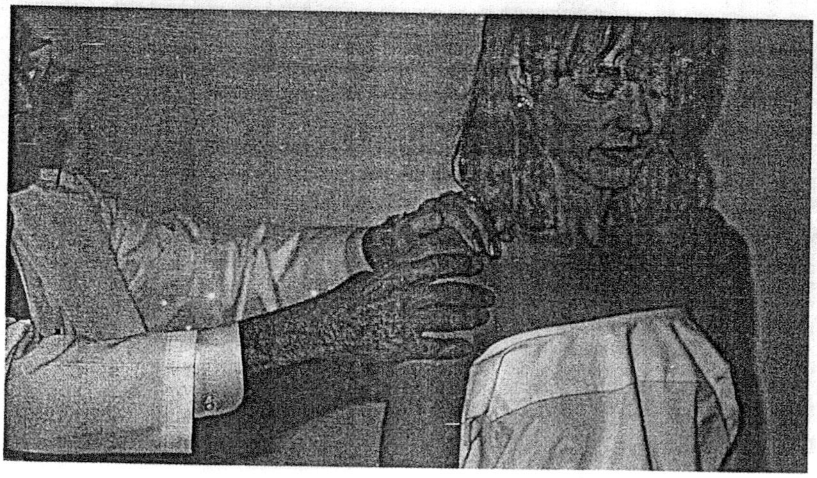

FIG. 1–12. The anterior-posterior drawer test, seated: With the examiner behind the patient, the left hand grasps the clavicle and scapular spine for stability while the right hand translates the shoulder anteriorly and posteriorly.

translate it anteriorly and posteriorly. Patients with hyperlaxity may move easily in either direction. Subtle instabilities are best elicited when the patient is supine and the arm is in some degree of abduction.

FORWARD FLEXION-INTERNAL ROTATION TEST FOR POSTERIOR INSTABILITY

The shoulder of the supine patient protrudes slightly beyond the edge of the examination table. The arm is brought into 90° of forward flexion and about 30° of internal rotation and slight adduction. The scapula is stabilized by its position on the examination table (Fig. 1–13). When pressure is exerted downward on the flexed elbow, the posterior restraints are stressed. Displacement beyond 50% of the humeral head occurs in the presence of pathologic laxity.

COMPRESSION TEST

This test is a variation of the apprehension test. The examiner's palm is placed firmly on the humeral head as the patient's arm is brought into abduction and external rotation. The pressure must be sufficient to restrain the head from translating anteriorly in the patient with instability (Fig. 1–14A). Apprehension may be noticeably overcome by this maneuver. The patient therefore may permit a range of motion wider than that allowed when the head is unsupported. When the examiner's palm is slowly removed, the head begins to slide anteriorly and apprehension returns (Fig. 1–14B). This test must be performed carefully because release of the anterior support may trigger a dislocation in the unstable shoulder. The test can be quite helpful in differentiating primary impingement from impingement secondary to instability. In both instances, the patient may have classic impingement signs, with shoulder pain developing as the arm is elevated. A subacromial injection of local anesthetic eliminates the impingement pain in both primary and secondary impingement; however, the patient with instability continues to demonstrate the findings of instability when the anterior capsule is stressed.

The patient with impingement secondary to instability is generally unable to

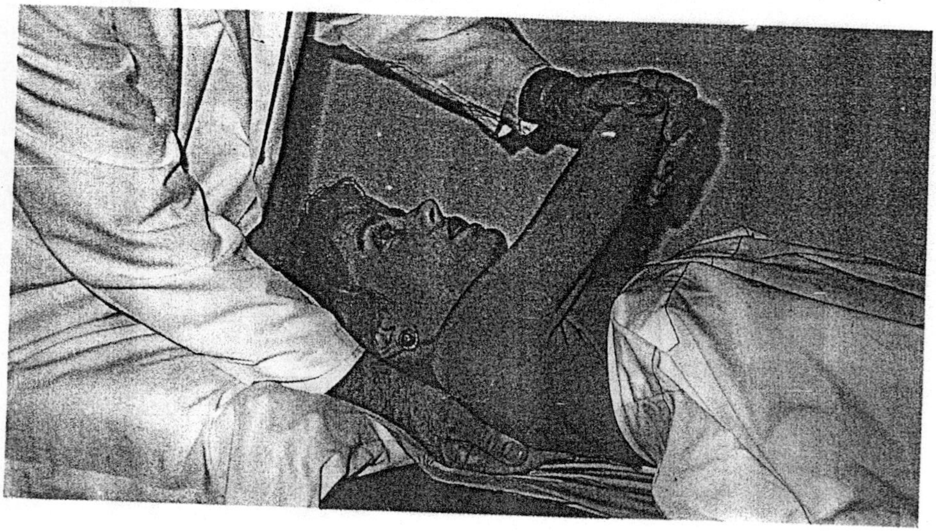

FIG. 1–13. Forward flexion-internal rotation test for posterior instability: The shoulder is flexed to 90°, adducted, and internally rotated. The table stabilizes the scapula while downward pressure is exerted on the flexed elbow to displace the joint posteriorly.

A
B
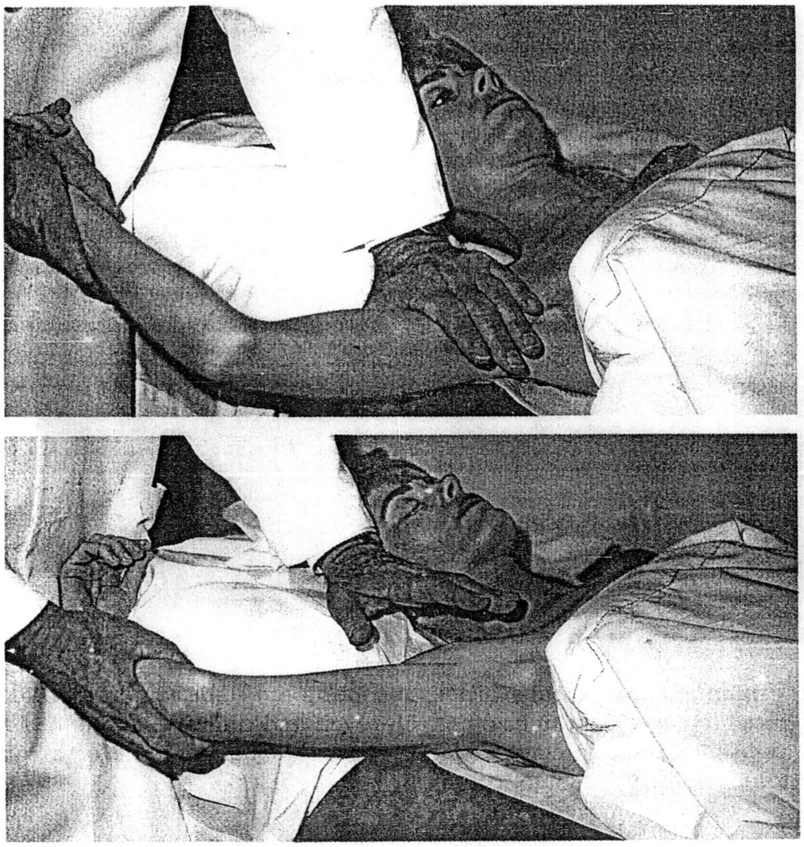

FIG. 1–14. Compression test. A, Compression is maintained against the humeral head as the arm is abducted and externally rotated. A patient with anterior instability feels more secure and loses some apprehension.
B, When the hand is lifted, the release of anterior stabilization permits the head to slide forward rather abruptly. Apprehension returns quickly. The test must be performed carefully to avoid inadvertent anterior dislocation.

pinpoint the exact origin of discomfort and may simply state that the shoulder becomes painful with elevation. The patient may fail to mention the sensation of slipping or loosening unless a direct inquiry is made. Elimination of pain in the subacromial region allows the patient to isolate the remaining discomfort caused by the instability alone. Quite often, that pain is located in the posterior aspect of the joint as the shoulder subluxates anteriorly. The patient with instability may be able to abduct and externally rotate without symptoms during the compression test, but when the examiner's palm is released, symptoms reappear.

SULCUS SIGN

The sulcus sign is elicited by pulling downward on the arm held at the side (Fig. 1–15). A definite sulcus appears below the lateral border of the acromion in patients with inferior subluxation. The sign is generally positive in patients with multidirectional instability. The sign is positive regardless of whether the primary instability is anteroinferior or posteroinferior. In many cases of multidirectional instability, the instability is global. The degree of inferior subluxation may be documented by a plain radiograph taken with the patient standing relaxed with a 10-pound weight tied around the wrist.

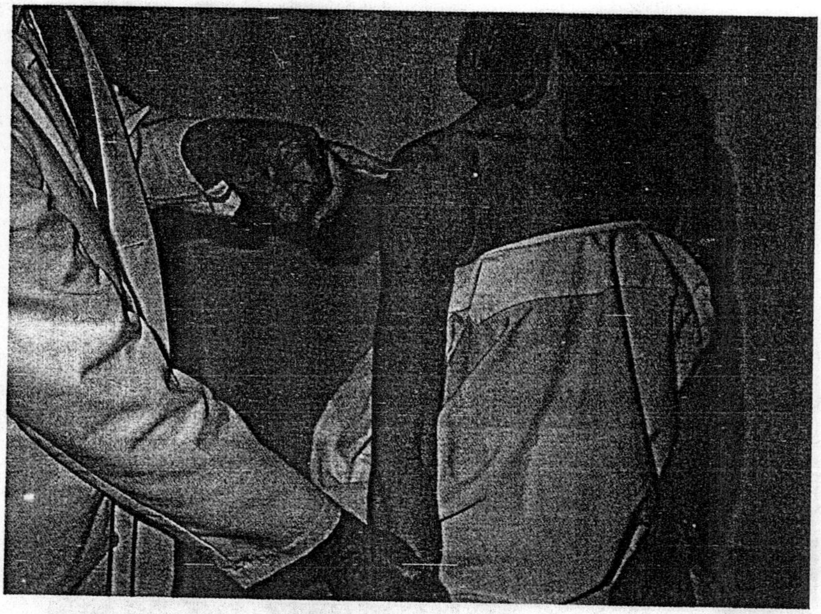

FIG. 1–15. Sulcus sign: Pulling downward on the relaxed arm held at the side may produce a definite sulcus below the lateral border of the acromion in patients with abnormal laxity.

DIAGNOSTIC IMAGING

Various techniques are available to confirm the clinical impression of instability. Instability is a clinical diagnosis, however, and clinical correlation is required to validate the interpretation of a magnetic resonance image or a computerized tomography arthrogram that describes a labral lesion.

RADIOGRAPHS

A plain radiograph showing a dislocation is the most direct method of demonstrating both the degree and the direction of displacement. The presence of a posterior dislocation may be missed if radiographs are not taken in the axillary or tangetial scapular "Y" projection, as well as in the anteroposterior (AP) projection (Fig. 1–16).

The *Hill-Sachs'* lesion may be demonstrated in a plain radiograph (Fig. 1–17). This impression fracture of the posterosuperior aspect of the humeral head is produced by contact with the anteroinferior glenoid when dislocated. A corresponding osseous defect in the labrum may occur through the same mechanism. Osseous labral defects are best seen when West Point axillary and Stryker notch views are added to radiographic studies of suspected instability.

A *stress x-ray* may capture the degree of displacement (Fig. 1–18). This study is most valuable when an axillary view demonstrates the degree of anterior or posterior displacement. The sulcus sign can be documented in the AP projection with a 10-pound weight tied to the patient's wrist.

DOUBLE-CONTRAST COMPUTERIZED TOMOGRAPHY (CT) ARTHROGRAM

Labral lesions may be defined with a double-contrast CT-arthrogram in the axial reconstruction. Any labral defect that extends well into the lower half of the

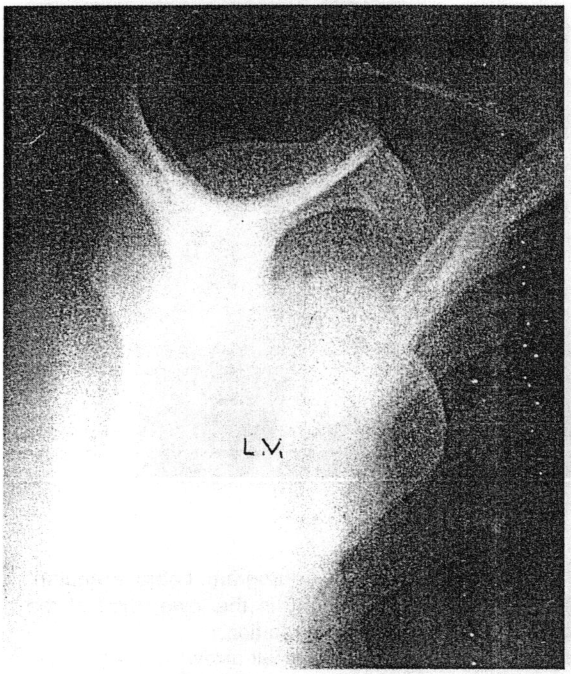

FIG. 1–16. Tangential (Y) view of the scapula shows anteroinferior dislocation of right shoulder.

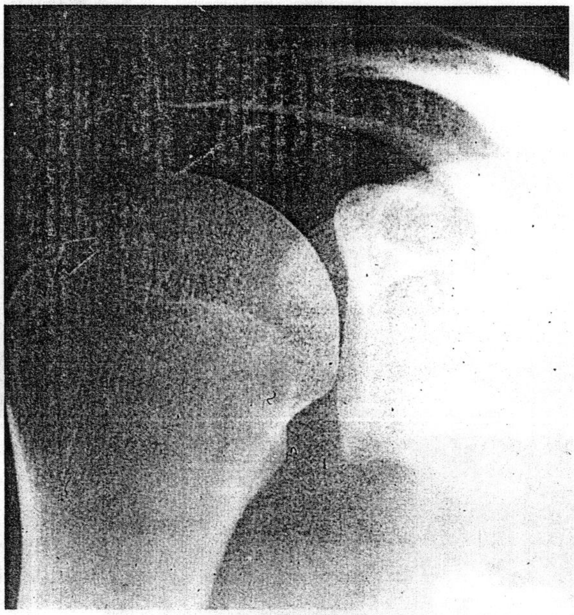

FIG. 1–17. Hill-Sachs' lesion is demonstrated on a plain radiograph in internal rotation.

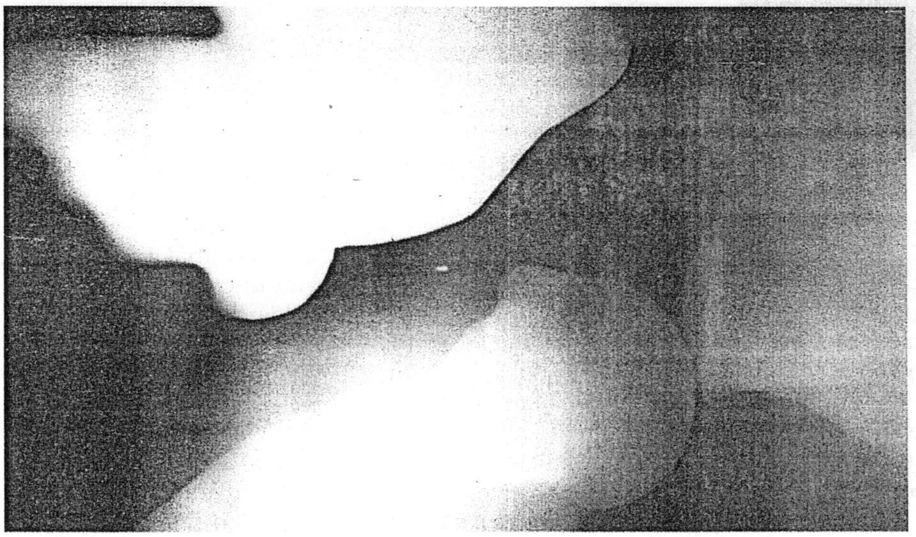

FIG. 1–18. Axillary stress x-ray: Posterior stress is exerted by a lead-gloved hand. Approximately 50% posterior displacement is demonstrated in this lax shoulder.

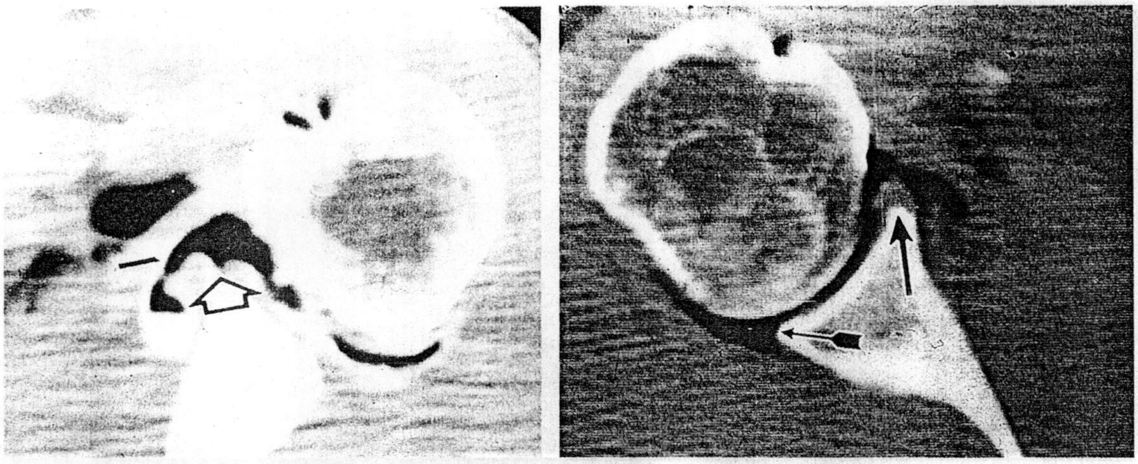

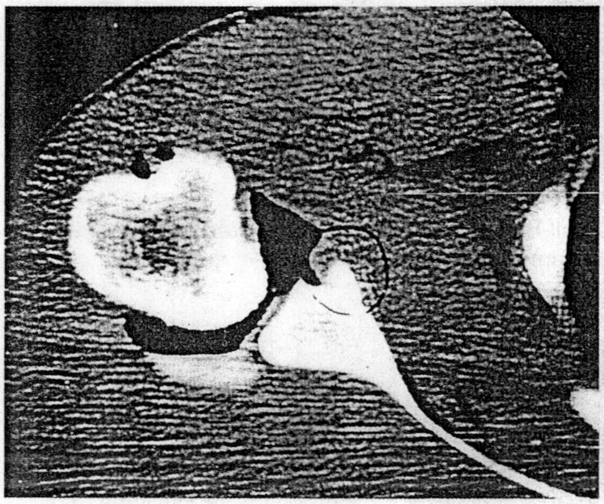

A B
C

FIG. 1–19. A, Double-contrast CT-arthrogram: Labral irregularity (arrow) is demonstrated anteriorly in the lower third of the glenoid with the humerus in internal rotation.
B, The posterior labrum is absent (small arrow with tail), while the anterior labrum appears normal (regular arrow).
C, The anterior lip of the glenoid has fractured during an anterior dislocation (bony Bankart lesion).

glenoid is considered clinically significant (Fig. 1–19). A CT-arthrogram should be taken with the arm in both internal (palm down) and external (palm up) rotation positions to define the capacity of the capsule and uncover any pathologic changes. The palm-down position places the shoulder in some internal rotation and compresses the air and dye anteriorly, thereby distending the anterior capsule. A pathologically capacious capsule may be seen inserting well down on the neck of the glenoid rather than arising more directly from the region of the labrum. The palm-up position places the arm in more external rotation and distends the posterior capsule. Clinical correlation is essential to the diagnostic significance of these images.

MAGNETIC RESONANCE IMAGING (MRI)

Quality scanners are capable of demonstrating labral lesions, but significant expertise is required to differentiate pathologic conditions from normal variations. Again, the level of the axial scan must be below the equator to have clinical significance (Fig. 1–20). Osseous irregularities in the glenoid and subtle Hill-Sachs' lesions can be seen well with MRI studies (Fig. 1–21).

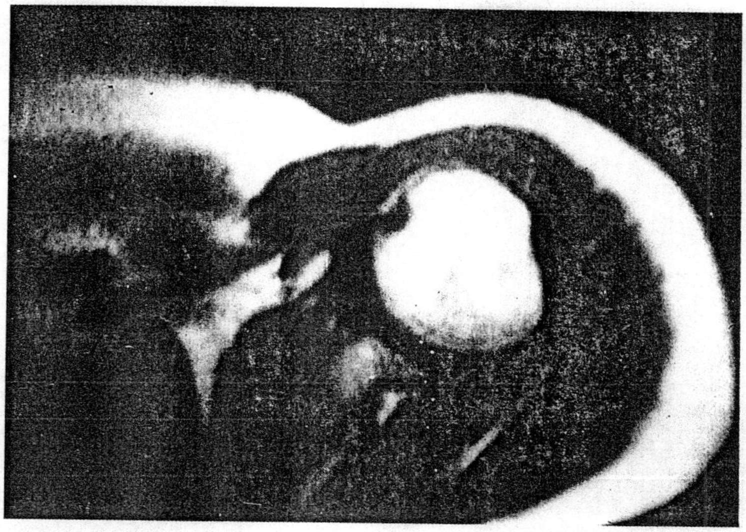

FIG. 1–20. MRI study shows anterior labral irregularity (Bankart lesion).

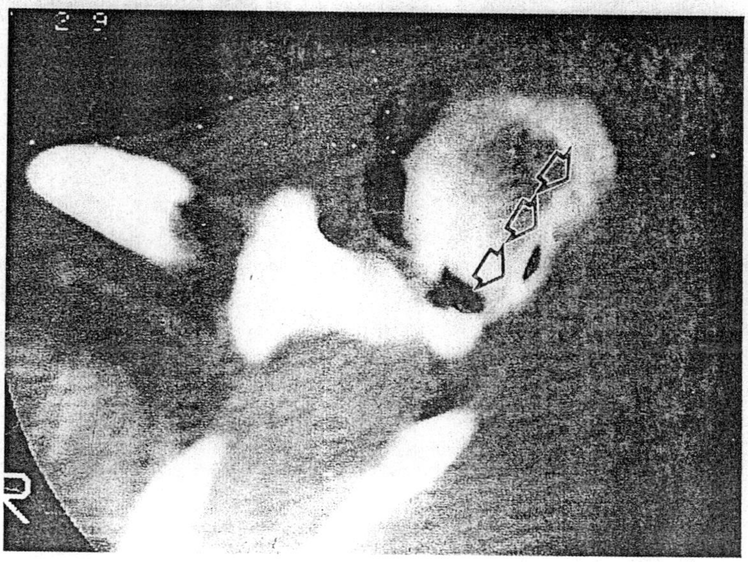

FIG. 1–21. MRI study shows flattening of superoposterior aspect of humeral head consistent with Hill-Sachs' lesion (open arrows).

EXAMINATION UNDER ANESTHESIA

Examination under anesthesia may be performed with or without fluoroscopy. An assistant should be enlisted to obtain maximum stabilization of the scapula while glenohumeral translation is examined. The glenoid must be loaded by compressing the humeral head against it during examination to elicit labral clicks and appreciate anterior or posterior displacement. The examination should be performed with the arm abducted at 60°, 90°, and 135° while externally rotated (Fig. 1–22A). The anterior and posterior drawer tests should be performed bilaterally to determine the patient's normal degree of laxity (Fig. 1–22B). Posterior displacement of up to 50% may be normal, whereas the head

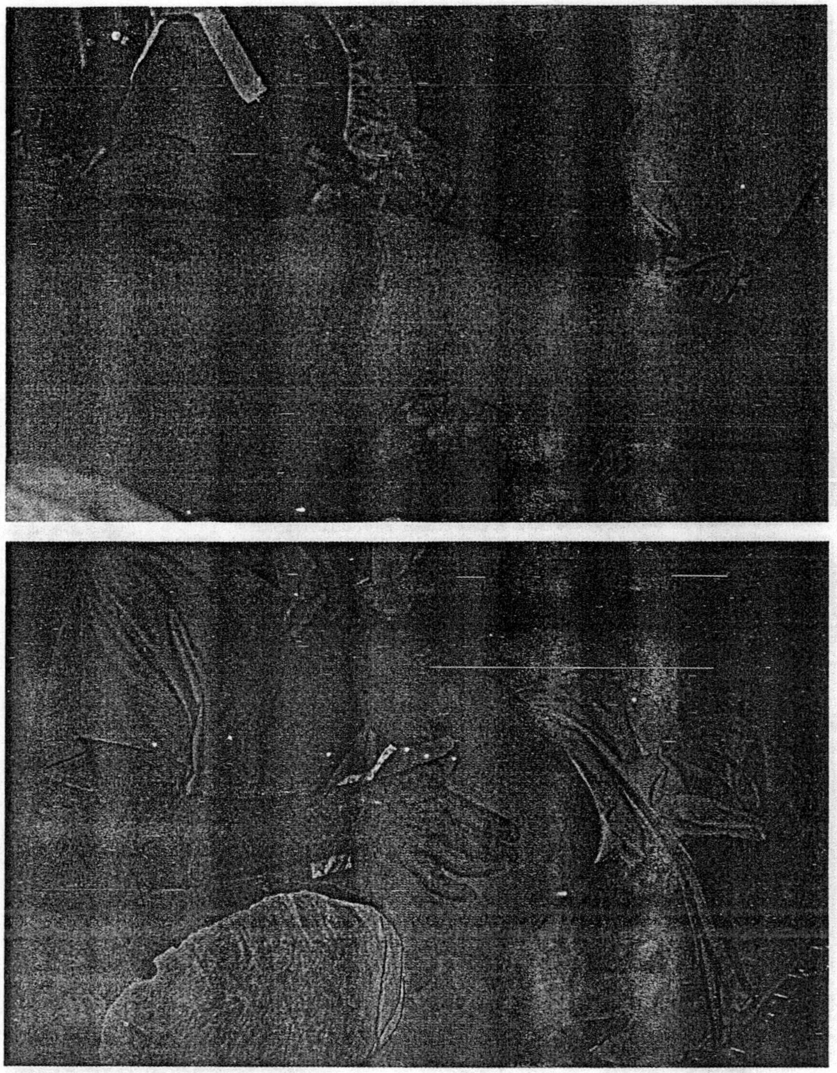

FIG. 1–22. A, Examination under anesthesia: The arm is brought into varying degrees of abduction with external rotation while loading the glenohumeral joint.
B, Posterior instability is tested by flexing the adducted arm to 90° while internally rotating and applying pressure in the posterior direction.

may translate anteriorly up to 25%, and at times 33%, in otherwise normal individuals.

Fluoroscopic control greatly enhances the value of examination under anesthesia. Examination under anesthesia should be performed to confirm the degree and direction of displacement prior to surgical repair of instability.

DIAGNOSTIC ARTHROSCOPY

Diagnostic arthroscopy clearly demonstrates the presence or absence of a capsulolabral disruption. A true Bankart lesion always involves the lower aspect of the glenoid (Fig. 1–23A). The inferior detachment may extend superiorly to eventually detach the entire anterior labrum. An isolated minor detachment or anatomically normal oval window in the superior half of the labrum should not be misinterpreted as an instability lesion (Fig. 1–23B).

Part of the stability of the shoulder is controlled by a vacuum-like effect. When air enters during posterior capsular penetration, the seal is broken and joint laxity increases. This characteristic must be considered when evaluating translation of the humeral head in relation to the glenoid in patients with suspected anterior or posterior subluxation. Athletes involved in sports that require throwing frequently demonstrate labral irregularities both anteriorly and posteriorly.

A subtle Hill-Sachs' lesion may be identified arthroscopically and should not be confused with a normal "anatomic bare patch" (Fig. 1–24). Labral osseous lesions are quite evident on arthroscopic evaluation.

Preoperative arthroscopic evaluation is hardly necessary in patients with well-documented evidence of recurrent dislocation or with an otherwise confirmed diagnosis as to the degree or direction of the displacement. A preoperative or intraoperative inspection with an optical catheter (MedDynamics) permits inspection of the glenoid before the capsule is opened. This procedure helps to determine whether the capsule should be incised vertically near the labrum for a Bankart repair or horizontally and near the humeral attachment for a capsular reefing. The patient with severe multidirectional instability may not have labral lesions. The capsule in such patients is simply so lax that the humeral head moves freely without disturbing the glenoid.

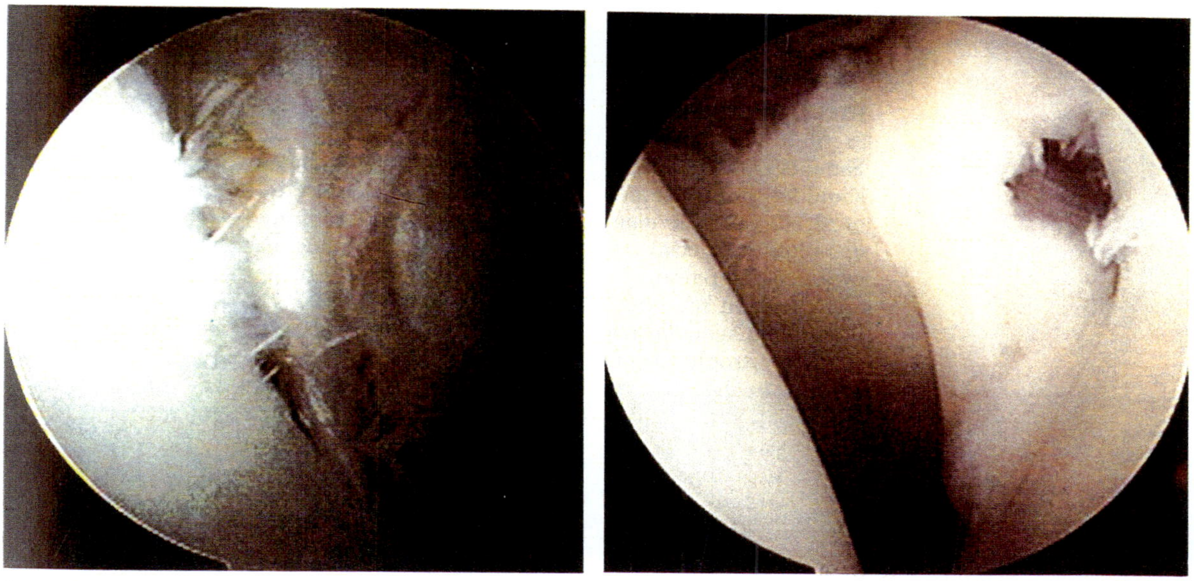

A B

FIG. 1–23. A, Capsulolabral separation (Bankart defect) involving the anteroinferior aspect of the labrum.
B, Normal anatomic variation in attachment of middle glenohumeral ligament leaves an oval window in the superior labrum.

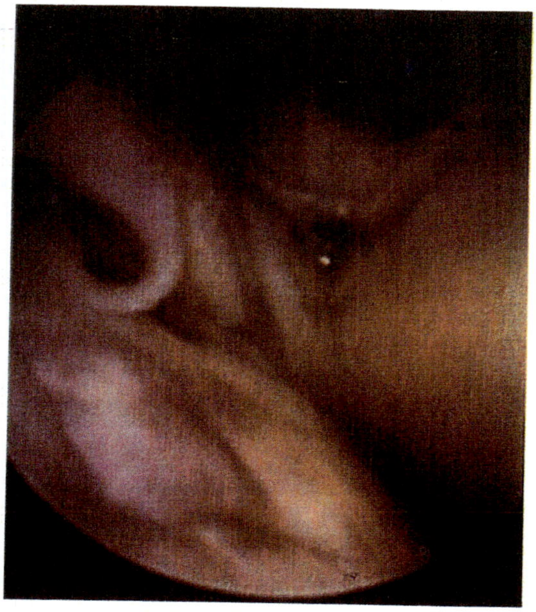

FIG. 1–24. A, subtle Hill-Sachs' lesion is identified arthroscopically at the superoposterior aspect of the humeral head.

GLENOHUMERAL ARTHRITIS

RHEUMATOID ARTHRITIS

Patients with rheumatoid arthritis rarely come to the orthopedic surgeon with a shoulder that is the primary joint involved. Because of the polyarticular nature of this disease, the diagnosis has usually been established by the time the shoulder requires special consideration. The typical patient is a frail woman who is experiencing painful restriction of shoulder motion. Her skin appears atrophic, and the joint may be warm and somewhat boggy to palpation because of the underlying synovial reaction. The regional musculature is diffusely wasted as a result of atrophy from disuse. The radiograph often already shows destructive changes in the humeral head and glenoid. The rotator cuff is vulnerable to the erosive effects of pannus formation, and a high incidence of rotator cuff tears accompanies the later stages of rheumatoid disease in the shoulder. Involvement of the subacromial bursa may initially give the impression of impingement syndrome, but when the joint is examined more closely, pain is found at the limits of motion in *every* direction. In the later stages of the disease, when the capsule is contracted and bony changes have developed, glenohumeral mobility becomes severely impaired, and the arm is moved only by combined scapulothoracic motion. When the rotator cuff has eroded, scapulohumeral rhythm is further impaired. The shoulder merely shrugs when elevation is attempted. The arm that is passively elevated falls uncontrollably (drop-arm sign).

Integrity of the cuff must be assessed prior to total shoulder replacement. Strength evaluation in the midrange of residual shoulder motion can be carried out by asking the patient to exert maximal effort despite discomfort. A double-contrast arthrogram not only confirms a tear if present, but gives some indication of the quality (thickness) of the remaining cuff tissue. The functional result of shoulder arthroplasty is quite limited in the absence of a repairable cuff.

Other inflammatory arthritides that affect the shoulder include lupus, ankylosing spondylitis, and polymyalgia rheumatica. Diagnostic and therapeutic considerations are included in Chapter 16, entitled Glenohumeral Arthritis.

OSTEOARTHRITIS

Patients with osteoarthritis characteristically complain of diminished mobility with pain at the limits of motion. The onset is insidious, and patients may be unaware of the problem until shoulder mobility has been reduced below the customary range used for activities of daily living. By this time, the radiograph may show a surprising amount of incongruity and loss of articular surface (Fig. 1–25). Osteoarthritic patients are more apt to be male and muscular than are their rheumatoid counterparts.

Atrophy may be inconsequential until the condition is quite advanced. Motion is primarily scapulothoracic and may be accompanied by a coarse crepitus. The joint eventually becomes fixed in internal rotation. From this position little movement can be made in either internal or external rotation. The rotator cuff is seldom torn. The factors that promulgate the development of osteoarthritis generally require an intact cuff.

POST-TRAUMATIC ARTHRITIS

Post-traumatic arthritis that develops following proximal humeral fracture or dislocation appears at an earlier age, and accompanying soft tissue involvement may be quite significant. Soft tissue examination may reveal atrophy and induration. The degree of soft tissue injury negatively affects the results of reconstruction arthroplasty.

AVASCULAR NECROSIS

The clinical findings associated with avascular necrosis of the humeral head may seem similar to those associated with osteoarthritis. Suspicion for avascular

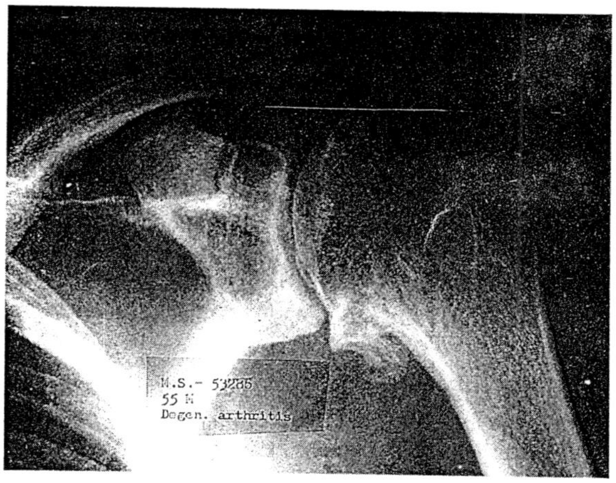

FIG. 1–25. Advanced degenerative joint disease.

necrosis is raised when the patient has a history of steroid ingestion for rheumatoid arthritis or lupus, or has been undergoing dialysis treatment. Scuba diving or excessive alcohol consumption present additional clues that point toward this diagnosis. Except in patients with rheumatoid arthritis, the cuff and associated soft tissues may be well preserved.

CHONDROMALACIA SIMULATING IMPINGEMENT SYNDROME

Chondromalacia and cartilaginous defects are signs of degenerative joint disease that develop long before joint narrowing or spur formation. The early symptoms of pain may simulate impingement syndrome. Indeed, if the joint is being subjected to repetitive stressful overhead activities (weight-lifting, throwing, or heavy labor), some degree of tendinitis may accompany chondromalacia. Ellman and colleagues have reported on 18 patients in whom an initial diagnosis of impingement syndrome was made by either the referring physician or the authors.[3] Although a more precise diagnosis was subsequently established, the presence of, as well as the extent of, early degenerative joint disease was quite unexpected. The pain ablation test relieved pain in many of these patients and was therefore unreliable in the differential diagnosis. In retrospect, some of these patients had slight joint narrowing that was not appreciated because a true AP radiograph (30° to coronal plane) had not been obtained. The plain radiograph in external rotation may also show as one of the earliest signs of degenerative joint disease a slight blunting or protuberance at the inferior portion of the

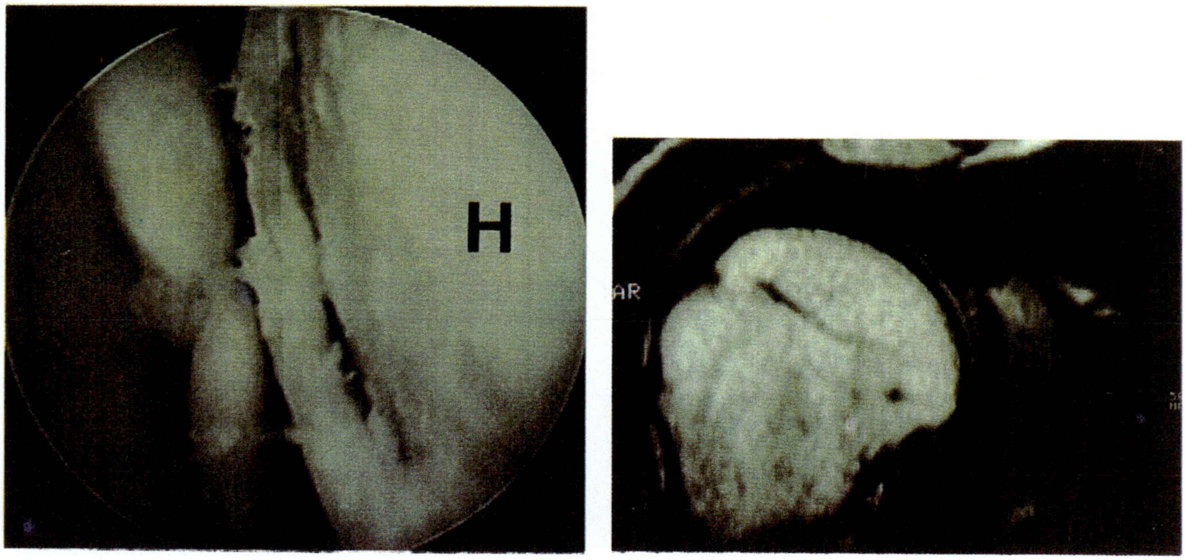

A B

FIG. 1–26. A, Unexpected degree of chondromalacia involving the humeral head (H) in a patient with impingement syndrome. Note two cartilaginous loose bodies.
B, MRI study of shoulder shown in Figure 1–26A. Small arrows indicate suspected area of chondromalacia.

humeral head where it joins the calcar (Fig. 1–26A). MRI studies failed to disclose articular loss in more than one half of the studies made, but this percentage improved when clinical suspicion alerted the radiologist to the possibility of chondromalacia (Fig. 1–26B).

The "compression-rotation" test was of some clinical value (Fig. 1–27).[3] The patient is placed in the lateral recumbent position on the unaffected side. The affected arm rests on the body with the elbow bent. The examiner presses firmly downward on the shoulder with both hands to load the glenohumeral joint. The patient is asked to rotate the joint internally and externally while firm compression is maintained. The compression-rotation test is positive if pain or crepitus is elicited. The test is most informative when performed after a subacromial injection of local anesthetic has eliminated any pain of subacromial origin.

A

B

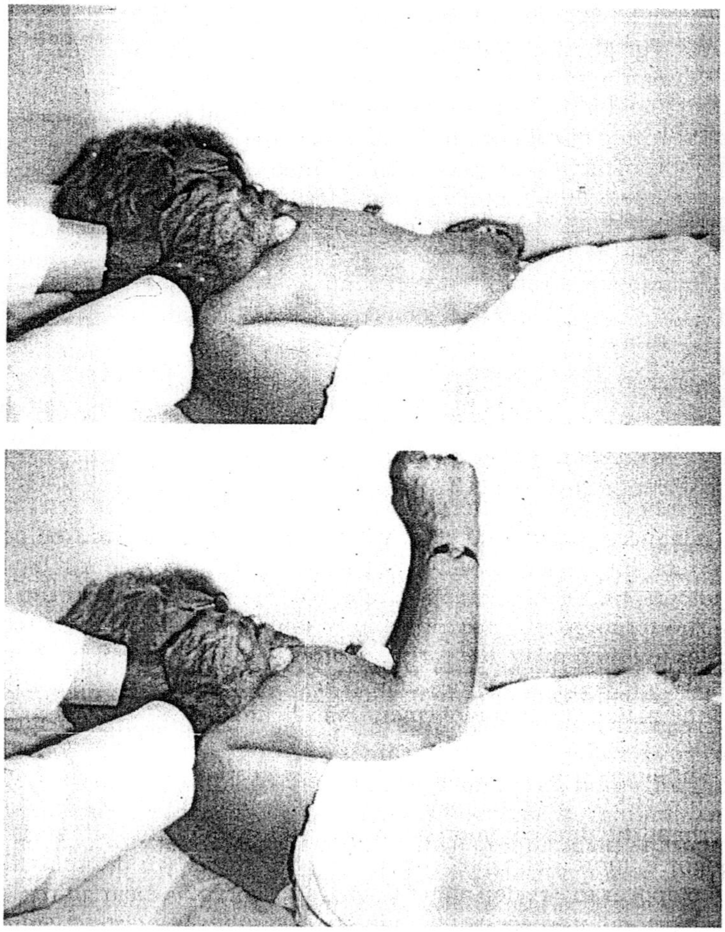

FIG. 1–27. Compression-rotation test. A, Patient in lateral recumbent position with arm at side and elbow bent. The examiner loads the glenohumeral joint by applying firm downward pressure.
B, Patient rotates the arm externally and internally. Crepitation or pain is considered positive for chondromalacia.

MISCELLANEOUS AFFECTIONS

With the exception of adhesive capsulitis, all the miscellaneous affections described in this section are local manifestations of a systemic disorder that may involve any other joint as well. Though shoulder involvement is uncommon, each condition must be considered in the diagnostic evaluation of shoulder pain.

ADHESIVE CAPSULITIS (FROZEN SHOULDER)

Adhesive capsulitis is a distinct clinical entity and must be differentiated from a "stiff, painful shoulder." Restricted motion and pain accompany both conditions, but the stiff, painful shoulder can result from a variety of disorders, such as injury, rotator cuff disease, arthritis, shoulder-hand syndrome, or a myriad of miscellaneous affections. *Primary* adhesive capsulitis (frozen shoulder) is a specific shoulder disorder of obscure cause. The clinical course is relatively predictable. The physical findings at various stages are characteristic.

At onset, the symptoms of adhesive capsulitis are indistinguishable from "bursitis" or "tendinitis" of the rotator cuff or bicipital tendon. Patients complain of chronic aching discomfort in the shoulder that often has been present for weeks or months before the physician is consulted. The pain is accompanied by a progressively diminishing range of shoulder motion in elevation and rotation (Fig. 1–28). Restriction of external rotation invariably accompanies adhesive capsulitis, and this isolated finding is one of the most helpful differential clues. Individuals with chronic impingement syndrome frequently demonstrate painful restriction of both forward flexion and external rotation when examined in the seated position.

When external rotation is tested while supine, however, a nearly normal degree of motion in spite of discomfort is possible in patients with impingement syndrome. The patient with adhesive capsulitis simply cannot externally rotate beyond perhaps 10 or 20° because of fixed periarticular contracture. Pain may not occur until this contracture is actively stretched at the limit of motion. Only two other clinical entities produce such a profound loss of external rotation. One is advanced glenohumeral arthritis, and the other is a missed posterior dislocation of the shoulder. Although both of these conditions have characteristic radiographs, the radiograph of adhesive capsulitis appears normal.

The response to subacromial injection of local anesthetic (impingement test) helps to differentiate the early symptoms of impingement from adhesive capsulitis. Whereas the local anesthetic relieves pain and restores considerable motion to the patient with impingement, hardly any benefit accrues to the patient with adhesive capsulitis.

Shoulder-hand syndrome following a heart attack or reflex sympathetic dystrophy (RSD) associated with trauma may result in intractable shoulder stiffness. Perhaps the final common pathway that leads to joint stiffness is similar, but the origin is more definable in patients with these two disorders than in patients who appear to develop adhesive capsulitis for little apparent reason. Subtle clinical observation suggests that adhesive capsulitis is a distinct entity. The vascular findings associated with RSD (pallor, coolness, or hyperhidrosis in the distal extremity) are absent in adhesive capsulitis. The pain in adhesive capsulitis seldom travels lower than the elbow, whereas aching and paresthesias may involve the forearm and entire hand of the patient with RSD.

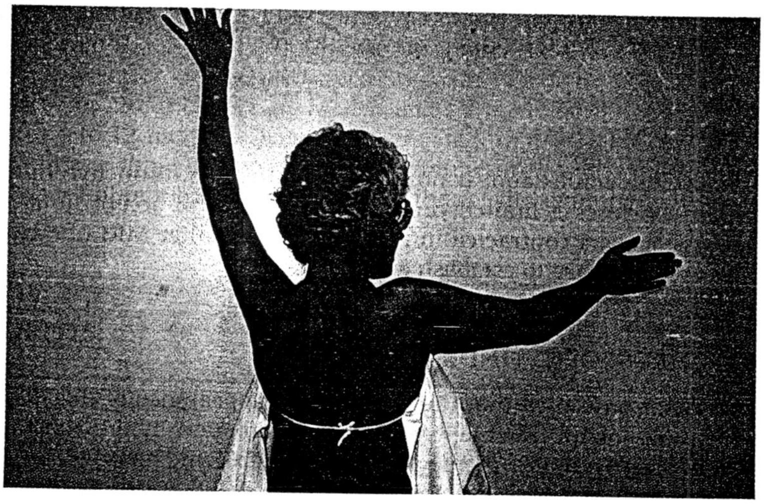

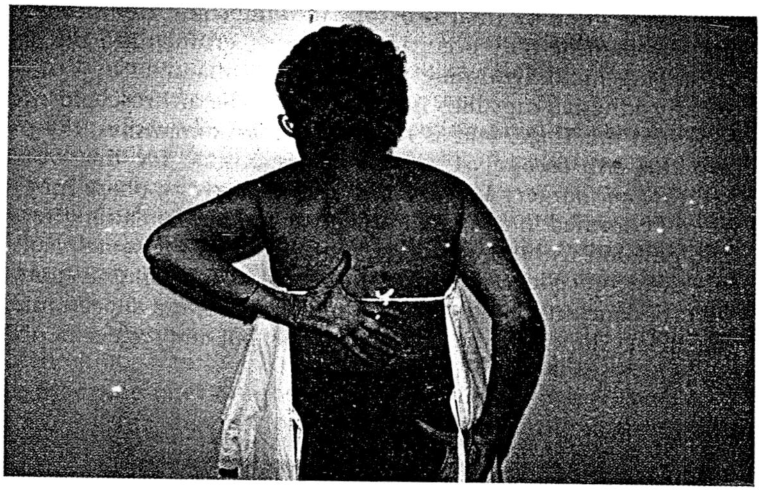

A

B

FIG. 1–28. Adhesive pericapsulitis: 50-year-old woman with a 4-month history of progressive pain and diminishing motion. Elevation (A) and rotation (B) are limited.

Demographic observation suggests that individuals with true adhesive capsulitis cluster around the age of 50 and are predominantly female. The patient with diabetes mellitus is a notable exception. The incidence of adhesive capsulitis is much higher in insulin-dependent diabetic persons than in the population in general, and response to treatment is often prolonged in the diabetic patient.

The clinical course of patients with adhesive capsulitis follows a somewhat bell-shaped curve over a period of 12 to 18 months. Symptoms appear to worsen progressively for 3 to 6 months. This period has been called the *freezing phase.*[4] Thereafter, a plateau is reached. Pain is absent except at the limits of motion, but stiffness persists *(frozen phase).* Efforts to mobilize the joint are more tolerable in this phase, and gradual improvement is observed over many subsequent months *(thawing phase).* The examiner must determine the phase of the disease to direct appropriate treatment. Well-intentioned but overly strenuous efforts to actively mobilize the joint during the freezing phase produce more pain and provoke resistance from the patient. Gentle measures used to reduce pain and mobilization allowed only to the point of stretch discomfort are more effective approaches. Premature intervention by manipulation or arthroscopic intervention during the freezing phase may be disastrous. With proper timing, either form of intervention may reduce morbidity.

DIAGNOSTIC IMAGING

Plain radiographs appear normal. MRI offers no distinctive findings. An arthrogram discloses a limited capacity of the joint to accept fluid, and the inferior recess appears contracted in most patients. Neither MRI nor arthrographic studies are necessary to establish a diagnosis.

ARTHROSCOPIC FINDINGS

Neviaser has noted that the arthroscopic appearance of this disorder varies with the stage of the disease. Synovial inflammation in the subscapular or axillary recess has been documented in the early "freezing phase" (Fig. 1–29).[4] Later, the inflammation fades and fibrotic bands may be seen in the subscapular recess. The introduction of an arthroscope into the contracted shoulder is difficult, and articular damage may occur. A premature, erroneous arthroscopic intervention for impingement syndrome that discloses inflammatory synovitis characteristic of early adhesive capsulitis is unfortunate. The arthroscopic intervention is of no benefit at this stage, and as range of motion diminishes, the patient may implicate the arthroscope as the agent responsible for the worsening condition. Arthroscopic surgery in the late frozen or thawing phase may shorten disability when performed in conjunction with closed manipulation. Because a well-timed manipulation without arthroscopy may achieve the same result, the value of the combined procedure is difficult to assess at this time. Hypothetically, debridement of contractures in the subscapular recess and subacromial bursa would be beneficial. Clinical studies are in progress, but end results are difficult to assess.

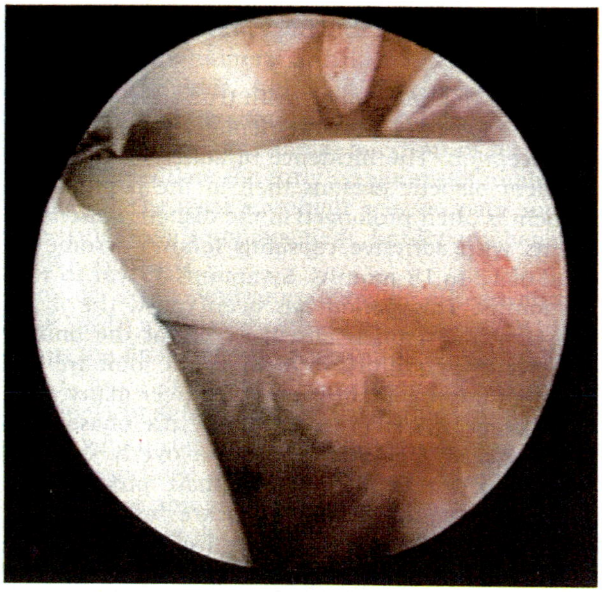

FIG. 1–29. Adhesive pericapsulitis: Freezing phase. Extensive synovitis is seen when looking downward from the horizontal long head of the biceps into the subscapular recess.

We have found that conservative management is generally quite satisfactory in the treatment of adhesive capsulitis. The patient must understand the prolonged course of this disorder. Gentle stretching exercises performed by the patient and assisted by the therapist gradually yield a functional range of comfortable motion in 6 to 12 months. Diabetic patients take considerably longer to recover and often have some degree of residual contracture. Additional studies have confirmed that full motion in comparison to that of the opposite extremity is not always restored.

SEPTIC ARTHRITIS

The adult shoulder seldom develops septic arthritis based on hematogenous spread from other areas. Notable exceptions to this statement are patients with immunosuppressive disorders or those on chronic steroid therapy who develop foci of sepsis elsewhere in the body. When septic glenohumeral arthritis develops, both pain and swelling are prominent. The pain becomes unremitting and only incidentally aggravated by motion. In rare instances, the subacromial bursa, rather than the glenohumeral joint, is involved primarily. The diagnosis in this instance is apt to be missed during the early stages.

A more likely cause of shoulder sepsis, either subacromial or glenohumeral, is direct contamination following diagnostic/therapeutic injection or arthroscopy. Unfortunately, low-grade sepsis is often present for weeks (occasionally months) before a diagnosis is established. The overlying musculature may mask local swelling, and the systemic febrile response is minimal. Leukocytosis and a shift may be minimal in these instances also, but the sedimentation rate is generally elevated. (If sepsis develops following an initial subacromial injection, the subsequent injection of additional steroids may further mask the condition.) Nosocomial infection apparently occurs less frequently following shoulder arthroscopy than following knee arthroscopy. This finding may be related to the increased vascularity of the shoulder or may simply reflect the fact that fewer interventions are being performed on the shoulder than on the knee.

Diagnostic aspiration for possible shoulder sepsis should be performed selectively. The subacromial space should be aspirated first. The possibility of cross-contamination can be avoided by using a different aspiration tray to enter the glenohumeral joint. Portals, either anterior or posterior, should be placed to avoid the subacromial bursa when aspirating the glenohumeral joint.

Arthroscopy is effective in the treatment of shoulder sepsis. The technique is described in Chapter 17.

SYNOVIAL CHONDROMATOSIS

This uncommon disorder has no predilection for the shoulder over any other articulation. Many small cartilaginous loose bodies may develop before the joint becomes symptomatic. Synovial distention produces pain at the limit of motion. Joint restriction may eventually simulate adhesive capsulitis. As the cartilaginous loose bodies enlarge, locking episodes occur. The initial radiographs are negative, but with time, the metaplastic cartilage ossifies and the diagnosis is apparent. Arthroscopic visualization confirms the diagnosis (Fig. 1–30). Arthroscopic removal of loose bodies and synovectomy are the treatment of choice.

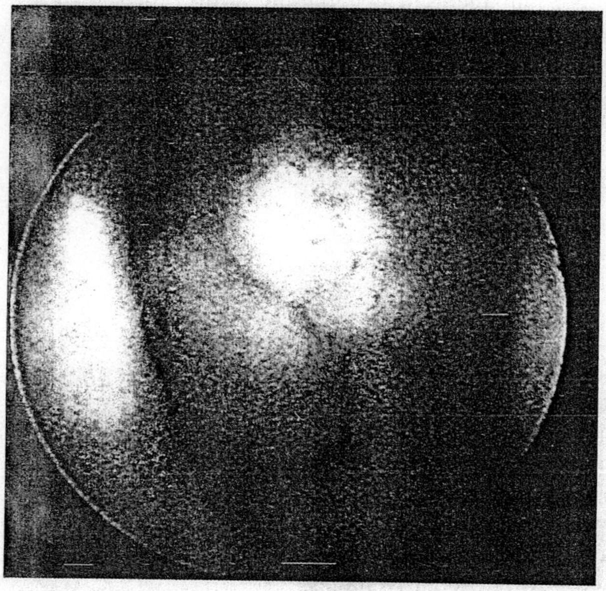

FIG. 1–30. Synovial osteochondromatosis: This 31-year-old woman was diagnosed as having "frozen shoulder" for 2 years. Many of the cartilaginous loose bodies seen in the region of the axillary recess were confluent.

PIGMENTED VILLONODULAR SYNOVITIS

This condition rarely affects the shoulder. Mild pain, swelling, and limited motion develop. Arthrographic findings in the shoulder are less distinctive than those seen when the condition affects the knee. Arthroscopic synovectomy is tedious but possible.

ADDITIONAL ARTHROPATHIES

Several other systemic disorders deserve consideration in the evaluation of shoulder pain.

Both gout and *pseudogout* may have shoulder manifestations. The symptoms are similar to those in other peripheral joints. Synovial fluid examination establishes a diagnosis based on identification of either urate crystals in gout or birefringent calcium pyrophosphate crystals in pseudogout.

Ochronosis (alkaptonuria) is an inherited condition caused by an absence of the enzyme homogentisate oxygenase. Ochronotic arthritis develops when homogentisic acid accumulates in cartilage. The desposits have a characteristic brown-black pigment that can be seen on arthroscopic inspection (Fig. 1–31).

Amyloid deposits may cause a destructive arthropathy (Fig. 1–32). This disorder may be seen in patients with chronic kidney disease who are undergoing dialysis.

Hemophilic arthropathy is recognized as a late stage of the disease and follows repeated episodes of intra-articular bleeding. The diagnosis is rarely in question.

The role of arthroscopy in the diagnosis and management of these various disorders is discussed further in Section IV, entitled The Arthritides and Miscellaneous Affections.

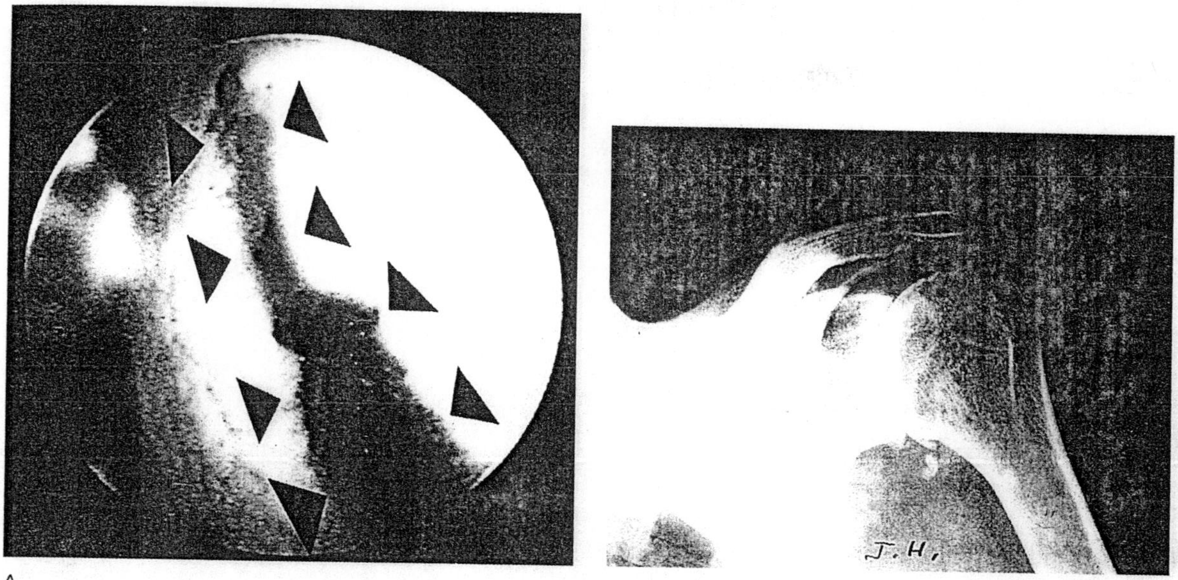

A B

FIG. 1–31. A, A white band of homogentisic acid stains the humeral head. The area is outlined by multiple short arrowheads.
B, X-ray of patient in Figure 1–31A.

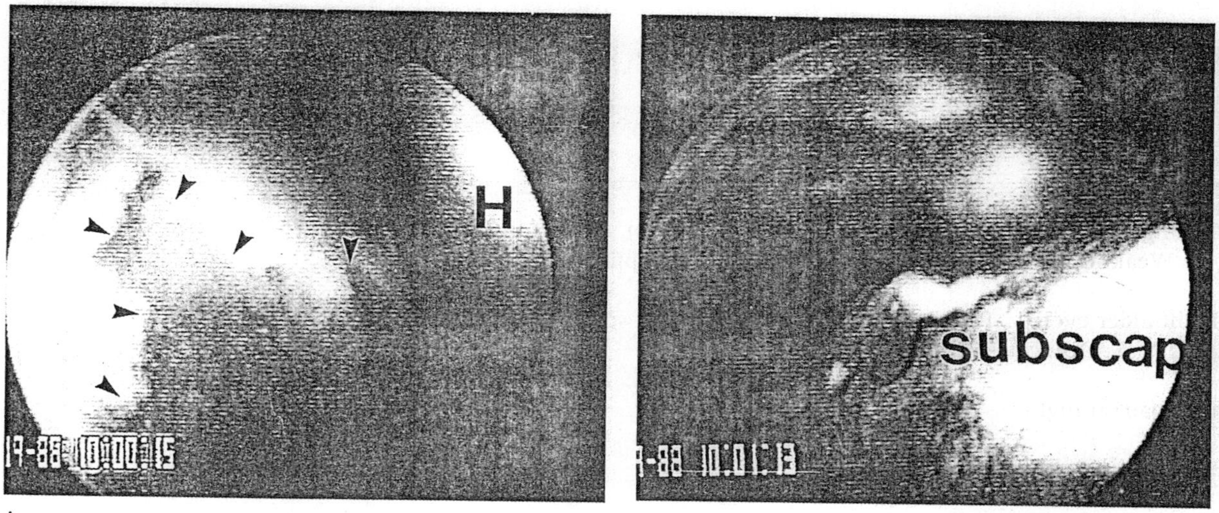

A B

FIG. 1–32. A, Extensive arthropathy (arrowheads) associated with chronic renal failure.
B, Note whitish amyloid deposits throughout the joint.

APPENDIX I

COMPREHENSIVE SHOULDER QUESTIONNAIRE

This questionnaire is designed to assist in the evaluation of your shoulder problem. Please circle or mark an X where indicated. Fill in the narrative spaces briefly. There will be plenty of time to discuss your symptoms in detail during the consultation.

Date: ____________________

Name: ____________________

Age: ____________________

Date of Birth: ______________

Sex: M ____ F ____

Are you *right* or *left*-handed? (circle one)

Which shoulder is involved? Rt ____ Lt ____ Both ____

How long have you been having trouble with your shoulder? Days ____ Weeks ____ Months ____ Years ____

Briefly describe how your shoulder problem started and what symptoms you are currently having. __________

____

____

Are you having any of these symptoms? (circle all that apply)
1. Pain 2. Weakness 3. Loss of motion 4. Catching, popping, or clicking

Does your shoulder ever: 1. Feel loose? 2. Slip in or out of socket? 3. Get "stuck" or "lock"? 4. Go "dead"? 5. Dislocate? (circle all that apply)

Do you have pain at night? Yes ____ No ____

Does lying on the side cause pain? Yes ____ No ____

Would you describe your pain as: Intermittent ____ Constant ____ ?
Is the intensity or severity of your pain: Mild ____ Moderate ____ Severe ____?

Which would best describe the character of your pain? Sharp ____ Dull ____ Aching ____ Other __________

Does movement of your arm cause pain? Yes ____ No ____
If "yes," which of these movements causes pain?
1. To shoulder height or above ____
2. Reaching behind back ____
3. Other ____

Are your symptoms increased with:

1. Daily activities ____
2. Work activities ____
3. Dressing ____
4. Lifting ____
5. Other ____________________

Does the pain travel down your arm? Yes ____ No ____

Does the pain travel into your fingers? Yes ____ No ____
If "yes," circle which finger: Thumb - Index - Long - Ring - Little

Do you have any pain in your neck? Yes ____ No ____

Does turning your head from side to side or looking up or down cause any pain to travel into your shoulder or down your arm? Yes ____ No ____

Do you have any numbness or tingling in your hand Yes ____ No ____
If "yes," does holding your arm overhead make the numbness or tingling: Better ____ Worse ____?

Have you any loss of hand dexterity, or do you drop things? Yes ____ No ____

Did your symptoms come on *gradually* or *suddenly*? (circle one)

Was the onset of your pain related to a specific injury Yes ____ No ____

If "no," go to next section .

If "yes," enter date of injury: ____________________
Mo Day Yr

Was the injury: Trivial ____ Moderate ____ Severe ____?
Describe what happened. ____________________

____

____

Was the injury work-related (injured on job)? Yes ____ No ____
How soon after injury did you consult a doctor? ____________

DIAGNOSTIC TESTS: If you have had any of the following tests, please enter the approximate date and what you were told of the results.

	Approximate Date	Results
X-RAYS	____________	____________________
ARTHROGRAM	____________	____________________
MRI	____________	____________________
EMG (ELECTROMYOGRAM)	____________	____________________

Have you had this problem before? Yes ____ No ____

If "no," go to next section.

If "yes," enter doctor's name (optional) and briefly describe the treatment (non-surgical) you received (rest, exercises, physiotherapy, injections).

	Doctor's Name	Approximate Date	Treatment
1.	____________	________	____________________
2.	____________	________	____________________
3.	____________	________	____________________

What is the total number of shoulder injections you have received? ____

If you have had shoulder surgery, enter date of surgery and describe briefly what was done.
Date ________ ____________________

____

ACTIVITY LEVEL:

What is your occupation? ____________________

Does your work require repetitive *overhead* activity? Yes ____ No ____

Are you required to pull, push, or lift heavy objects? Yes ____ No ____

What sports do you play? ____________________

How often do you play? ____________________

Are your sports activities: Recreational ____ Competitive ____?

Do you "work out" with weights or machine? Yes ____ No ____

How often? ____________________

Has your shoulder problem caused you to stop ____ or modify ____ work?

Has your shoulder problem caused you to stop ____ or modify ____ sport?

If "yes," how long ago did you stop work ________ or sport ________ ?

Add any additional history or pertinent information here: ____________________

____

____

____

____

OPERATING ROOM SETUP

The shoulder arthroscopist basically depends on the performance of a variety of sophisticated mechanical instruments. These devices should be arranged within the confines of a rather large operating room in a fashion that facilitates the procedure without entangling the participants in a Gordian knot of electrical cords, optical cables, and plastic tubing. Although the arrangement may be varied to accommodate an individual's preference, the basic setup of the required instruments can be described and illustrated.

SPECIFIC INSTRUMENTS

MECHANICAL INSTRUMENTS

Various mechanical devices are available to operate suction shavers and burs. The full-radius synovial resector (4.5 mm) and the serrated shaver (4.5 mm) seem to be the most valuable for debriding frayed or partially torn surfaces (Fig. 2–1). For more aggressive debridement, the 4.5-mm Synovator (Dyonics) is quite effective. Disposable instruments ensure maximum efficiency with initial use. Gas sterilization is advisable if instruments are reused. Round or oval burs are required in different circumstances (size 4.0 to 5.5 mm). The mechanical driver should permit variable speed and suction control.

ELECTROSURGICAL GENERATOR AND ELECTRODES

The ability to utilize both electrocoagulation and cautery within a fluid medium was one of the important breakthroughs in shoulder arthroscopy. Hemostasis is essential to visualization. Capillary oozing is readily controlled by hemostatic pressure within the glenohumeral joint when the initial catheter penetrations are preserved. The bleeding associated with extensive synovectomy requires pinpoint control of small bleeders to effectively remove a large amount of hyperemic synovium under direct visualization. The surgical electrode is required when procedures within the subacromial space are performed (Fig. 2–2). Beyond the hemostatic function of the coagulation current, the cutting electrode allows precise release of the coracoacromial ligament at a point near its inser-

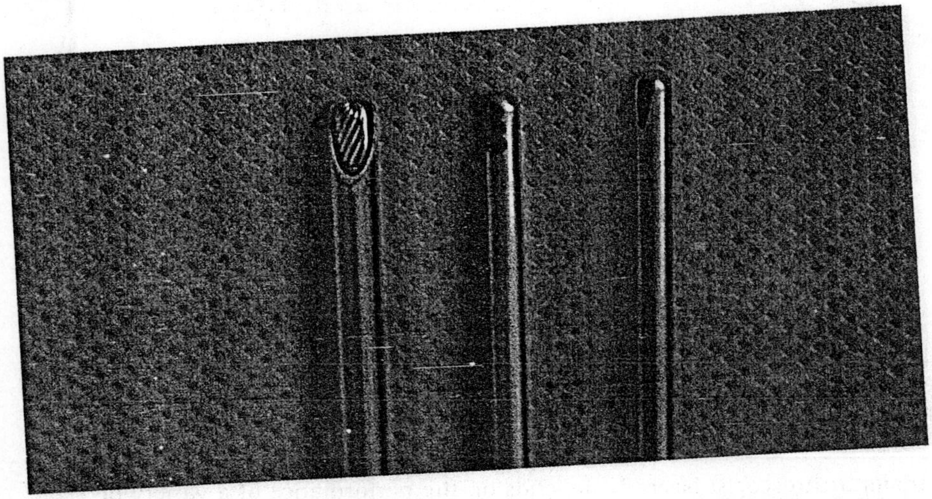

FIG. 2–1. Three mechanically driven instruments. Left, Full-radius resector. Center, Serrated shaver. Right, Oval bur.

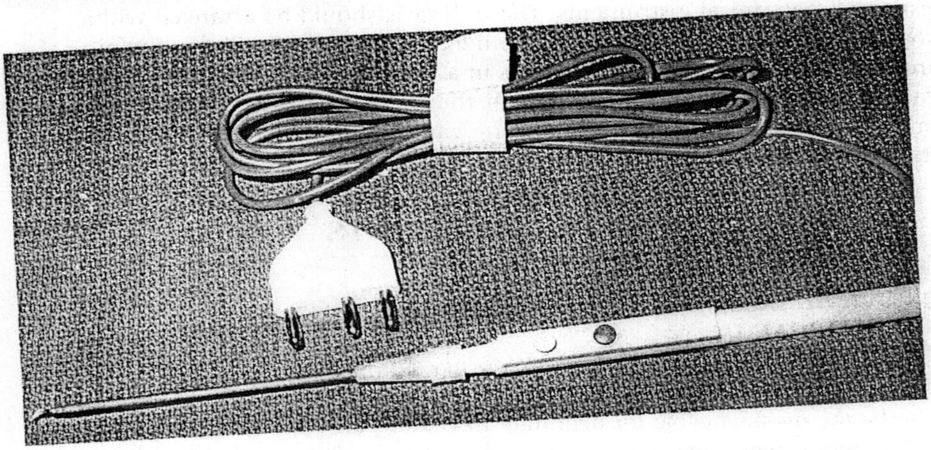

FIG. 2–2. Surgical electrode is used to release coracoacromial ligament and to control bleeding.

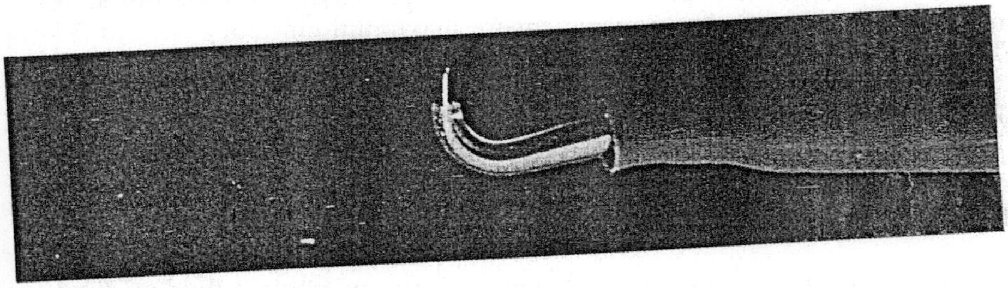

FIG. 2–3. Plastic-coated right-angled meniscectomy electrode permits both cautery and coagulation within a normal saline medium.

tion. When fibers of deltoid are inadvertantly invaded, the significant bleeding that results is readily controllable. If a branch of the coracoacromial artery is severed during shaving or burring, the resultant torrential-appearing hemorrhage can be controlled. The inability to control such bleeding may cause the procedure to be terminated.

The plastic-coated right-angled meniscectomy electrode developed by Concept, Inc., has allowed electrosurgery to be performed within a normal saline medium (Fig. 2–3). No other special irrigating fluids are required. A small right-angled electrode is insulated with plastic down to the tip. This design permits both coagulation and cutting to be carried out at the point of contact.

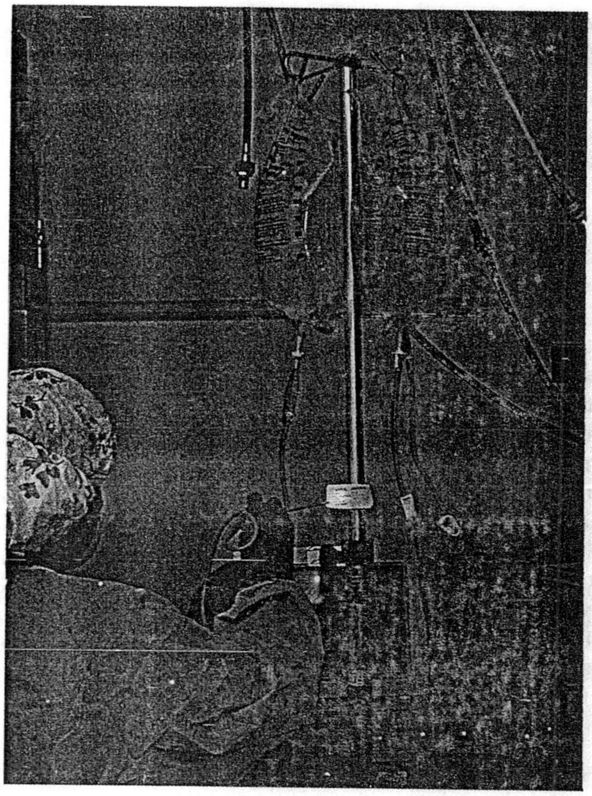

FIG. 2–4. Two 3000-ml bags of normal saline are suspended on an IV standard and are connected to cystoscopy Y-tubing.

HYDROSTATIC IRRIGATION SYSTEM

Shoulder arthroscopy requires continuous distention with a fluid medium. Normal saline solution is preferred over any other irrigating solution. This physiologic solution has demonstrated no untoward effects on articular cartilage or deriving from systemic absorption when extravasated into the surrounding tissues. Although the original technique for arthroscopic subacromial decompression required a switch to distilled water or some other nonconductive medium to allow the use of electrosurgical cutting and coagulating equipment, this change is no longer necessary when a plastic-coated surgical electrode is used.

Hydrostatic pressure must be sufficient to both distend the joint and retard capillary bleeding for efficient shoulder arthroscopy. Static or gravity-assisted fluid inflow can be effectively used in shoulder procedures. The hydrostatic pressure achieved is related to the height of the fluid irrigant in relation to the shoulder. Two 3000-ml bags of normal saline solution are suspended on a sturdy IV standard (Fig. 2–4) and are connected to a cystoscopy Y-tube that leads to a fluid-ingress cannula (see Appendix at the end of this chapter). An additional 1000-ml bag of normal saline solution that will be connected with cystoscopy tubing to the sheath of the arthroscope is also hung. The bottoms of the bags should be approximately 2 feet above the level of the shoulder. The base of the IV standard is reinforced with small sandbag weights to prevent it from toppling during the procedure. A 10-inch step stool placed nearby can help a short individual to change bags easily or to elevate the pole when necessary. An electrically operated IV pole is commercially available (Appendix). Its base is weighted and quite sturdy, and the bags can be raised and lowered with an electrical control.

ARTHROSCOPY PUMP

Numerous arthroscopy pump systems are available. The pumps are designed to control irrigation and distention of the joint by automatically maintaining selected pressure and fluid flow rates. The optimum system controls pressure and fluid flow independently. This feature requires a system that automatically monitors the actual pressure within the joint or subacromial bursa and may be adjusted to maintain variations in either flow rate or pressure reliably. We have used the 3M pump system since it was introduced and regard it as a valuable adjunct to shoulder arthroscopy (Appendix) (Fig. 2–5). This system automatically decreases flow as the pressure increases 10% over the preset value. When the pressure increases 20%, the pump automatically stops, and fluid may be drained to relieve excess pressure, thereby diminishing the risk of dangerous extravasation. When pressure returns to the desired range, the pump can automatically restart to avoid loss of distention. When properly utilized, the pump can improve visibility by suppressing capillary oozing or, when more aggressive bleeding occurs, by increasing flow while suction is carried out, thereby maintaining distention pressure. The saline bags can be kept at an accessible level when the pump is used in place of gravity.

HAND INSTRUMENTS

Several manually operated instruments are used in shoulder arthroscopy. The rack of hand-operated instruments routinely used in knee arthroscopy is placed on the back table to allow the surgeon to select a favorite instrument as may be required. The three instruments most frequently used are the basket forceps, grasping forceps, and open curette (Fig. 2–6). The basket forceps trims remnants of ligament or periosteum attached to the acromion, and may be used to resect a portion of the coracoacromial ligament after it has been released. The basket forceps is also used in the glenohumeral joint to resect labral flap tears, assist in synovectomy, and obtain material for biopsy. The grasping forceps is used to remove loose bodies and, on occasion, to extract foreign material that may be incidental to equipment failure. The grasping forceps also helps to assess the mobility of a torn rotator cuff. A small open curette (ring curette) (Appendix) effectively removes the thickened bursal tissue from the undersurface of the acromion to expose the bone for subsequent burring. This curette also works well to trim the loosened cartilaginous margins in areas of chondromalacia. The ordinary cup-shaped curette with a long handle is also helpful in these circumstances and may be used to remove calcific deposits from the interstitial region of a cuff tendon.

TRANSFER RODS

Two types of transfer rods are used (Fig. 2–7). One sturdy blunt-tipped portal rod, commonly referred to as a Wissinger rod, is used to pass through the

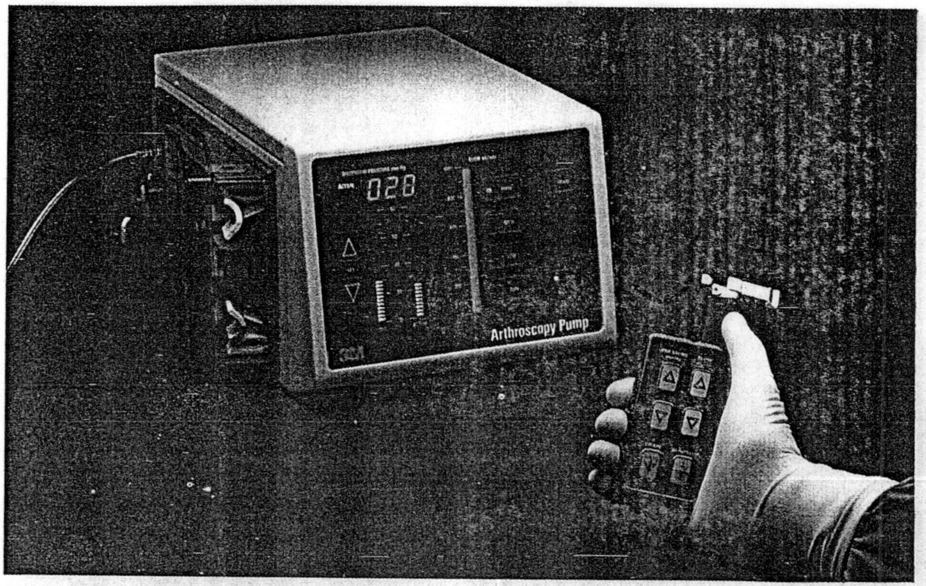

A

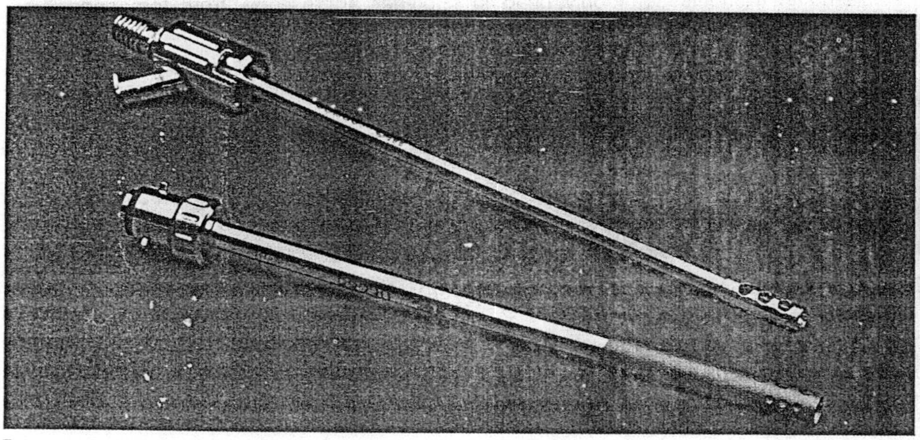

B

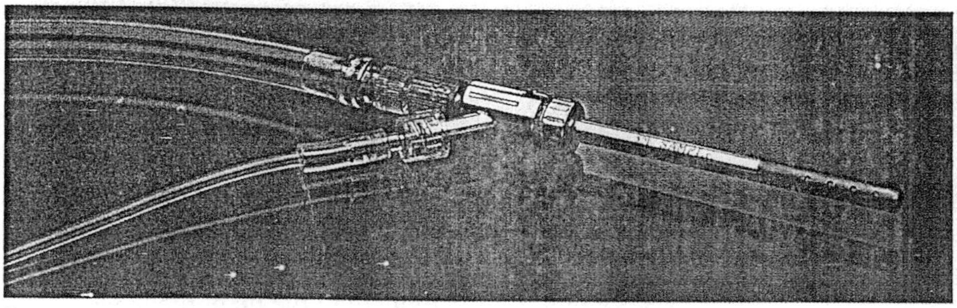

C

FIG. 2–5. A, Arthroscopy pump control box (3M).
B, Fluid ingress flow adapter.
C, Pump sensor attached to fluid ingress cannula.

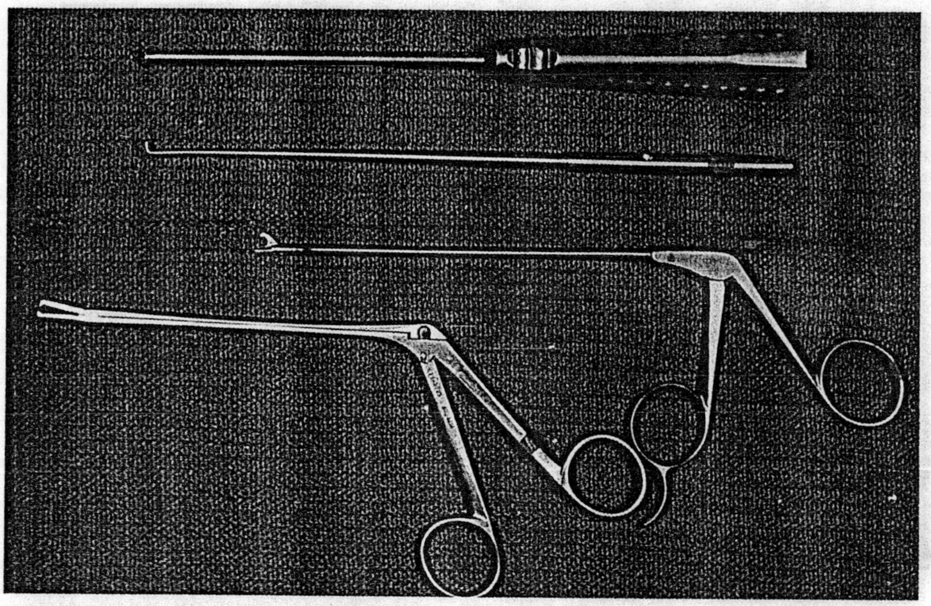

FIG. 2–6. Hand instruments commonly used in shoulder arthroscopy, from top: open curette, bent-arm probe, basket forceps, grasping forceps.

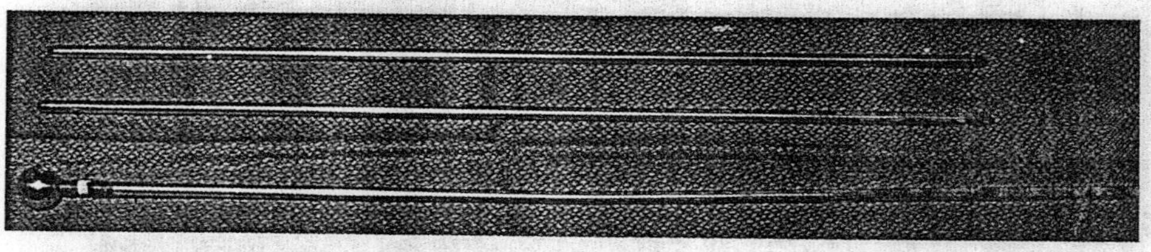

FIG. 2–7. Two types of transfer rods. Top, Wissinger rod. Bottom, Two switching sticks.

arthroscopic sheath posteriorly to penetrate the anterior capsule and exit the front of the shoulder superior and lateral to the tip of the coracoid. This rod becomes a guide over which the anterior portal cannula is introduced. One end of this rod generally is attached to a round ball-shaped handle that allows one to apply pressure comfortably. The other type of rod is called a switching stick. These rods are shorter and bluntly rounded at both ends. A pair of these sticks should be available. They are placed through the lumen of an established arthroscopic sheath or cannula to preserve the portal when the position of the arthroscope or operating cannula is changed from one side to another.

ARTHROSCOPIC CANNULAS

Various cannulas are used in shoulder arthroscopy. In general, the use of a nonfenestrated cannula is best because a minor misplacement of the tip of the fenestrated cannula would permit unnecessary extravasation of fluid into the soft tissue.

The fluid-ingress cannula is either a standard 5-mm metal cannula or a cannula specifically designed for use with the arthroscopy pump.

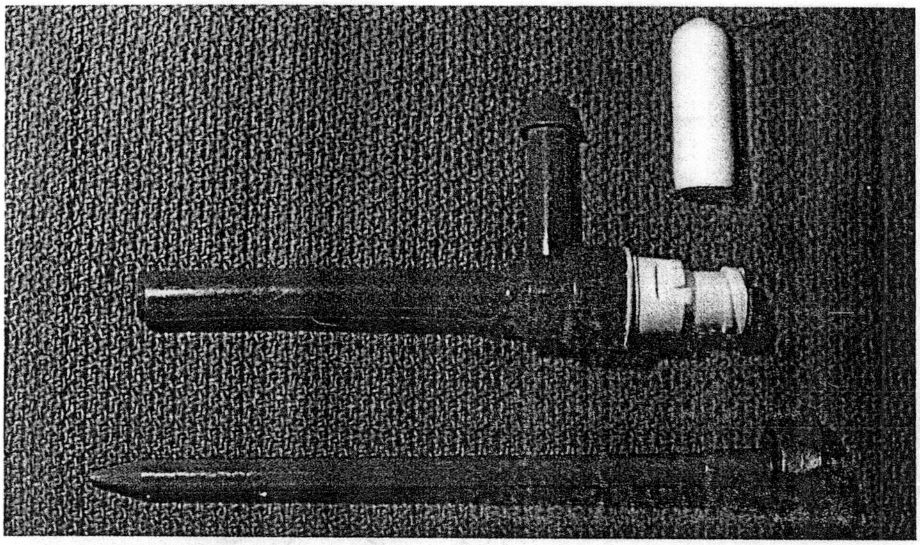

FIG. 2–8. Plastic surgical cannula with plastic diaphragm. The orange obturator is used to introduce the cannula.

The surgical cannula is made of plastic to allow electrosurgery without risk of conducting current and contains a diaphragm to maintain distention when instruments are removed and reintroduced (Fig. 2–8). Both blunt and sharp obturators are available for use during introduction of the cannula.

Special cannulas have been designed to introduce various larger instruments for specific procedures. They will be described later in the appropriate section.

ARTHROSCOPE

The standard arthroscope for use in the shoulder should have a 30° angled lens, a sheath that permits high-volume flow, and arms for both fluid inflow and suction outflow. An accessory 70° angled lens should be available for special circumstances.

POSITIONING EQUIPMENT

The positioning of equipment within the operating theater may vary with the preference of the surgeon and the confines of the operating room. We believe the following placement of equipment is most effective when performing shoulder arthroscopy in the lateral recumbent position (Fig. 2–9).

The arrangement for surgery to be performed on the right shoulder is described. The personnel and certain pieces of equipment are moved to the opposite side for surgery on the left shoulder.

The *television monitor* is placed at the head of the table, regardless of whether surgery is being performed on the right or left shoulder. The monitor should be situated 3 to 4 feet from the head of the table and elevated into a position where it can be easily viewed by the surgical team.

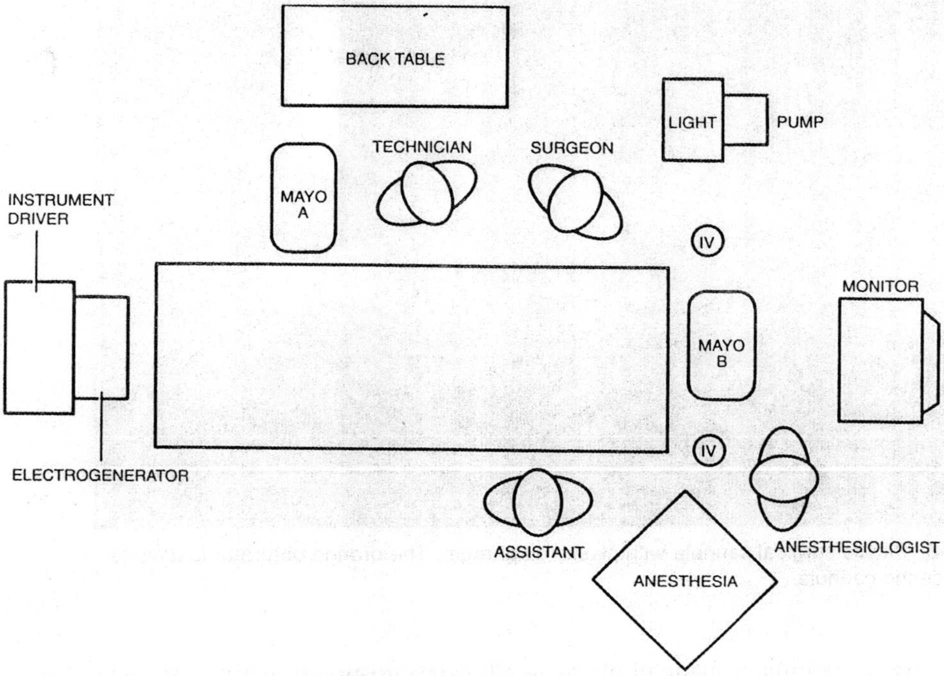

FIG. 2–9. Position of equipment for shoulder arthroscopy.

The *mechanical instrument driver* and *electrosurgical generator* are always placed at the foot of the table.

The *anesthetic equipment* and the anesthesiologist are always on the side facing the patient.

The *light source* (and the *arthroscopy pump*) are positioned behind the patient, close to the monitor.

IV poles are positioned at the head of the table on either side of the monitor. The pole situated behind the patient (on the same side as the light source and arthroscopy pump) holds 2 bags containing 3000 ml each of normal saline fluid and 1 bag containing 1000 ml of fluid.

Two *Mayo stands* are used for this procedure (Fig. 2–10). *Mayo stand A* is controlled by the scrub nurse and is positioned over the lower half of the table (Fig. 2–10A). This Mayo stand holds the following equipment:

1. Marking pen.
2. Scalpel with No. 11 blade.
3. 60-ml syringe (and extension tubing with 18-gauge 3½ inch spinal needle) filled with normal saline.
4. 20-ml syringe (with 25-gauge needle) filled with 0.25% bupivacaine (Marcaine) with adrenaline.
5. Arthroscope sheath with dual stopcock arms.
6. Fluid-ingress cannula, either
   a. For gravity inflow: 5-mm cannula (nonfenestrated) with dull and sharp trocars and an infusion adapter, or
   b. For arthroscopy pump: special cannula with sensor.

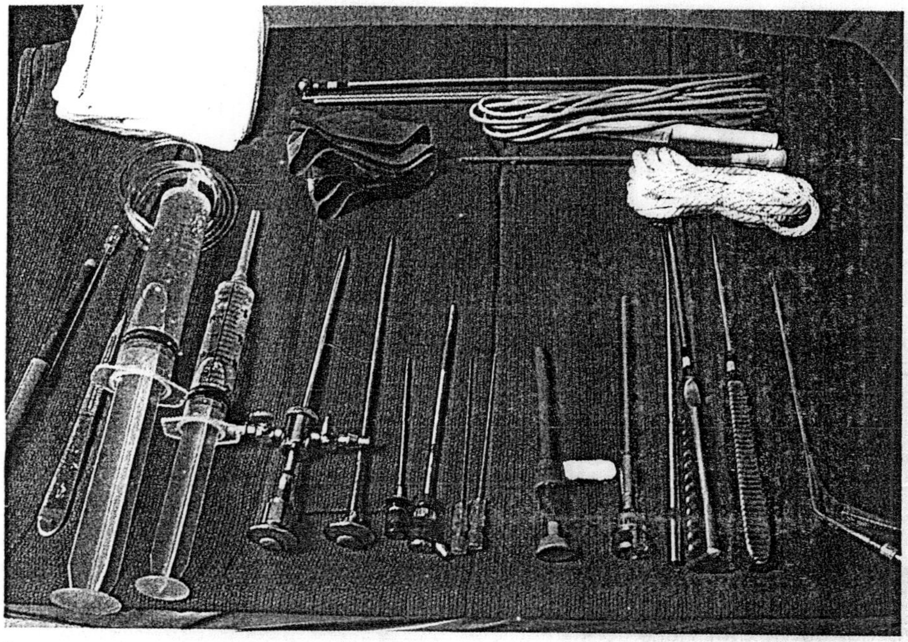

A

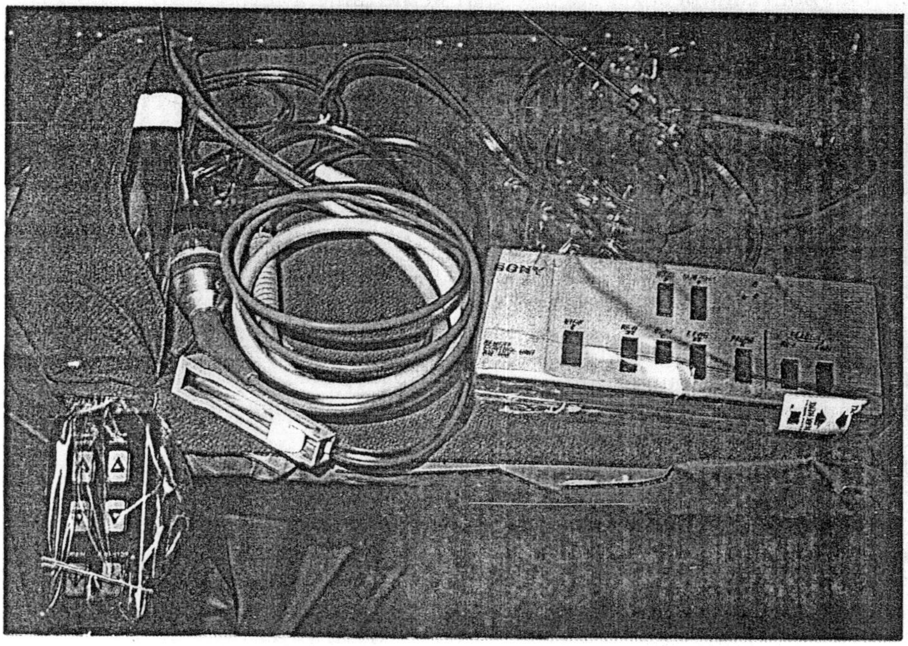

B

FIG. 2–10. A, Contents of Mayo stand A described in text are illustrated counterclockwise from the lower left.
B, Contents of Mayo stand B.

7. Two 20-gauge lumbar puncture needles.
8. Plastic operating cannula.
9. Hand instruments, including probe, curettes, basket forceps.
10. Two switching sticks and Wissinger (portal) rod.
11. Surgical electrode with cord.
12. Light handle covers.
13. Sterile rope for traction.

Mayo Stand B is positioned between the head of the table and the TV monitor after the patient has been draped (Fig. 2–10B). This Mayo stand contains:

1. Camera.
2. Light leads.
3. Suction tubing: two sets, one for arm of arthroscope sheath and the other to connect to motorized instrument driver.
4. Fluid ingress tubing.
   a. Gravity flow: cystoscopy Y-tubing from the 2 3000-ml bags of saline, or
   b. Arthroscopy pump tubing.
5. Cystoscopy tubing from 1000-ml bag of normal saline, to be connected to fluid ingress on arthroscopy sheath.
6. Control box for video deck.
7. Control for arthroscopy pump (if used).
8. N.B.: Both control boxes are placed in sterile camera covers.

This setup provides a dual fluid-ingress system. The tubing is connected to the bags of fluid and is "bled" to remove air bubbles from the system. The stopcock on the arthroscope closest to the head of the table is used for fluid ingress, and suction tubing is attached to the other stopcock.

When all the equipment is arranged, a final check is performed to ensure that everything mechanical is operational.

1. Test function of mechanical shaver (hand or foot control).
2. Be certain that suction is connected and working.
3. Check that electrosurgical generator is at proper settings for coagulation and cautery.
4. Verify that video monitor is on.
5. Verify that light source is on.
6. Connect light source to arthroscope and perform "white-out" to adjust color balance.
7. Record patient data at beginning of videotape or photodocumentation system.

The operating room is now ready for the patient.

LATERAL RECUMBENT POSITION

We routinely perform shoulder arthroscopy with the patient in the lateral recumbent position (Fig. 2–11A). This position best enables the surgeon to acquire skill in penetrating and exploring both the glenohumeral and the subacromial space. The semi-sitting (beach chair) position is described later in this chapter.

Positioning in the lateral recumbent position begins before the patient is

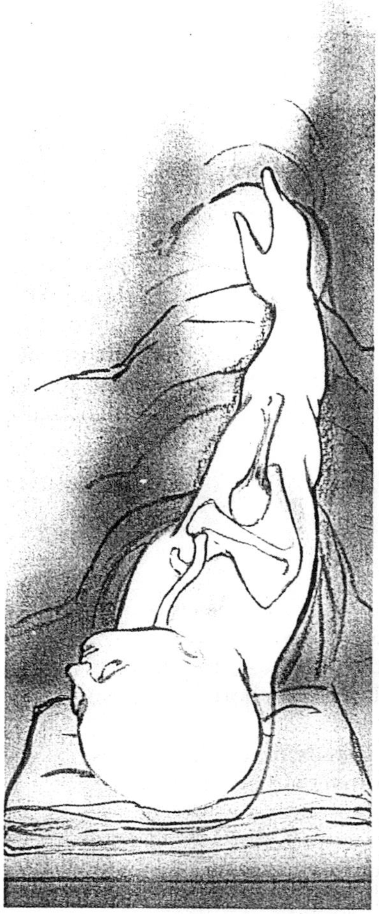

A

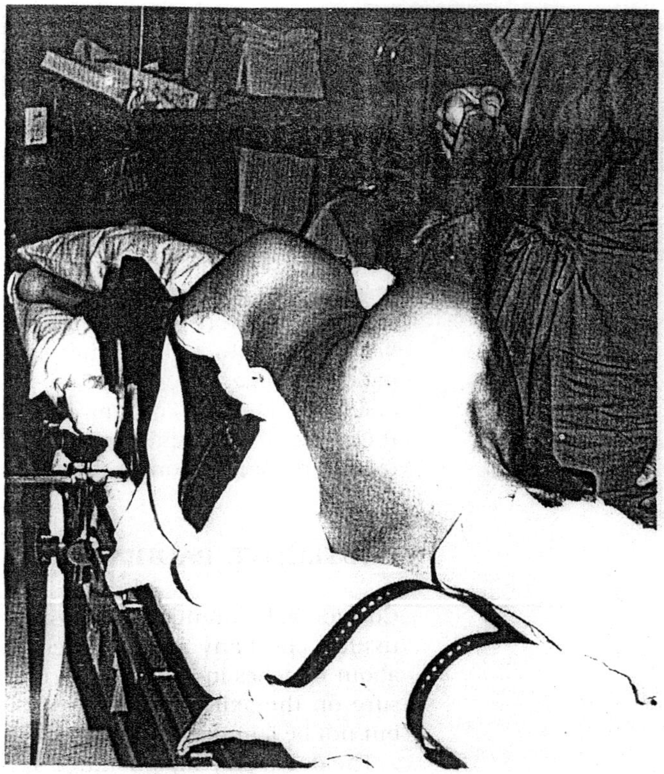

B

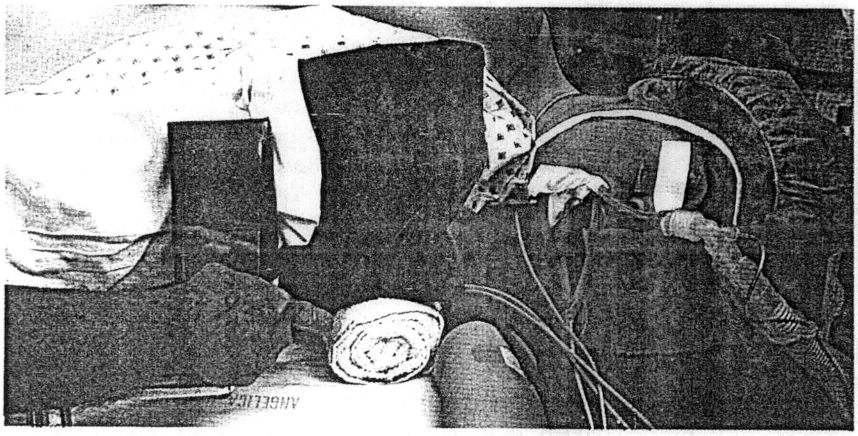

C

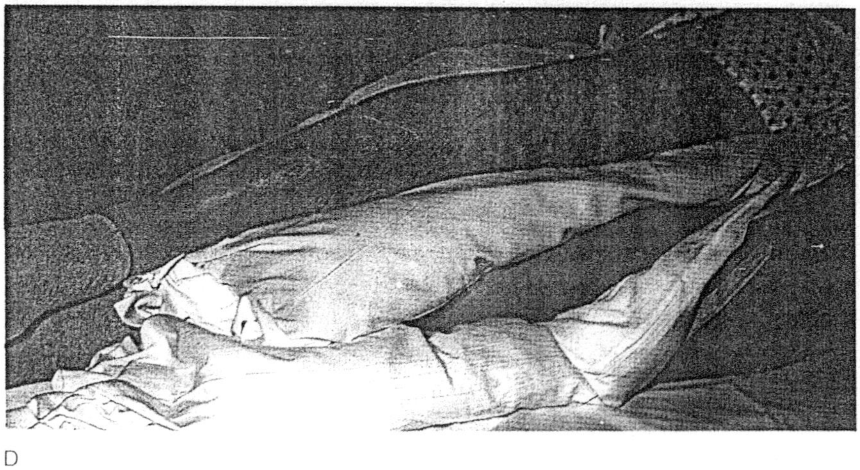

D

FIG. 2–11. Lateral recumbent position.
A, Sketch of patient in lateral recumbent position.
B, Patient in lateral recumbent position with suction support stiffened and reinforced by kidney rests.
C, Axillary roll in position to minimize pressure on axillary structures.
D, Peroneal nerves are protected by placing pillows beneath the lower leg and between the lower and upper leg.

placed on the operating room table. A vacuum-type beanbag (Appendix) is placed on the operating room table, and the particles are smoothed for even distribution. The patient is assisted onto the table and centered on the beanbag. The proximal end of the support should be level with the patient's axilla. After general endotracheal anesthesia has been established, both shoulders are examined for evidence of instability. The patient is then rolled over to lie on the unaffected side, making sure both the pelvis and shoulders are vertical to the table. The beanbag is gathered up and smoothed against the patient. At this point, the patient is rolled another 15 or 20° posteriorly, and the suction support is stiffened (Fig. 2–11B). Posterior inclination of the laterally recumbent patient places the plane of the glenohumeral joint in a near horizontal position, which facilitates joint penetration.

PROTECTIVE PADDING

Considerable attention is given to protecting the neurovascular structures, soft tissues, and bony prominences. An axillary roll made of a soft sheet or towel about 6 inches in circumference is placed just below the axilla to minimize pressure on the axillary structures (Fig. 2–11C). The roll must support the thorax, but not be jammed too high into the axilla.

The down-side hip and knee are moderately flexed to stabilize the lateral position. Both peroneal nerves, as well as the knees and malleoli, are protected by placing pillows beneath the lower leg and between the lower and upper leg (Fig. 2–11D). Breasts are also carefully padded to avoid pressure from the beanbag. Each pressure area is checked by the surgeon. Kidney rests, pelvic straps, or broad adhesive tape are used to stabilize this position further.

The cervical spine must be supported throughout the procedure to avoid any hyperextension or lateral angulation that might provoke cervicobrachial radiculopathy in older patients. The anesthesiologist is asked to tape the endotracheal tube on the side of the mouth away from the surgical side.

PREP AND DRAPE

The shaved area includes the shoulder, the upper outer quadrant of the thorax anteriorly and posteriorly, and the arm to the elbow. Prior to skin preparation, a sterile adhesive U-drape is placed to screen the shoulder region (Fig. 2–12A). The operating area should not be constrained by this drape. The "U" should be attached to the side and back of the neck just below the hairline. Wide access to the shoulder is obtained posteriorly by affixing the drape along the vertebral border of the scapula and anteriorly by positioning the drape just lateral to the nipple line.

The skin area outlined is washed and painted with an iodine-based preparation (or other scrub solution preferred by the surgeon). The area of preparation includes the entire arm and hand (Fig. 2–12B). Sterile drapes are then applied with care to avoid encroaching on the operative area. Commercially available paper shoulder packs containing two large U-shaped tails are quite convenient. The drapes are arranged first with the tails up and then with the tails down (Fig. 2–12C and D). The Kimberly-Clark shoulder drape pack (see Appendix) includes a fluid-containment device that fits nicely around the shoulder and seals the

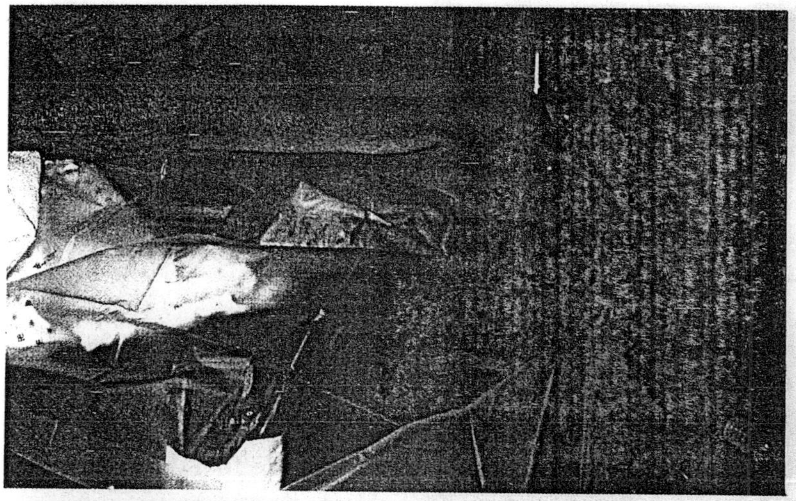

A

FIG. 2–12. A, A sterile U-drape is placed to allow wide access to the shoulder region.
B, The shoulder and entire arm and hand are prepped.
C, Shoulder pack (Kimberly-Clark) provides two adhesive-backed U-shaped split sheets. The first is placed from below upward.

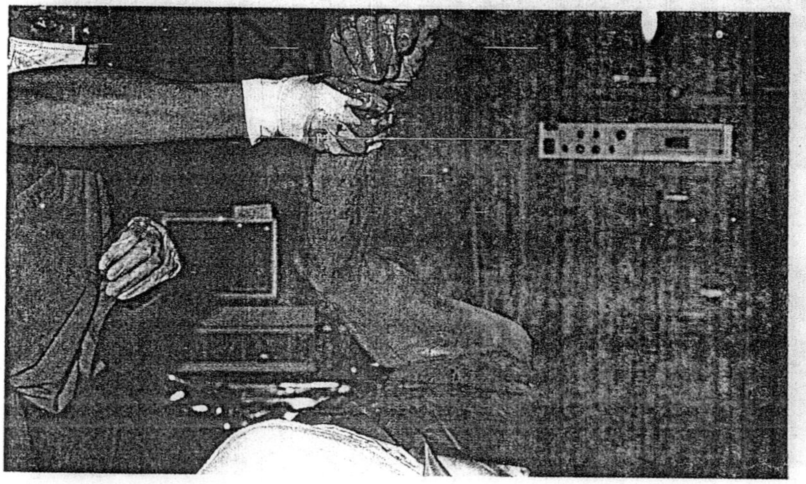

B

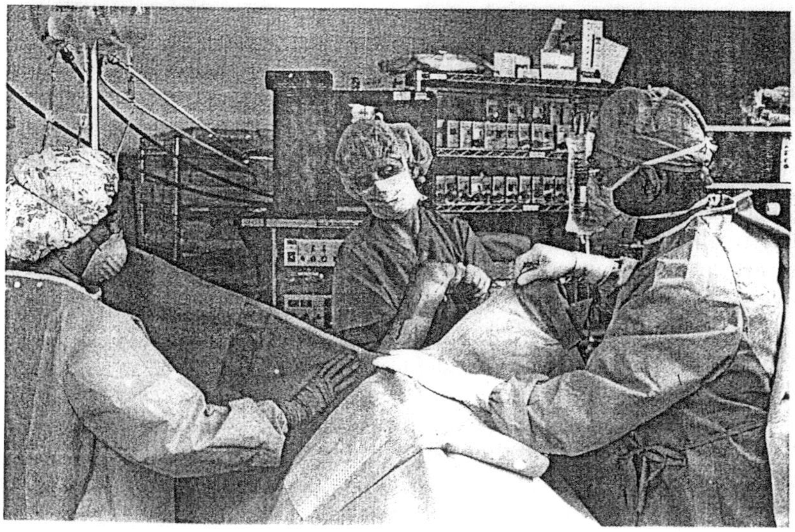

C

FIG. 2–12. (Continues)

FIG. 2–12. (Continued)
D, The tails of the second split sheet are applied from above downward.
E, The superior drape includes a fluid-containment device that seals the area and is channeled to gravity drainage.

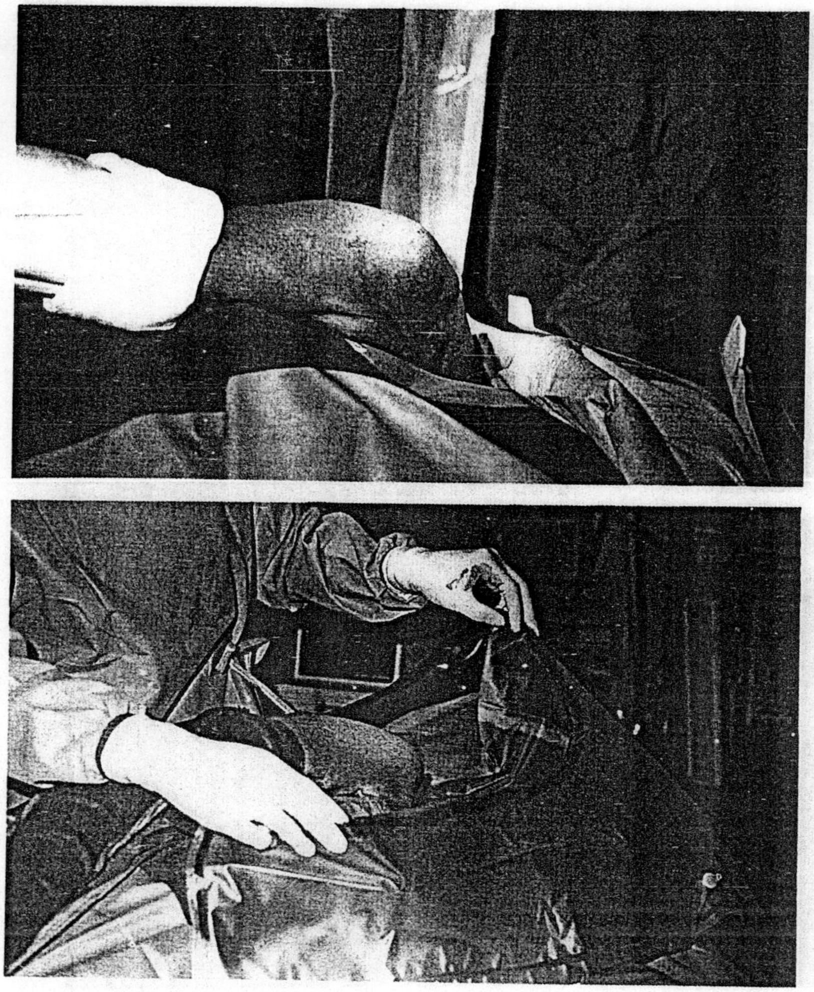

D

E

area (Fig. 2–12E). Excess fluids are collected neatly and channeled to gravity drainage. The forearm is then placed in traction.

TRACTION

Traction to the arm may be applied in various fashions. Commercial traction sleeves are available. Some are based on the Buck's extension principle with adhesive strips affixed to the forearm. A simple device composed of padded plastic-lined tubular stockinette includes a cloth loop at the end with a sterile hook and rope attached (Appendix). The device is held to the forearm with Coban or elastic bandages (Fig. 2–13A).

For many years, we encased the arm in plastic-lined tubular stockinette held by sterile elastic bandages and then padded the wrist with a 4-inch roll of sterile cast padding. A roll of 3- or 4-inch sterile gauze was then used to place a loop around the wrist, which was then attached to a weighted pulley system.

SKY HOOK TRACTION

We have attached a sturdy fixture hook to the operating room ceiling (Fig. 2–13B). A rope with a pulley attached is suspended from this "sky hook," and a second loop of rope passes through the pulley to a weight carrier (Fig. 2–13C and D). The operating room table is arranged in relation to the sky hook, so that the arm is suspended in 15 to 20° of abduction and 15 to 20° of forward flexion (Fig. 2–13E).

The sterile rope, or tails of the sterile roller gauze attached to the padded arm sleeve, is then tied to the traction rope at a point distal to the operating table, thereby preserving sterility along the entire extremity.

The table is angled in relation to the sky hook to accommodate either a right or a left arm. A line drawn on the operating room floor facilitates the positioning of the table before the procedure begins.

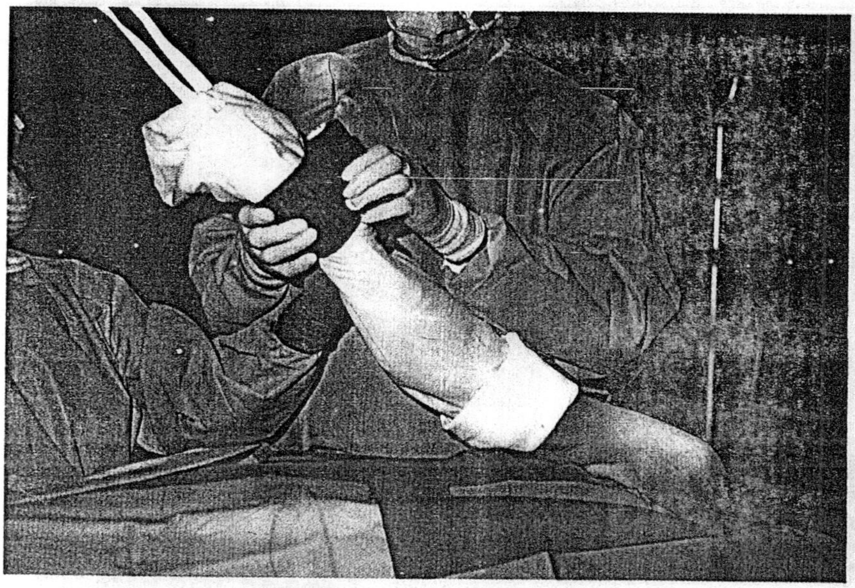

FIG. 2–13. A, The arm is encased in a plastic-lined tubular stockinette and is held in position with Coban. B, A sturdy fixture hook is attached to the ceiling, and a rope with pulley attached is suspended.

A
B

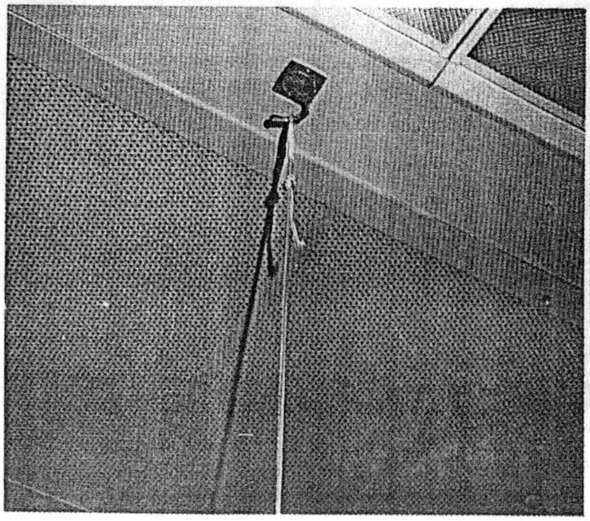

FIG. 2–13. (Continues)

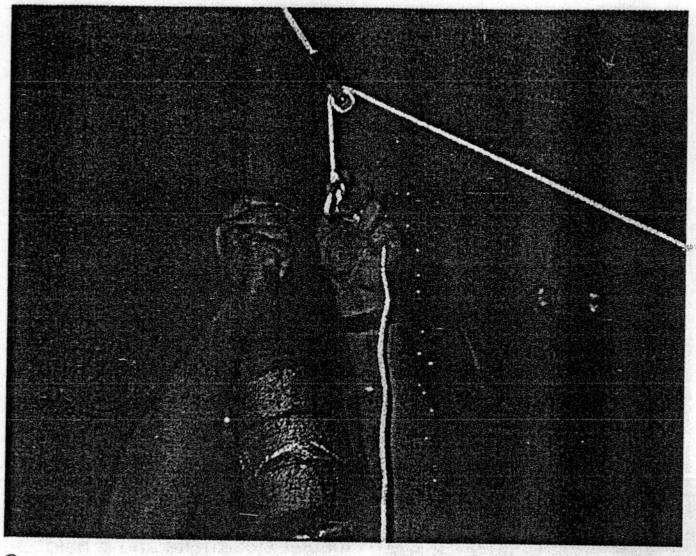

C

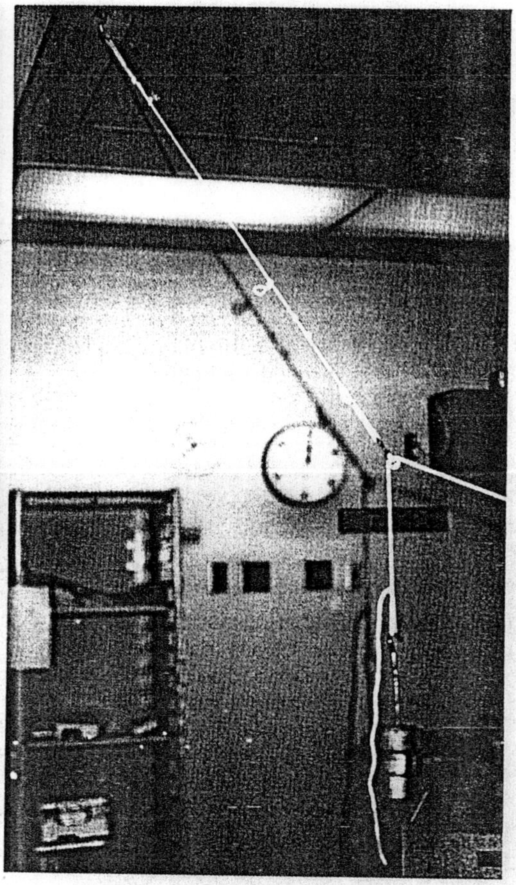

D

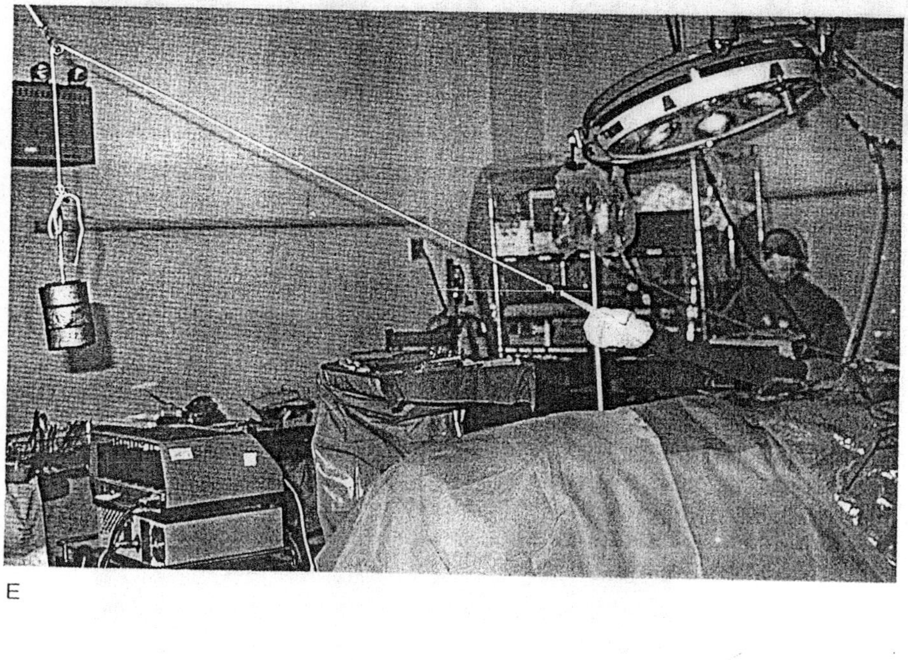

E

FIG. 2–13. (Continued)
C, The traction rope passes through the pulley suspended from the ceiling, and 10 to 15 pounds of traction are applied.
D, The vector of forces in "sky hook" traction setup.
E, The arm is suspended in 15 to 20° of abduction for arthroscopic surgery in the lateral recumbent position.

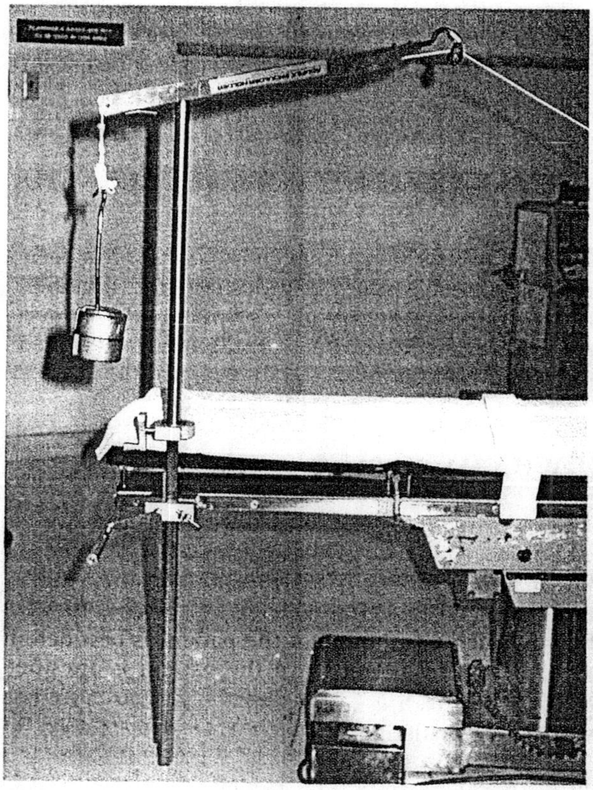

FIG. 2–14. A sturdy traction device is attached to the table.

OTHER TRACTION DEVICES

Numerous traction devices that attach directly to the table are available (Fig. 2–14). Most of them, however, are designed to hold the arm at 45° or more of abduction, which is too much abduction for this type of procedure. The tuberosity encroaches on the subacromial space as abduction is increased, thereby making instrumentation in the area quite difficult. A shoulder holder that can be adjusted for as little as 20° abduction should be selected. Most of these attached shoulder holders encroach on the area above the table. Care must be taken to avoid compromising sterility. A bulky but effective traction device may also be constructed from the materials used for an overhead bed frame.

TRACTION TIPS

Neurovascular structures may be compromised by sustained traction. The greater the abduction, the more the brachial plexus is at risk. Traction weight should not exceed 15 pounds. For smaller individuals, a weight of 10 pounds is adequate. The arm should not be suspended from a fixed point. Minor changes in position of the patient or table could provoke serious traction neuropathy.

Peripheral nerves should be protected also. The dorsal cutaneous branch of the superficial radial nerve to the thumb is in jeopardy when traction is applied at the wrist area. Padding is required from the metacarpophalangeal level of the thumb to a point proximal to the radial styloid to protect this nerve.

Traction is ineffective when the rope hangs up at the corner of the pulley or when a knot rests directly against the pulley. The weights must not be allowed to rest on the floor. Weights should be tied securely. Slippage may cause injury to the patient or personnel.

SEMI-SITTING (BEACH CHAIR) POSITION

The semi-sitting or beach chair position has been adopted by some as preferable to the lateral recumbent position for shoulder arthroscopy. We employ the beach chair position on all *open* shoulder surgery. When an open procedure is probable, but diagnostic arthroscopy is indicated to confirm the diagnosis, the patient is set up in the beach chair position.

BEACH CHAIR SETUP

The key to achieving a true beach chair position for shoulder surgery is the horizontal positioning of the thighs, with the knees slightly bent, while the trunk (torso) approaches the vertical. Whether the operating room table and the manipulation of the controls by the anesthesiologist or circulating nurse will allow such positioning of the patient is best determined *before* the patient enters the operating room. Once the patient is anesthetized, it is too late to discover that the controls are not functioning properly or that neither the anesthesiologist nor the circulating nurse has a clear idea of the position you wish to achieve.

The head must be stabilized when the backrest is elevated. We usually use the neurosurgical headrest for shoulder surgery in the beach chair position (Fig. 2–15). The device must be positioned as far as possible toward the affected side to maximize overhang of the shoulder. A kidney rest or pelvic strap is added to prevent the patient from falling. The backrest should be elevated before the head is taped to the support. The neck should be maintained in as anatomically neutral a position as possible. The position of the head and neck should be checked after even slight adjustments in position. Slippage could be catastrophic. A contoured foam rubber cushion instead of the neurosurgical headrest may be used to support the head. This cushion, however, may not allow as much access to the shoulder if the device is too bulky. The head must be taped securely in every case.

Specially designed beach chair supports are available and may be attached to a standard operating table. These supports offer secure fixation and good access to the shoulder.

PROBLEMS WITH THE BEACH CHAIR POSITION

Although the weight of the arm provides distraction when the patient is in the beach chair position, additional traction may be required. Arthroscopic acromioplasty may be quite difficult in a muscular patient without sustained traction. This procedure, therefore, is best accomplished in the lateral recumbent position with attached weights operated through a pulley system.

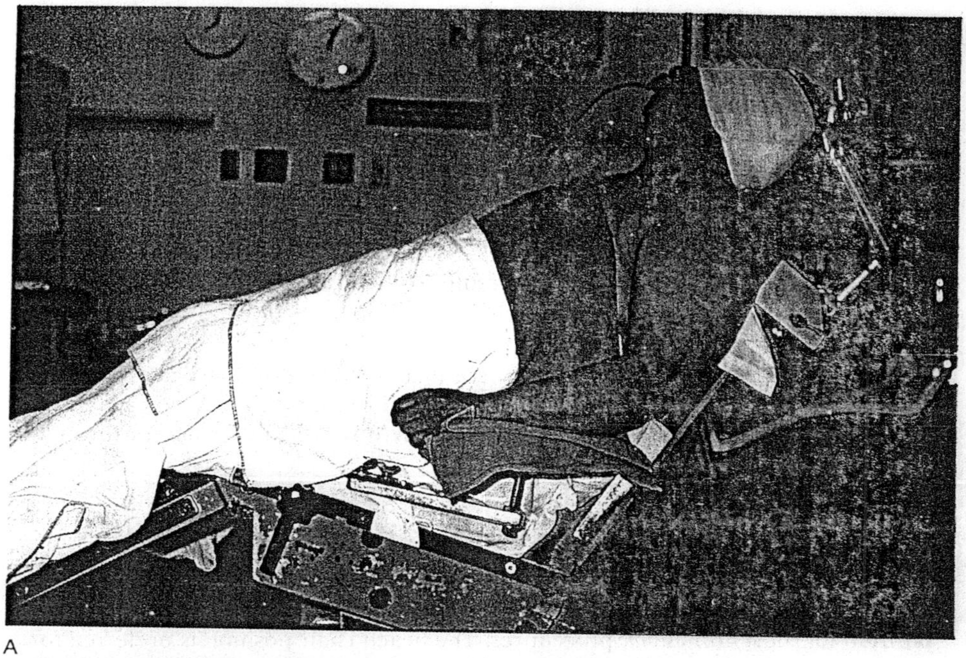

A

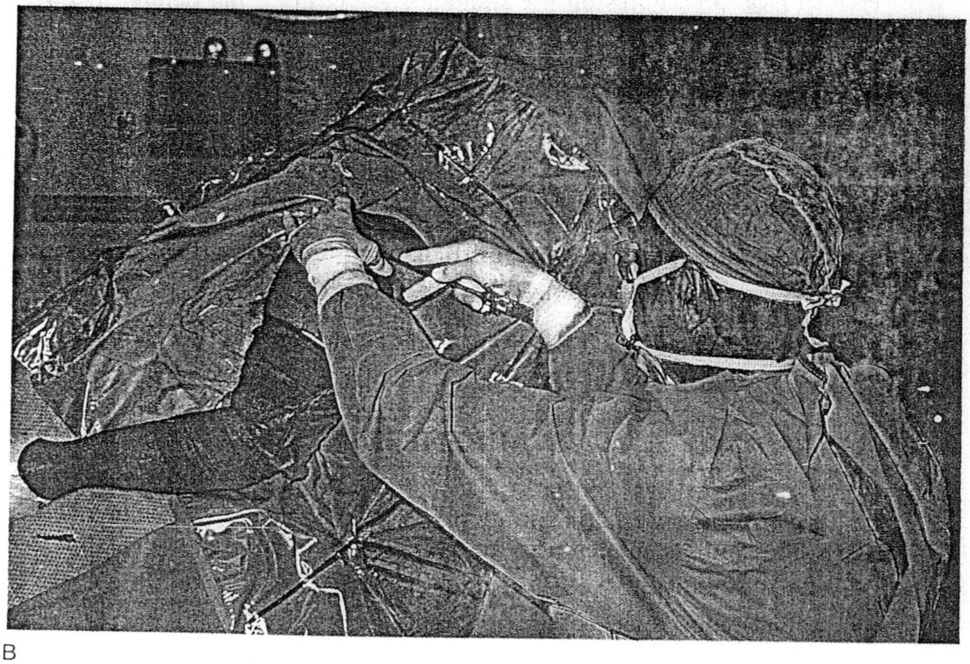

B

FIG. 2–15. Beach chair or semi-sitting position.
A, Backrest is elevated, and head is stabilized in the neurosurgical headrest.
B, The surgeon is behind the patient, who is in a semi-sitting position. The arthroscope is being introduced.

Hypotension may develop in the anesthetized patient as the head is elevated to the beach chair position. The backrest should be raised slowly and the blood pressure monitored during the process.

Most proponents of the beach chair position advocate regional anesthesia with a scalene block. We have found that the ability to achieve this block varies with the skill of the anesthesiologist. Induction of the block takes longer than endotracheal anesthesia. When either depth of anesthesia or patient apprehension requires supplemental general anesthesia, an awkward and potentially dangerous situation develops. Preservation of an adequate airway is difficult in a sitting position should supplemental inhalation or intravenous anesthesia be required. In some instances, the procedure may have to be interrupted while the patient is intubated.

Failure to elevate the patient's back to a near-vertical position places the surgeon in an awkward position. When sufficient back elevation is not achieved, the surgeon must crouch and work from below upward to gain access through the posterior portal.

POSITIONING TIPS

For many of the reasons noted in this chapter, we prefer the lateral recumbent position for most *arthroscopic* procedures. The beach chair position is preferred for most *open* surgical procedures on the shoulder. We position the patient in the beach chair position for diagnostic arthroscopy when the probability is high that open intervention will follow. A common example involves the patient with instability. Following examination under anesthesia, the arthroscope sometimes is introduced to evaluate labral capsular integrity and to search for Hill-Sachs' or other osteocartilaginous abnormalities (see Chap. 13). The findings may either negate further intervention or confirm the indication for open stabilization (Bankart or capsular reefing) or arthroscopic surgery. Another example occurs when the repairability of a cuff tear is in question. In principle, the arthroscope is not used as a routine diagnostic instrument but rather as a tool to augment or negate the clinical diagnosis after the patient has been brought into the operating room for intervention. The decision to position the patient in either the lateral recumbent or the beach chair position depends on the probability that the preoperative diagnosis is correct. Either position can be changed when indicated.

APPENDIX

The basic arthroscopy equipment referred to in the text is listed below. This list reflects the authors' preference, and no endorsement is intended. In most instances, various manufacturers supply comparable equipment.

1. Full-radius resectors
   4.5-mm (Smith & Nephew United, Inc./Dyonics #3443)
   4.2-mm (Linvatec/Concept #9247A)
2. Serrated shavers
   Turbotrimmer, 4.5-mm (Smith & Nephew United, Inc./Dyonics #3529)
   Meniscal cutter, 4.2-mm (Linvatec/Concept #9761A)
3. Aggressive shavers
   Synovator, 4.5-mm (Smith & Nephew United, Inc./Dyonics #3826)
   Gator aggressive meniscal cutter, 4.2-mm (Linvatec/Concept #9761A)

4. Round or oval burs
   Acromionizer, 4.0-mm (Smith & Nephew United, Inc./Dyonics #3452)
   Acromionizer, 5.5-mm (Smith & Nephew United, Inc./Dyonics #3453)
   Abrader (spherical bur), 4.0-mm (Smith & Nephew United, Inc./Dyonics #3450)
   Oval bur, 4.0-mm (Linvatec/Concept #9759)
   Spherical bur, 4.5-mm (Linvatec/Concept #9774)
5. Electrosurgical equipment
   Electrosurgical arthroscopy generator (ESA) (Linvatec/Concept)
   Meniscectomy electrode, 165-mm, 6.5-inches-long (Linvatec/Concept #9735B)
6. Irrigation tubing
   Cystoscopy/bladder irrigation set, 2-meter (Baxter Healthcare Corp., #264040)
7. Fluid bag elevation
   Power lifter (Ditmore Co.)
8. Cannulas
   Fluid ingress cannula set (includes 4.5-mm cannula, two obturators, trocar set, and infusion adapter) (Smith & Nephew United, Inc./Dyonics #3707)
   Plastic surgical cannula, shoulder, without fenestration, 7-cm × 5.5-mm (Linvatec/Concept #9718)
   Plastic cannula, 7-cm × 7-mm (Acufex #012420)
9. Patient support
   Vac-Pac vacuum beanbag (Olympic Medical)
10. Draping
   Shoulder arthroscopy pack (Kimberly–Clark Corp., #88592)
11. Shoulder suspension
   Shoulder suspension kit, 7-foot sterile rope with S hook, and impermeable drape (Smith & Nephew United, Inc./Dyonics #3583)
   Coban, 4-inch-wide 3M Health Care
12. Pump
   Arthroscopy pump system 3M Health Care

GLENOHUMERAL JOINT ARTHROSCOPY: NORMAL ANATOMY AND VARIATIONS

3

Shoulder arthroscopy encompasses both the glenohumeral joint and the subacromial space. Both regions must be entered and inspected independently, except when a rotator cuff rupture rolls back the roof of the glenohumeral joint, thereby establishing free communication between the two regions.

This chapter describes in step-by-step detail the technique for penetrating the glenohumeral joint, inspecting its surfaces, and establishing the portals necessary for intra-articular surgery. Normal anatomy, as well as borderline variations, is described and illustrated. The techniques of subacromial space surgery, including arthroscopic subacromial decompression, are covered subsequently.

BONY LANDMARKS

The procedure begins with the anesthetized patient in the lateral recumbent position. After traction has been established, the bony landmarks are outlined. The location of the acromion, clavicle, acromioclavicular joint, coracoid process, and coracoacromial ligament should be precisely outlined at the onset of the procedure. A right shoulder is illustrated as viewed from the head of the table (Fig. 3–1).

Begin with the *posterior angle of the acromion.* This angle can be palpated even in the most muscular or obese patients. Pinch the angle with the thumb and index finger and mark the area with a marking pen (Fig. 3–1A). The angle formed is slightly obtuse.

Place your index finger just below the *spine of the scapula* and move upward along the inferior border. Extend the line medially (Fig. 3–1B).

Next, press your thumb into the *supraclavicular fossa* behind the most lateral portion of the clavicle. The curvilinear outline of your thumb defines the medial aspect of the acromion, as well as the posterior end of the clavicle (Fig. 3–1C).

Search for the *anterior subcutaneous border of the clavicle* (Fig. 3–1D). This border is readily palpable when you begin medially below the sternoclavicular joint. Outline the landmark laterally.

Now, to define the *lateral margin of the acromion,* snug the index finger up from below the lateral border of the acromion and extend the line forward to the anterolateral corner of the acromion. Then, connect the anterior border of the

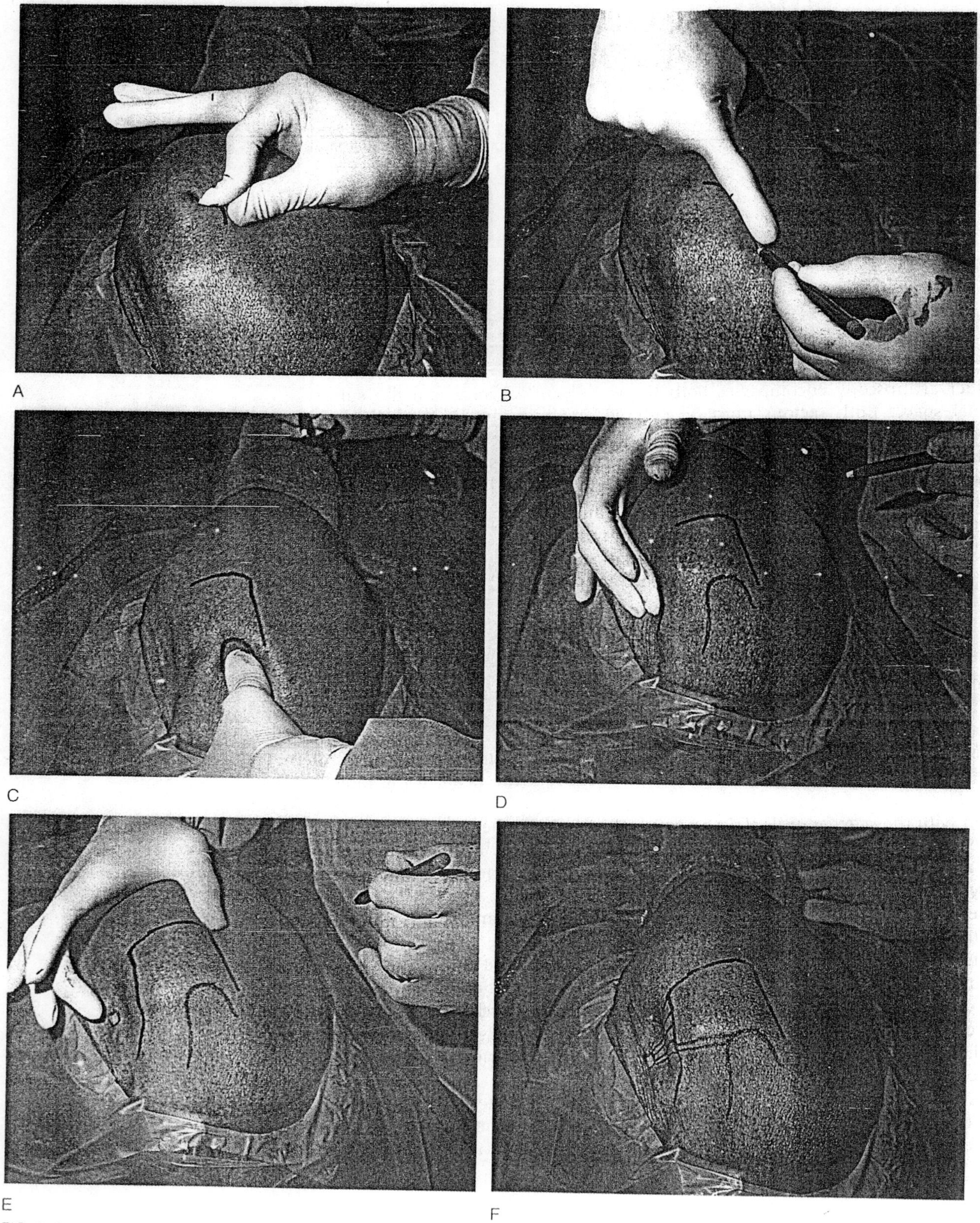

A B C D E F

FIG. 3–1

◀ FIG. 3–1. Bony landmarks of a right shoulder in the lateral recumbent position are outlined. The surgeon is behind the patient, and the view is from above.
A, Posterior angle of acromion is palpated and marked.
B, Finger just below spine of scapula.
C, Thumb in supraclavicular fossa defines medial aspect of acromion and posterior border of clavicle.
D, Marking anterior subcutaneous border of clavicle.
E, Lateral and anterior margins of the acromion have been added. Tip of coracoid is being palpated.
F, The location of the acromioclavicular joint and coracoacromial ligament are drawn to complete the bony landmarks.

clavicle to the corner of the acromion. Define the *posterior border of the clavicle,* and then extend the outline of the scapular spine along its posterosuperior border (Fig. 3–1E).

Mark the *acromioclavicular joint,* and then palpate and circle the tip of the coracoid. Draw in the *coracoacromial ligament* to complete the bony landmarks (Fig. 3–1F).

MARKING THE PORTALS

The four potential portals for shoulder arthroscopy are the posterior, posterolateral, anterolateral, and anterior portals. Their locations are marked at this time.

POSTERIOR PORTAL

The posterior portal, which is the primary portal for shoulder arthroscopy, is used initially to penetrate the glenohumeral joint and explore its contents. Later, this same portal is used to direct instruments into the subacromial space.

The posterior portal is marked approximately 2 cm (1 thumbbreadth) distal and 2 cm medial to the posterior angle of the acromion (Fig. 3–2A). This point represents the location of a soft spot between the infraspinatus and teres minor overlying the posterior border of the glenohumeral joint.

POSTEROLATERAL PORTAL

This portal is marked approximately 1.5 cm below the posterior angle of the acromion (Fig. 3–2B). During subacromial space surgery, the arthroscope is directed through this portal. In a small individual, this portal is moved 1 cm anteriorly to allow more room for manipulation of the instruments without any collision.

ANTEROLATERAL PORTAL

This portal is marked no more than 3 cm lateral to the anterolateral corner of the scapula *in a direct line with the anterior margin of the acromion* (Fig. 3–2C). A plastic operating cannula must enter through this portal to perform surgery within the subacromial space (see Chapter 5).

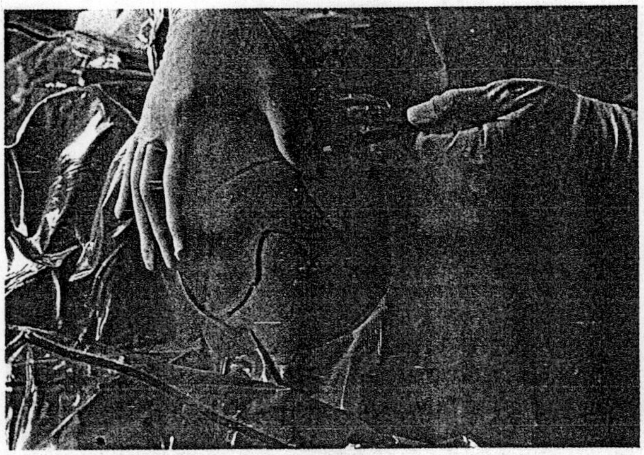

A

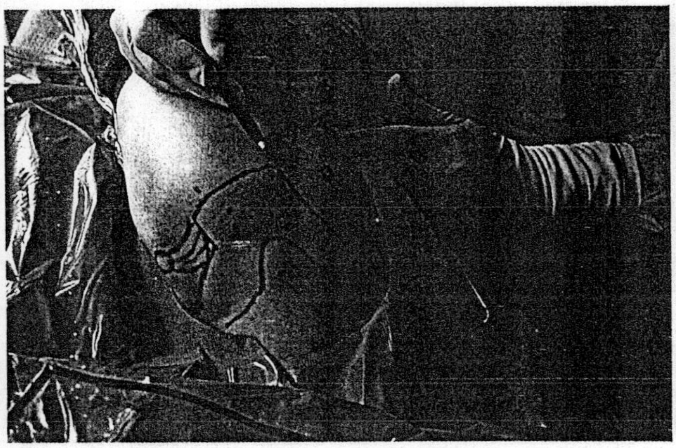

B

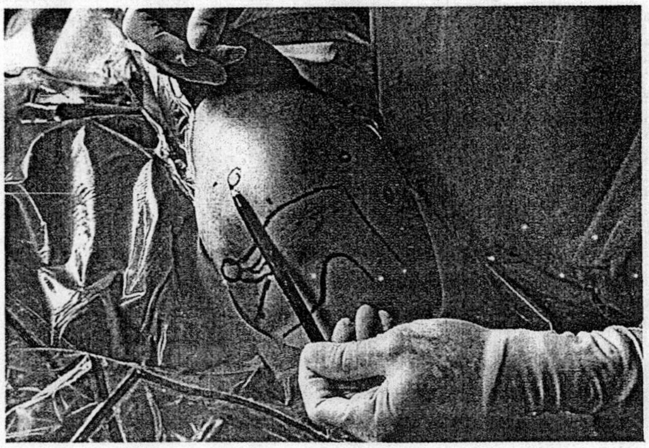

C

FIG. 3–2. Marking the portals.
A, The superior portal is located 2 cm (1 thumb-breadth) distal and 2 cm medial to the posterior angle of the acromion.
B, The posterolateral portal is approximately 1.5 cm below the posterior angle of the acromion.
C, Anterolateral portal marked 3 to 4 cm distal to acromion in a direct line with anterior edge.

ANTERIOR PORTAL

The frequently used anterior portal is located just above and slightly lateral to the tip of the acromion process. This portal is established from within the joint, as described subsequently.

Before proceeding, recheck your outline of the bony prominences and portals carefully. Make any corrections necessary to ensure the accuracy of your drawing. Poorly defined landmarks invariably plague the procedure.

A 10-ml syringe filled with bupivacaine (Marcaine) and adrenaline is used to infiltrate the portals. Both subcutaneous and deeper structures are injected to reduce portal bleeding and diminish postoperative discomfort.

GLENOHUMERAL INSPECTION

Every shoulder arthroscopy begins with a systematic inspection of the glenohumeral joint. The joint is entered through the posterior portal, which has been previously marked. A relative soft spot can be palpated approximately 1 thumb-breadth (2 cm) inferior and 1 thumb-breadth (2 cm) medial to the posterior angle of the acromion. The humeral head can be grasped from behind and translated anteriorly and posteriorly in relation to the stabilized scapula (Fig. 3–3). The precise location of the posterior joint line is established in this fashion. An actual sketch of the contour of the humeral head and glenoid drawn directly on the patient's skin may help to better appreciate the relationships. Remember that the glenoid surface is relatively anteverted about 30° in relation to the trunk. Tilting of the patient (or of the table) about 30° posteriorly places the glenoid surface in a relatively horizontal position (Fig. 3–4).

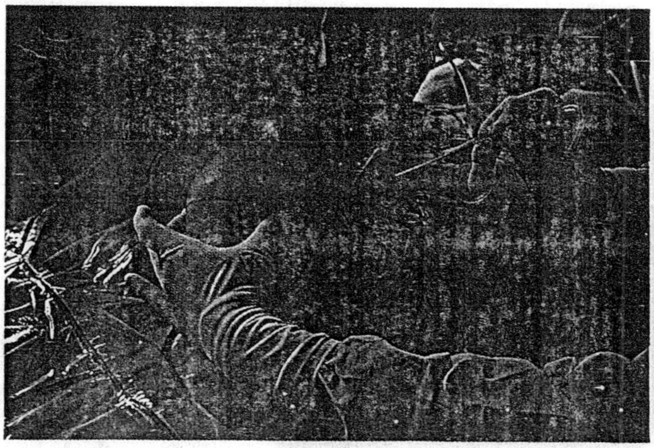

FIG. 3–3. The humeral head is grasped and translated anteriorly and posteriorly to identify posterior soft spot.

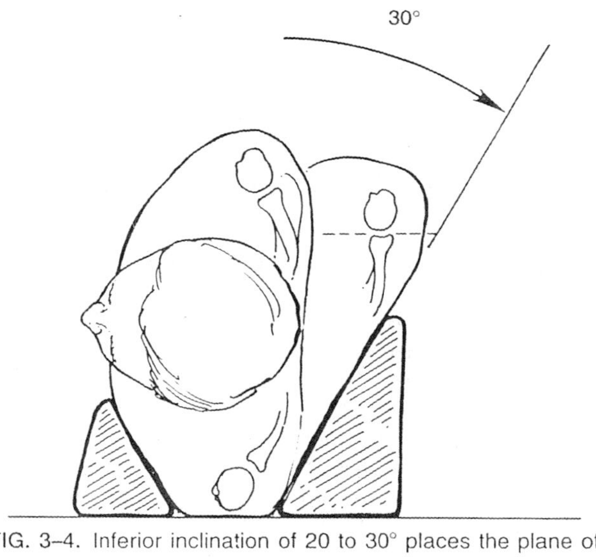

FIG. 3–4. Inferior inclination of 20 to 30° places the plane of the glenohumeral joint in a relatively horizontal position.

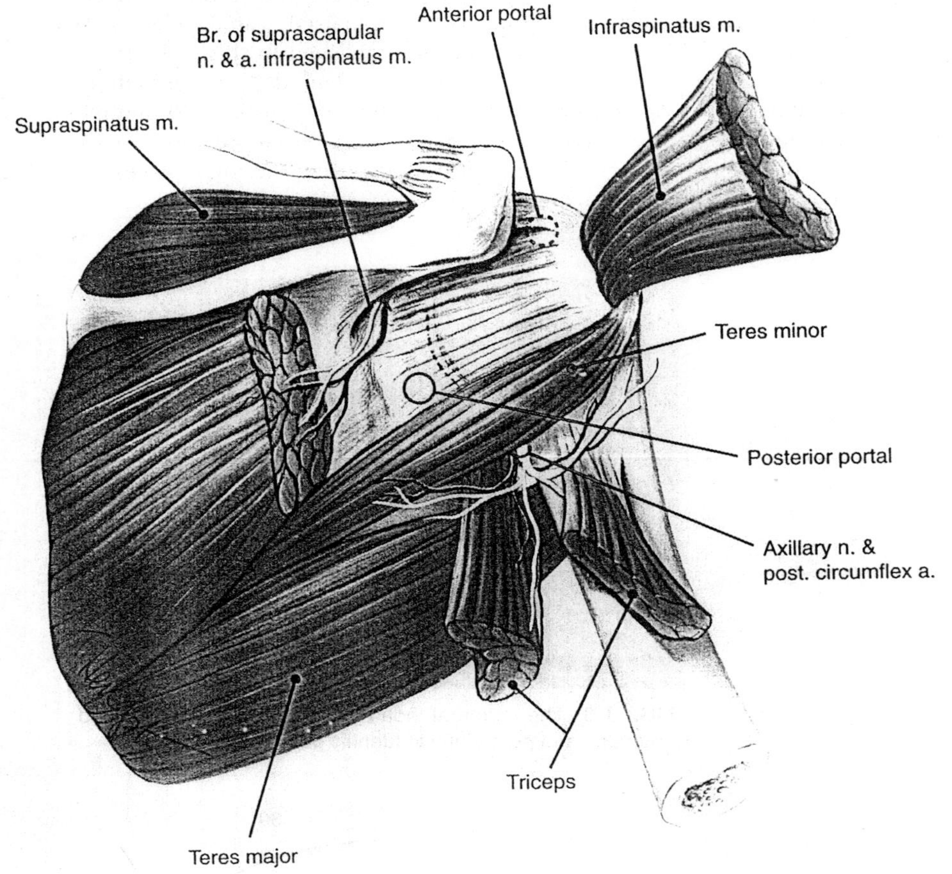

FIG. 3–5. Posterior portal anatomy. Posterior portal location in relation to contiguous structures. Note that teres minor separates the posterior portal from the axillary nerve and the posterior circumflex artery as they emerge from the quadrangular space. Also observe proximity of the infraspinous branch of the subscapular nerve.

POSTERIOR PORTAL ANATOMY (FIG. 3–5)

The optimum location for posterior joint penetration lies between the inferior margin of the infraspinatus and the superior margin of the teres minor at the joint line. The width of the teres minor separates this portal from the axillary nerve as it exits the quadrangular space. Branches of the suprascapular nerve to the infraspinatus are located 1.5 to 2 cm from the joint line along the posterior aspect of the glenoid neck. Thus, both the axillary and the suprascapular nerves are close to the posterior portal. Great care must be exercised to avoid injury to these nerves when establishing this portal.

PREINSUFFLATION

The glenohumeral joint is preinsufflated with 30 to 40 ml of normal saline prior to introducing the arthroscope. An 18-gauge needle with flexible plastic tubing

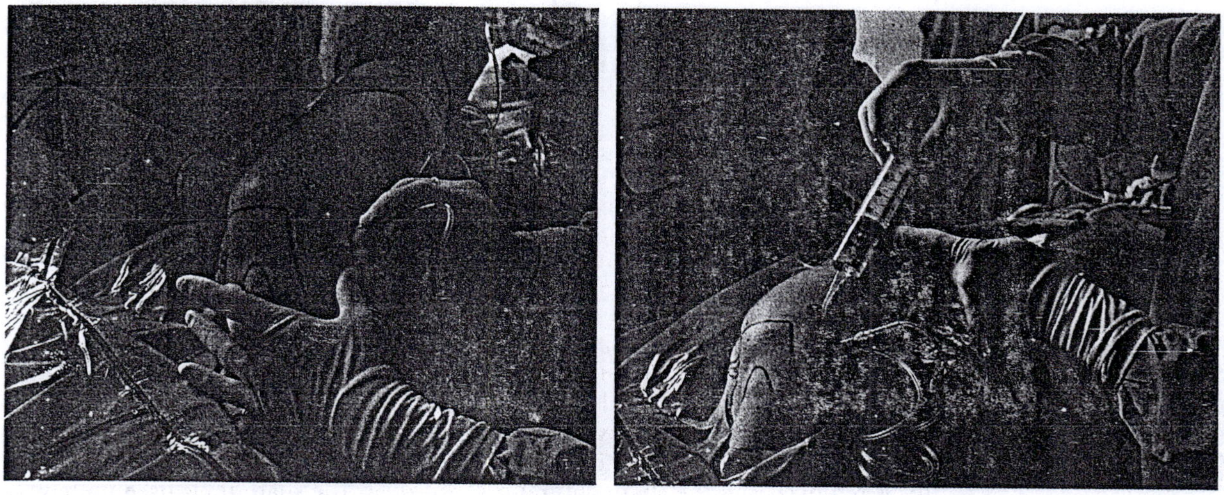

A B

FIG. 3–6. A, An 18-gauge lumbar puncture needle is placed into the joint through the posterior portal.
B, The joint is preinsufflated with normal saline. A normal joint holds about 35 ml.

is attached to a 60-ml syringe holding normal saline. The needle penetrates the previously marked posterior portal and attempts to enter the joint (Fig. 3–6A). If bone is encountered, gently rotate the humeral head. If the needle is placed too far laterally, the movement of the head can be appreciated. If the pin touches bone and does not move with humeral rotation, the pin is embedded into the neck of the scapula too far medially. In this fashion, simple adjustments can be made to determine the precise planes of the joint surfaces. With the patient angled 25 to 30° posteriorly, the plane of the joint should be nearly horizontal.

When the needle is within the joint, fluid can be introduced with relative ease. In the intact joint, fluid can be withdrawn after 15 or 20 ml have been introduced to confirm proper positioning. The normal joint holds about 35 ml of fluid before offering resistance (Fig. 3–6B). The joint capacity is much reduced in cases of adhesive capsulitis. Conversely, a great deal more fluid may be introduced when a full-thickness tear of the rotator cuff is present. The fluid simply drains from the glenohumeral region into the subacromial space when the cuff is torn. The principle here is the same as that applied when an arthrogram is performed. Indeed, the surgeon can suspect the presence of a full-thickness tear when more than 35 ml of fluid are admitted without tension. The subdeltoid region of the subacromial space may become palpably distended during preinsufflation when the cuff is torn.

The position of the spinal puncture needle should be observed carefully before it is withdrawn. It is a reliable guide for introduction of the arthroscope.

INTRODUCING THE ARTHROSCOPE

The posterior portal is infiltrated with bupivacaine, and a skin incision approximately 5 mm in length is made along Langer's lines with a No. 11 blade (Fig. 3–7A). Only the skin and subcutaneous tissues are penetrated. The arthroscopic sheath is introduced initially with a sharp trocar (Fig. 3–7B). A finger is placed over the tip of the coracoid process, and the instrument is aimed from behind toward this point. If the arthroscope sheath is allowed to stray inferior to the coracoid, serious injury may result. The index finger should be extended along the sheath as the instrument travels to the level of the posterior joint space (Fig. 3–7C). This positioning of the index finger prevents plunging too deeply.

Once the level of the posterior joint space has been reached, a change is made from the sharp to the blunt trocar (Fig. 3–7D). The assistant then widens the joint space by performing a simple maneuver. A fist is placed just below the axilla, and pressure is applied downward on the elbow while the arm is maintained in traction. This action levers the joint surfaces apart, and the dull obturator palpates the lips of the widened joint (Fig. 3–7E). The instrument is again aimed toward the tip of the coracoid, and with the finger extended along the sheath to control the depth of penetration, an attempt is made to enter the joint using the dull obturator. When the capsule cannot be penetrated without undue force, the sheath is maintained in position at the back of the capsule while the dull obturator is removed and the sharp obturator substituted. The sharp tip is used merely to penetrate the joint capsule, and it is then removed. Penetration can be confirmed because fluid can be observed as it escapes through one of the stopcocks if it has been left open. At this point, the dull obturator is reintroduced and the joint is entered. The arthroscopy sheath should not be introduced with the sharp obturator. Articular surfaces are easily injured by the sharp tip. Even the dull instrument creases the joint surfaces at times.

ALTERNATE METHOD

A 3- or 4-mm transfer rod may be used to facilitate introduction of the scope. This smaller-diameter blunt rod may be easier than the fully assembled scope sheath to introduce into the joint. Once the transfer rod has entered the joint, the sheath of the arthroscope may be guided over it; then the rod is removed.

The examiner now can insert the camera, attach fluid-ingress and suction tubing to the double stopcock arms, and begin inspection of the glenohumeral joint (Fig. 3–7F).

FIG. 3–7. A, A 5-mm skin incision is made at the posterior portal. ▶
B, A sharp trocar is used to penetrate through the deltoid to the level of the posterior capsule.
C, The tip of the instrument is directed toward the coracoid process. The index finger is extended along the shaft of the arthroscope to avoid any sudden or uncontrolled penetration.
D, Change from sharp to blunt trocar before penetrating the joint to avoid injury to intra-articular structures.
E, The assistant widens the joint space by placing a fist near the axilla and pressing downward upon the elbow to lever the joint surfaces apart. The instrument then is pressed gently into the joint.
F, Fluid and suction tubing are attached, and the arthroscope is introduced.

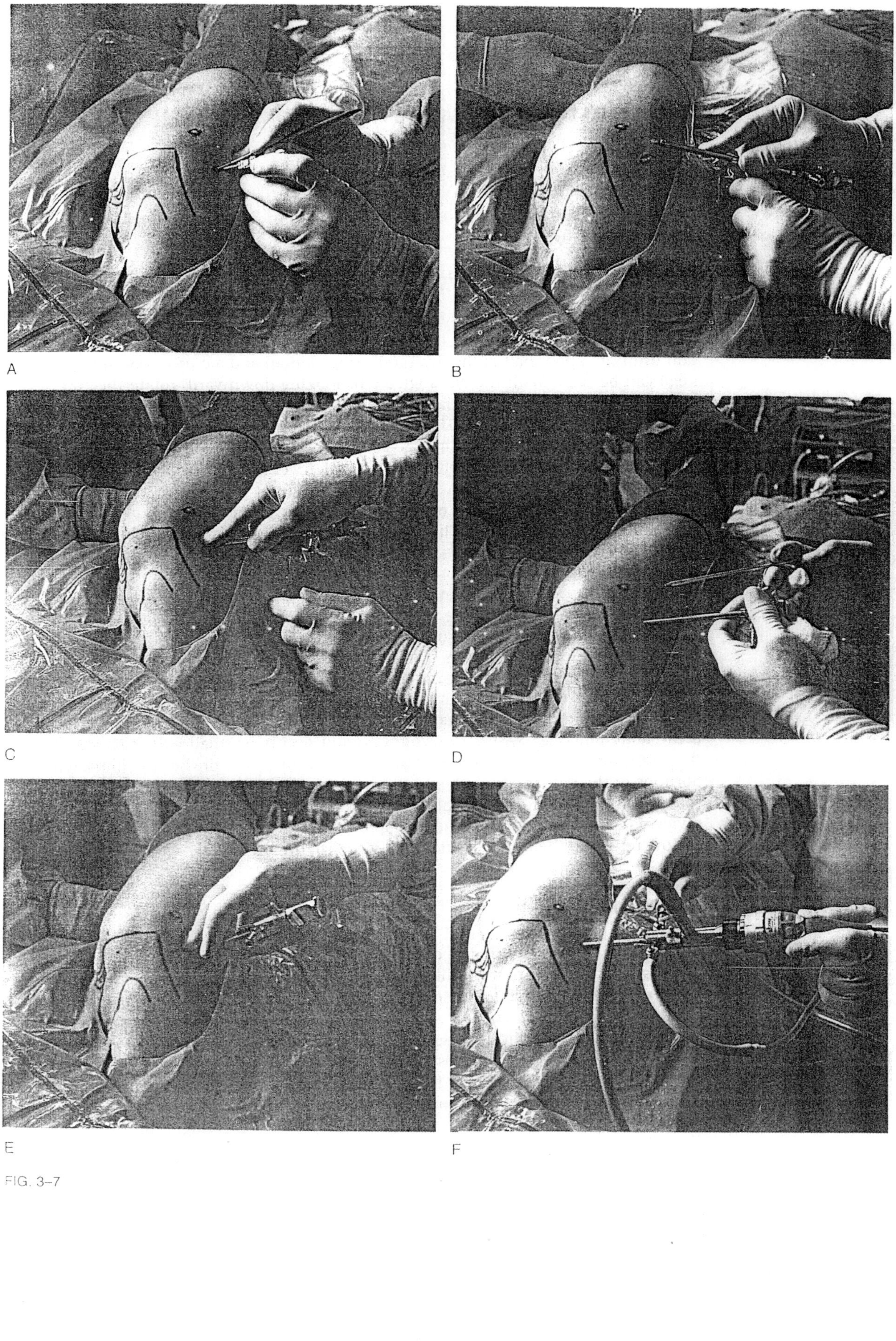

FIG. 3–7

NORMAL AND VARIANT ANATOMIC FINDINGS

Glenohumeral joint inspection is carried out in a systematic fashion. The routine is simple and should be repeated in every shoulder arthroscopy. A right shoulder is illustrated, as viewed through the posterior portal (Fig. 3–8).

LONG HEAD OF THE BICEPS

Begin by visualizing the long head of the biceps (LHB) at the point of insertion into the supraglenoid tubercle (Fig. 3–8A). Back away from this point of insertion until the upper half of the oval-appearing glenoid and a crescent of humeral head can be seen. With the 30° angled lens looking downward, rotate the camera until the LHB appears horizontal and the opposing glenohumeral cartilaginous surfaces appear vertical. The relationship of the glenoid and biceps has the appearance of an inverted Q. This site is considered the "home" position. Return home for orientation after each foray, and then set out again to inspect other nooks and crannies of the joint.

Now move back closer to the point of LHB insertion. The tendon should appear round and glistening. The tendon appears to insert into the fibrous ring of the superior labrum (Fig. 3–8B). In individuals over the age of 40, a slight beard-like fraying may project a few millimeters downward at the most inferior point of attachment. The tendon can be followed laterally to its point of exit into the intertubercular sulcus (Fig. 3–8C). A slight amount of injection may be noted on the superior surface of the tendon just before it departs the joint in some cases of bicipital tendinitis (Fig. 3–8D). The tendon should not be adherent to the structures superior to it. Such adherence sometimes happens in the later stages of adhesive capsulitis or in the rare instance that a superior vincula is present. The superior structures may seem to encroach upon the tendon without being adherent (Fig. 3–8E). This configuration occurs in small cuff tears when the subacromial space has become distended with fluid and presses the impacted portions of the cuff and underlying capsule downward. Partial and full-thickness rotator cuff tears are quite apparent. Biceps tendon and rotator cuff lesions are reviewed extensively in subsequent chapters.

Now return to the home position and visualize the inverted Q again.

GLENOID LABRUM

The glenoid labrum is a ring of dense fibrous connective tissue that attaches to the osseous glenoid rim. A thin transitional zone of fibrocartilage may be demonstrated at the point of osseous attachment. Significant variations in labral structure have been described.[5-7] These variations may be readily observed during arthroscopy. The labrum is described as wedge-shaped or triangular in cross-section, with a free edge that is directed toward the center of the glenoid. A well-developed glenoid labrum is approximately 3 mm high and 4 mm wide. Hyaline cartilage may underlie this wedge out to its point of osseous attachment. Detrisac and Johnson have noted that this wedge-shaped configuration may be present in only a segment of the glenoid ring, e.g., superiorly, posteriorly, anteriorly, or anterosuperiorly.[7] A probe can pass between the overlapping labrum and articular cartilage in each of these circumstances, whereas the remainder of

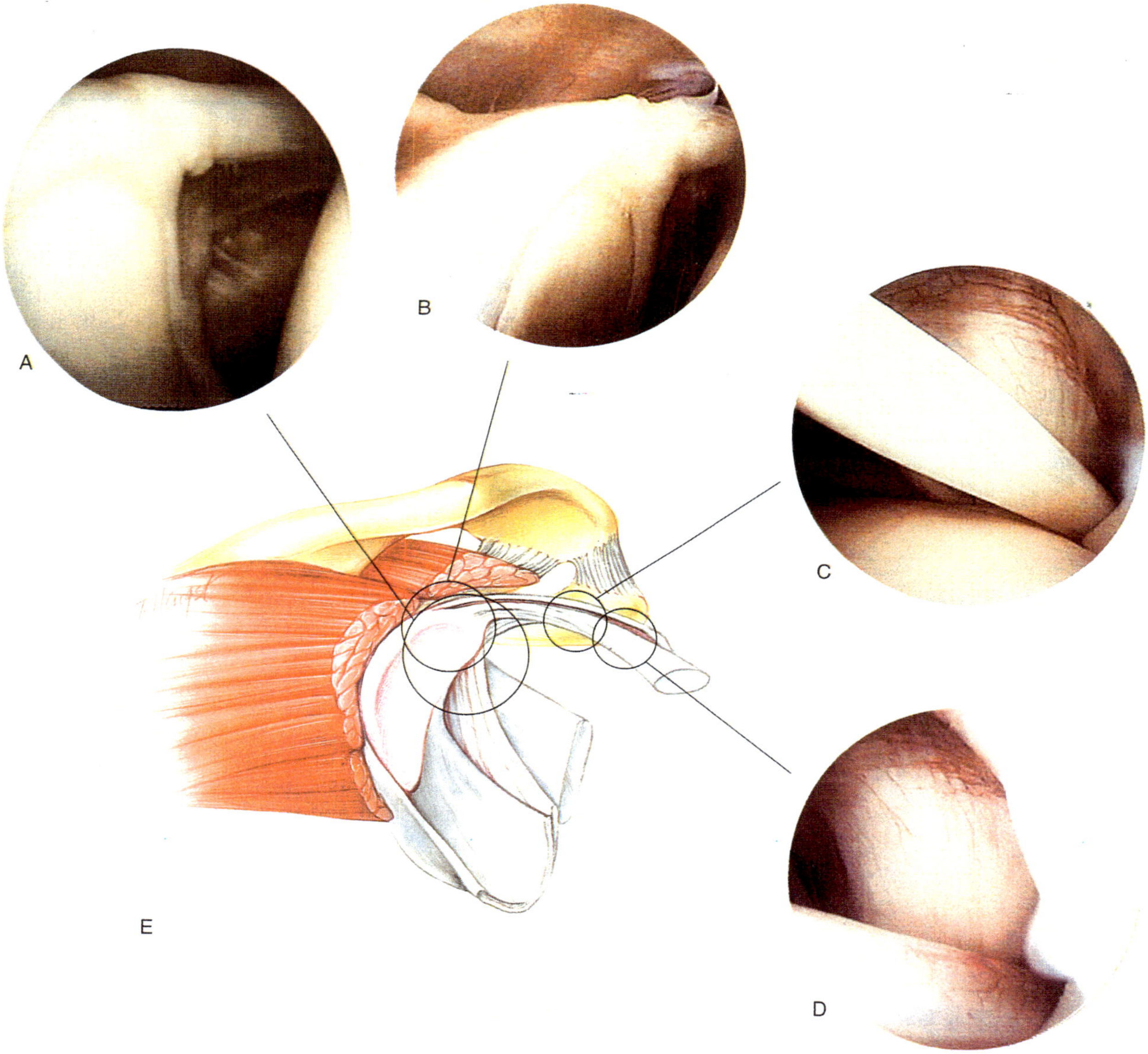

FIG. 3–8. A, Home position. The relationship of the glenoid and biceps has the appearance of an inverted Q.
B, The tendon inserts into the fibrous ring of the superior labrum.
C, The tendon is followed laterally to its point of exit into the intertubercular sulcus.
D, Note slight injection on superior surface of tendon as it exits joint.
E, Orientation sketch of glenohumeral joint as viewed from posterior portal.

the labrum is attached firmly to the glenoid. The anterior band of the inferior glenohumeral ligament (IGHL) arises from the anteroinferior half of the labrum and blends with the labrum as it extends superiorly. The biceps tendon and superior glenohumeral ligament (SGHL) also merge with the labrum at its superior aspect. The labrum deepens the glenoid socket and, according to many examiners, adds stability to the shoulder.

LABRAL INSPECTION

Return to the home position and begin to inspect the anterior labrum just below the insertion of the LHB (Fig. 3–9A). Follow the labrum inferiorly as you inspect the quality of the labral tissue and its attachment to the glenoid (Fig. 3–9B). Make your initial inspection all along the anterior border of the glenoid down to the 6 o'clock position. Mentally mark the delineation point between the superior and inferior halves of the glenoid, and then go back for a further look at the superior half of the anterior glenoid. Determine whether the labrum appears wedge-shaped or atrophic. Is hypertrophy or fraying evident? The question of superior labral detachment requires special consideration and a knowledge of a common variation from normal. The middle glenohumeral ligament (MGHL) attaches on the neck of the scapula and upper half of the glenoid. A foramen of varying size may be present between this ligament and the glenoid labrum (Fig. 3–9C). This foramen communicates with the subscapularis bursa (Fig. 3–9D). Careful examination shows that the labrum, which contains superior projections of the IGHL, is indeed still attached to the glenoid. This foramen, therefore, is bordered by the MGHL and the labrum and superior extension of the IGHL.

Isolated pathologic detachments involving only the superior labrum are rarely encountered. Pathologic detachment of the superior labrum frequently develops as an extension of a pre-existing inferior labral detachment caused by traumatic anterior dislocation. Less commonly, an anterosuperior labral detachment is associated with a posterosuperior labral detachment (SLAP lesion) (Fig. 3–10A). The IGHL and its anterior band normally attach to the inferior half of the anterior labrum and send its superior band upward as it blends with the labrum. The anteroinferior labrum may appear quite stout and well developed (Fig. 3–10B). In other instances, the labrum may appear rather thin and almost insignificant, although the IGHL is attached. Scuffing, fraying, and even flap-like tears may be observed as a consequence of shoulder subluxation or recurrent dislocation (Fig. 3–10C).

Bankart described a complete disruption of the labral-capsular attachment from the anteroinferior glenoid as the "essential lesion" in shoulder instability. The Bankart lesion is readily identified and is considered a cardinal sign for the diagnosis of recurrent anterior dislocation of the shoulder (Fig. 3–10D). The presence of an old healed glenoid fracture in this location is described as a "bony Bankart lesion." Arthroscopic evaluation immediately following the reduction of an acute anterior shoulder dislocation has disclosed anterior capsular ruptures, as well as both types of Bankart lesions.

The resultant healing of an acute traumatic lesion may leave the anterior capsule patulous to such a degree that recurrent anterior dislocation may occur without evidence of a labral lesion. The microstretching of the anterior capsule associated with injuries caused by throwing may lead to significant instability. This type of chronic subluxor is more apt to reveal scuffing, fraying, and attenuation of the anterior labrum and may have flap tears. Posterior labral injury is also common in athletes involved in sports that require throwing (Fig. 3–10E).

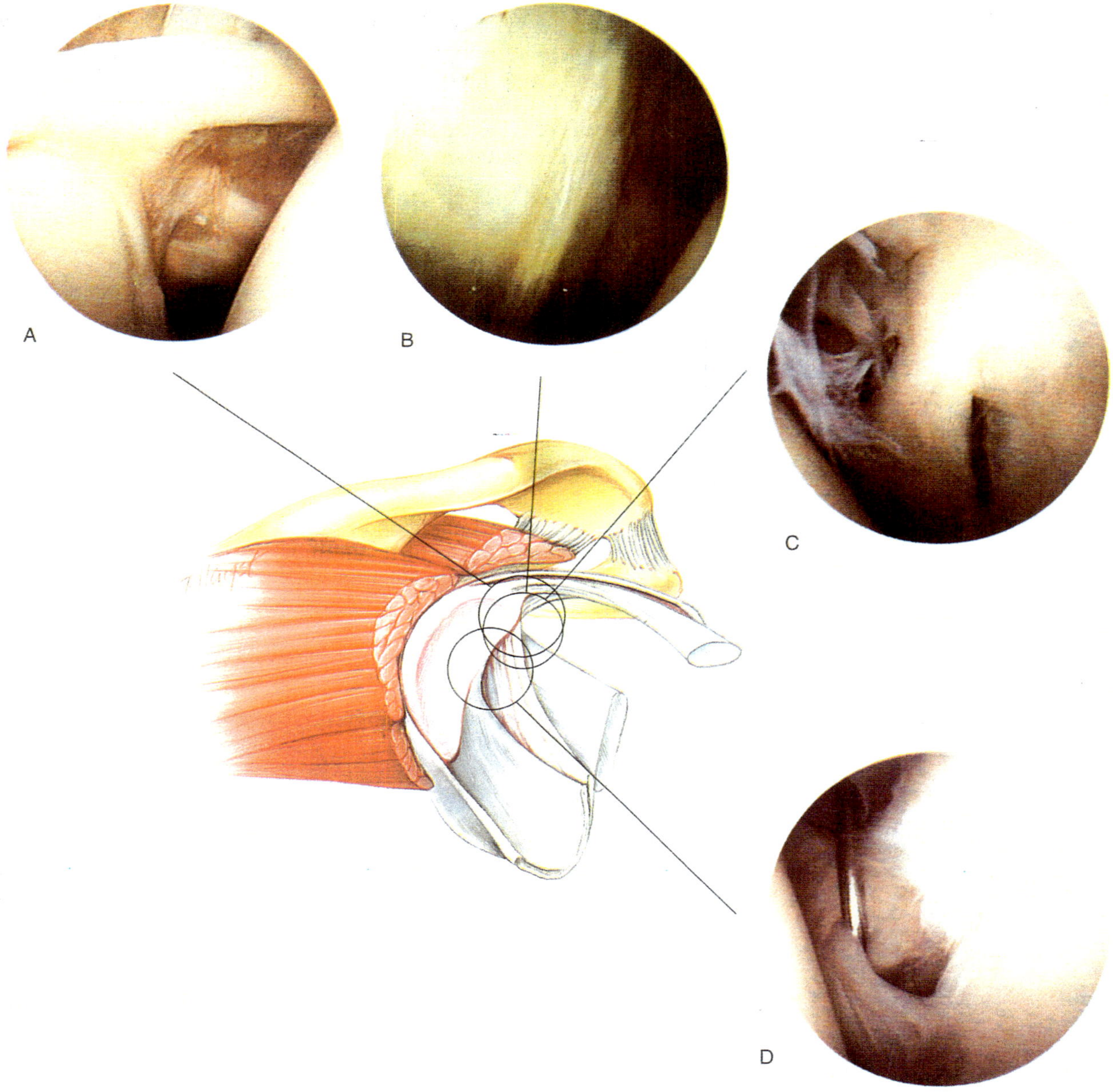

FIG. 3–9. A, Return "home" to inspect anterior labrum. Note normal cleft in the anterosuperior half of the labrum.
B, Follow labrum inferiorly. A normal marginal cleft is less apparent.
C, The superior labral foramen visualized is a common variant.
D, The superior foramen communicates freely with the subscapularis bursa.

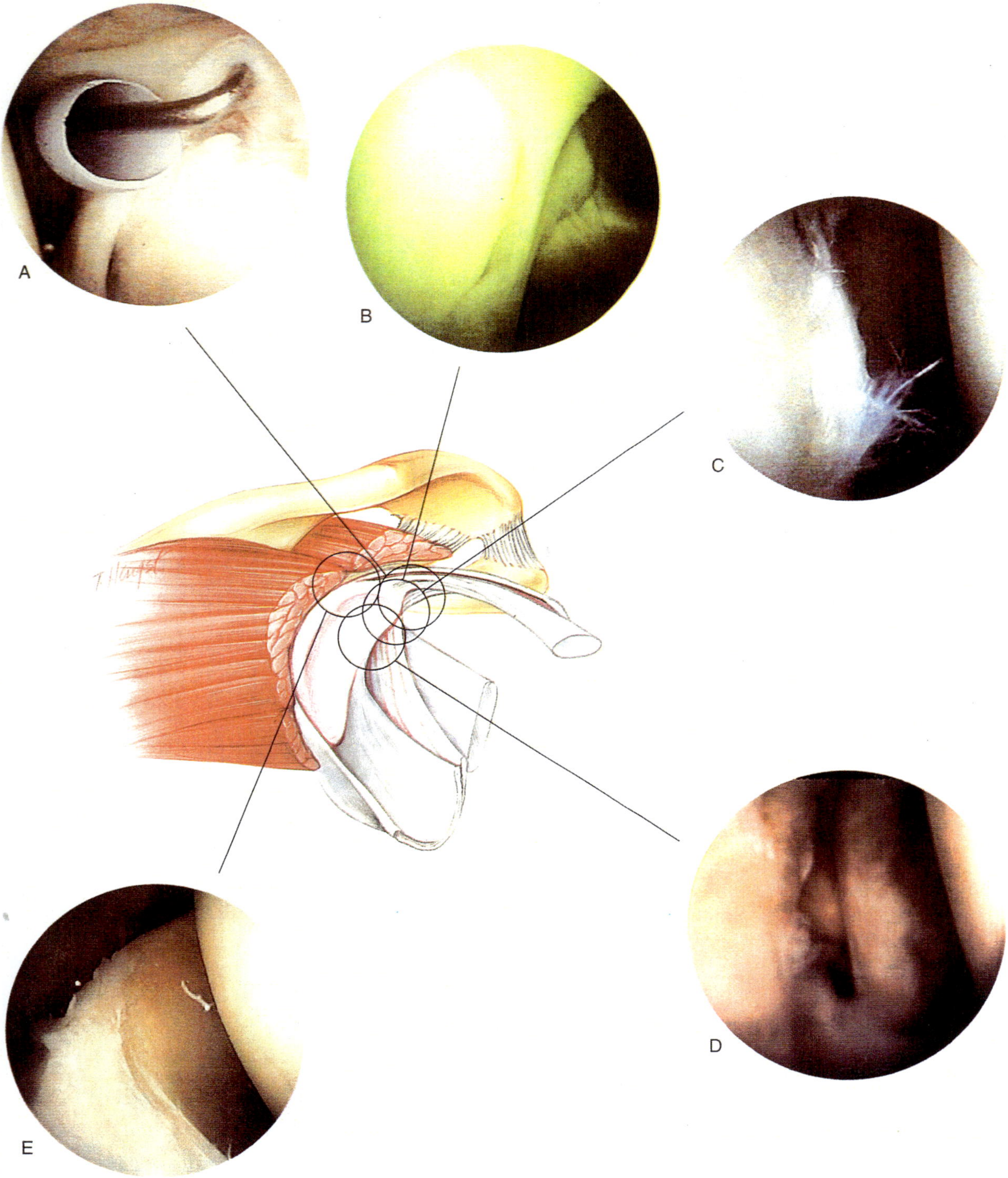

FIG. 3–10. A, The labrum is detached superiorly and, to some extent, anteriorly and posteriorly (SLAP lesion).
B, The anterior labrum appears quite stout with a normal cleft near the glenoid insertion.
C, Scuffing, fraying, or flap-like tears of the anteroinferior labrum are signs of instability.
D, The entire capsulolabral complex has been torn away from the labrum (Bankart lesion).
E, Posterior fraying or attenuation is a common finding in athletes involved in sports that require throwing.

Not surprisingly, the hyperlax individual with multidirectional instability shows few labral abnormalities. The joint is simply so capacious that scuffing does not occur.

Labral inspection is completed by sweeping around from the 6 o'clock position along the posterior margin of the glenoid until the arthroscope is returned to the home position. Be careful to avoid slipping out and losing the posterior portal during posterior labral inspection.

ARTICULAR SURFACE EVALUATION

Articular surface evaluation begins with the glenoid surface. Look for fibrillation, frank loosening, or color changes. Areas of chondromalacia may be encountered unexpectedly. These small rounded areas of denuded cartilage with undermined fragmenting cartilage at the periphery are the earliest signs of degenerative joint disease (Fig. 3–11A). Do not mistake these lesions for the normal pitted area seen frequently in older individuals (Fig. 3–11B). This shallow round or oval area, less than 10 mm in circumference, is located just below the equator in the central portion of the glenoid. Although subchondral bone is exposed centrally, the cartilaginous margins are quite smooth and appear normal in thickness.

The articular surface of the humeral head is examined next. Particular attention should be devoted to a search for a cartilaginous or osseous Hill-Sachs' lesion. This lesion is located in the posterosuperior aspect of the humeral head. The lesion should not be confused with the intercapsular portion of the humeral neck, an area that has been termed the anatomic bare patch. The humeral head

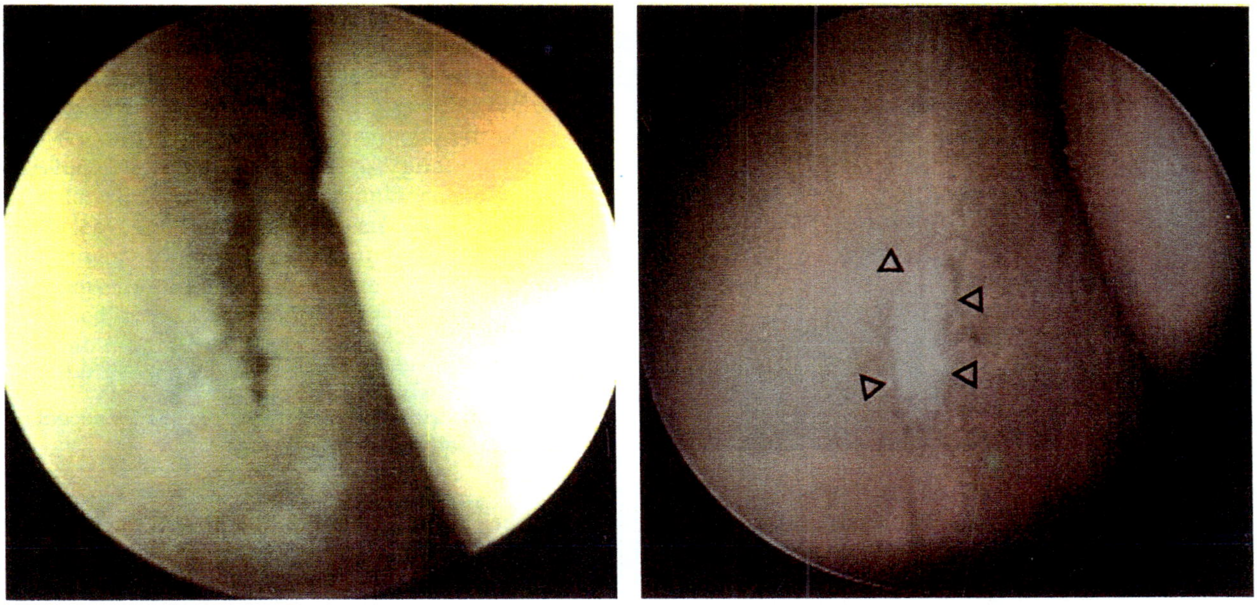

A B

FIG. 3–11. A, Chondral defect in the central region of the glenoid is irregular. Note undermined fragments of cartilage at periphery.
B, Normal oval-shaped pitted area in similar region of glenoid is surrounded by arrowheads.

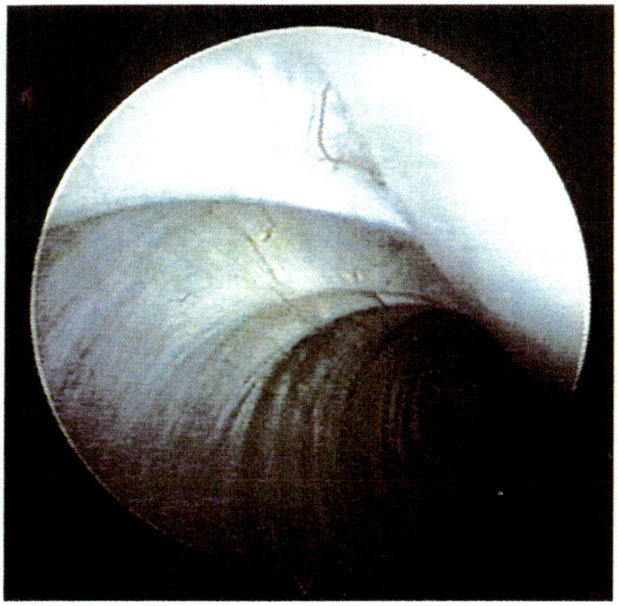

A

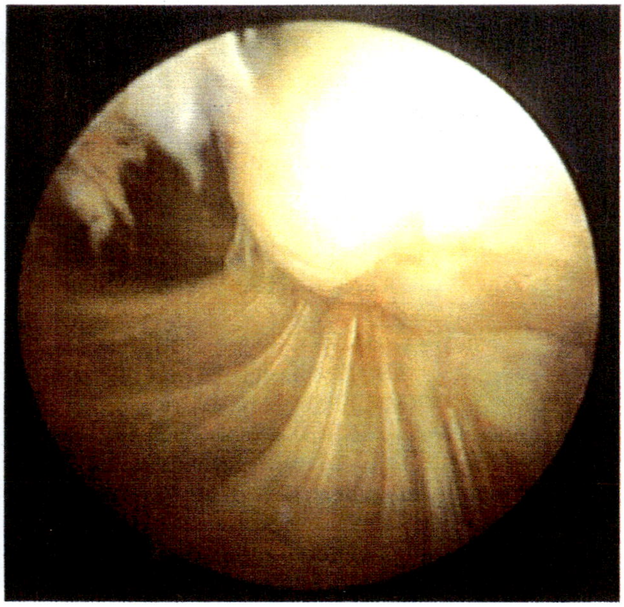

B

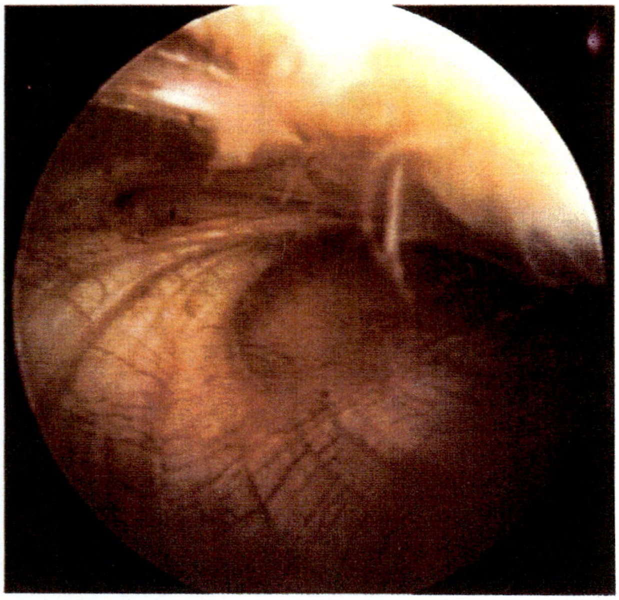

C

FIG. 3–12. Variations in axillary recess.
A, Normal axillary recess.
B, A small spur is developing at the inferior aspect of the humeral head.
C, The axillary recess is injected, and the inferior aspect of the acromial head shows chondromalacia.

may be rotated while the scope performs a thorough inspection. When areas of chondromalacia are encountered, the size and location of the lesions are noted. When inspection of the head is completed, return to the home position.

AXILLARY (INFERIOR) RECESS

As inspection of the humeral head ends, take a peek into the inferior recess to disclose any cartilaginous or osseous loose bodies or evidence of synovitis (Fig. 3–12). Then glance upward at the most inferior aspect of the humeral head for any signs of early spur formation arising as a small bulge near the junction of the articular surface of the head with the calcar region.

SUBSCAPULAR RECESS

Return to the home area and look directly ahead into a roughly triangular-shaped area that is bounded by the LHB above, the upper half of the glenoid on one side, and the curvilinear surface of the humeral head on the other (Fig. 3–13A). The most prominent structure is the cord-like upper margin of the subscapularis. This margin runs roughly parallel to the LHB and is commonly mistaken for that structure before one becomes oriented to the glenohumeral joint (Fig. 3–13B). This intra-articular portion of the subscapularis travels laterally to insert into the lesser tuberosity. The articular surface is covered only by the relatively thin anterior capsule of the shoulder, which billows out superiorly to become the "rotator interval," which is the gap between the superior border of the subscapularis and the nearby anterior border of the supraspinatus. The subscapularis insertion may be as much as 4 to 5 cm wide when measured from the superior aspect to the inferior border. Only the upper tendinous portion of this insertion is seen arthroscopically. On occasion, this portion of the tendon may be torn (Fig. 3–13C). The lower aspect becomes more muscular than tendinous. This region is obscured by the attachment of the IGHL, which is described in a subsequent section. On a precise anatomic basis, the recess lies between the articular surface of the subscapularis and the neck of the glenoid. When the IGHL leaves a foramen between the anterosuperior glenoid and its point of attachment (as described previously), this foramen may be considered a second and more inferior entrance to the subacromial recess. When reactive changes are provoked in the synovium, for a variety of reasons, the chronic synovitis appears quite abundant in this recess. The region is a popular nesting place for intra-articular loose bodies.

GLENOHUMERAL LIGAMENTS

These ligaments are variable thickenings within the capsule of the shoulder and are described as anterior, middle, and inferior according to their location.

The superior glenohumeral ligament (SGHL) is the most difficult glenohumeral ligament to visualize arthroscopically. The SGHL originates from the region of the supraglenoid tubercle somewhat anterior to the LHB. This ligament courses laterally above the LHB to its point of insertion to the medial tubercle of the intertubercular sulcus. When viewed from the posterior portal, the SGHL not

(Text continues on page 76)

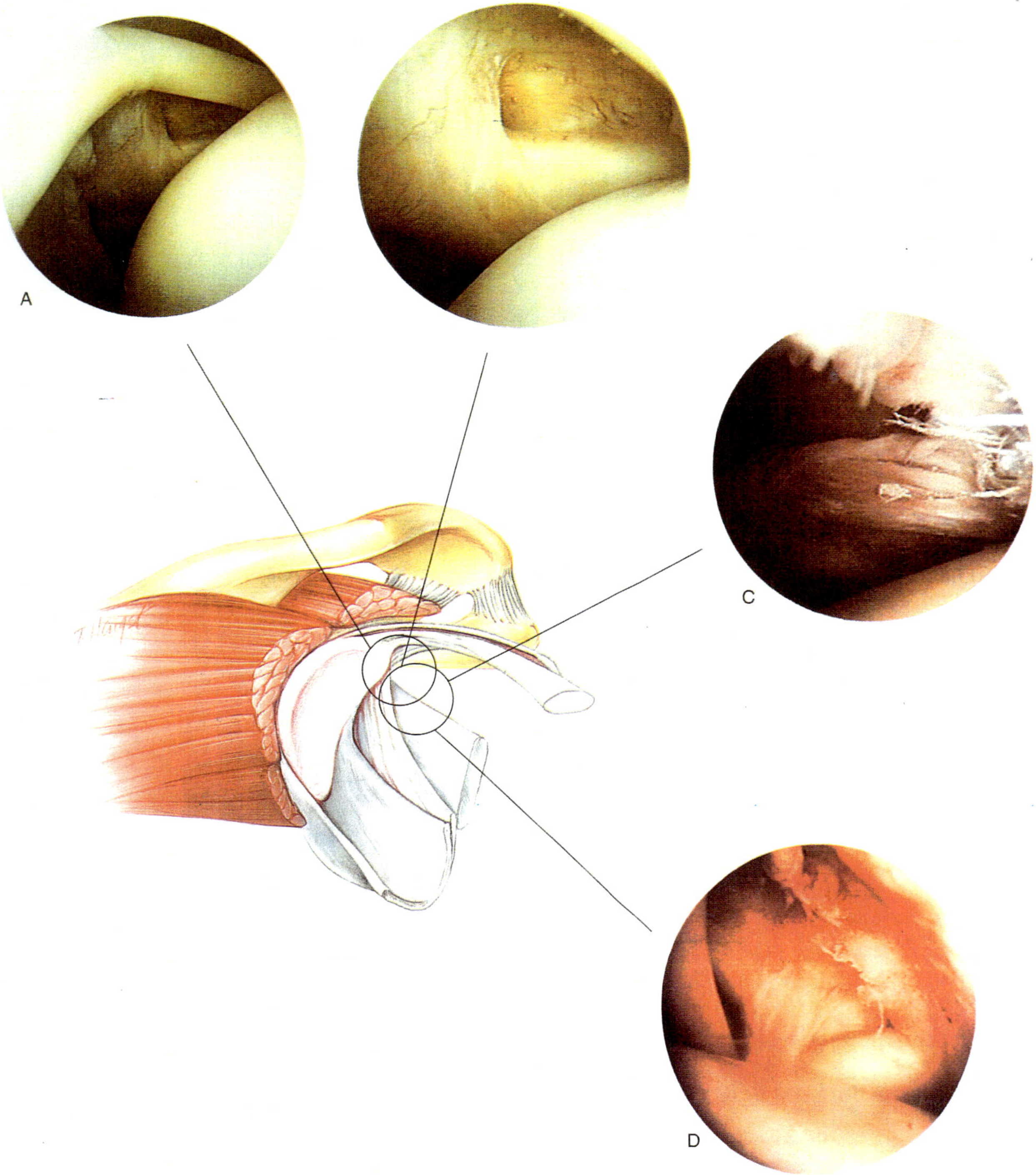

FIG. 3–13. A, Looking into the subscapularis recess bounded by the long head of biceps, head of humerus, and glenoid.
B, The cord-like upper margin of the subscapularis crosses the recess.
C, The cord-like superior surface of the subscapularis is partially torn laterally.
D, Chronic synovitis involves the suprascapular recess.

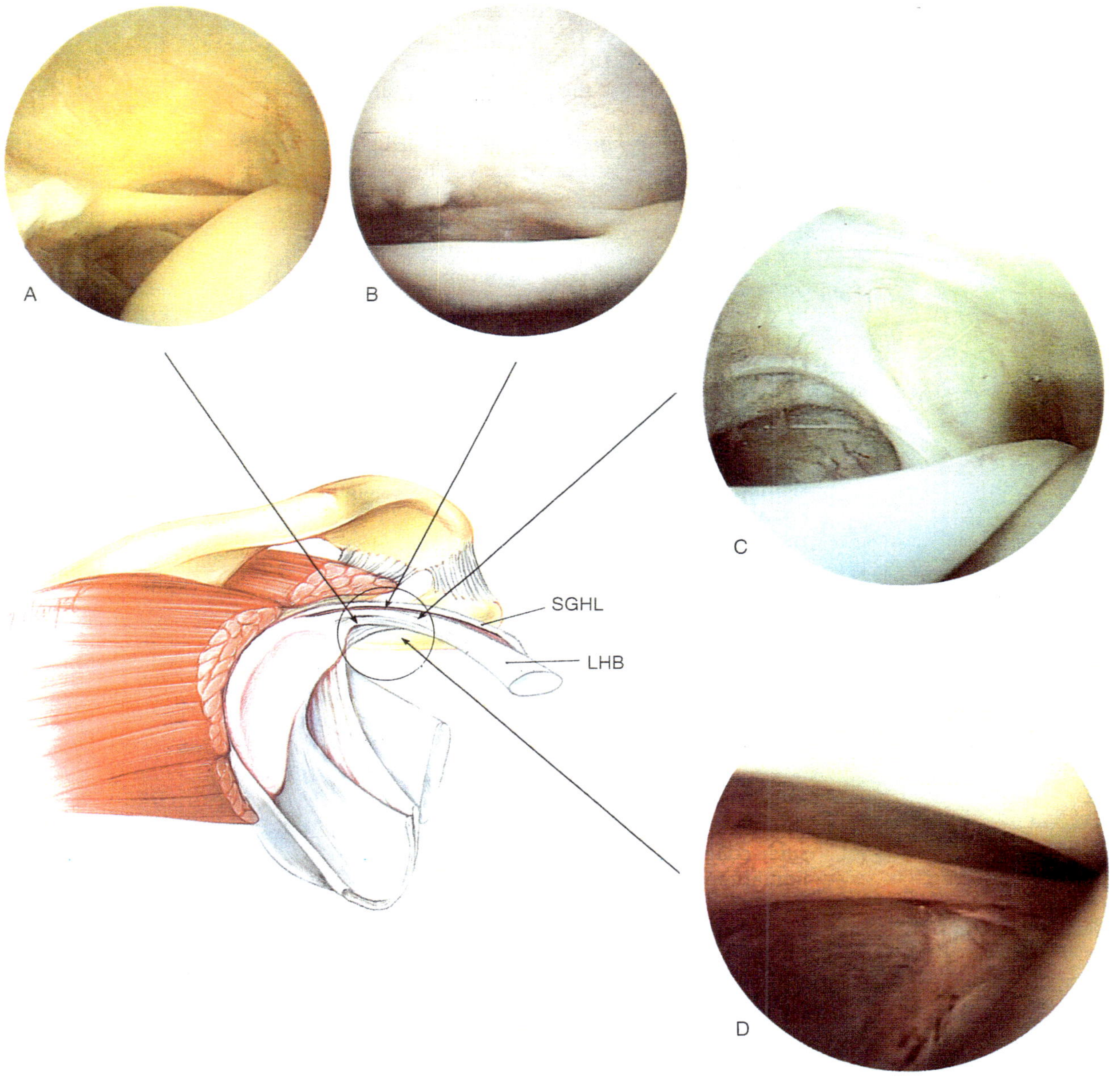

FIG. 3–14. Superior glenohumeral ligament (SGHL): Variations of normal.

A, The SGHL commonly appears as an ill-defined thickening in the capsule above the long head of the biceps.

B, SGHL appears as a more discrete thickening partially obscured by the long head of the biceps (LHB).

C, Fibers of the SGHL appear to be reinforced by descending fibers from the coraco-humeral ligament to create an unusually thickened band of attachment into the anterior wall of the intertubercular sulcus.

D, The SGHL forms an unusually discrete band in this photograph. The LHB tendon is above, in the foreground.

only may be obscured by the biceps tendon, but also may be too thin to be evident on inspection. The common appearance and variations of normal are shown in Figure 3–14. Unlike the "emperor's new clothes," anatomic dissections have confirmed that the SGHL is a constant structure that aids in humeral suspension.

The *middle glenohumeral ligament* (MGHL), though variable in size, usually can be demonstrated arthroscopically. The MGHL passes the upper border of the subscapularis in an obliquely vertical fashion to attach to the superior glenoid in most persons. It appears to be 3 or 4 mm in width and relatively thin. This ligament is the most variable in appearance (Fig. 3–15) and seems to be attenuated or absent in patients with significant anterior capsular insufficiency (subluxors and recurrent dislocators). In other patients, the MGHL may appear to be quite thick and substantial as it slopes upward to obscure the more medial portion of the upper border of the subscapularis. Again, the appearance of a superior foramen is created when a well-developed ligament seeks insertion on the superior aspect of the glenoid and neck, but leaves a space between its medial border and the labrum.

The *inferior glenohumeral ligament* (IGHL) is the most constant and clinically significant of the capsular ligaments. Bowen and colleagues have greatly extended our knowledge of this ligament.[8] The ligament functions as a suspensory sling that both supports and stabilizes the glenohumeral joint. A thick anterosuperior band of the ligament is easily identified in the normal shoulder (Fig. 3–16A). When the shoulder is inspected in 15 to 20° of abduction, the band appears to arise lazily from the inferior recess and slope upward toward the middle third of the glenoid (Fig. 3–16B), where it merges with the labrum as it extends upward. As the shoulder is abducted, the superior band moves superiorly to a more horizontal position in relation to the glenoid, consequently leading the IGHL upward as this suspensory sling tightens to support the humeral head anteroinferiorly (Fig. 3–16C). A similar unobserved process occurs posteriorly as the posterosuperior band accompanies its anterior counterpart during abduction (Fig. 3–16D). The IGHL inserts into the labrum and through that structure into the glenoid, thus giving rise to the term "labrocapsular complex." Disruption of this labrocapsular complex insertion (commonly called a Bankart lesion) usually occurs during anteroinferior dislocation of the shoulder. The disruption may extend upward to include the entire anterior labrum, but the lower half must be involved to be considered the essential lesion associated with anterior instability (Fig. 3–16E).

FIG. 3–15. Middle glenohumeral ligament (MGHL): Variations of normal.
A, The MGHL is visualized crossing the cord-like upper border of the subscapularis in a vertical direction. The width shown here is relatively common.
B, The MGHL is quite thin and attenuated in this patient with capsular laxity
C, The MGHL is quite broad and stout, thus obscuring the more medial border of the subscapularis as it gains attachment to the anterior neck of the glenoid.
D, A broad MGHL appears confluent with the inferior glenohumeral ligament (IGHL). The MGHL attaches to the superior rim of the glenoid labrum, thereby leaving a small oval window.
E, Complete absence of the MGHL. This joint was quite lax despite a relatively normal-appearing glenoid labrum.

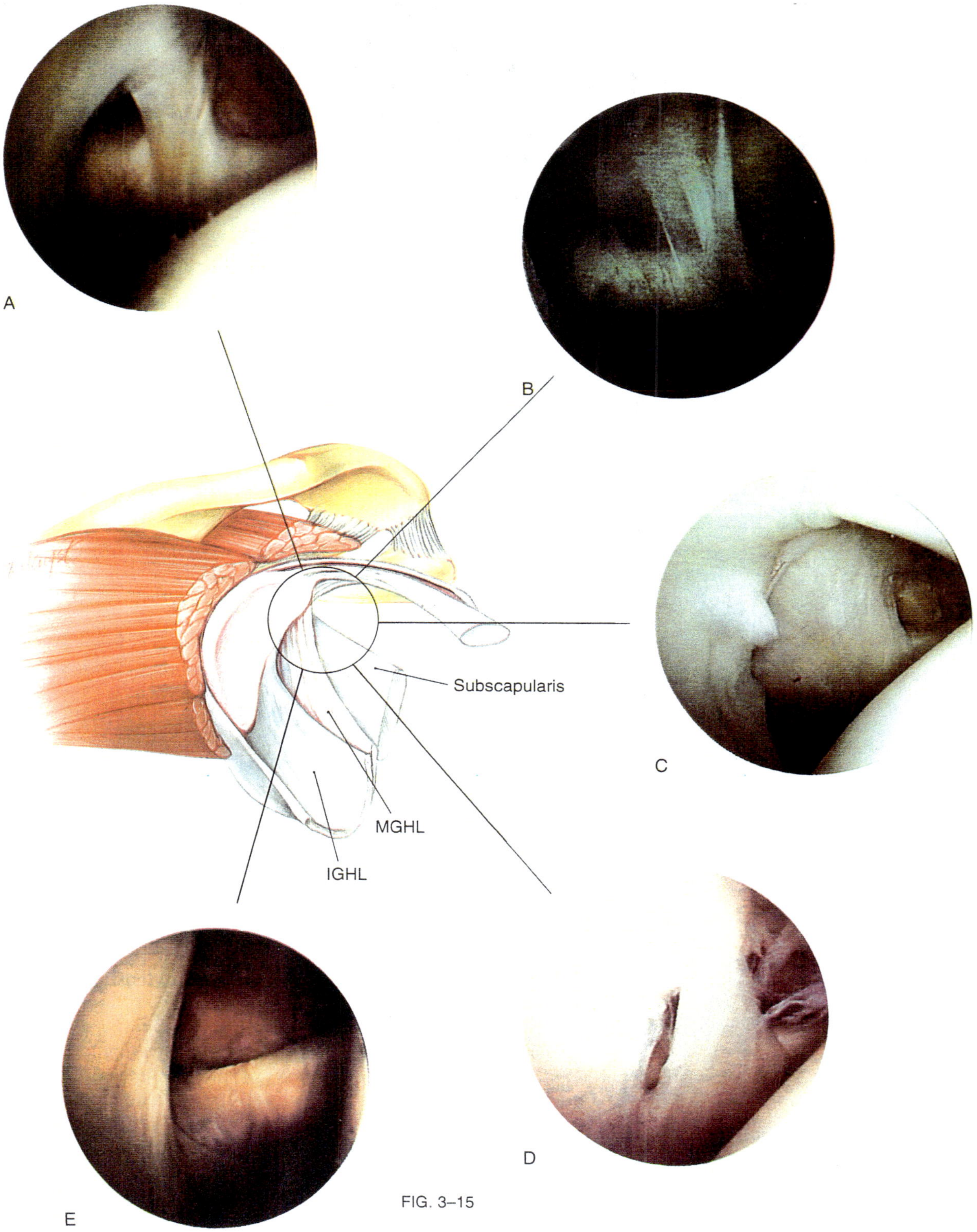

FIG. 3–15

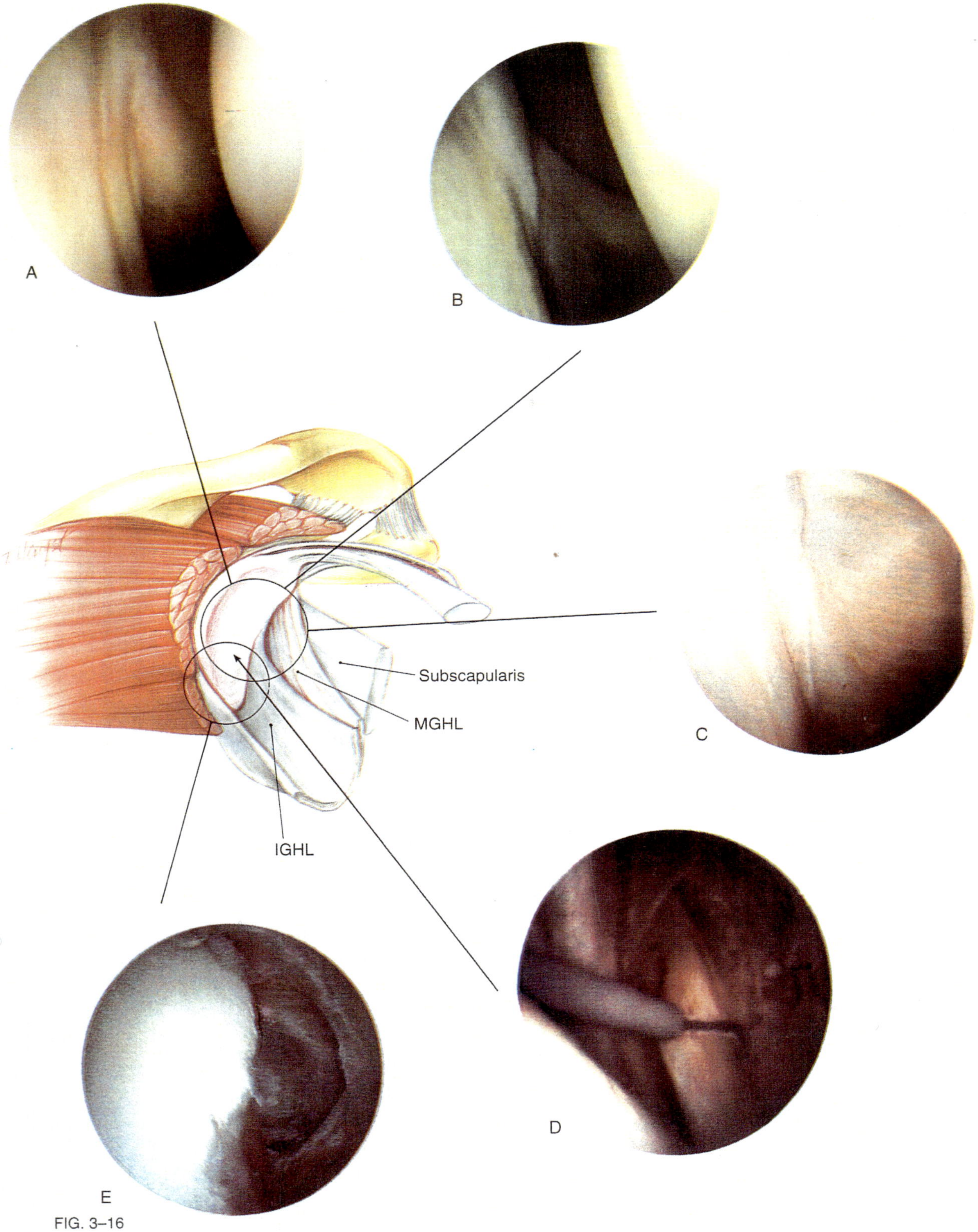

FIG. 3–16

◀ FIG. 3–16. Inferior glenohumeral ligament (IGHL): Normal and Bankart lesion.
A, The thick anterior band of IGHL is sloping downward from its origin on the labrum.
B, As the shoulder is abducted, the band appears to arise lazily from the inferior recess. The IGHL appears broader.
C, With further abduction, the normal IGHL moves upward to afford broad support against anteroinferior instability.
D, The posterior band of the IGHL is being probed. The portals are reversed, because this photograph was taken through the anterior portal, looking backward.
E, A complete disruption in the labrocapsular attachment has created a Bankart lesion along the full anterior border of the glenoid.

The axillary recess, described earlier, is actually a loose outpouching below the inferior portion of the humeral head. This normally lax structure is a portion of the IGHL suspended between the antero- and posterosuperior bands. The laxity of the inferior pouch permits an extensive range of glenohumeral motion. It tightens as the joint is fully elevated. Adhesions within the inferior recess, which may occur with adhesive capsulitis, significantly restrict glenohumeral motion.

ROTATOR CUFF INSPECTION

Return to the home position to inspect the rotator cuff musculature. The cord-like superior border of the subscapularis already has been viewed. Only the upper portions of this muscle can be seen arthroscopically and its integrity confirmed. Although isolated ruptures of the subscapularis are rarely encountered, the tendinous insertion into the lesser tuberosity is frequently torn in association with an anterior dislocation of the shoulder in individuals over the age of 50. In this circumstance, the subscapularis is usually torn along with the insertions of both the supra- and the infraspinatus, thereby producing a massive avulsion of the musculotendinous cuff. Rupture of the subscapularis allows the LHB to dislocate anteriorly, and when one of these disruptions is encountered, the other should be suspected.

The tendons of the supraspinatus, infraspinatus, and teres minor insert into the superior and posterior aspects of the greater tuberosity. Their relative position is recalled from the anatomy lab mnemonic: The three muscles SIT on the tuberosity from above downward. The supraspinatus occupies the superior facet, the infraspinatus the middle, and the teres minor the inferior facet. The articular capsule is adherent to the undersurface of these tendons, and the borders of the individual tendons cannot be identified arthroscopically.

In the normal shoulder, the LHB delineates the most anterior margin of the supraspinatus. Follow the LHB tendon laterally to its exit and begin inspection of the supraspinatus insertion (Fig. 3–17A). Increasing abduction and a slight amount of external rotation may facilitate inspection. The normal supraspinatus insertion is adjacent to the articular border of the humeral head, where it appears to enter the sulcus between the humeral head and the tip of the tuberosity (Fig. 3–17B). The insertions of the infraspinatus and teres minor are located more posteriorly and inferiorly. These two tendons attach somewhat more lateral to the articular surface of the humeral head, thereby exposing a portion of the intracapsular neck of the humerus (Fig. 3–17C). This intracapsular portion of humeral neck has been called the anatomic bare patch, and the region

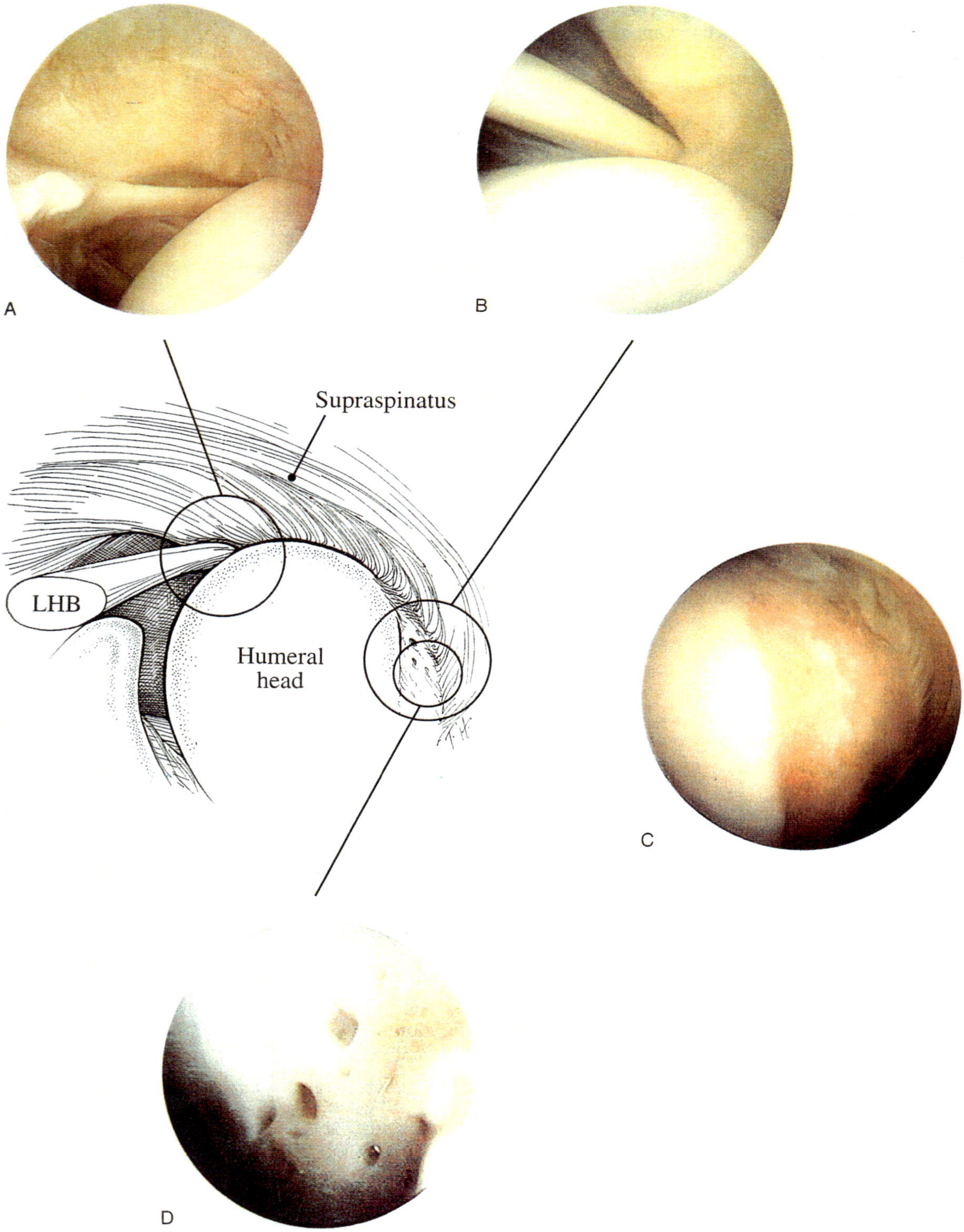
A
B
Supraspinatus
LHB
Humeral
head
C
D

◀ FIG. 3–17. Normal rotator cuff insertion.
A, Orientation view shows long head of biceps, humeral head, and insertion of supraspinatus.
B, The long head of biceps marks the anterior margin of the supraspinatus insertion. The insertion of the supraspinatus hugs the articular cartilage.
C, Intracapsular portion of humeral neck (bare patch) exposed. Fibers of the infraspinatus and supraspinatus insert posteriorly at some distance lateral to the articular cartilage.
D, Small pitted fenestrations for nutrient arteries are characteristically seen in the bare patch.

is characterized by the appearance of several small pitted openings for nutrient arteries (Fig. 3–17D). This bare area should not be confused with a Hill-Sachs' lesion. The insertions of all three tendons can be inspected through the posterior portal. During inspection, the scope sweeps from the superior aspect of the shoulder down its posterior aspect to end in the region of the inferior recess. External rotation facilitates this maneuver.

Rotator cuff failure is a progressive disorder, and the earliest separation of insertional fibers can be seen. Partial tears involving both the articular and the bursal surfaces of the rotator cuff can be visualized arthroscopically. Chapter 6, entitled Treatment of Partial-Thickness Rotator Cuff Tears: Arthroscopic and Mini-Open, deals comprehensively with this subject.

ANTERIOR PORTAL

Although a thorough glenohumeral inspection can be carried out through the posterior portal, diagnostic arthroscopy often requires the establishment of an anterior portal (Fig. 3–18). The posterior labrum and capsule can be examined more thoroughly through the anterior portal. A probe, shaver, or biopsy forceps may be introduced through the anterior portal when required.

The anterior portal is established by the use of a long portal rod (Wissinger rod). The area selected for anterior capsule penetration is above the intra-articular border of the subscapularis and below the LHB tendon (Fig. 3–19A). The most lateral aspect of this triangular-shaped region is selected so that the rod can exit superior and slightly lateral to the tip of the coracoid process. A rod directed inferior or medial to the coracoid could potentially wreak havoc on the structures within the axillary sheath.

The scope is advanced to press against the anterior capsule in the proper location (Fig. 3–19B). While the sheath is held in position, the lens is removed and the long transfer rod is inserted and pressed forward through the capsule and soft tissue to tent the skin as it bulges anteriorly. The skin in this area is infiltrated with bupivacaine with adrenaline and then is incised along the line of skin cleavage to allow the rod to pass through from behind (Fig. 3–19C). The incision is widened to admit the operating cannula. Because the portal rods are only 3 or 4 mm in diameter, the capsular opening should be enlarged somewhat before attempting to introduce the 5.5-mm plastic surgical cannula. We do this by removing the 5-mm bur from its sheath and passing this metal sheath into the joint over the transfer rod before attempting to insert the plastic surgical cannula (Fig. 3–19D, E, and F).

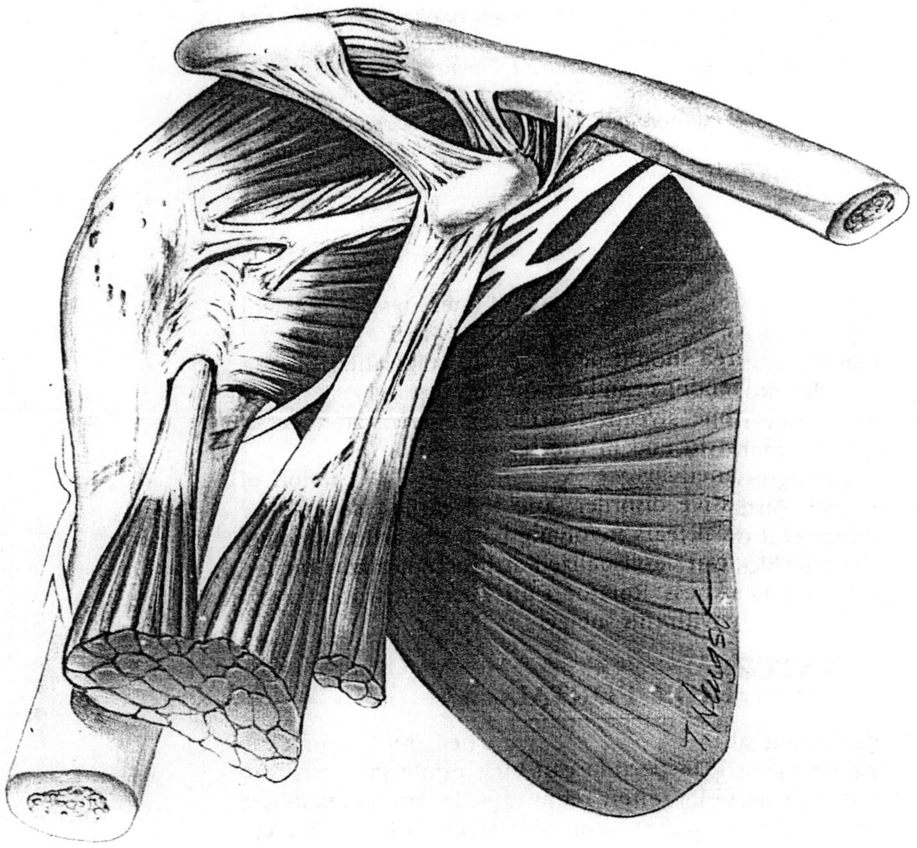

FIG. 3–18. The anterior portal, just lateral to and slightly above the coracoid, is indicated on this anatomic drawing of the shoulder.

FIG. 3–19. Establishing the anterior portal. A, The Wissinger rod should penetrate the capsule at the most superolateral margin of the triangle formed by the undersurface of the long head of the biceps, the humeral head, and the superior aspect of the subscapularis.B, The scope is advanced to the anterior capsule in proper location under direct vision and is held firmly in place while the camera is removed and the Wissinger rod is inserted.

C, Great care is taken to ensure that the anterior portal is established superior and somewhat lateral to the coracoid process before a skin incision is made and the rod is passed through. *Under no circumstances should the rod be directed inferior and medial to the coracoid.*

D, The capsular opening is enlarged by passing the metal sheath from the 5-mm bur over the Wissinger rod.

E, The 5.5-mm plastic cannula is shown immediately before it is introduced into the joint.

F, After the tip of the cannula has been placed well into the joint, the Wissinger rod is removed.

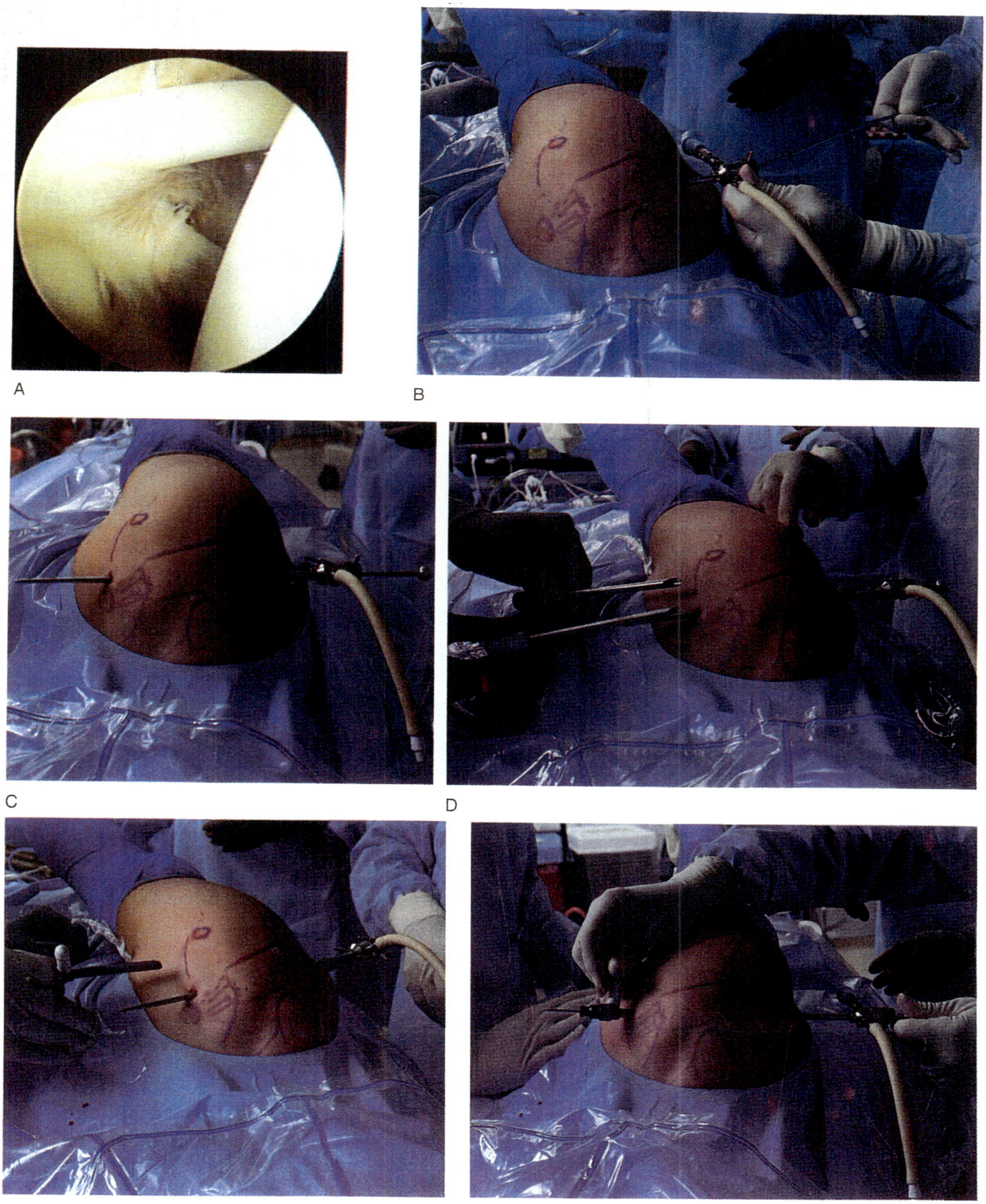

A B C D E F

FIG. 3–19

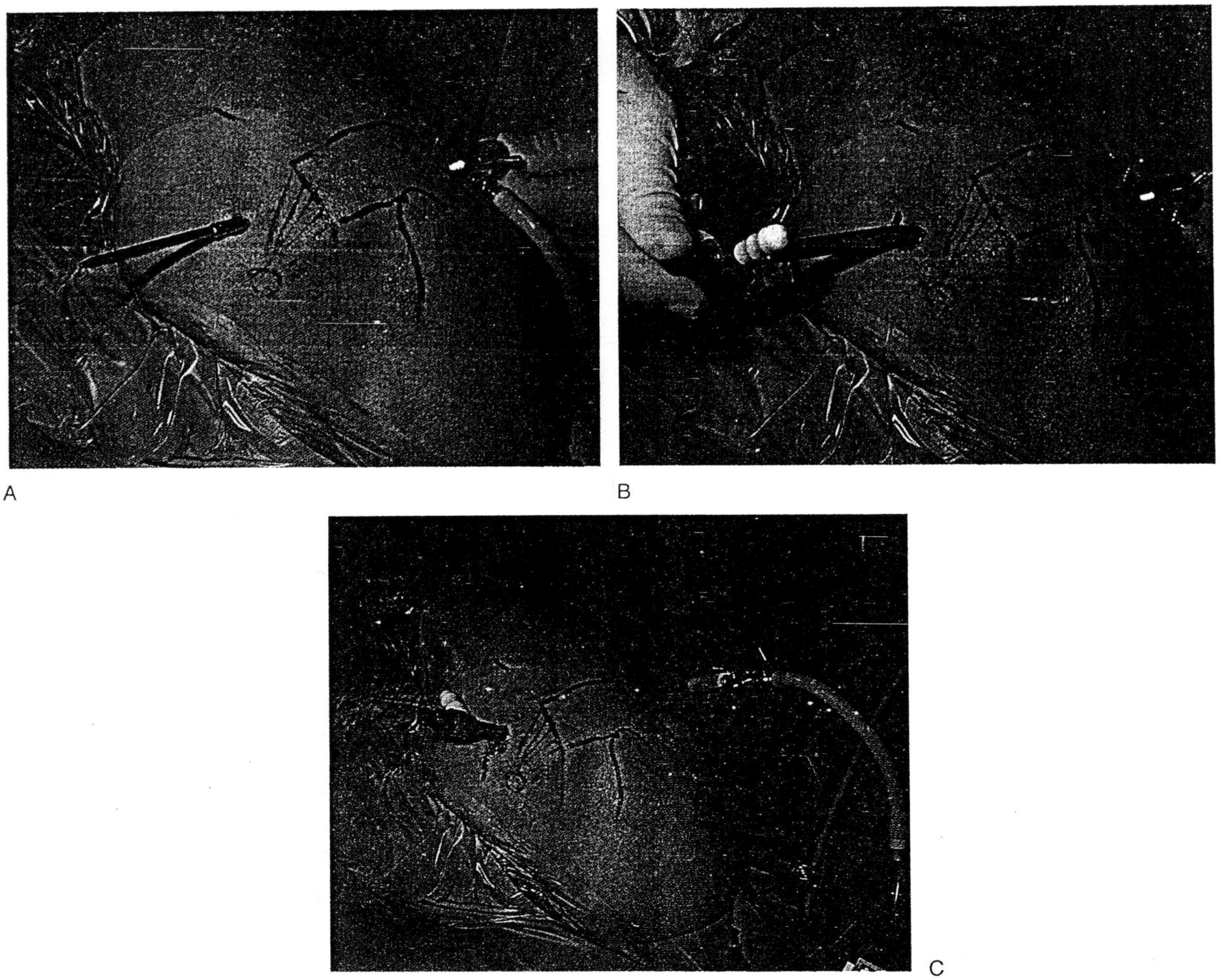

FIG. 3–20. Alternate method for introducing cannula through anterior portal.
A, If the shoulder is not too large, the sheath of the arthroscope can be advanced over the Wissinger rod to exit the joint anteriorly.
B, The 5.5-mm plastic cannula is fitted snugly over the tip of the arthroscopic sheath.
C, The tip of the cannula is moved into the center of the joint before the Wissinger rod is removed and the instruments are uncoupled.

If the shoulder is not too large, the arthroscope sheath may simply be pushed anteriorly around the portal rod until the tip exits the skin (Fig. 3–20A). The plastic cannula is fitted directly over the arthroscope sheath (Fig. 3–20B). The ends of both instruments are then moved together into the middle of the joint. The rod is withdrawn and the instruments uncoupled (Fig. 3–20C). Although a metal cannula could be introduced directly over the rod to accomplish anterior joint penetration, we prefer a plastic cannula with a diaphragm so that the joint distention can be maintained.

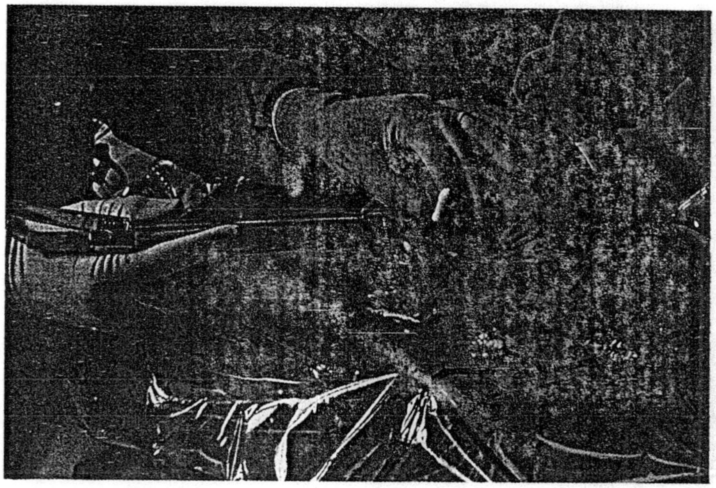

FIG. 3–21. The suction shaver is one of a variety of instruments that can be passed through the cannula.

As the anterior cannula is introduced, the tips of both the arthroscopic sheath and the anterior cannula must be within the joint before withdrawing the transfer rod. Unnecessary capsular penetration must be avoided to ensure that undue extravasation of fluid does not occur during shoulder arthroscopy.

A 3-mm bent-arm probe may be introduced through the anterior portal to facilitate examination of the labral attachment or cartilaginous defects. Fraying may obscure partial or complete lesions of the rotator cuff or LHB. A suction shaver passed through the anterior portal is used to debride these lesions and augment evaluation (Fig. 3–21). Transfer rods are used to maintain portals when reversing the position of the arthroscope and operating cannula. Joint debridement, synovectomy, removal of loose bodies, and capsular stabilization are all performed through the anterior portal.

The subacromial space is routinely examined following glenohumeral arthroscopy. Instruction on subacromial space arthroscopy, including the technique of arthroscopic subacromial decompression, is located in Chapter 5.

SECTION

ROTATOR CUFF DISORDERS

PATHOGENESIS AND CLINICAL EVALUATION OF ROTATOR CUFF DISEASE

The management of rotator cuff disease requires an understanding of the histopathology and pathomechanics of rotator cuff failure as well as the ability to establish an accurate diagnosis. Only after the nature and extent of fiber failure have been established can appropriate treatment be applied to the individual patient.

CONTROVERSY IN CUFF TREATMENT

The first published description of a rotator cuff tear appeared in 1835.[9] A British anatomist, John G. Smith, described the dissection of a massive cuff avulsion "in the body of a man brought to the dissecting room, under the old system of violation of the grave. . . ." It seems that some controversy surrounded the method by which this original specimen had been obtained. In 1927, nearly 100 years later, E.A. Codman published a paper entitled, "Obscure lesions of the shoulder; rupture of the supraspinatus tendon."[10] This "obscure lesion" is now mentioned frequently on the nightly news and in the sports pages of our newspapers. Codman regaled his colleagues when he noted that "ruptures of the supraspinatus are seldom recognized and promptly and efficiently treated." His experience with chronic neglected tears brought him to regard the surgical reconstruction "as difficult, convalescence as trying, and the results only good, not perfect." His admonition was to "recognize this very disabling lesion early and perform a really easy and satisfactory operation promptly." In the years that followed, techniques for imaging rotator cuff tears developed, and methods of surgical reconstructions were refined.[1,11-33]

Other investigators have advocated conservative, nonoperative treatment of these tears.[34-37] They document diminished pain and return of function without surgical treatment following some full-thickness tears. Early anatomists described a communication between the glenohumeral joint and subacromial space. This communication was so prevalent that what we now know to be a small tear in the supraspinatus was then considered a normal variant. All rotator cuff tears are not symptomatic. Most examiners have had the experience of observing a documented tear in a shoulder that functioned well. Shoulder elevation is possible even with a large tear when the humeral head migrates superiorly and medially to develop a pseudoarticulation below the coracoacromial arch.

The cuff invariably shows signs of wear before it tears. Further, once torn, the defect may widen and extend. This situation creates a dilemma. The moderate tear may be tolerated, but with further degenerative changes and trivial trauma, the disruption extends until the patient develops a serious disability with a large defect in the musculotendinous cuff surrounded by tissue of poor quality—truly an irreparable cuff.

Arthroscopic treatment bridges the gap between conservative and open surgical treatment. Debridement of the irregular, fibrotic margins of the torn cuff and accompanying synovial reactive changes in conjunction with anterior acromioplasty relieve the pain associated with rotator cuff failure. This relief can be accomplished with either open or arthroscopic surgical techniques.[38-41] Strength may appear to improve when pain is relieved, but the ultimate degree of recovered strength is proportional to the extent of the tear. When a cuff rupture is not repaired, the relative weakness persists even though pain has been relieved by debridement and decompression.

When mechanical impingement is present, acromioplasty appears to retard the progression of cuff failure. This statement is made with increasing clinical conviction based on 20 years of observation following the introduction of Neer's technique of anterior acromioplasty. No scientific end-result study, however, has been presented to confirm this hypothesis. Degeneration with aging continues regardless of an acromioplasty, and further fiber failure surely follows stressful activity that produces mechanical overload, whether by micro- or macrotrauma. The decision to debride rather than to repair a torn rotator cuff should not be made lightly, and the consequences of each technique should be shared with the patient. The current protocol and rationale for its application are presented with the conviction that both indications and techniques will continue to evolve.

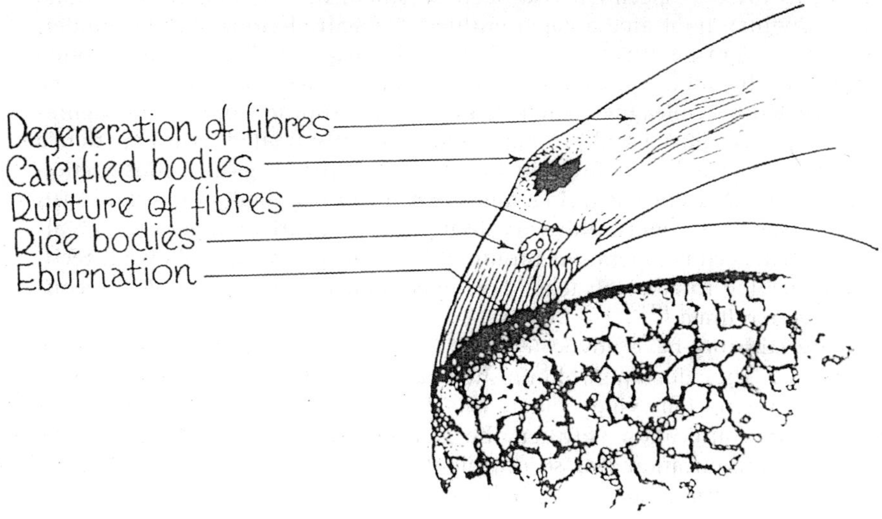

FIG. 4–1. Various changes involving the rotator cuff insertion have been described. Note small articular surface rupture.

HISTOPATHOLOGY

With the exception of a rare traumatic avulsion through normal tissue, Codman and Akerson observed that degenerative changes in the tendinous insertion of the rotator cuff were the earliest signs of fiber failure (Fig. 4–1).[42] They described incomplete tears of the articular surface at the synovial reflection ("rim-rents"), bursal surface tears (craters, "straps"), and degeneration of interstitial fibers. As the articular surface tear of the supraspinatus extends, the sulcus between the tuberosity and articular surface widens, and bony changes develop. Areas of sclerosis interspersed with cystic changes may be seen. Codman described these findings as "craters and volcanoes" (Fig. 4–2).[11] This process of progressive insertional failure has been termed "enthesopathy."[43] A similar process of deepening fiber failure can be observed from the bursal surface within 1 cm of tendinous insertion.[44] Codman observed crater-like erosions of the bursal surface and described superficial "strap"-like fibers of eroded tendon (Fig. 4–3). He commented that "they seem to be worn, as from friction."[11] In time, these partial tears become complete, and an *en masse* extension may occur. These full-thickness ruptures usually develop first in the supraspinatus insertion and then extend to involve an increasing portion of the infraspinatus, teres minor, and even subscapularis.

Normal shoulder elevation results from a "force-couple" action between an intact rotator cuff and deltoid. As the rotator cuff fails, shoulder dynamics alter. Extension and retraction of a tear involving the supraspinatus and infraspinatus permit the humeral head to migrate progressively upward until it articulates with the acromion. This "boutonniere" deformity is stabilized anteriorly by the subscapularis and posteriorly by the teres minor as long as they remain intact. Eventually, the humeral head develops degenerative changes in its superior surface. The classic "shoulder shrug" of a massive rotator cuff tear is observed clini-

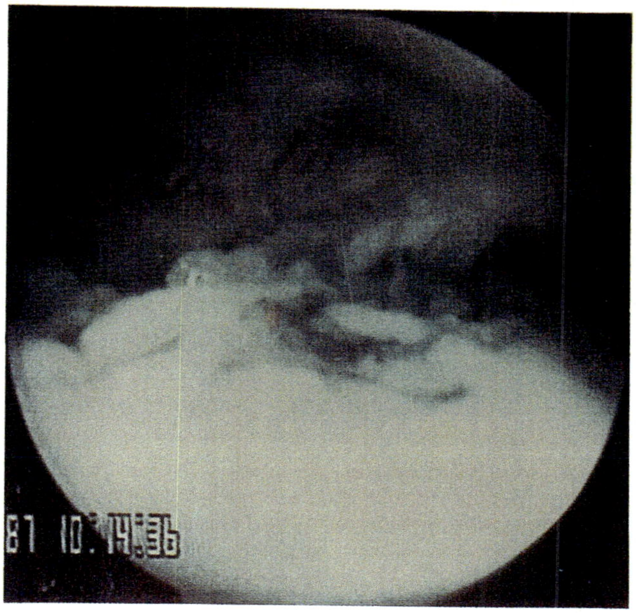

FIG. 4–2. "Volcanoes and craters" develop between humeral head and tuberosity (below) as cuff fibers fail and retract (above).

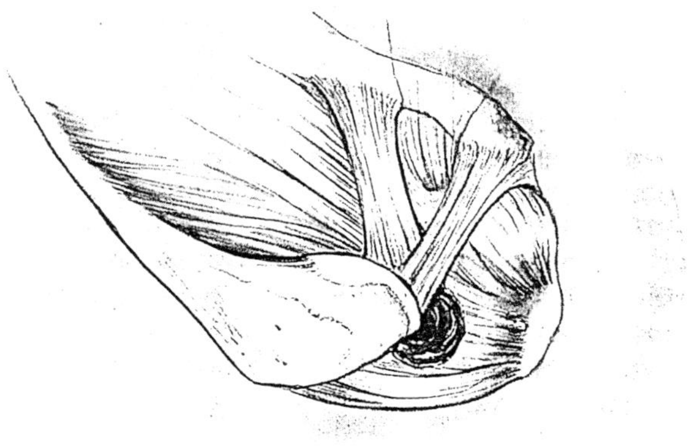

FIG. 4–3. Crater-like erosion develops directly under the anterior acromion as a result of friction.

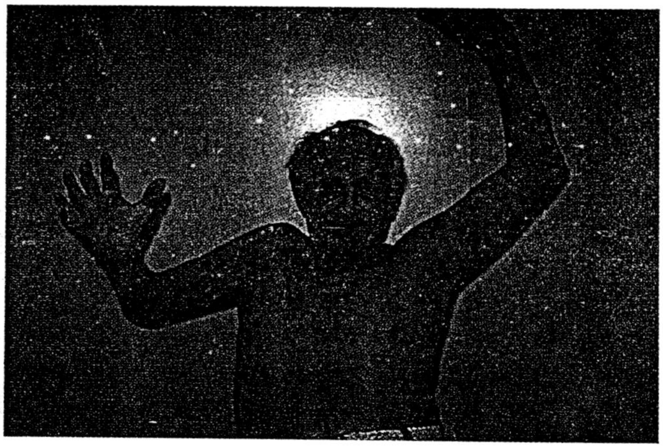

FIG. 4–4. Classic "shoulder shrug" associated with massive rotator cuff tear.

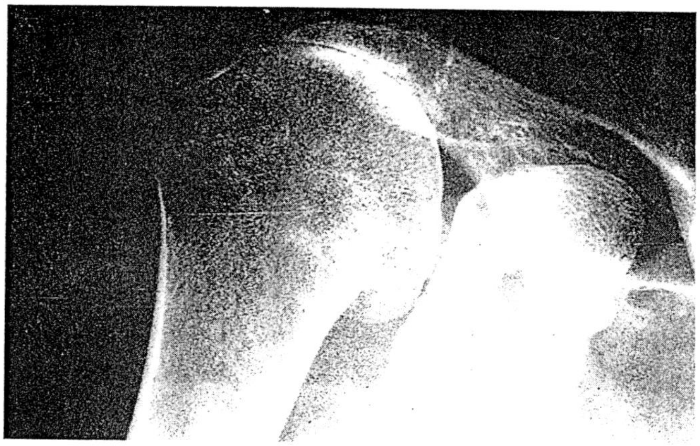

FIG. 4–5. High-riding humeral head and reduced acromiohumeral distance in patient with chronic massive rotator cuff tear.

cally (Fig. 4–4). Plain radiographs taken in 15 to 20° of attempted abduction show the distance between the undersurface of the acromion and the superior aspect of the humeral head (acromiohumeral distance) to be 3 mm or less. The greater tuberosity erodes and loses its prominence (Fig. 4–5). In some patients, an adaptive pseudoarticulation may develop (see Chap. 8). The tuberosity rounds down to the contour of the humeral head, and the patient with good deltoid strength and no significant pain is able to elevate the cuffless extremity to 90° or more as the superiorly and medially directed humeral head is stabilized beneath the coracoacromial arch.

CUFF ARTHROPATHY

The most unfortunate result of end-stage rotator cuff disease is the development of cuff arthropathy.[45] The condition is characterized by chronic synovitis with effusion, often hemorrhagic. Instability develops, and eventually collapse of the humeral head occurs. Crystalline deposits have been observed. The condition appears to be similar to that described as "Milwaukee shoulder" in the rheumatology literature.[46] The instability appears to be related to capsular stretching associated with chronic distention, as well as to rupture of the subscapularis. Loss of the anterior stabilizing effect of the subscapularis eliminates any hope for the development of a pseudoarticulation that might provide even limited function.

PATHOMECHANICS

Various factors contribute to the development of a rotator cuff tear. These factors may be intrinsic, extrinsic, or secondary.

INTRINSIC FACTORS

DEGENERATION WITH AGE

The relationship of age to rotator cuff rupture is widely appreciated. DePalma studied the shoulders of 96 patients (age 18 to 74 years) who had no recorded complaint of shoulder dysfunction.[47] He found partial ruptures of the supraspinatus in 37% of the shoulders. He observed a gradual increase in the size of the tears with each subsequent decade. The tears were most often seen in the sixth and seventh decades. Lohr and Uhthoff reported similar findings from their examination of 306 rotator cuff tears at autopsy.[43] The age of these specimens ranged from 26 to 95 years; 32% had partial tears, and 19.9% had full-thickness tears. The incidence of partial tears increased in the 50- and 60-year-old groups, whereas the incidence of complete tears was highest in those aged 70 years or older.

VASCULAR DEFICIENCY

Lindblom[48] and Moseley and Goldie[49] described an area of relative avascularity in the supraspinatus tendon adjacent to its insertion. Moseley and Goldie termed this area the "critical zone" and believed it represented an area of anastomosis between the tendinous blood supply arising from the osseous insertion laterally and from the muscle belly medially. Rothman and Parke believed this "critical zone" was related to advancing age.[50] MacNab and Rathbun conducted microvascular studies of the supraspinatus tendon and suggested that the apparent avascularity is related to a "wringing out" of the vessels by compression as they travel over the top of the humeral head when the arm is in the adducted position.[51] Regardless of the mechanism for production of relative avascularity, this region within 1 cm of the insertion of the supraspinatus tendon is the principal location of cuff failure.

OVERUSE (REPETITIVE MICROTRAUMA)

Repetitive microtrauma appears to be a factor in the relatively premature development of articular surface rotator cuff tears among athletes involved in sports that require throwing or the use of racquets. Andrews and colleagues reported on 18 partial articular tears that occurred in a group of patients between 18 and 22 years of age.[52] The relationship between acromial slope and instability is not established in this study. Repetitive overhead activities, whether vocational or avocational, are frequently implicated in the development of rotator cuff disease. This etiologic concept is tempered, however, by the high incidence of bilateral involvement in 55% of patients with cuff tears as determined by a positive ultrasound study on the opposite side.[53]

MAJOR TRAUMA

An isolated major trauma can assuredly avulse the cuff tendons; however, age and its accompanying degenerative changes certainly play a role. Consider the findings associated with acute anterior dislocation of the shoulder. The patient between 18 and 40 years of age is more apt to fracture the greater tuberosity than to avulse the supraspinatus when the shoulder dislocates. As the age of a patient with acute antero-inferior dislocation of the shoulder extends beyond 40 years, the probability of an associated rotator cuff tear increases. Indeed, even the subscapularis may avulse from the lesser tuberosity rather than the labrum detaching from the glenoid.

In most patients, the history discloses that the trauma associated with a rotator cuff tear was trivial rather than significant, thus indicating that the rupture occurred through an area of prior degeneration. As often as not, the elderly patient who appears with an acute rotator cuff tear has suffered an extension of a pre-existing smaller tear.

CALCIFIC TENDINITIS

Calcareous deposits are a common form of intrinsic tendinopathy. In the most promising theory, proposed by Uhthoff and colleagues,[54] calcium deposition begins with a fall in oxygen tension (PO_2), and, with the mediation of chondrocytes, sizable foci of intratendinous calcium develop. After a variable period of time, this chronic deposit may go through a phase of resorption. Vascular infiltration accompanies an increase in oxygen tension, and the calcium may disappear entirely. This tendinopathy is often self healing. When quiescent, the sheer bulk of the calcium within the tendon may cause a relative narrowing of the supraspinatus outlet and accompanying impingement-type symptoms. At other times, most probably when resorption begins or the calcium ruptures into the subacromial space, an extremely painful condition develops. The released calcium acts as though it were a "chemical boil." Once the calcification has resolved, the tendon appears to reconstitute itself.

EXTRINSIC FACTORS

The structure of the coracoacromial arch may mechanically encroach upon the rotator cuff, either primarily or secondarily, and thereby produce injury. We are indebted to Neer for his description of the impingement syndrome and of the role of anterior acromioplasty in the treatment of this condition.[1]

ACROMIAL SLOPE

Acromial structure has been classified into three types based on the curvature as viewed from the lateral projection (Fig. 4–6).[55] Type I is flat. Type II is curved to the extent that the undersurface is essentially parallel to the convexity of the underlying humeral head. In type III, the anterior portion is hooked downward. This downcurving is accentuated by the development of a traction spur at the point of coracoclavicular ligament insertion.

Acromial structure can be demonstrated radiographically on a tangential view of the scapula centered at the level of the acromion. This projection is quite similar to the "trauma" or "Y" view originally described by Neer and has been termed the supraspinatus outlet view (Fig. 4–7).[56]

The incidence of rotator cuff disease increases in type II and III acromions.[55] In a retrospective study by Ellman of consecutive patients who had undergone arthroscopic acromioplasty for impingement syndrome, not one type I acromion was found.

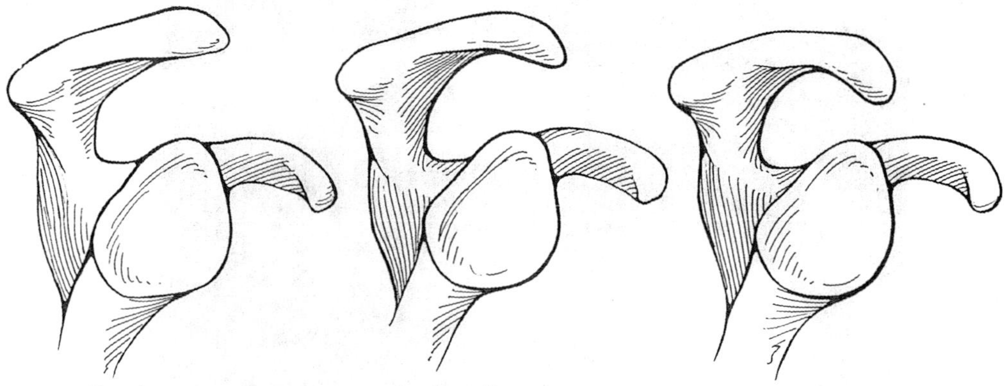

FIG. 4–6. Classification of acromial morphology into three types: I = flat; II = curved; III = hooked.

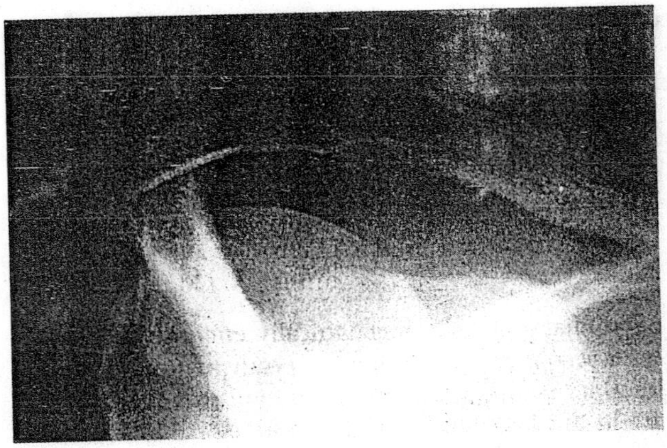

FIG. 4–7. Supraspinatus outlet view (arch view).

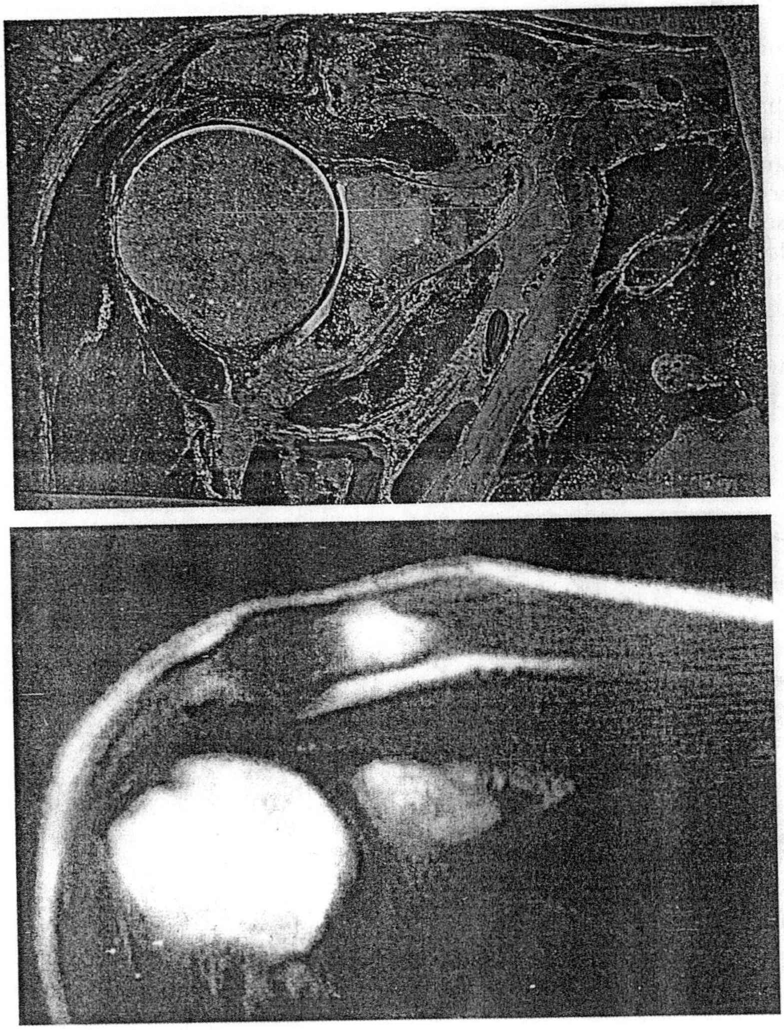

A
B

FIG. 4–8. A, Microcryosection of right shoulder in frontal plane. Note pressure exerted on supraspinatus tendon by the undersurface of the outer end of the clavicle.
B, MRI: Frontal oblique view shows similar downward pressure on the supraspinatus directly below a bulbous acromioclavicular joint.

CORACOACROMIAL LIGAMENT

The coracoacromial ligament provides a firm ligamentous cover to complete the coracoacromial arch. Anatomic purists do not consider this structure a true ligament, because it stretches between two bony prominences on the same bone rather than from one bone to another. This ligament creates a rigid obstruction to the bursa and underlying rotator cuff insertion, particularly when the elevated arm is adducted and internally rotated. This ligament is released or partially resected in all procedures designed to decompress the subacromial space.

ACROMIOCLAVICULAR SPURS

Hypertrophic spurs arise from the contiguous borders of the undersurface of an arthritic acromioclavicular joint. Downward-protruding spurs encroach upon the musculotendinous junction of the supraspinatus when the arm is at the side (Fig. 4–8). Elevation and rotation cause these spurs to impinge more laterally. Petersson and Gentz consider acromioclavicular spurs to be more of a culprit in the production of mechanical impingement than is the acromion itself.[57]

SECONDARY CAUSES

Various secondary causes may place the cuff at a mechanical disadvantage and thereby provoke undue strain on its insertion.

INSTABILITY

Instability is the most common cause of secondary impingement. Joint laxity permits an abnormal translation of the humeral head not only anteriorly and posteriorly but superiorly as well. Throwing, or racquet sports requiring similar movement, may stretch the anterior as well as the posterior capsular structures. Failure of the anterior capsular restraints produces instability. Strengthening of the muscular stabilizers may be insufficient to overcome this instability. Consequently, cuff lesions develop in the athlete who throws, plays racquet sports, or swims. Certain activities related to weight training, such as the behind-the-head military press and the maneuver designed to strengthen the pectoral musculature, commonly called "flys," may unduly stretch the anterior capsule. This form of secondary impingement can be overcome only by correcting the instability; however, at times, the cuff lesion progresses to such a degree that it also must be treated.

INTRINSIC OVERLOAD

Weakness in the rotator cuff musculature provoked by overuse during strenuous activities may cause the cuff muscles to become vulnerable to injury. This situation differs from repetitive microtrauma because fatigue with associated weakness is the offender.

CLASSIFICATION OF ROTATOR CUFF TEARS

Failure of the insertional fibers of the rotator cuff may vary from minute to massive. The following classification enables us to stage the degree of fiber failure in an orderly fashion. This classification describes the degree of fiber failure and permits outcome studies of the various groups based on the method of treatment. The system combines the Ellman classification of partial-thickness tears[58] with the Matsen system for staging degenerative tears of the rotator cuff.[59]

Partial Tear. Partial tear of the rotator cuff usually involves the supraspinatus muscle. Partial tears of the supraspinatus may be observed on either the articular or the bursal surface. The partial tear is divided into three grades, depending on the depth of the tear (Fig. 4–9).

Grade 1. Only capsule or superficial fibers are involved. The depth of the tear is less than 3 mm, as measured by a bent-arm probe or the known circumference of a shaver. This grade of tear involves less than one-fourth the thickness of the cuff.

Grade 2. Less than one-half the thickness of the cuff is involved. The depth of the grade 2 tear is never greater than 6 mm.

Grade 3. More than one-half the thickness of the cuff attachment is torn.

The description of the tear should indicate whether the articular (A) or bursal (B) surface is involved. In addition, the base of the tear and the width of retraction are measured and expressed in mm^2. Although this system provides at best a clinical estimate rather than an exact measurement of the extent of the defect, the grading system is far superior to a mere statement that a partial tear is present.

Full-Thickness Tear. Matsen's classification of full-thickness rotator cuff tear is based on the extent to which the musculotendinous insertion of the rotator cuff has failed.

Stage 1. Full-thickness defect of the supraspinatus.

Stage 2. Defect involves all the supraspinatus and at least part of the infraspinatus.

Stage 3. Full-thickness defect involving the supraspinatus, infraspinatus, and subscapularis.

Stage 4. Rotator cuff arthropathy.

This system of staging may be correlated with the more traditional method of describing tears as small, medium, large, and massive. The cuff is weakened when fibers of insertion fail, regardless of how far the torn cuff is retracted. The borders of the individual cuff muscles at their point of insertion are difficult, if not impossible, to distinguish. The size of the tear is related to the number of muscles that are disrupted. A full-thickness tear that appears no more than 2 cm in width does not involve more than the supraspinatus, and, thus, is a stage 1 tear. The full-thickness tear that extends from 2 through 4 cm certainly requires involvement of at least a portion of the infraspinatus (stage 2). Any tear that involves the supraspinatus, infraspinatus, and subscapularis is more than 5 cm and is truly massive (stage 3). Measuring the base of the tear and the depth of retraction in cm^2 is valuable in calculating the *extent* of the defect.

The ability to repair the cuff is influenced by the quality of the tissue, as well as by the area of the defect. Rupture of a thin, attenuated cuff may provide poor tissue for reconstruction, whereas the *en masse* extension of a small tear into relatively healthy tendon can be readily repaired if done promptly. The duration of the tear becomes a factor in repairability. In time, the retracted muscle becomes atrophic with disuse. The muscle belly is fibrotic and relatively inelastic, thus challenging efforts at mobilization. With progressive cuff failure, the retracted cuff margins are ground away as the humeral head rises to articulate with the acromion, thereby creating an extensive defect.

The surgeon's ability to discern the extent and repairability of rotator cuff fiber failure by astute clinical evaluation determines the optimal treatment for the individual patient.

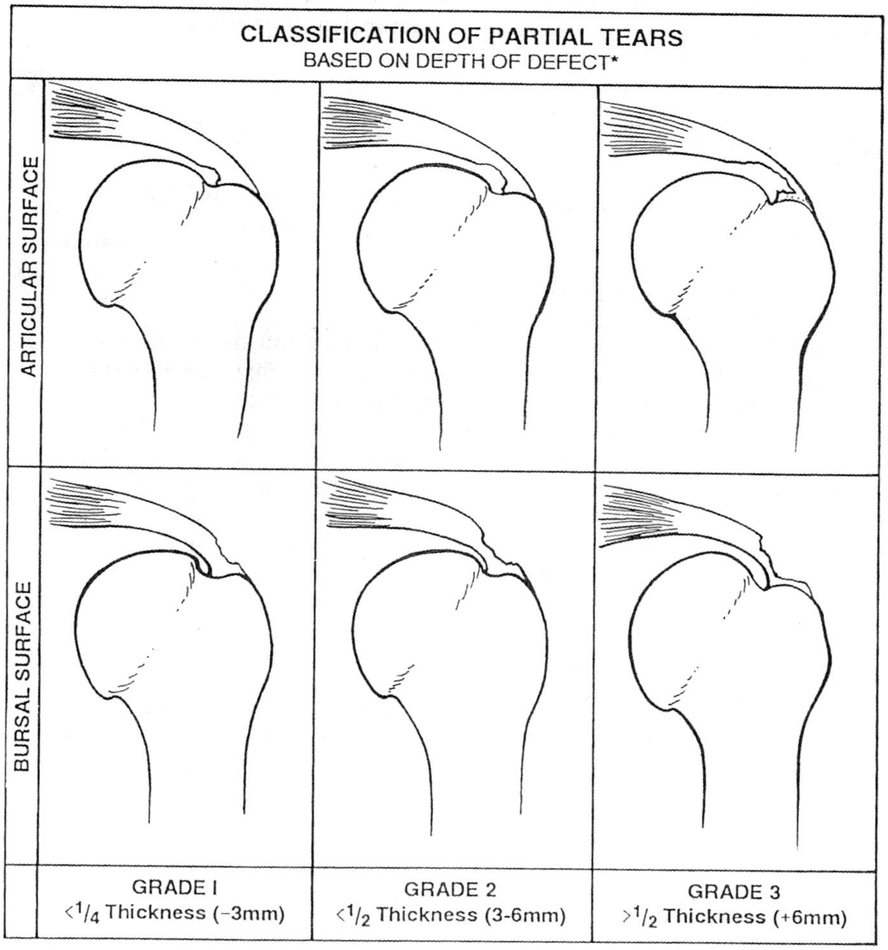

*Indicate AREA OF DEFECT: Base of tear × maximum retraction = mm^2

FIG. 4–9. Ellman classification of partial-thickness rotator cuff tears (stage P).

CLINICAL EVALUATION

The clinical evaluation of rotator cuff disease combines history and physical findings with diagnostic imaging. The goal is to define both the nature and the extent of cuff involvement.

HISTORY

Age, handedness, and *level of activity,* both vocational and avocational, must be clearly defined at the outset. Each of these factors has a bearing on the patient's functional requirements and relates directly to the goals of rehabilitation.

The *duration of symptoms* and the *role of trauma,* whether trivial or significant, must be defined. The type of previous treatment, including multiple steroid injections, and the response to that treatment should be established. The position in which pain is provoked should be recorded. The effect of night pain on the patient should be noted. Pain arising from rotator cuff disease is commonly referred to the upper outer third of the humerus.

PHYSICAL FINDINGS

The three stages of the impingement syndrome described by Neer are based on a progression of histopathologic changes within the cuff,[60] as follows:

Stage I: Edema and hemorrhage.
Stage II: Fibrosis and tendinitis.
Stage III: Rotator cuff tear; bony changes.

Stage I generally involves a younger group of patients, and the changes are reversible. Stage II encompasses a somewhat older group of individuals in whom structural changes in the cuff are more advanced. Patients with a stage III rotator cuff tear are usually older than 40 years. The bony changes are considered a consequence of the cuff tear and develop later. Neer has pointed out that the *clinical signs are the same in all three stages of the impingement syndrome.* Pain occurring during the arc of forward elevation of the shoulder accompanies various disorders (see Chap. 1). Physical findings associated most directly with cuff disease, however, are reviewed in this chapter.

TENDERNESS

Tenderness is usually present in the region of the tuberosity insertion or beneath the coracoacromial ligament near its point of attachment to the anterior edge of the acromion (Fig. 4–10A). Because bicipital tendinitis is commonly associated with rotator cuff disease, tenderness may also be found at the proximal portion of the intertubercular sulcus.

CREPITUS

Crepitus arising from the subacromial region is invariably found in the presence of a rotator cuff tear. A chronically inflamed bursa or partial-thickness bursal tear, however, may produce considerable crepitus without a full-thickness

A
B

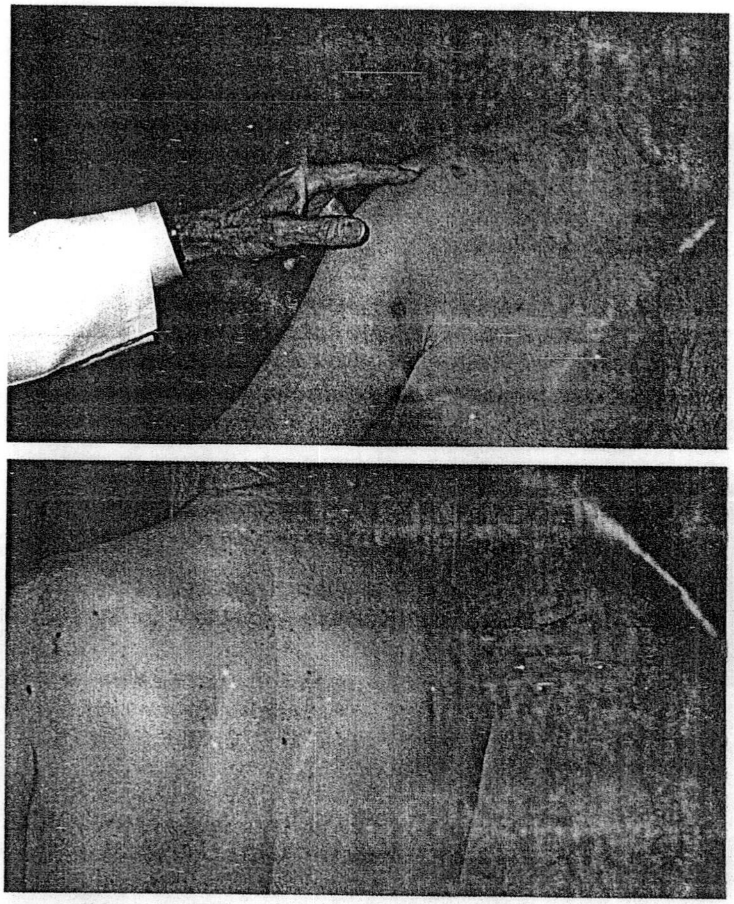

FIG. 4–10. A, Tenderness usually occurs in region of greater tuberosity or beneath coracoacromial ligament.
B, Selective atrophy in large chronic rotator cuff tears.

lesion. At times, the crepitus may be quite audible. Auscultation with a stethoscope reveals subacromial pops and clicks with sometimes alarming magnification.

ATROPHY

Selective atrophy of the supraspinatus or infraspinatus is seen in large chronic rotator cuff tears (Fig. 4–10B).

IMPINGEMENT SIGNS

The classic impingement sign is produced by stabilizing the scapula with the palm of the examiner's hand while the patient's arm is elevated in the forward plane. The humerus should be internally rotated during elevation (Fig. 4–11A). In the presence of cuff disease, pain develops at about 70° and continues

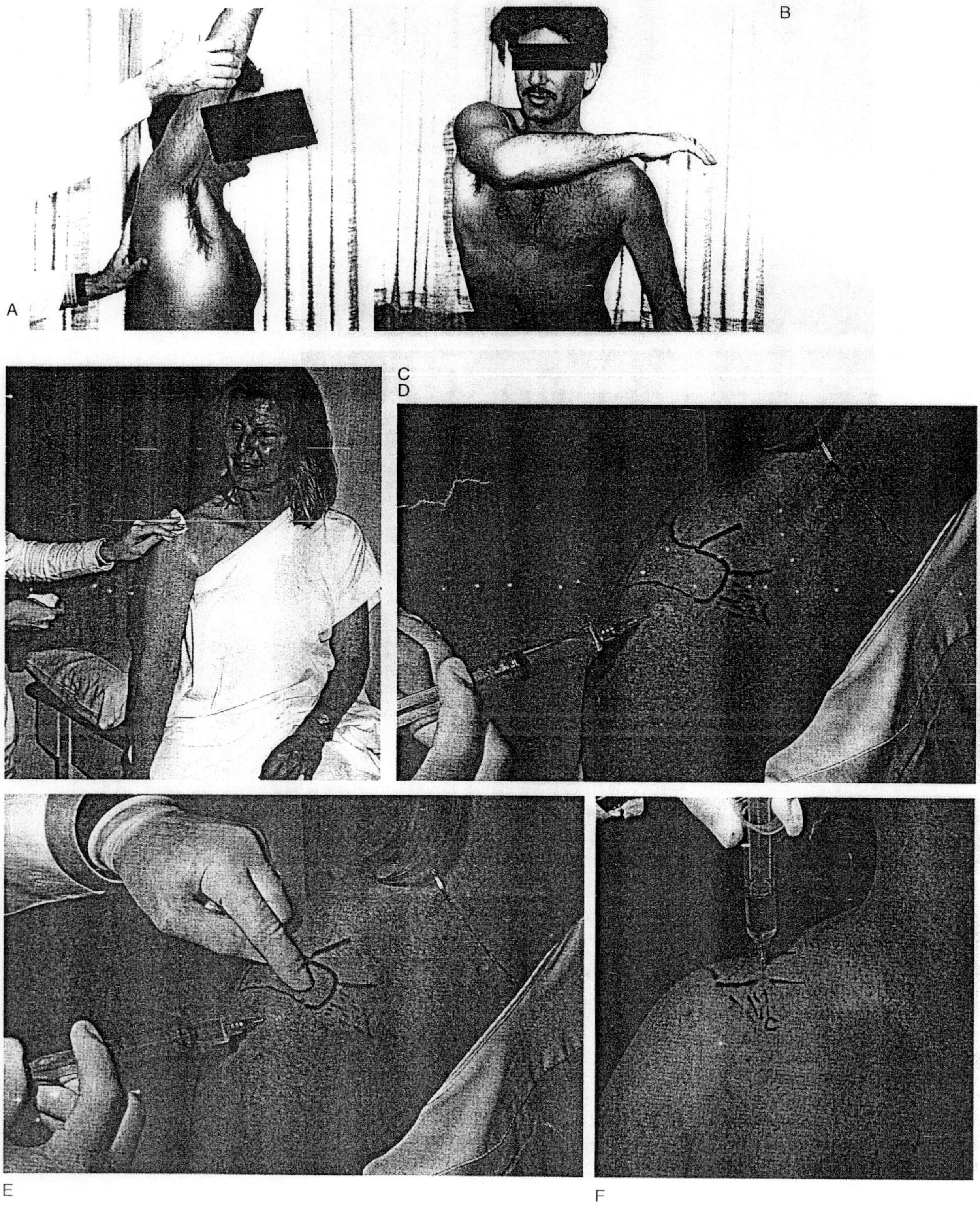
A
B
C
D
E
F

FIG. 4–11. A, Impingement sign: Forward elevation with the forearm pronated and the scapula stabilized.
B, Impingement sign II: Forward elevation to 90° combined with internal rotation and adduction.
C through F, Impingement test. The seated patient is turned slightly to allow arm to dangle freely (C). Injection begins just below lateral border of acromion about 2 cm posterior to the anterolateral margin (D). Needle is advanced to lie directly beneath the anterior one third of the acromion (E). Acromioclavicular joint injection (F): In some patients, a selective injection of local anesthetic is made directly into the acromioclavicular joint to determine whether symptoms are arising from the subacromial space or from the acromioclavicular joint.

through the entire arc of elevation. If the scapula is felt to move unduly upward as the arm is elevated, adhesive capsulitis or advanced degenerative joint disease should be considered more likely than cuff involvement to be the cause of pain.

Another provocative maneuver for cuff disease is called the *impingement sign II.* The arm is elevated to shoulder level and then internally rotated while being adducted across the chest (Fig. 4–11B).[61] This maneuver squeezes the supraspinatus against the anterior acromion and coracoacromial ligament, consequently provoking pain in the patient with rotator cuff disease. Forceful cross-chest adduction at shoulder level also compresses the acromioclavicular joint, and pain associated with hypertrophic arthritis or osteolysis may be provoked with this test. The patient may be able to indicate whether the pain comes primarily from the subacromial space or the acromioclavicular joint during this maneuver. A selective injection of local anesthetic may be even more helpful in determining whether the pain is originating in the subacromial space or the acromioclavicular joint, because the acromioclavicular joint, as well as the anterior acromion, has been implicated in producing cuff disorders.

IMPINGEMENT TESTS

The ablation of pain in the shoulder following the injection of 10 ml of local anesthetic into the subacromial space is considered presumptive evidence of an impingement disorder. The test is performed in the following fashion: While seated on an examination table, the patient is turned just enough to let the arm dangle freely at the side (Fig. 4–11C). The lateral border of the acromion is identified by palpation. Following appropriate preparation of the skin, a 22-gauge needle attached to a 10-ml syringe full of local anesthetic solution is injected into the subacromial space. The point for injection is just below the lateral border of the acromion, about 2 cm posterior to the anterolateral margin (Fig. 4–11D). The medication should not be placed into the substance of the rotator cuff. We prefer 0.25% bupivacaine (Marcaine) without adrenaline for this injection. The needle is then advanced to lie directly beneath the anterior one third of the acromion (Fig. 4–11E). The needle may be adjusted a bit posteriorly or anteriorly through the same puncture wound to distribute the medication evenly in the subacromial space. An apprehensive patient may have to be reminded to relax and permit the weight of the extremity to open the subacromial region to simplify the injection. Following the injection, the patient is asked to lie down for a few minutes to allow the local anesthetic to infiltrate the region. This routine also diminishes the incidence of syncopal reaction among the approximate one third of the population that is estimated to be belonophobic (Gr. *belon*—needle).

After about 5 minutes, the impingement maneuvers are repeated. A well-placed injection completely eliminates the pain provoked by mechanical impingement. When acromioclavicular joint disease is suspected, forced cross-chest adduction is repeated to determine if pain arising from the acromioclavicular joint persists. If so, a selective injection of the acromioclavicular joint can be made (Fig. 4–11F). These selective injections can be quite helpful in determining whether symptoms are arising from either the subacromial space or the acromioclavicular joint. Both range of motion and strength may improve following this pain-ablation test. The significance of this observation is considered in the following sections.

RANGE OF MOTION

Mobility is influenced by pain as well as by the weakness that accompanies rupture of the cuff tendons. Range of motion of the shoulder is measured in forward flexion (Fig. 4–12A), abduction, and external rotation with the arm at the side (Fig. 4–12B). These movements are carefully measured with a goniometer and recorded numerically as right/left. Internal rotation is measured by the anatomic level achieved by the patient's thumb (Fig. 4–12C), for example, the level of thoracic or lumbar spinous process, the sacroiliac joint, or the greater trochanter. Recognition that the inferior tip of the scapula usually lies adjacent to the seventh dorsal vertebra is helpful. Again, the comparison is recorded as right/left. Internal and external rotation may also be measured with the arm abducted 90° in the coronal plane.

The reciprocal relationship between range of motion and strength may preclude *active* elevation when a large cuff tear is present, yet a full range of motion can be achieved with passive assistance. The passive range of motion in each parameter also should be recorded when it exceeds the active range.

A popular misconception is that capsulitis does not accompany rotator cuff ruptures. Some degree of stiffness often accompanies chronic tears of long duration. This type of painful stiff shoulder can usually be differentiated from true adhesive capsulitis by testing external rotation while the patient is supine. The classic "frozen shoulder" is more firmly fixed in internal rotation than is the shoulder with cuff rupture. Even when the tear is so massive that the patient cannot externally rotate against gravity, a significant degree of passive motion can be produced while supine. The shoulder cannot achieve full overhead elevation unless it is externally rotated.

When measuring forward flexion the forearm should be supinated until the palm faces upward. The patient should be seated to minimize body motion. The arms of the goniometer should be placed down the central axis of the trunk and the proximal humerus. Surprisingly few adults achieve 180° when measured in this fashion. Constant and Murley have documented an age-related decrease in range of motion and have established normal values for the various decades.[62]

Abduction must also be performed in external rotation (palm upward) to achieve full potential. When abduction is performed while the humerus is internally rotated, the greater tuberosity becomes locked beneath the lateral acromion at about 90°, and further motion is purely scapulothoracic. External rotation unlocks the joint and permits full elevation.

If the impingement test successfully ablates the patient's pain, the accompanying improvement in range of motion should be noted.

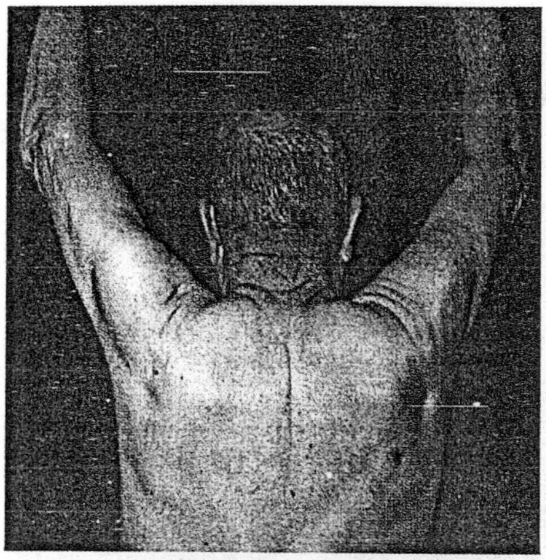

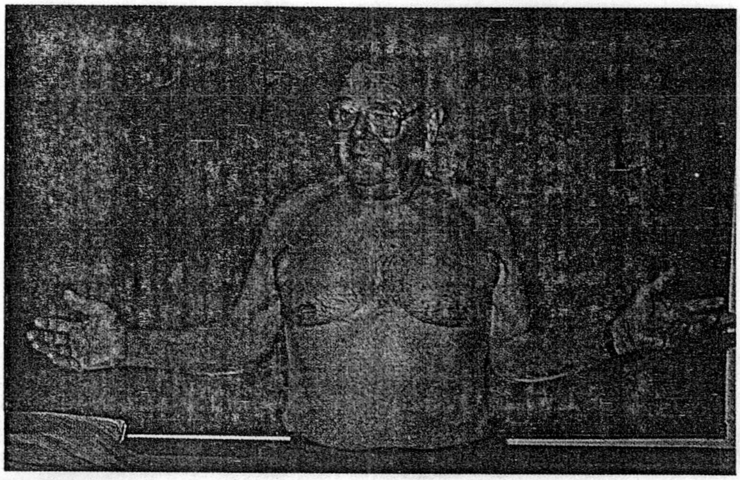

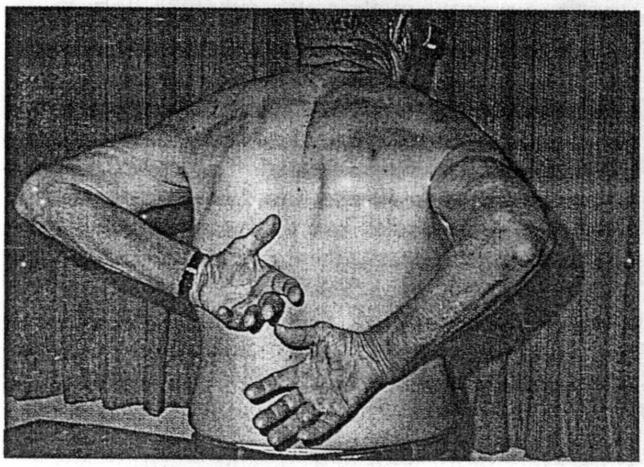

A B
C

FIG. 4–12. A, Range of motion measured in forward flexion.
B, Range of motion measured in external rotation with arms at side.
C, Anatomic level achieved with patient's thumb measures extent of internal rotation.

STRENGTH

Strength evaluation is the astute clinician's most valuable index in assessing the degree of cuff fiber failure. *Pain must be ablated by local anesthetic to make an accurate assessment of strength.* The patient with Neer's clinical stage I or stage II impingement may "give way" as strength is tested because of pain, even though the cuff is quite intact. The injection of a local anesthetic into the subacromial space may restore strength to the level of that in the opposite extremity. *Weakness following pain ablation is the cardinal sign of cuff rupture.* In general, the degree of weakness varies with the size of the tear.[28]

Manual muscle testing is graded on a scale from 0 to 5:

GRADE		DEGREE OF STRENGTH
0 : Zero	=	Paralysis
1 : Trace	=	Muscle contracts but does not move
2 : Poor	=	Able to move with gravity eliminated
3 : Fair	=	Able to overcome gravity but no resistance
4 : Good	=	Moves against gravity and moderate resistance
5 : Excellent	=	Normal strength

Strength is individually graded in forward flexion, abduction, and external rotation (Fig. 4–13). The supraspinatus muscle may be tested selectively by elevating the arm to 90° in a position midway between forward flexion and abduction. This position corresponds roughly to the scapular plane. While in this position, the arm is pronated as though one is emptying the contents of a cup. This maneuver brings the supraspinatus to a position directly on top of the humeral head. If the patient is unable to resist the downward pressure applied by two fingers of the examiner, a supraspinatus tear is likely.

A small full-thickness tear of the supraspinatus may produce little or no weakness. Again, weakness increases in direct proportion to the size of the tear.

When weakness in abduction and forward flexion is combined with weakness in external rotation, the tear involves the infraspinatus as well as the supraspinatus and, therefore, is quite large (stage 2). At times, the weakness may be so profound that the seated patient cannot maintain the arm in external rotation when it is passively placed in this position with the elbow bent. The extremity simply swings backward toward the midline, thereby indicating a complete rupture of the external rotators. The classic "shoulder shrug" indicates an extensive tear. The scapular elevators and deltoid contract simultaneously; as the scapula elevates, the patient's body tilts to the opposite side in a vain effort to elevate the arm.

The "drop-arm sign" can usually be elicited when a shoulder shrug is present. When the weakened arm is passively placed into a position of full elevation, the scapula usually can rotate enough to balance the humeral head on the glenoid, much as a golf ball rests on a tee. The trapezius, latissimus, and pectoralis all help the deltoid and scapular rotators to maintain this position. As the arm is lowered toward the horizontal, this coalition of musculature cannot maintain the arm against gravity in the absence of the rotator cuff, and the arm falls precipitously. Later in the course of rotator cuff disease, the medial and superior migration of the humeral head may permit the development of a pseudoarticulation, as was mentioned earlier. In this circumstance, the patient with a strong deltoid and accessory musculature can control both descent and ascent of the arm surprisingly well. Nevertheless, the telltale shrug of cuff deficiency can be observed. More importantly, considerable weakness persists. The patient normally cannot elevate more than 3 to 5 pounds repetitively, and the 2-finger resistance test demonstrates significant weakness, particularly when performed with the arm a few degrees below horizontal. The manual evaluation of strength is at best a gross assessment tempered by the examiner's subjectivity. These clinical precepts serve well for diagnosis.

DIAGNOSTIC IMAGING

Current advances in the technology of diagnostic imaging now enable further evaluation of the quantity of the defect and the quality of the residual tissue. With these factors in mind, a rational therapeutic decision can be made. Various methods for imaging defects in the rotator cuff are available. The value of each method varies in relation to the technique and interpretation available.

PLAIN RADIOGRAPHS

The plain radiograph is of inestimable value. Films are routinely taken in the anteroposterior (AP) plane of the joint, in internal and external rotation, and in

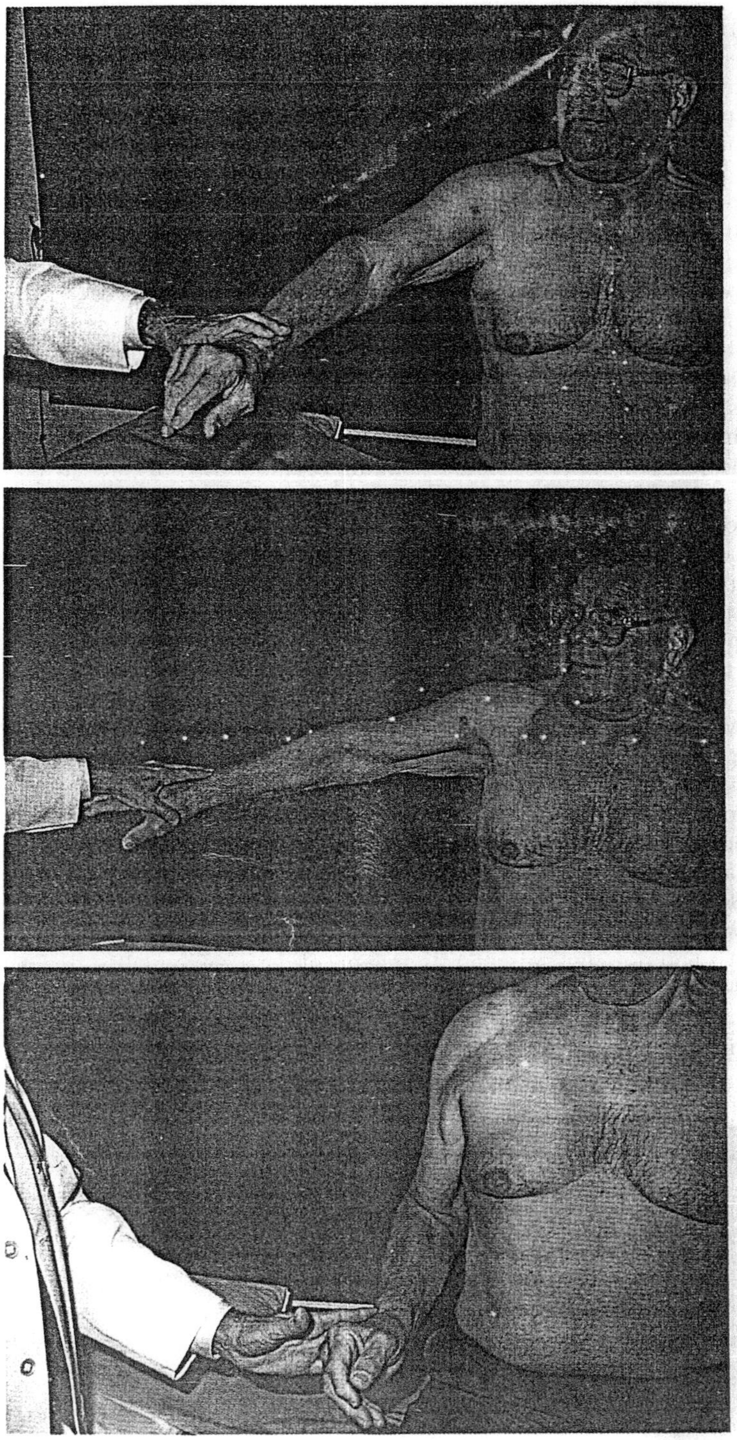

A B C

FIG. 4–13. Strength evaluation is performed in forward flexion (A), abduction (B), and external rotation (C).

axillary and supraspinatus outlet (arch view) projections. Numerous changes suggesting cuff degeneration may be evident. The *notch* between the tuberosity and articular surface of the humeral head may show subchondral cystic changes interspersed with areas of sclerosis. This telltale sign of enthesopathy (the craters and volcanoes described by Codman) develops after the cuff fibers have peeled away from their insertion. The thin mantle of cortical bone in this region loses its stimulation and undergoes degenerative changes. The adjacent *tuberosity* may appear sclerotic or become rounded as the head drifts upward in response to the weakened supraspinatus. The *acromion* may respond to compression from below by developing a well-demarcated line of sclerosis along its undersurface (Fig. 4–14). As a cuff tear widens, or perhaps as an intact cuff thins with atrophy and partial tearing, the distance between the undersurface of the acromion and the superior articular surface of the humeral head narrows.

This *acromiohumeral interval* (AHI) varies somewhat, depending on whether the film is taken with the patient supine or standing, because the weight of the arm distracts the interval in the standing position. This distraction is overcome when the standing patient actively abducts the arm a mere 15 or 20°. Fukuda and colleagues have described a weight-bearing view that makes this measurement even more constant.[63] He asks the seated patient to use both hands to push upward from the chair while a radiograph of the joint is taken in the AP projection. Various studies of the acromiohumeral distance, without reference to any specific weight-bearing views, have been published.[64-66] These studies conclude that the normal AHI is between 12 and 14 mm (Fig. 4–15A). A high incidence of full-thickness rotator cuff tears is found when the distance is 7 mm or less. We have observed that the tear is massive and the quality of residual tissue quite poor when the distance is narrowed to 3 mm or less (Fig. 4–15B).

Acromiohumeral arthritis often develops as a result of the articulation of the humeral head with the undersurface of the acromion. The superior articular surface becomes pebbled, and the prominence of the tuberosity becomes diminished and rounded. Increased acromial concavity appears to develop as a result of massive cuff disruption in this situation (Fig. 4–16).

Acromial spurs may be commonly seen with appropriate radiographic projection. An anterior spur arises in the region of coracoacromial ligament insertion (Fig. 4–17). The appearance is that of a traction spur that extends into the substance of the ligament, presumably as a result of a trampoline effect from the high-riding humeral head. Because the coracoacromial ligament spans two

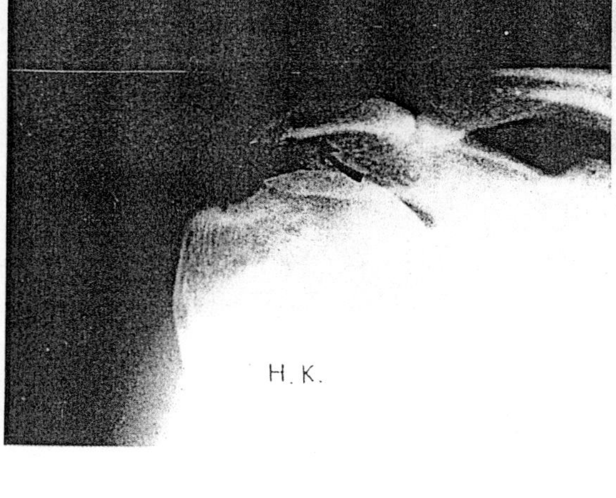

FIG. 4–14. Plain radiograph: Curved arrow points to sclerosis beneath the acromion. Note subchondral cyst and sclerosis between the rounded tuberosity and the humeral head (enthesopathy).

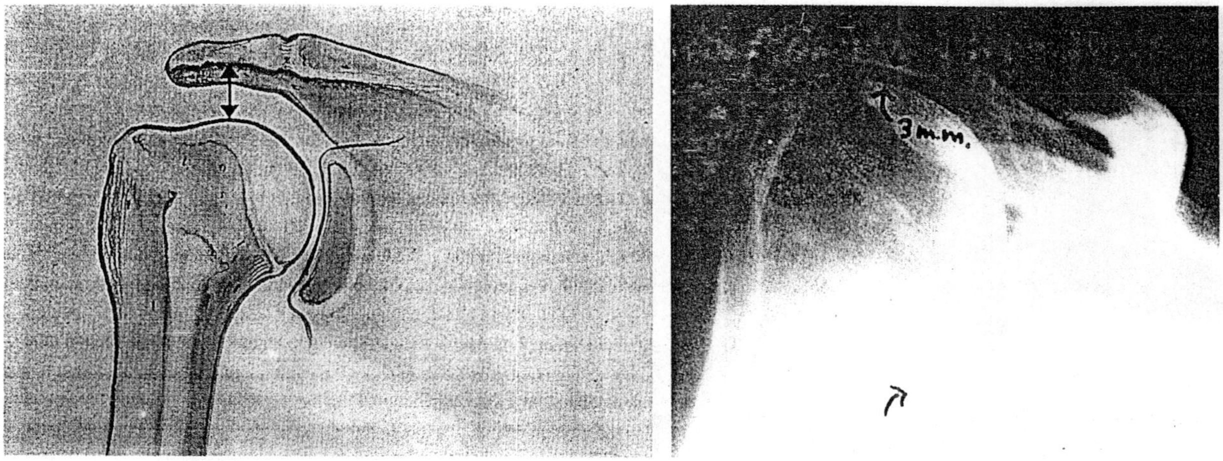

A B

FIG. 4–15. A, Acromiohumeral interval (AHI): The distance between the superior surface of the humerus and the undersurface of the acromion is between 12 and 14 mm. B, When the AHI is narrowed to 3 mm or less, the tear is massive.

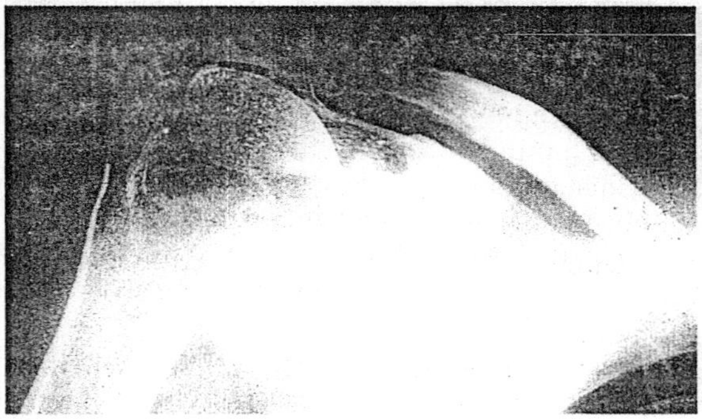

FIG. 4–16. Acromiohumeral arthritis associated with massive tear. The superior articular surface becomes pebbled, and the tuberosity is rounded.

points in the same bone, few other causes for this reaction have been suggested. An increase in acromial concavity has been noted in patients with cuff rupture. The incidence of rotator cuff tears is higher in patients with type 2 and type 3 configurations than in patients with the type 1 (flat) acromion.[55]

The *caudal tilt* projection, as seen in Figure 4–17A, has been popularized by Rockwood to demonstrate the projection of a downcurving acromion anterior to the anterior margin of the clavicle.[67] This view is taken 30° caudal to a standard AP view of the shoulder. The projecting portion of acromion is readily demonstrated.

The concavity of the undersurface of the acromion can be measured with variable accuracy utilizing the *supraspinatus outlet view (arch view)*. This view must precisely image the acromion in the sagittal plane to be reliable (Fig. 4–18A). The projection is essentially a tangential view of the scapula taken with 15° of caudal tilt. The tangential view of the scapula was described by Alexander in older radiology textbooks. This view is a minor modification of the "lateral trauma view" described by Neer.[68]

The technique for the supraspinatus outlet view is as follows. The patient is placed on the x-ray table in the lateral recumbent position and then is allowed

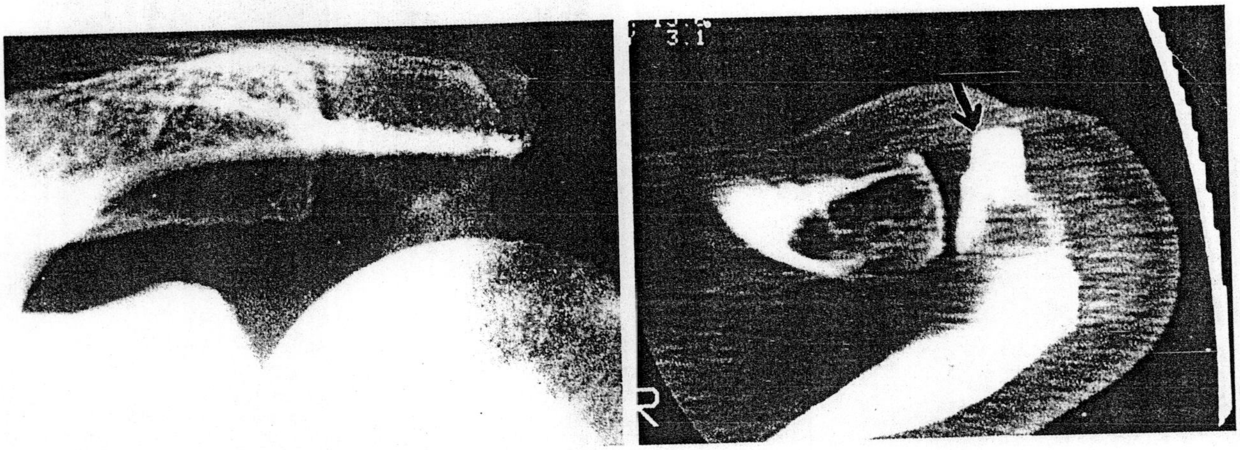

A B

FIG. 4–17. A, Large acromial spur arises from the anterior margin (anteroposterior radiograph taken with 30° caudal tilt).
B, The same spur as that shown in Figure 4–17A is seen in an axial CT scan (arrow).

to roll 30 to 45° toward the prone position (Fig. 4–18B, C, D). A large 45° foam rubber wedge supports the trunk in this position while the x-ray tube is directed downward along the axis of the scapula with 15° caudal tilt. An accurate projection is ensured by asking the patient to lie in this relatively comfortable position for a few minutes while the film is processed and reviewed. Minor adjustments can be made if a repeat view is necessary. We believe this recumbent position is superior to a standing view designed to accomplish the same goal. When standing, the patient invariably moves from the initial position after the film has been taken, and accurate repositioning is often difficult when a repeat film is required.

Acromioclavicular spurs projecting downward from the inferior aspect of both margins of the acromioclavicular joint have been implicated in the production of mechanically induced cuff tears (see Fig. 4–8). Their presence should be duly noted and treated in the course of any operative procedure designed to decompress the subacromial space.

The ossification centers of the acromion *(os acromiale)* are often the last to fuse in the human body, in some instances not until the age of 27. An axillary projection reveals these failures of ossification. Three patterns of failure of ossification centers have been reported by Neer (Fig. 4–19).[69] The *preacromion* outlines a relatively small anterior fragment of acromion. The *mesacromion* represents a failure of ossification through the midportion of the acromion. Both these anomalies permit the acromion to hinge downward and impinge on the rotator cuff. The *metacromion* traverses the most posterior aspect of the acromion and is less likely than the more anterior deficits to cause cuff disorders.

ARTHROGRAPHY

In 1927, Codman prophesied: "Some day, we shall inject air or nonradiable fluid into the bursa and diagnose these cases easily." Today we do both, and the single- or double-contrast arthrogram has been used widely for many years to demonstrate full-thickness tears of the rotator cuff.

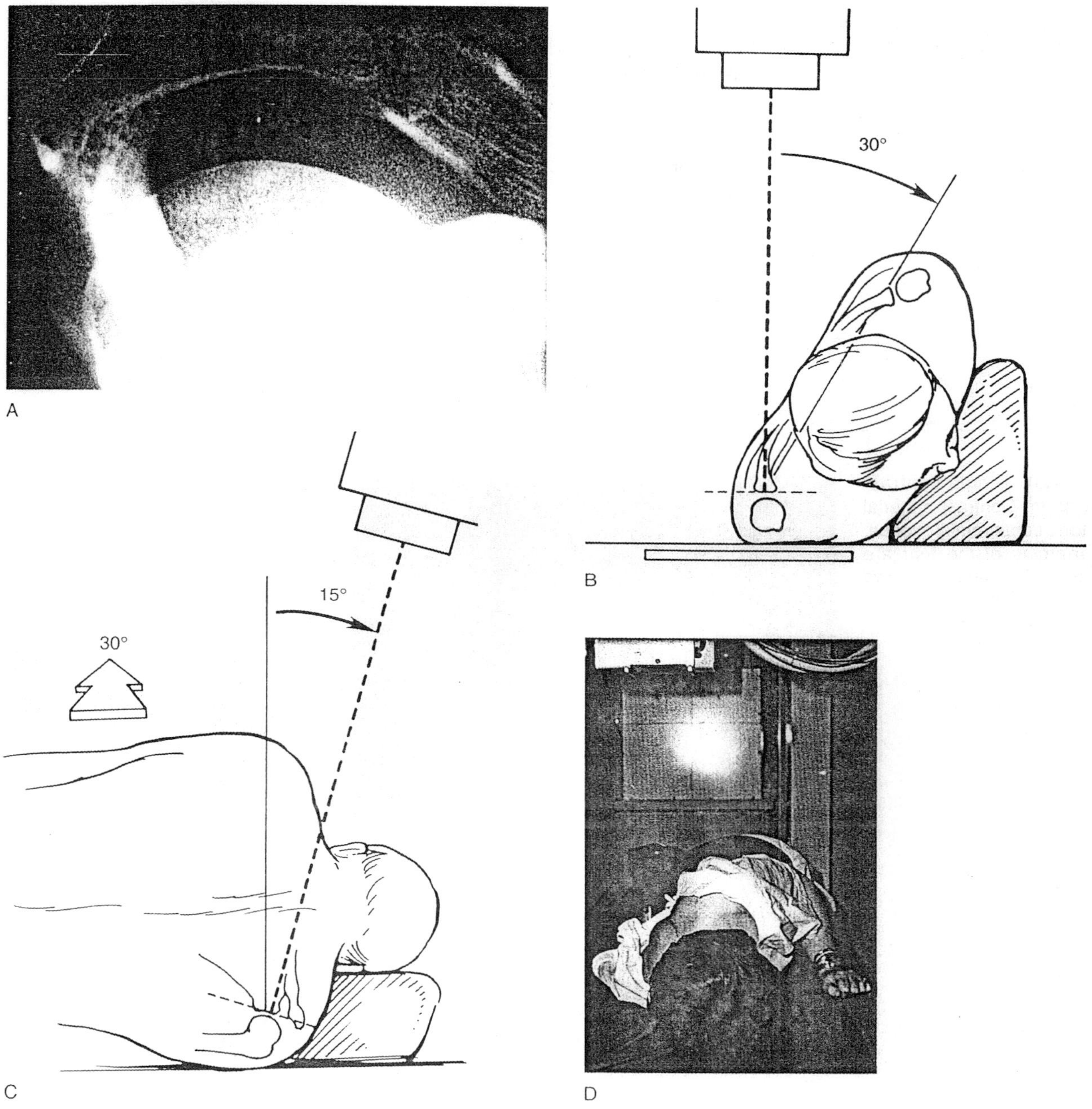

FIG. 4–18. A, Supraspinatus outlet view (arch view).
B, Patient lying in lateral recumbent position is rolled 30 to 45° anteriorly to obtain a tangential view of the scapula.
C, The x-ray beam is also directed 15° caudally to obtain the proper projection.
D, Patient lying in position for supraspinatus outlet (arch) view.

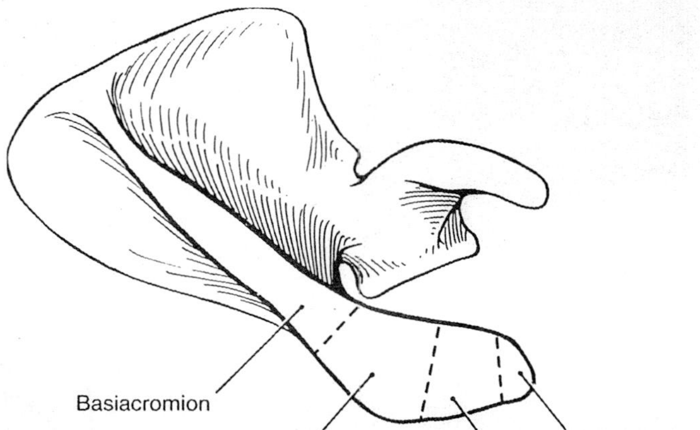

FIG. 4–19. Patterns of failure of ossification centers.

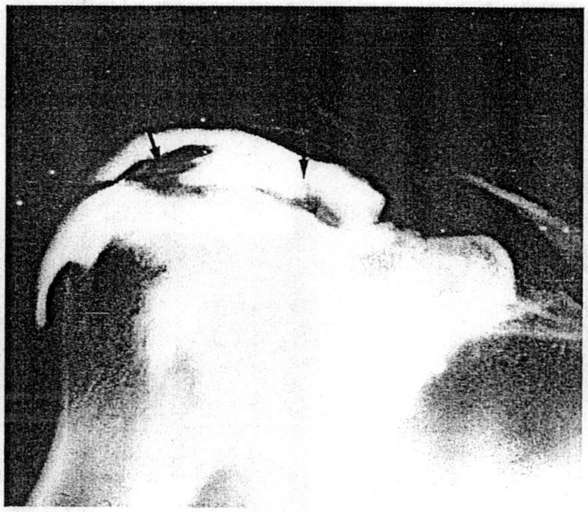

FIG. 4–20. Single-contrast arthrogram. Contrast material fills the subacromial space. The margins of the tear are indicated by small arrows while dye fills the defect.

The *single-contrast arthrogram* introduces radiopaque material into the glenohumeral joint through an anterior portal (Fig. 4–20).[70-72] A full-thickness defect in the rotator cuff permits this material to circulate into the subacromial space, thereby confirming the diagnosis. This test has been recognized as the "gold standard" for the diagnosis of rotator cuff tears.

Double-contrast shoulder arthrography (DCSA) has the capability of demonstrating the size of the rotator cuff tear as well as the quality of the tissue.[72,73] Injection of 2 or 3 ml of radiopaque material into the glenohumeral joint is accompanied by 10 ml of room air. Following a brief period of active exercise, slightly underexposed radiographs are taken in both internal and external rotation (Fig. 4–21A). A second set of films is taken in the same position, but is slightly overexposed (Fig. 4–21B). The small amount of dye injected coats the rotator cuff tear and glenohumeral articular surfaces. The air tends to rise superiorly and, in the presence of a full-thickness tear, may be seen within the subacromial space. The underexposed film helps to delineate the air that has

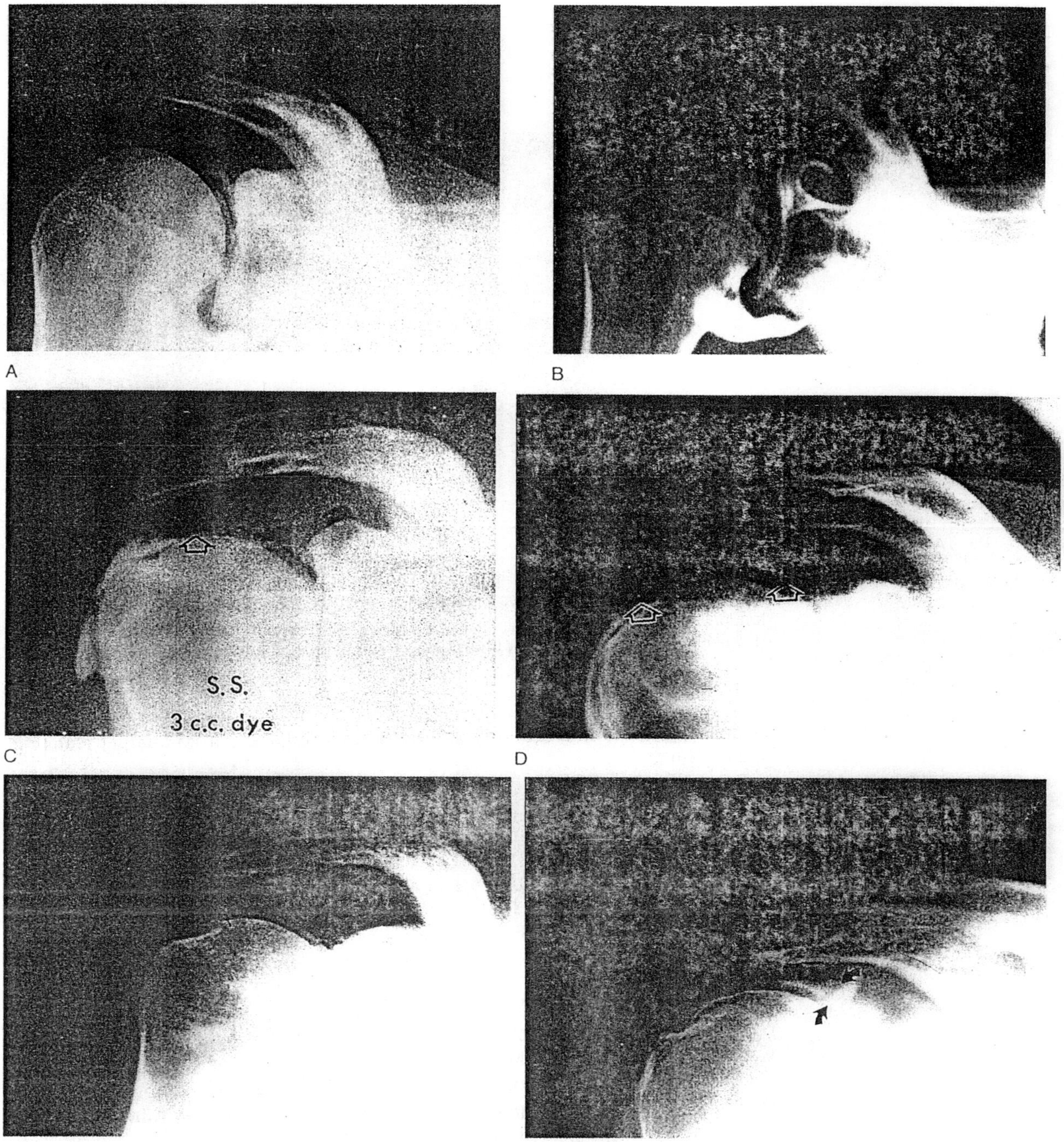

FIG. 4–21. Double-contrast shoulder arthrography (DCSA).
A, Normal DCSA. The radiograph is taken in internal rotation and is slightly underexposed to show dye accumulating beneath an intact cuff.
B, Normal DCSA, somewhat overexposed. The dye coats the articular surfaces and shows normal glenohumeral articular surfaces.
C, Small full-thickness tear. Open arrow marks retracted margin of thick rotator cuff tear.
D, Large tear. Open arrows mark the tuberosity and the severely retracted cuff.
E, A thin, attenuated cuff is outlined by small arrows. The quality of this residual tissue is quite poor.
F, The frayed, retracted margins of this large chronic tear show increased density as dye infiltrates the frayed margins.

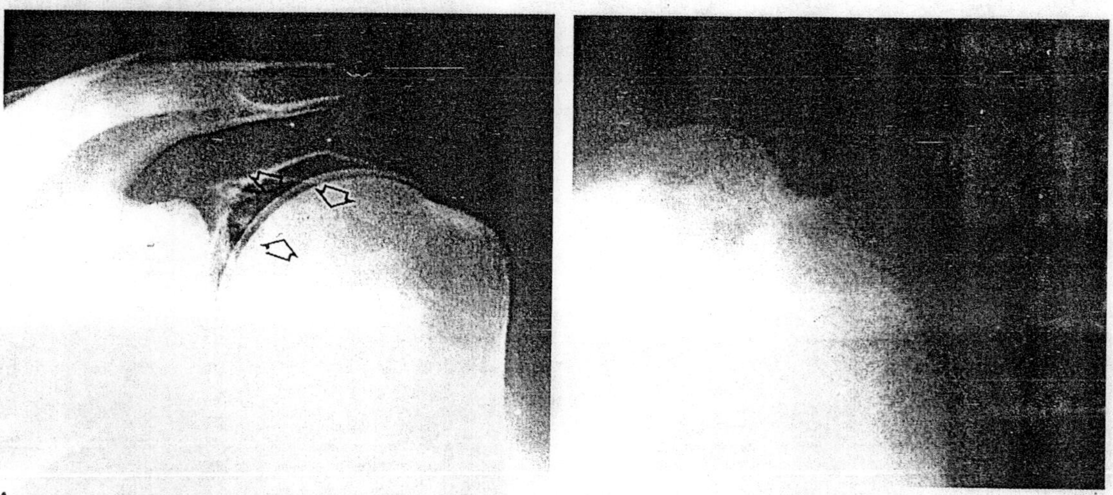

A B

FIG. 4–22. A, Intra-articular portion of the long head of the biceps seen within capsule distended by air. Two open arrows mark the top and one open arrow marks the bottom of the tendon.
B, Special bicipital groove view shows long head of biceps in normal position.

escaped upward and frequently differentiates a small tear from a larger tear (Fig. 4–21C and D).

DCSA can also delineate the quality of the residual cuff tissue (Fig. 4–21E). Figure 4–21F shows the thin, retracted elements of a chronically torn rotator cuff. The ability of this technique to demonstrate the quality of the torn edges of the tendon affects the selection of patients for surgical reconstruction. The thickness of the tendon may differentiate a relatively healthy tendon from a severely degenerated thin tendon. The torn edge that is frayed or laminated accepts an increased amount of dye. In one series, the actual site of the tear was visualized in 93% of 535 arthrograms.[74] Surgical confirmation of the size and quality of the tear in 27 patients "was never incorrect more than one grade." Although Ellman and associates did not find the predictive value of DCSA that significant in their report on rotator cuff tears,[28] the tear was clearly visualized in many studies and was helpful in the selection of appropriate management.

Lesions involving the long head of the biceps can be demonstrated with DCSA. The intra-articular portion of the tendon can be seen within the capsule distended by air (Fig. 4–22A). The erect external-rotation view is best. This lesion is easy to diagnose clinically and is often associated with tears of the rotator cuff. When torn, the shadow of the tendon is not visualized within the joint cavity or the sheath. The sheath may be distorted, especially when medial dislocation of the tendon from the intertubercular sulcus has occurred. This disorder is best seen in a special bicipital groove view (Fig. 4–22B).

Conventional double-contrast shoulder arthrography is combined with computerized arthrotomography to produce a technique best described as *CT-arthrography (CTA)*.[75] A somewhat smaller amount (1 to 2 ml) of radiopaque material is used. A double-contrast arthrogram is performed first, and the presence or absence of a rotator cuff tear is established. The CT scan is then performed with the patient in the supine position with both arms at the side and the shoulder in slight internal rotation to optimize distention of the anterior capsule and subscapular bursa. When posterior subluxation is suspected, an additional scan is taken with the shoulder in external rotation to force air around the posterior labrum (Fig. 4–23). This technique allows visualization of both the anterior and the posterior fibrous labrum, as well as of the capsular structures. Erosion, fraying, or a classic labral detachment involving the inferior half of the labrum (Bankart lesion) may be identified.

CTA is more valuable in demonstrating labral lesions than in demonstrating cuff tears. Technology permitting three-dimensional reconstruction of the CT scan suggests the potential for accurately visualizing and measuring a full-thickness rotator cuff tear with CT-arthrography.

BURSOGRAPHY

The injection of radiopaque material directly into the subacromial bursa has received little attention as a diagnostic technique for the assessment of rotator cuff lesions. The technique can demonstrate bursal surface tears. Fukuda and

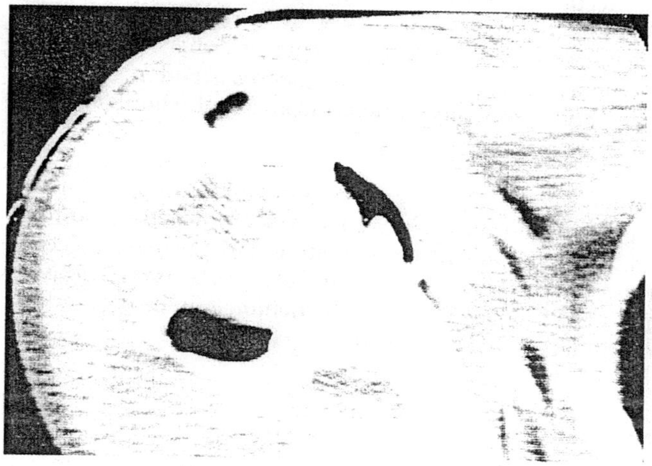

A

FIG. 4–23. A, CT arthrogram: Note normal outline of both anterior and posterior labrum.
B, Internal rotation view shows absent anterior labrum (arrow) in a patient with multidirectional instability.
C, External rotation view of same patient with multidirectional instability shows posterior labral defect (arrow).

B C

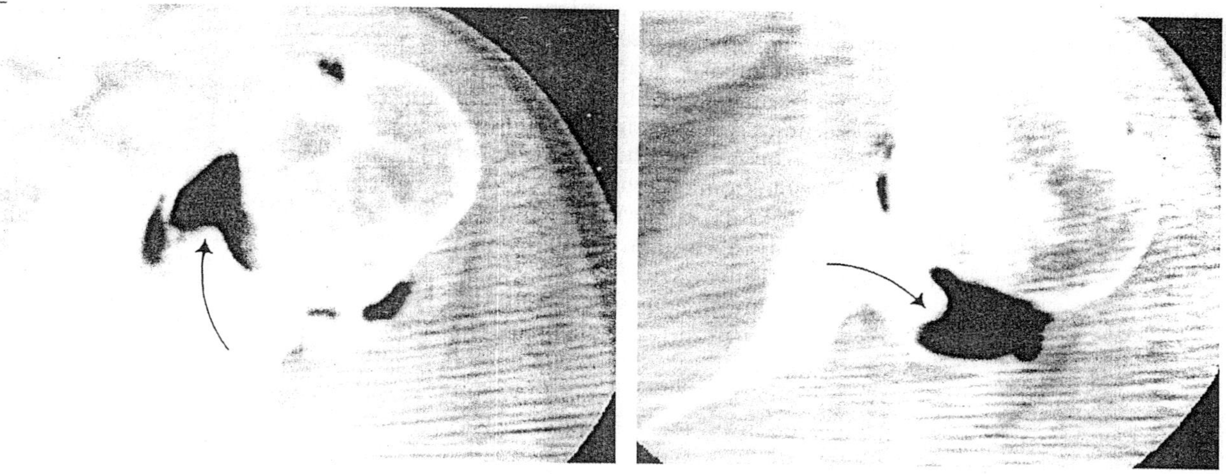

associates successfully identified incomplete bursal surface tears using subacromial bursography.[44] Subacromial bursography has not achieved wide clinical acceptance.

ULTRASONOGRAPHY

Ultrasonography utilizes images constructed from the echoes produced when high-frequency waves are projected onto the structure of interest. The development of high-resolution real-time instruments has produced a valuable method for diagnosing rotator cuff tears (Fig. 4–24). Full-thickness tears are best confirmed by demonstrating either focal discontinuity or nonvisualization of the cuff. Unfortunately, focal echogenicity is a less valuable finding and can be present in patients with small or partial tears, as well as in those with calcific tendinitis, surgical scarring, or impingement without any evidence of a rotator cuff tear. Therefore, small full-thickness tears are difficult to distinguish from these conditions with ultrasonography. Performance and interpretation of the test are operator dependent. The accuracy, sensitivity, and specificity achieved with ultrasonography were reported as greater than 90% by 3 separate groups of investigators.[76-78] Ultrasonography has definite advantages when used as a screening test. The technique accurately identifies an *abnormal* tendon. The test is inexpensive, noninvasive, and can be performed quickly. Both shoulders can be imaged for comparison.

Clinical Tip. The following protocol for using ultrasonography in the diagnosis of rotator cuff tears is suggested. If a technically good study is negative, no further evaluation is needed. If a definite tear of moderate to large proportions can be demonstrated, no further evaluation is needed. If the study is nondiagnostic or technically inadequate, or if echogenicity alone is demonstrated, proceed to either arthrography or magnetic resonance imaging.

MAGNETIC RESONANCE IMAGING

Magnetic resonance imaging (MRI) has become widely utilized for the diagnosis of rotator cuff disorders.[9-81] Moderate to large tears can be accurately imaged (Fig. 4–25A and B). Smaller (less than 2 cm) or partial-thickness tears are more difficult to define. Improved surface coils combined with enhanced equipment allow more reliable imaging of diagnostic quality in smaller lesions. An abnormal signal intensity within the supraspinatus tendon, in the presence of an otherwise normal-appearing supraspinatus muscle, suggests either a partial-thickness tear or a relatively small full-thickness lesion (Fig. 4–25C and D). These findings can be most evident on T_2-weighted images. Interstitial tears, not clinically visible from either the bursal or the articular surface, may light up the tendon in these T_2 studies. These interstitial abnormalities may accompany symptoms of advanced stage II impingement. In a sense, they represent the "fibrosis and tendinitis" described by Neer in the second stage of impingement. The presence of an increased high-intensity signal below the acromioclavicular joint may accompany chronic impingement (Fig. 4–25E).[82] The sagittal sections demonstrate the acromial arch accurately. Concavity can be graded and significant spurs visualized. The slope of the acromion may also be a factor in subacromial impingement.

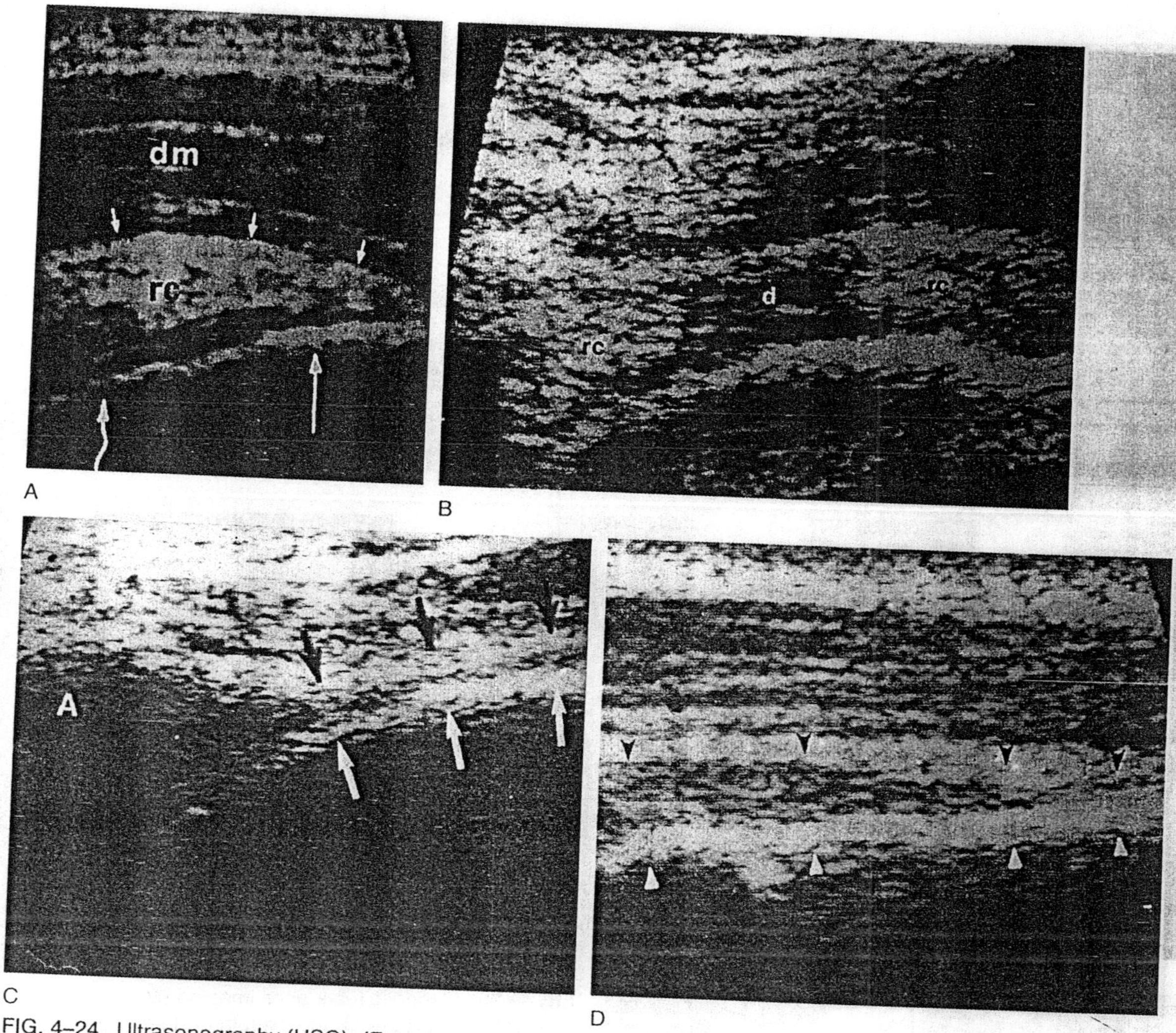

FIG. 4–24. Ultrasonography (USG). (From Middleton, W. D., et al.: Ultrasonography of the rotator cuff: Technique and normal anatomy. J. Ultrasound Med., *3*:549, 1984.)
A, Normal supraspinatus insertion. dm = deltoid muscle; rc = rotator cuff. The long white arrows indicate the cartilage overlying the humeral head.
B, USG demonstrates focal discontinuity in the supraspinatus tendon. rc = rotator cuff; d = defect.
C, Nonvisualization of rotator cuff. The superior structures (black arrows) rest directly on the humeral head (white arrows).
D, Focal thinning of rotator cuff near insertion is outlined by black arrows above and white arrows below.

The *coronal (frontal) oblique* view is established by placing the cursor precisely along the plane of the scapula. In this projection, the entire belly of the supraspinatus, as well as its musculotendinous junction, is visualized (Fig. 4–26). The healthy muscle belly appears quite homogenous, but with aging, both atrophy and fibrotic infiltrations may be seen. When a large tear is present, the extent of retraction can be accurately assessed. When the cuff is retracted to the

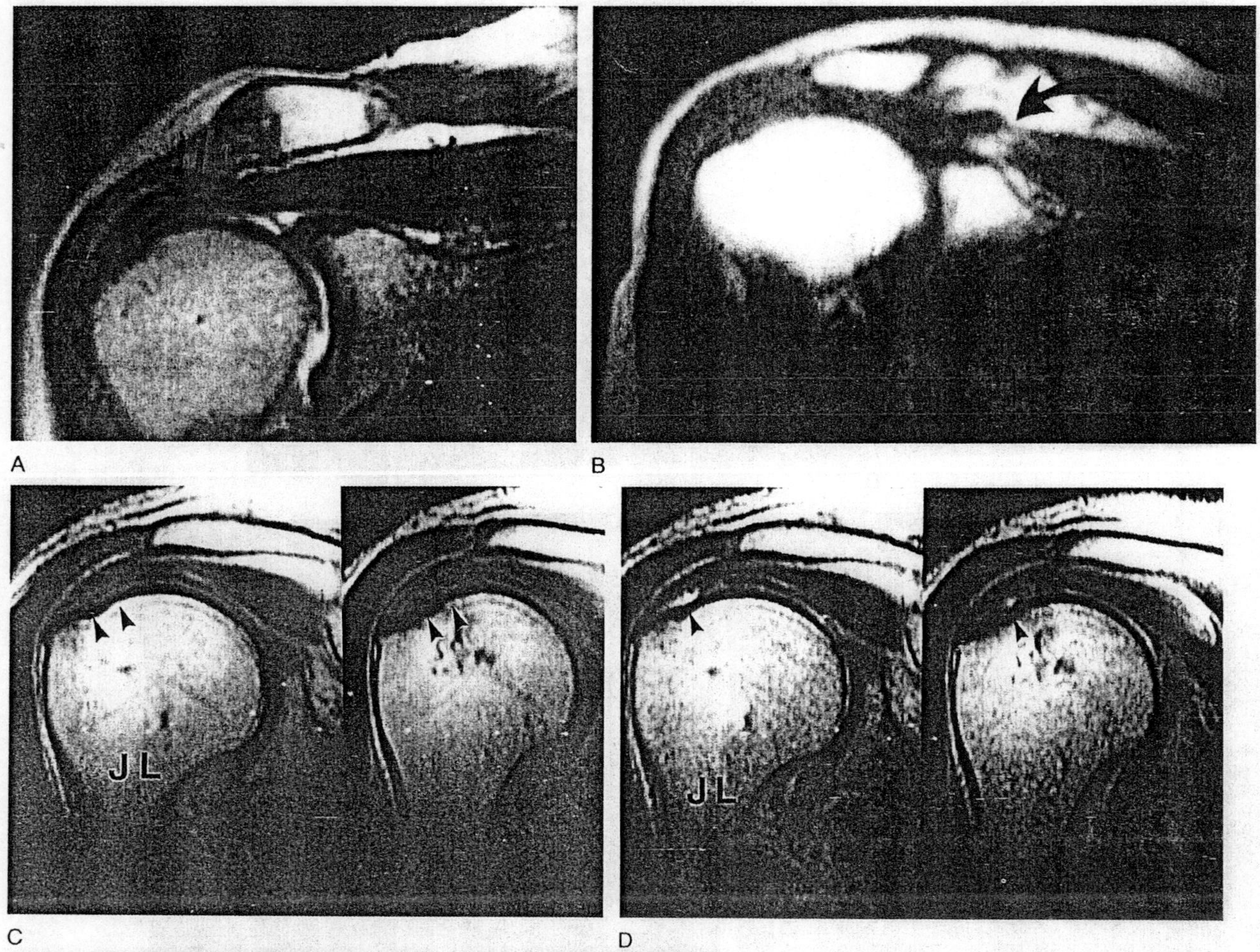

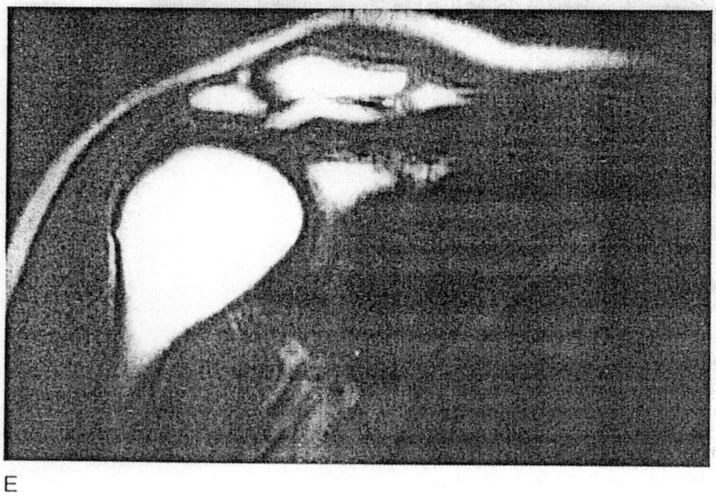

FIG. 4–25. Magnetic resonance imaging (MRI).
A, Woman, 76 years of age, with large tear. Two vertical marks indicate the acromial hook, which appears quite dark on the MRI.
B, Massive tear. Curved arrow points to retracted end of supraspinatus, which lies above the glenoid.
C, Partial tear, grade 3 articular. T_1 images of 2 adjacent cuts are shown. The double arrows indicate the region of grayish mixed image consistent with chronic impingement.
D, T_2 images of the patient in Figure 4–25C. A bright signal intensity is created by a grade 3 articular tear.
E, The extensive high-intensity signals beneath the outer acromion and acromioclavicular joint are considered signs of chronic impingement.

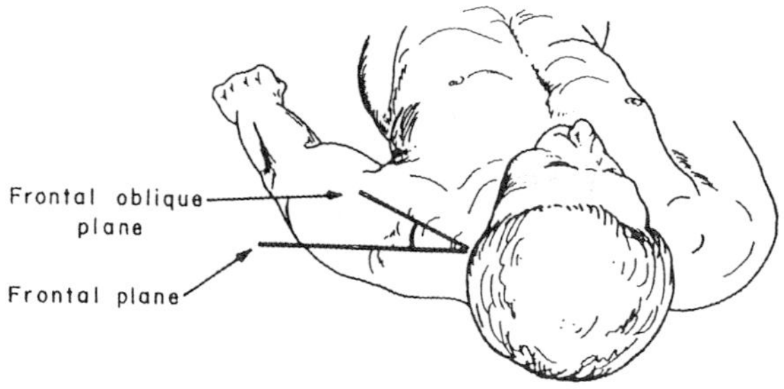

A

FIG. 4–26. A, Coronal (frontal) oblique view. Visualization of the full length of the supraspinatus tendon requires placing the cursor along the plane of the scapula.
B, Normal MRI in coronal (frontal) oblique projection. The muscle appears quite homogenous, and the tendinous insertion is black.
C, Microcryosection of elderly cadaver specimen in coronal (frontal) oblique plane. Note atrophy and fibrosis with fatty infiltration in the body of the muscle. The tendinous insertion is intact.

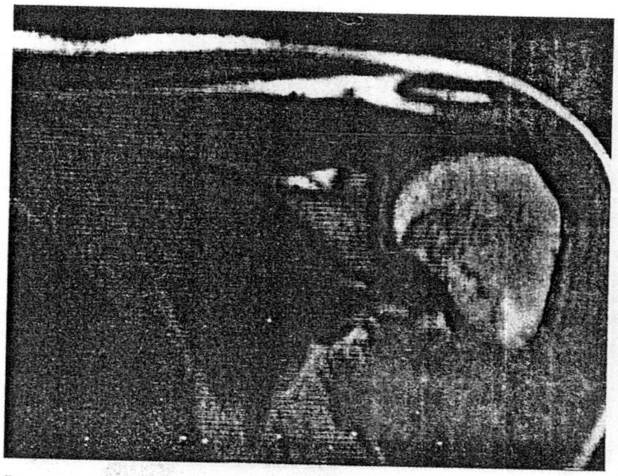

B

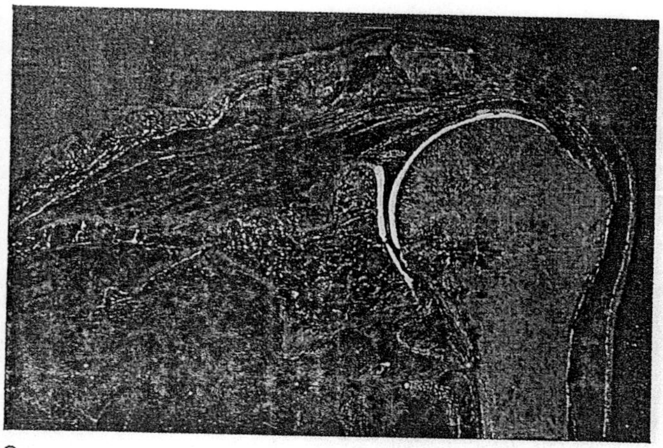

C

level of the glenoid and is atrophic as well as fibrotic, mobilization certainly is difficult, if not impossible. MRI imaging can be combined with third-dimensional reconstruction of the soft tissue to assess the cuff deficit accurately. Cineradiography can be combined with MRI to create a motion study. These procedures are likely to be economically impractical, however, because clinical evaluation in combination with standard imaging generally provides sufficient information for the therapeutic decision.

The diagnosis of rotator cuff disease as the primary source of a patient's symptoms should be established by the detailed clinical evaluation just concluded. In addition, the surgeon should have formed an opinion as to the extent of fiber failure that is present. When conservative management is inadequate, three surgical options are available: arthroscopic treatment, open surgical reconstruction, and combined arthroscopic and mini-open repair. The indications and techniques for each are reviewed in the next three chapters.

SUBACROMIAL SPACE ARTHROSCOPY: ARTHROSCOPIC SUBACROMIAL DECOMPRESSION

5

In 1972, Neer described the technique of open anterior acromioplasty for treatment of the chronic impingement syndrome.[1] Subsequent reports have documented the efficacy of this procedure.[83–87] The first arthroscopic subacromial decompression was performed by Ellman in 1983 as an alternative to open anterior acromioplasty.[88] Subsequent reports by various authors have confirmed that results comparable to the open procedure can be achieved with arthroscopic techniques.[39,89-96]

The operation requires the basic arthroscopic instruments and operating room setup described in Chapter 2. A mechanical suction shaver is used to perform a subtotal bursectomy to establish visualization within the subacromial space. The coracoacromial ligament is released with the surgical electrode. Electrocautery is also used to control bleeding and maintain visibility. The anterior acromioplasty is performed with a round or oval mechanical bur.

INDICATIONS

The indications for arthroscopic subacromial decompression are identical to those for open anterior acromioplasty. Pathologic changes in the rotator cuff should be based on extrinsic factors, such as abnormal acromial slope or spurs arising within the coracoacromial ligament or acromioclavicular joint that compromise the supraspinatus outlet.

Arthroscopic subacromial decompression is the keystone of arthroscopic treatment in certain stages of rotator cuff disease.

ADVANCED STAGE II IMPINGEMENT WITHOUT ROTATOR CUFF TEAR

The primary indication for use of this procedure is in patients with chronic impingement syndrome without rotator cuff tears who have failed to respond adequately to conservative measures for 6 months to 1 year. Conservative treatment should include rest, nonsteroidal anti-inflammatory drugs, and a rehabilitation program designed to strengthen the rotator cuff and restore normal scapulohumeral rhythm. No more than three steroid injections into the subacromial space should be given during the course of treatment.

PARTIAL-THICKNESS ROTATOR CUFF TEARS

Tears less than one-half the thickness of the tendon, involving either the articular or the bursal surface, are generally treated with arthroscopic subacromial decompression and cuff debridement. When partial ruptures exceed one-half the substance of the tendon, open techniques of reconstruction are often performed in active individuals. The technique for evaluation and treatment of partial-thickness tears is the subject of Chapter 6.

SELECTED FULL-THICKNESS ROTATOR CUFF TEARS

In general, we advocate open reconstruction of most reparable full-thickness rotator cuff tears. This recommendation is based on the superior results obtained following open reconstruction in comparison to those obtained by arthroscopic treatment. Certain *selected* circumstances related to age, activity level, handedness, and size of tear support the choice of arthroscopic decompression and debridement. Chapter 11 is devoted to patient selection and technique in this controversial area. The arthroscopic treatment of massive, irreparable tears is also covered in a subsequent chapter.

MINIMALLY DISPLACED GREATER TUBEROSITY FRACTURES

A superiorly displaced healed fracture of the greater tuberosity may provoke impingement pain with elevation. Subacromial decompression eliminates this pain by providing adequate clearance for minimally displaced fractures.

INTRINSIC TENDINOPATHY

Intrinsic tendinopathy associated with large, chronic calcareous deposits within the cuff tendon may require decompression in addition to calcium removal in some circumstances. The arthroscopic treatment of calcific tendinitis is the subject of Chapter 9.

CONTRAINDICATIONS

Pain occurring during the arc of shoulder elevation may result from many causes other than the mechanical impingement syndrome. Early rheumatoid synovitis may involve both the glenohumeral joint and the subacromial bursa. Chondromalacia associated with early degenerative or post-traumatic arthritis may simulate the impingement syndrome. Other less common causes for a painful arc include synovial chondromatosis, early avascular necrosis, ochronosis, and amyloidosis. The more *commonly* encountered contraindications are as follows.

ACROMIOCLAVICULAR ARTHRITIS OR OSTEOLYSIS

Pain originating in the acromioclavicular joint as a result of symptomatic acromioclavicular arthritis or osteolysis must be differentiated from mechanical impingement and treated independently (see Chap. 17).

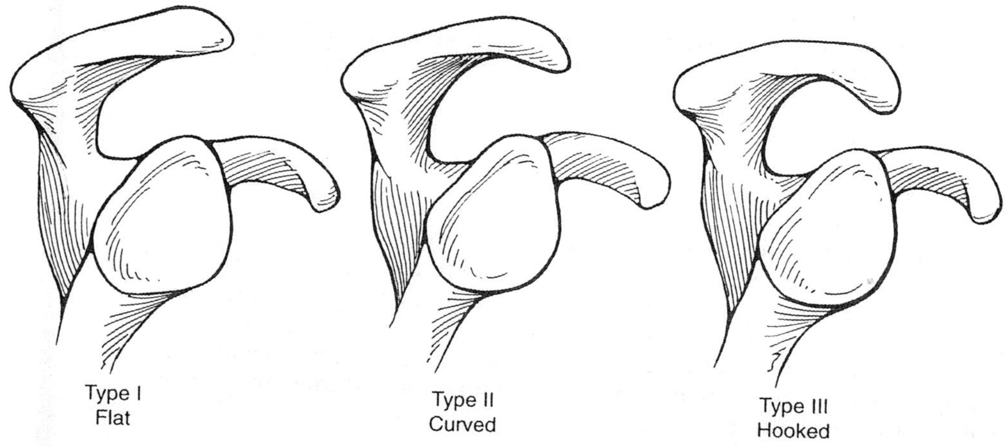

FIG. 5–1. Acromial morphology as viewed from the sagittal plane is divided into three shapes: type I–flat, type II–curved, and type III–hooked.

PRIMARY TENDON OVERLOAD

Excessive, repetitive stress may produce intrinsic scarring or even acute tendon rupture. Unless associated mechanical factors are present, acromioplasty fails to relieve the painful arc symptoms.

ACROMIAL STRUCTURE

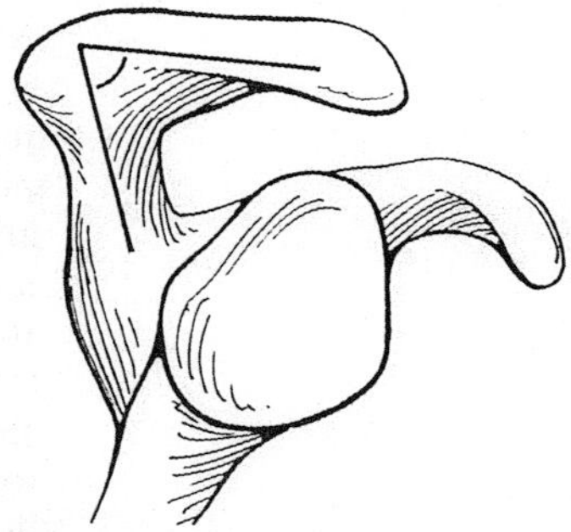

FIG. 5–2. An increase in the angle of acromial inclination narrows the supraspinatus outlet despite a type I (flat) acromion.

Acromial structure has been described as type I (flat); type II (curved); and type III (hooked) (Fig. 5–1).[55] The incidence of rotator cuff disease is greater in type II and type III. We performed a retrospective study of acromial structure in 44 patients who had undergone arthroscopic subacromial decompression for impingement syndrome. Type I acromions were not found in this group of symptomatic patients. We consider a type I acromion a relative contraindication to arthroscopic subacromial decompression unless a downward sloping angle of acromial inclination produces narrowing of the supraspinatus outlet in spite of a relatively flat acromion (Fig. 5–2).

BLEEDING TENDENCIES

Hemostasis is essential in this procedure. The patient is required to stop ingesting aspirin or related nonsteroidal anti-inflammatory medications 2 weeks prior to surgery. In addition to a complete blood count, tests for prothrombin time, partial thromboplastin time, and bleeding time are performed preoperatively. Acromioplasty should be avoided if abnormalities are discovered.

PACEMAKERS

The patient wearing a pacemaker presents a potential complication, particularly if the device is implanted in proximity to the affected shoulder. The surgical electrode may gravely affect the operation of the pacemaker. Precautions should include an arterial line and constant monitoring by the anesthesiologist. Medication should be instantly available to treat any arrhythmia. The surgical electrode should be used in brief 1-second bursts. The grounding pad is attached as far from the pacemaker as possible. A defibrillator is situated within the operating room.

ADHESIVE CAPSULITIS

Every effort should be made to avoid performing arthroscopic subacromial decompression on a patient who is developing adhesive capsulitis ("frozen shoulder"). The onset of this condition mimics bursitis and tendinitis. The relatively rapid development of restricted motion, particularly in external and internal rotation, helps the clinician to recognize this perplexing condition. Arthroscopic subacromial decompression is contraindicated during the active phase of this disorder.

IMPINGEMENT SECONDARY TO INSTABILITY

Impingement symptoms frequently develop secondary to instability in swimmers and in athletes involved in throwing or racquet sports. These activities may stress the static ligamentous restraints of the shoulder to such a degree that capsular stretching with instability results. The lax joint may translate excessively in an anteroposterior direction. The humeral head may also displace superiorly, thereby provoking impingement. Although the presenting complaints are generally those of impingement, examination readily discloses the associated instability. Some men and women with a tendency toward familial joint laxity may develop impingement syndrome following workouts with resistance equipment. Treatment for secondary impingement should be directed toward overcoming the instability, either by prolonged rehabilitation of the dynamic (muscular) stabilizers or, in some patients, by capsular stabilization. Acromioplasty usually fails unless instability has been overcome.

SURGICAL ORIENTATION

SUBACROMIAL SPACE

The subacromial space is a pseudoarticulation that permits gliding between the proximal humerus and the coracoacromial arch. Numerous bursae are described around the proximal humerus. Some anatomists describe the subacromial and subdeltoid bursae as separate structures. A distinct subacromial bursa has also been identified. At best, the bursal walls are flimsy structures with ill-defined borders (Fig. 5–3). Arthroscopic exploration has led us to regard this interstitial area as the "subacromial space," which reveals some well-defined borders when distended and cleared of hyperplastic tissue associated with chronic impingement. This space begins more than halfway forward from the back to the front of the acromion. Entry from behind requires penetration of a "posterior veil" to position instruments directly below the anterior acromion (Fig. 5–4). Both medial and lateral gutters can be defined when the space is pristine. The medial confines are below the acromioclavicular (AC) joint, and exposure of the lateral end of the clavicle requires resection of thick fibrofatty (and sometimes vascular) tis-

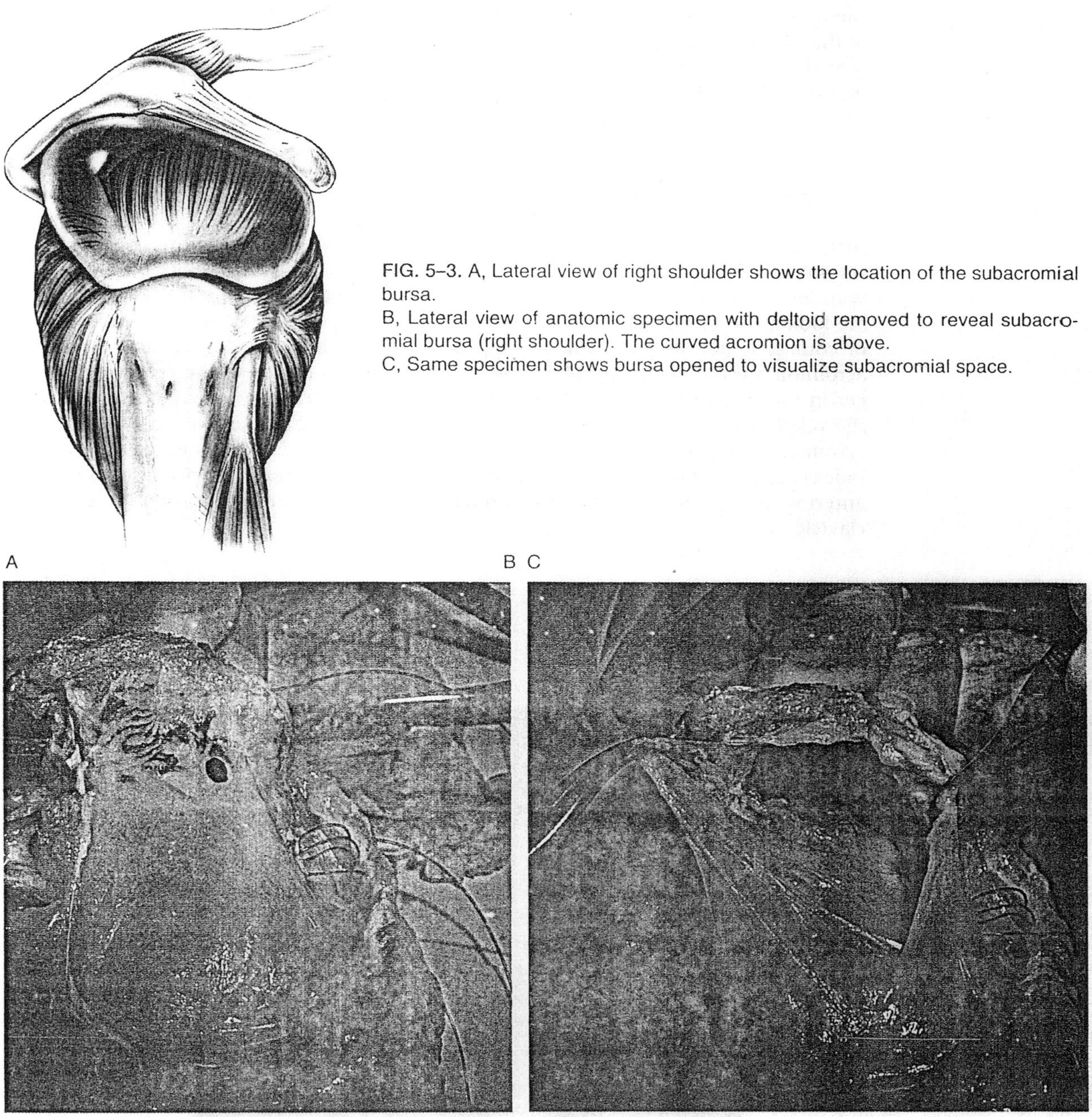

FIG. 5–3. A, Lateral view of right shoulder shows the location of the subacromial bursa.
B, Lateral view of anatomic specimen with deltoid removed to reveal subacromial bursa (right shoulder). The curved acromion is above.
C, Same specimen shows bursa opened to visualize subacromial space.

sue to achieve exposure of the AC joint. The lateral wall lies beyond the mound of the greater tuberosity. The coracoacromial ligament guards this space anteriorly (Fig. 5–5). Often the ligament is obscured by a hypertrophic bursal lining that must be debrided before the glistening, thinly packed fibers of ligament can be identified.

DIGITAL ANALOGY

Arthroscopic subacromial decompression is performed within the confines of the subacromial space. To develop some spatial concepts about this region, look at your left thumb in profile, with the distal phalanx slightly bent, and imagine you are looking at a right acromion from the lateral aspect (Fig. 5–6). The acromion, of course, is not so thick, but the length and breadth of the thumb and the acromion are rather similar. Now oppose the thumb to the tip of the index finger in the pinch position. When viewed from the side or top, you have defined the relationship of the AC joint and lateral end of the clavicle to the anterior acromion (Fig. 5–7). Allow the tip of the thumb to extend forward a bit past the index finger to simulate the relationship even more accurately, because the anterior edge of the acromion often protrudes beyond the anterior margin of the clavicle.

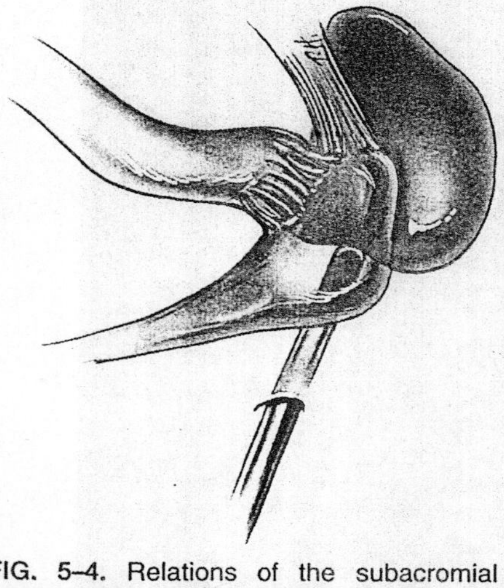

FIG. 5–4. Relations of the subacromial bursa when viewed from above the acromion. An instrument is positioned to penetrate the "posterior veil."

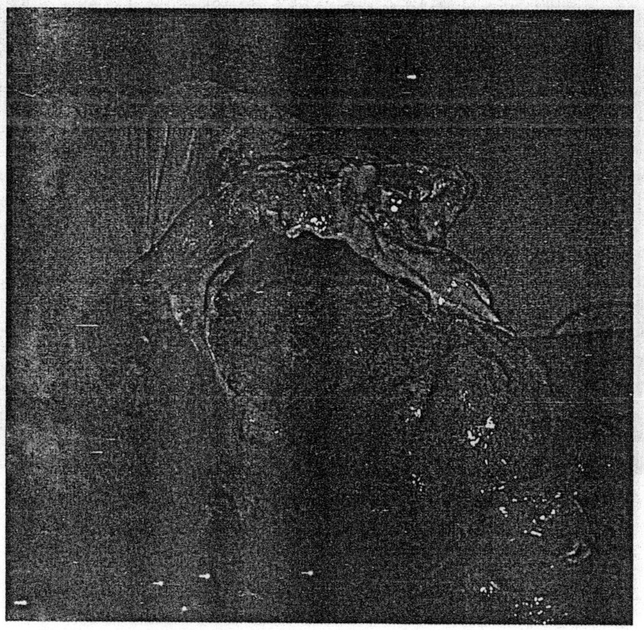

FIG. 5–5. Same specimen as that shown in Figure 5–3, B and C. The bursal wall has been removed. Note anterior location of thick coracoacromial ligament.

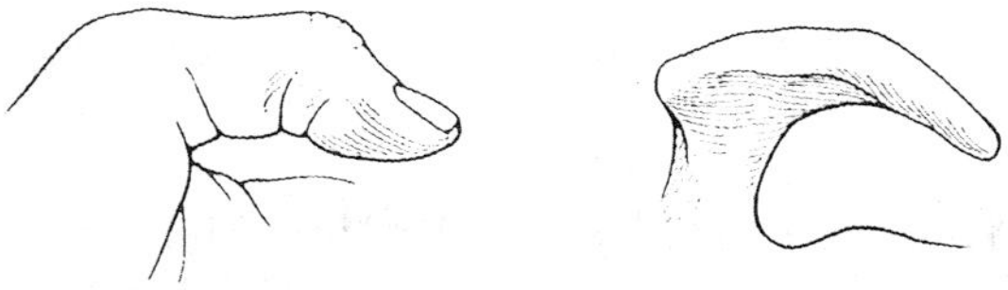

FIG. 5–6. Digital analogy compares a left thumb to the right acromion when viewed in profile.

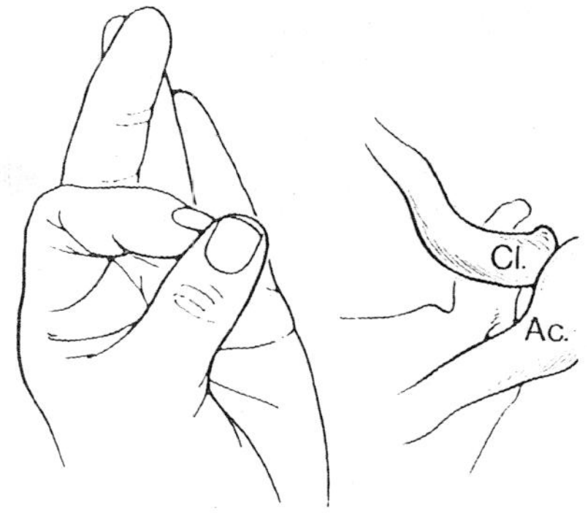

FIG. 5–7. Placement of the thumb and index finger into the pinch position defines the relationship of the acromion (Ac.) and clavicle (Cl.) meeting at the acromioclavicular joint.

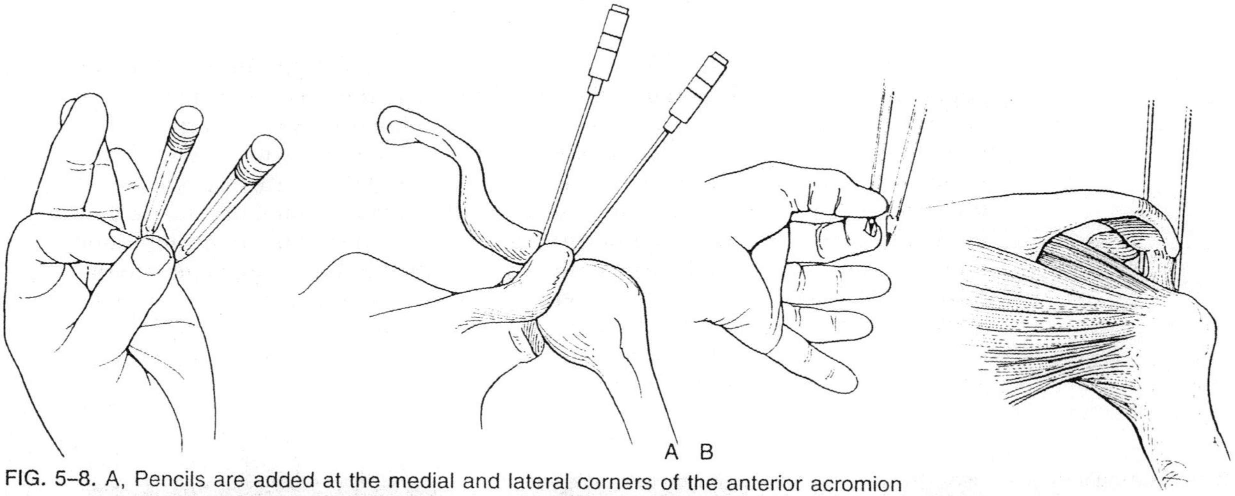

FIG. 5–8. A, Pencils are added at the medial and lateral corners of the anterior acromion to represent the position of marker pins placed for surgical orientation.
B, After supination of the wrist, the digital analogy is viewed from below. This view simulates the spatial relationships that are observed through the arthroscope when the subacromial space is viewed from the posterolateral portal, as depicted. (The right hand may be used to simulate a left shoulder in these digital analogies.)

The coracoacromial ligament attaches to the anterior edge of the acromion and appears to extend posteriorly as it merges with the periosteum investing the undersurface of the acromion. The introduction of marker pins to outline the area of coracoacromial ligament attachment provides an invaluable orientation aid for the surgeon throughout the subacromial arthroscopic procedure.

Consider the digital analogy again to understand better the placement of these pins and their appearance from within. Hold a pencil or pen in front of the AC joint (thumb/index junction) and direct the point vertically to represent the medial marker pin. The pin protrudes into the subacromial space, thus marking the anteromedial corner of the acromion. Now add another pencil or pen at the anterolateral aspect of your thumb to indicate the lateral pin that marks the anterolateral aspect of the acromion (Fig. 5–8A). Now supinate your wrist and look at this arrangement from below. The view simulated in this model is spatially similar to the arthroscopic field seen from the posterolateral portal in a right shoulder (Fig. 5–8B).

The thumb and index finger of the right hand are used to simulate spacial concepts in a left shoulder.

ELLMAN TECHNIQUE OF ARTHROSCOPIC SUBACROMIAL DECOMPRESSION

Every shoulder arthroscopy begins with glenohumeral inspection through the posterolateral portal. The diagnosis may be confirmed or altered by this evaluation (see Chap. 3).

POSTERIOR FLUID-INGRESS PORTAL

After glenohumeral inspection, the arthroscope is withdrawn from the posterior portal (Fig. 5–9A). This portal is then used to insert the accessory fluid-ingress cannula. A nonfenestrated cannula is preferred for gravity flow. The arthroscopy pump systems provide a special pressure-sensing cannula with fenestrations. Either cannula is introduced with a blunt obturator (Fig. 5–9B) that is directed through the space between the undersurface of the acromion and the rotator cuff until the tip lies below the anterior acromion (Fig. 5–9C). The tip of the obturator is directed upward to avoid injury to the cuff, but the tip should not penetrate the thick bursal tissue underlying the anterior acromion. Waggling the cannula medially and laterally within the subacromial space helps to clear the area of obstruction to flow. Figure 5–9D and E show the posterior fluid-ingress cannula as it appears within the bursa and when viewed from the top.

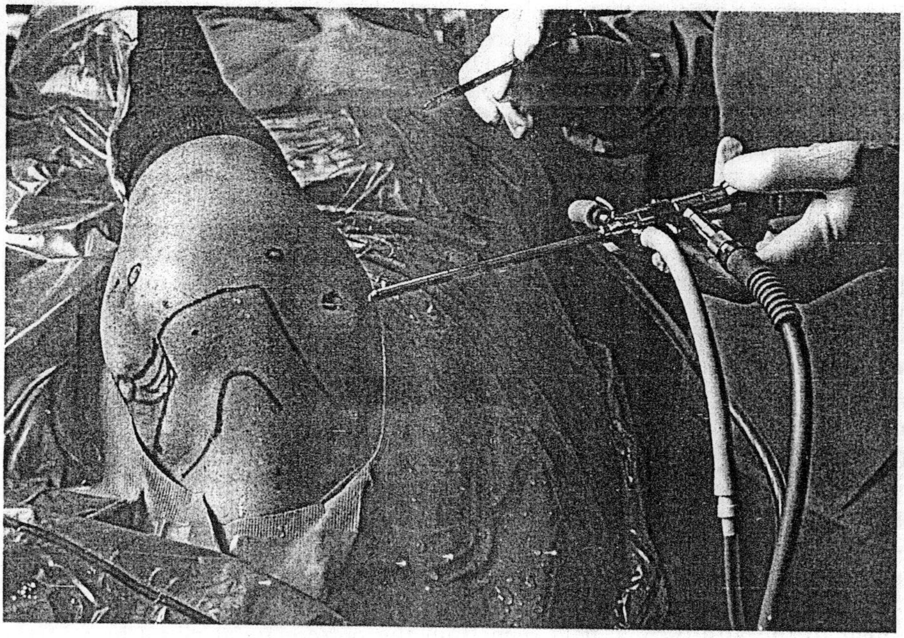

FIG. 5–9. A, The right shoulder of a patient in the lateral decubitus position viewed from the cephalic end of the table. The arthroscope has just been removed from the posterior portal at the conclusion of glenohumeral arthroscopy.

(continued)

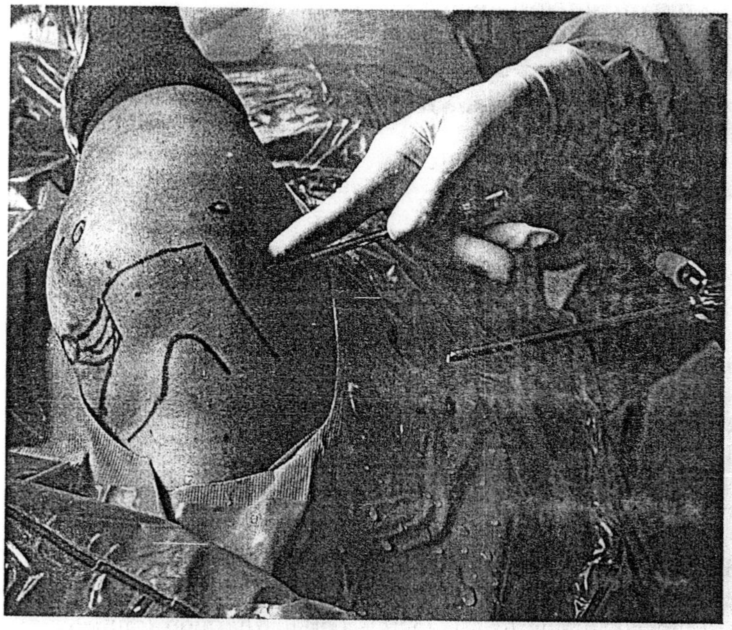

B

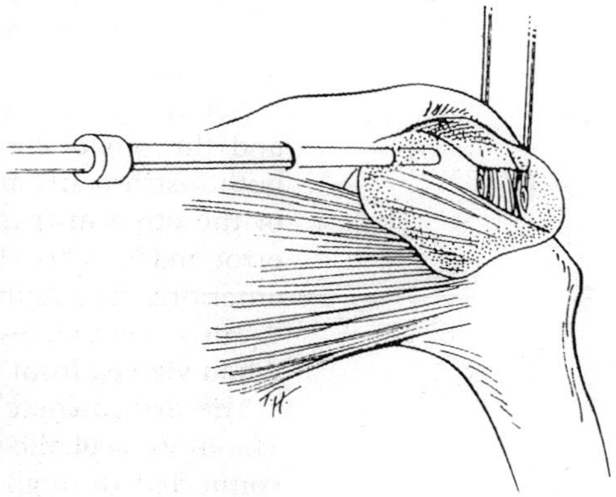

D

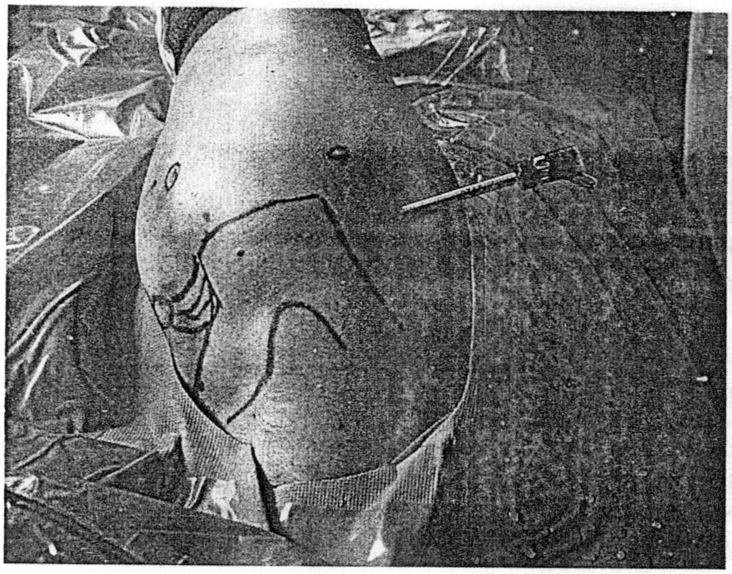

C

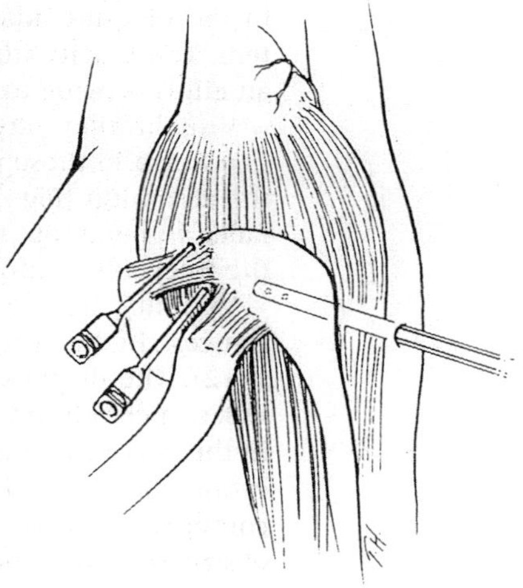

E

B, The accessory fluid-ingress cannula is introduced through the posterior skin incision and is directed upward and anteriorly into the subacromial space.
C, The posterior fluid-ingress cannula has been placed in its final position.
D, The posterior fluid-ingress cannula as it appears within the bursa.
E, Relative position of the fluid-ingress cannula when viewed from above.

POSTEROLATERAL ARTHROSCOPIC PORTAL

The posterolateral arthroscopic portal is then established. This portal, as previously marked, lies 1.5 cm inferior and slightly anterior to the posterolateral angle of the acromion. The small skin incision is made along Langer's lines (Fig. 5–10A). The scope is carefully aimed so that the tip lies below the midportion of the anterior acromion. A sharp obturator may be used in the scope sheath to penetrate the deltoid, but this instrument is replaced by a dull obturator before the scope is advanced anteriorly. Again, the instrument is aimed superiorly to avoid cuff injury, but the soft tissue adherent to the acromion also must not be penetrated (Fig. 5–10B).

Before the lens of the arthroscope is inserted, manipulate both the cannula and the scope sheath together gently. This "fencing" maneuver ensures that both instruments are in the same compartment. If contact cannot be made, one or the other instrument should be repositioned at this time. The most common error made is the failure to advance one instrument or the other far enough anteriorly. The blunt probe is removed, and the arthroscopic lens is inserted (Fig. 5–10C). Figures 5–10D and E show the relative position of both instruments when viewed from within the bursa and from the top.

The arthroscopic sheath contains two openings for fluid ingress and egress. The more cephalic portal is used for fluid ingress. A 3-L bag of normal saline is connected through a section of tubing to this ingress portal. The more caudal portal is attached to suction. Stopcocks on the portals control fluid ingress and suction. The tubing should be connected directly to the portals to avoid the confusion of using adapters, which often add a second set of stopcocks to the system. The gravity inflow portal is opened, and as the subacromial space distends, an effort is made to identify the position of the accessory fluid cannula.

Visualization may be difficult in patients with advanced stage II impingement. The bursa in these patients is hypertrophic directly beneath the anterior third of the acromion (Fig. 5–11). Visibility is even less clear when the instruments have failed to penetrate the posterior veil of the bursal region and thus remain within the thick adventitious tissue beneath the posterior two thirds of the acromion.

Visibility may be good within the bursa in two diametrically opposed circumstances. In the first, the normal subacromial space may appear pristine (Fig. 5–12). The diagnosis of impingement syndrome should be seriously questioned when such a bursa is encountered. At the other extreme, visibility may be good in the presence of a full-thickness rotator cuff tear (grade 3). The free communication of joint fluid between the glenohumeral and subacromial regions may compress or wash away the flimsy bursal stroma (Fig. 5–13). The primary obstruction to visibility may be a mass of fibrotic margins of torn cuff tissue.

FIG. 5–10. A, Posterolateral arthroscopic portal, 1.5 cm inferior and slightly anterior to the posterior angle of the acromion. Skin incision placed along Langer's line. ►
B, The arthroscope has been introduced with the dull probe.
C, The lens and camera are attached. Irrigating fluid enters through the proximal arm of the arthroscopic sheath, and suction (blue adapter) is attached to the distal portal.
D, Relative position of fluid-ingress cannula and arthroscope when viewed from within the bursa.
E, Fluid-ingress cannula and arthroscope when viewed from the top.

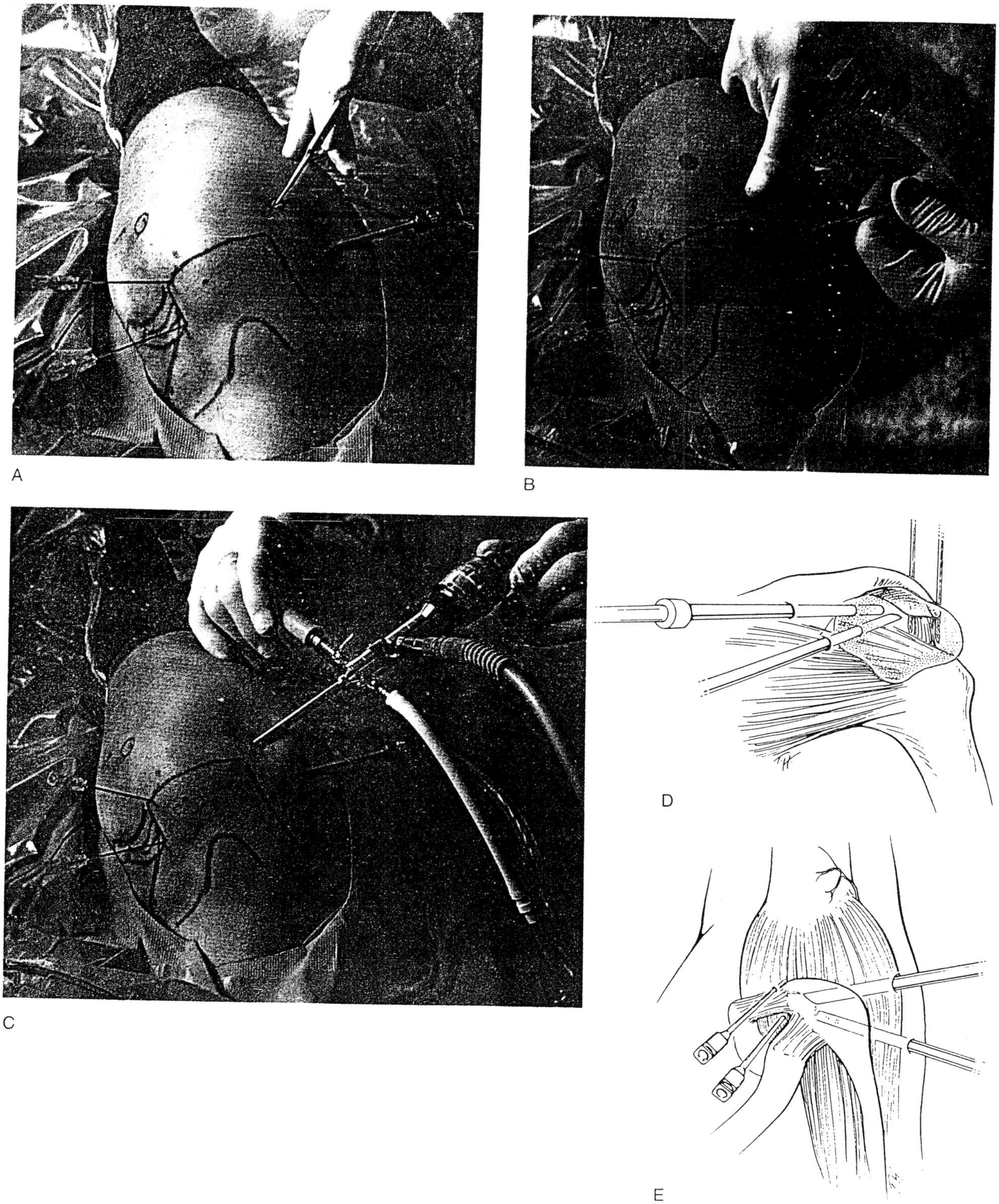

A B C D E

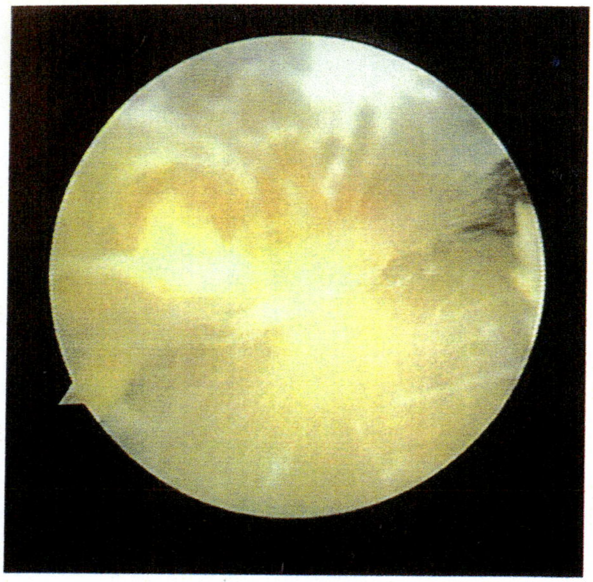

FIG. 5–11

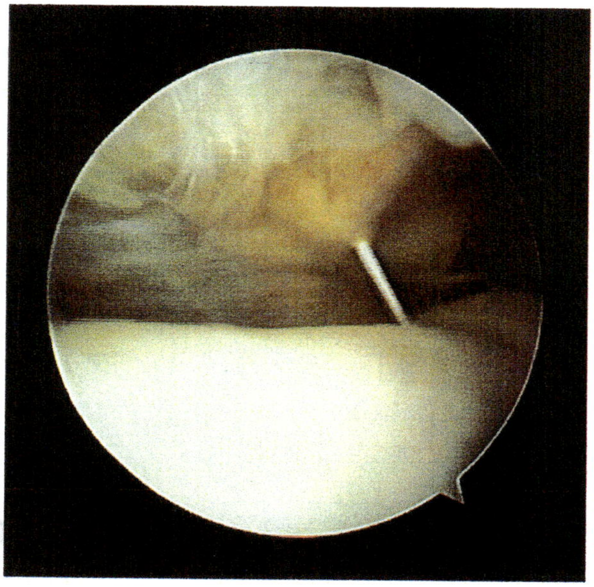

FIG. 5–12

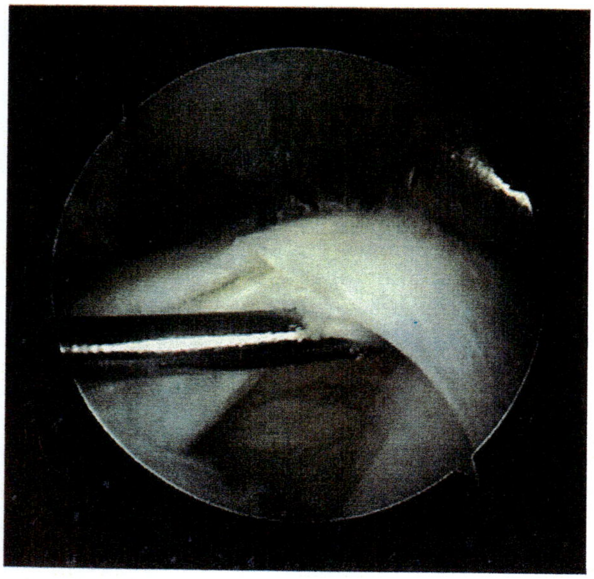

FIG 5–13

FIG. 5–11. Bursal hypertrophy obscures visibility in advanced stage II impingement.

FIG. 5–12. Normal subacromial space appears pristine when viewed through the posterolateral portal. A lumbar puncture needle has been introduced from above to mark the anterolateral corner of the acromion.

FIG. 5–13. Visibility within the bursa (above) may be quite good when joint fluid flows freely through a full-thickness rotator cuff tear (being held open by a probe) into the subacromial space.

After a proper position below the anterior third of the acromion has been achieved, the accessory fluid-ingress cannula is opened. For gravity flow, the bags of fluid should be elevated 2 or 3 feet above the level of the patient's shoulder. The fluid pressure increases 22 mm Hg for every 1 foot of elevation during gravity flow. When an arthroscopy pump system is used, the pressure sensor is attached to the ingress cannula provided by the manufacturer (Fig. 5–14). In this situation, the height of the fluid bags is immaterial. The accessory fluid system is opened at this point, and additional distention of the subacromial space is achieved.

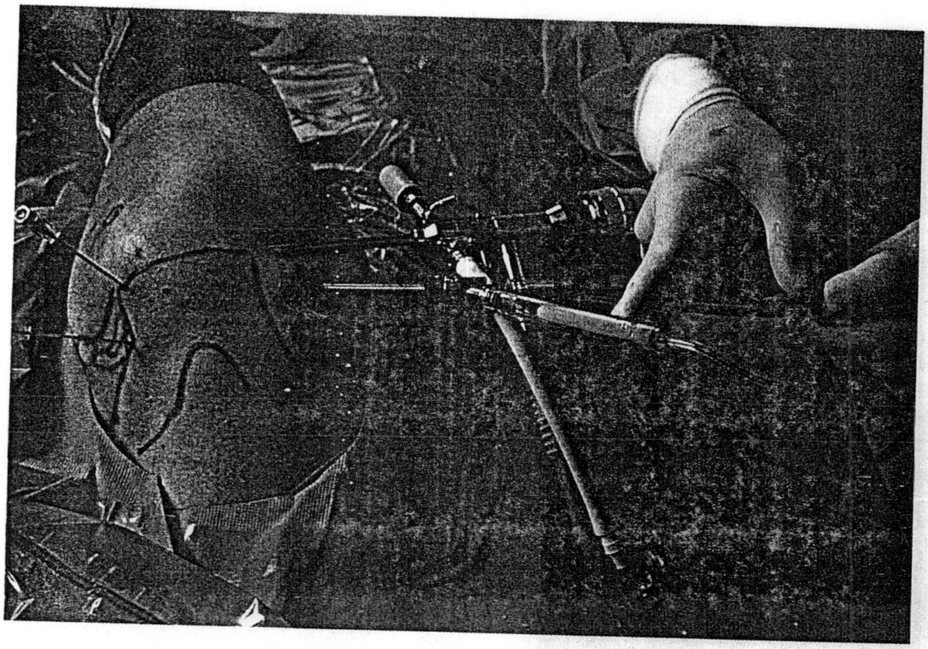

FIG. 5–14. A finger points to the pressure sensor for the arthroscopy pump system, which has been attached to the posterior fluid-ingress cannula.

MARKER PINS

Two 20-gauge lumbar puncture needles are used to mark the attachment of the coracoacromial ligament. The stylets are not removed. The needles are oriented vertically into the subacromial space. The tips may converge slightly. The *lateral marker* enters precisely at the anterolateral corner of the acromion (Fig. 5–15A). The vertically directed needle may palpate the bone lightly to ensure its proximity to bone before it is pushed down and into the subacromial space.

The *medial marker pin* enters just anterior to the AC joint, and the tip descends to the level of the rotator cuff (Fig. 5–15B). The two pins should be roughly parallel (Fig. 5–15C).

Because some fibers of the coracoacromial ligament insert into the capsule of the AC joint, this medial marker pin must be placed in front of the AC joint rather than at the anteromedial border of the acromion.

ANTEROLATERAL OPERATING PORTAL

The operating cannula is now introduced. The portal lies approximately 3 to 4 cm lateral to the anterolateral corner of the acromion *in a direct line with the 2 marker pins* (Fig. 5–16). This configuration ensures placement at the anterior margin of the acromion. The operating cannula is made of plastic and contains a diaphragm. Plastic is preferable to metal because electrocautery is performed through this cannula. The diaphragm ensures maintenance of the distention as the instruments used for shoulder arthroscopy are introduced and withdrawn.

FIG. 5–15. A, A lumbar puncture needle is introduced to mark the anterolateral corner of the acromion.
B, Another needle is placed immediately in front of the acromioclavicular joint.
C, These marker pins outline the attachment of the coracoacromial ligament to the anterior margin of the acromion.

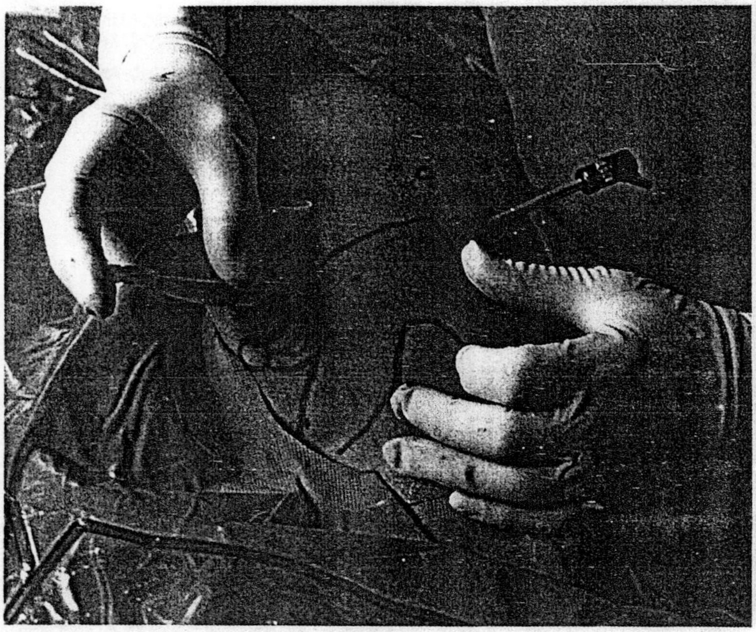

A

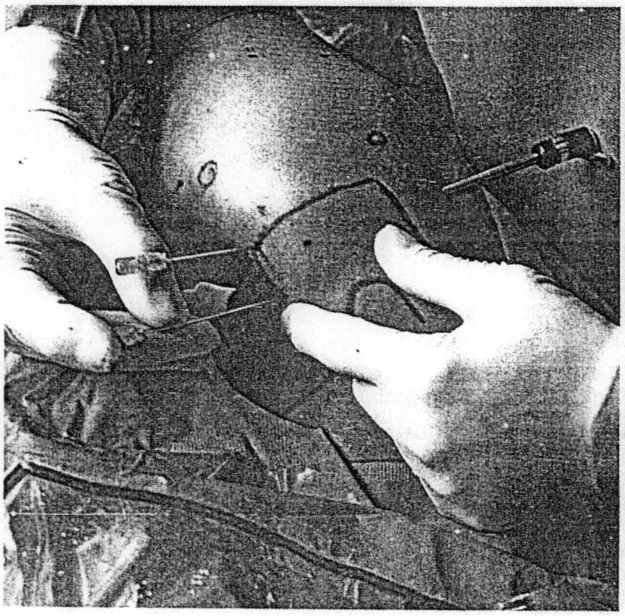

B

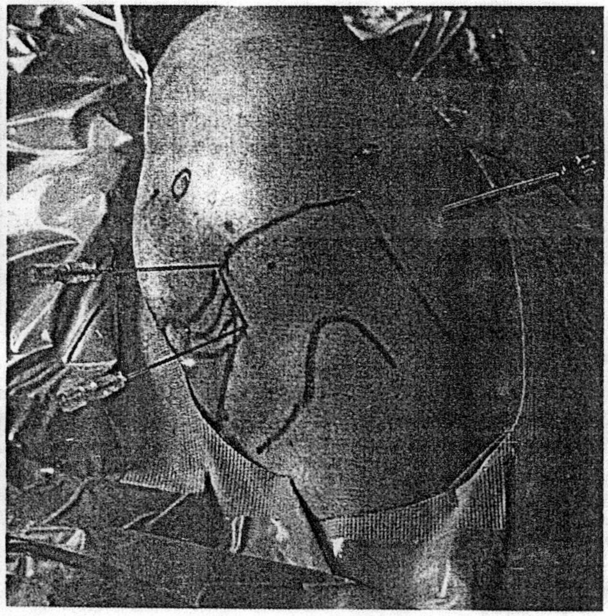

C

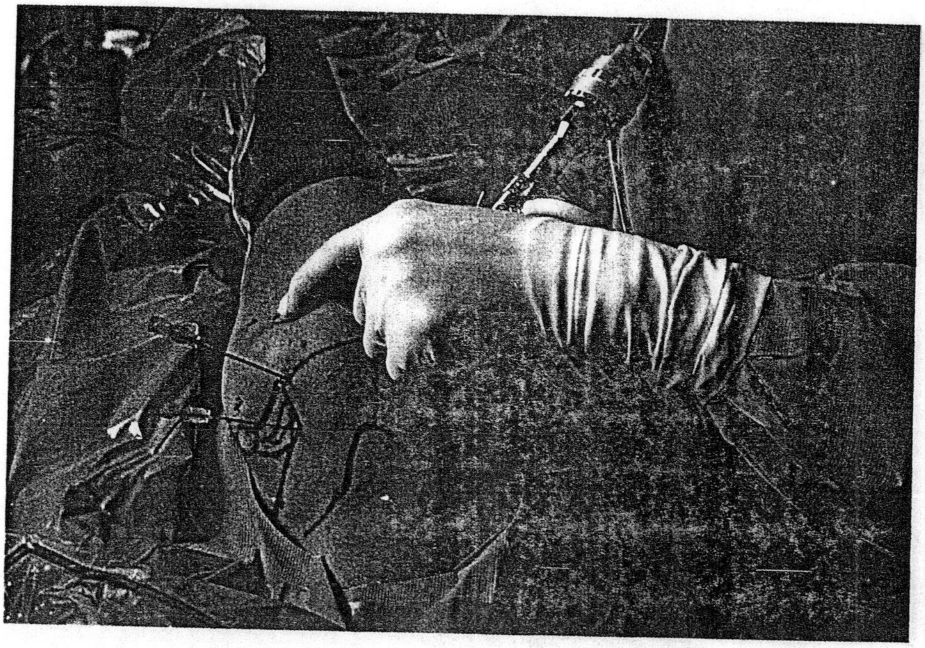

FIG. 5–16. The location of the anterolateral portal is indicated. The portal lies 3 to 4 cm lateral to the anterolateral corner of the acromion in a direct line with 2 marker pins.

AXILLARY NERVE RELATIONSHIPS

Improper placement of the anterolateral portal puts the axillary nerve in jeopardy. After crossing over the lower portion of the subscapularis from the front (Fig. 5–17A), the axillary nerve passes through the quadrangular space posteriorly and divides into a superior and an inferior division (Fig. 5–17B). The superior division accompanies the posterior circumflex humeral artery as it winds around the neck of the humerus under the deltoid muscle in a horizontal fashion about 4 to 5 cm below the acromion and gives off numerous stout twigs that enter the deltoid (Fig. 5–17C). A few fine fibers pierce the deltoid and end in the skin that covers the middle third of that muscle. The inferior division divides into a lateral cutaneous branch, which supplies the skin covering the lower third of the deltoid, and a muscular branch, which is distributed to the teres minor and lower posterior part of the deltoid.

PLACEMENT OF SKIN INCISION

The nerve is in jeopardy if the anterolateral portal is placed too far distal to the acromion. A skin incision is made along Langer's lines no lower than 3 to 4 cm (depending on the size of the patient) below the anterolateral margin of the acromion. This distance is usually no more than 2 to 2 1/2 fingerbreadths beyond the anterolateral pin (Fig. 5–18A). The incision is placed along the direct line that would be formed if the two pins that mark the anterior border of the acromion were connected. Only the skin and subcutaneous tissue are incised (Fig. 5–18B).

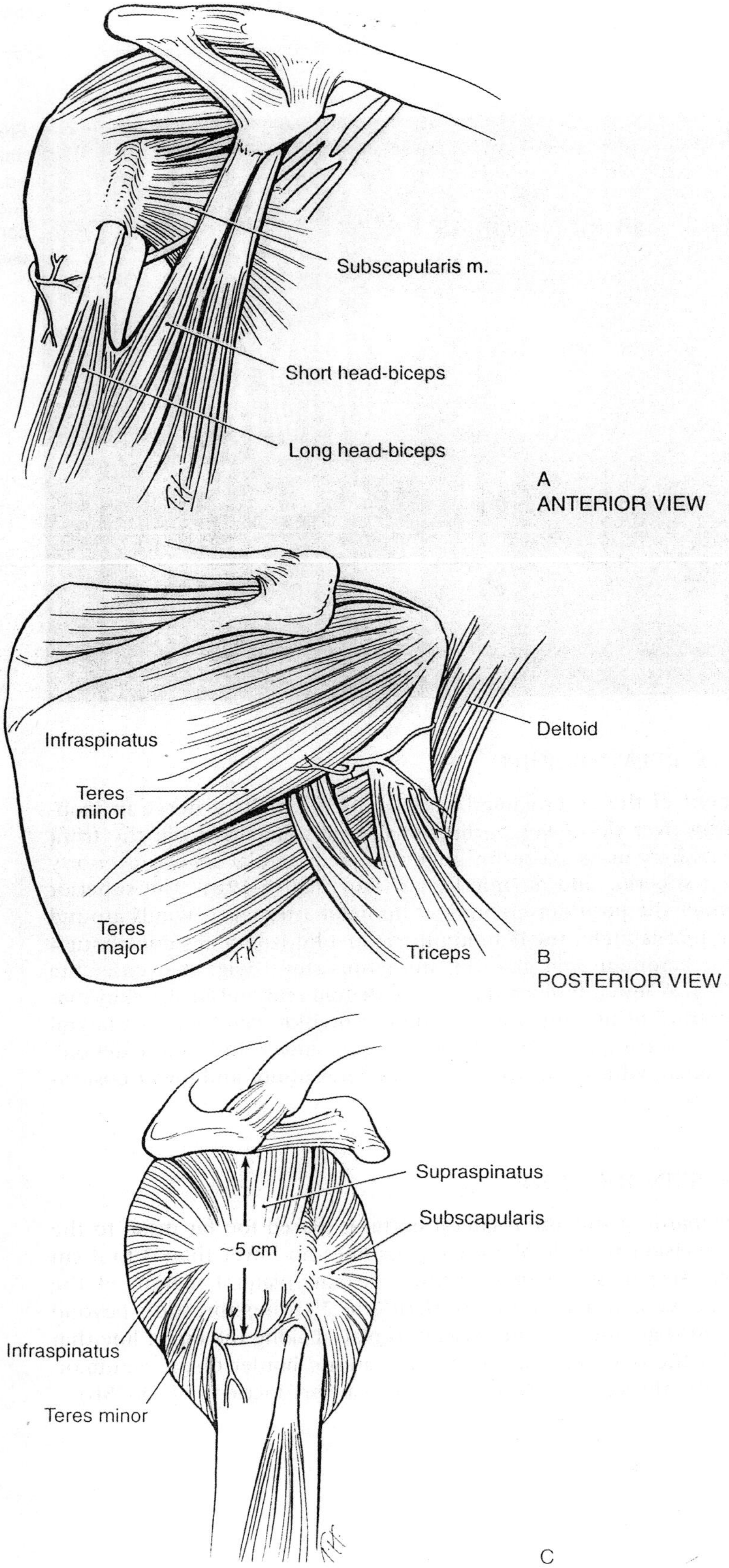

FIG. 5–17. Axillary nerve relationships.
A, Anterior view of axillary nerve as it crosses over the lower aspect of the subscapularis to enter the quadrangular space.
B, Posterior-view. The axillary nerve passes through the quadrangular space and divides into a superior and an inferior division.
C, The superior division winds around the neck of the humerus under the deltoid muscle in a horizontal fashion, about 5 cm below the acromion, and gives off twigs to the deltoid.

CANNULA INSERTION

A cannula with a round-tip obturator is initially directed slightly downward toward the tip of the greater tuberosity, and the deltoid is split by blunt dissection (Fig. 5–18C). Once the firm bony contour of the tuberosity has been reached, the tip of the obturator is directed more superiorly and pushed medially to enter the subacromial space just lateral to the lateral marker pin (Fig. 5–18D). If the cannula enters medial to this lateral pin, instruments introduced through this portal cannot reach the more lateral portions of the acromion. The obturator should not be allowed to damage the cuff or to penetrate the undersurface of the acromion when it is introduced. As with the other portals, the point of entry

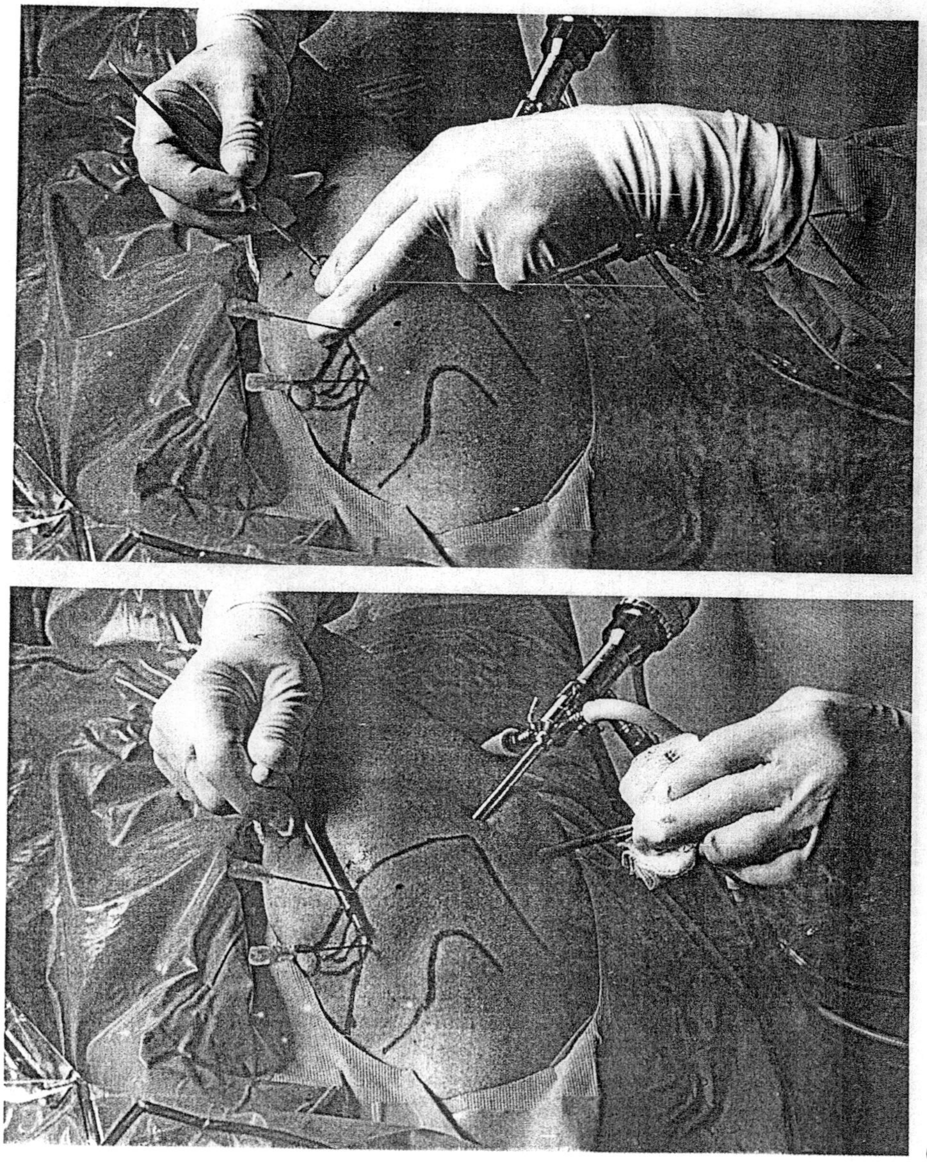

FIG 5–18 A, Skin incision for anterolateral portal, placed 2 fingerbreadths (3 to 4 cm) below the anterolateral margin of the acromion.
B. Incision along a direct line formed by connecting the two pins that mark the anterior border of the acromion.

A

B

(continued)

Fig. 5–18 (continued)

C, Blunt obturator directed medially and slightly downward to split deltoid fibers and contact greater tuberosity.
D, Cannula then is directed superiorly and medially to enter subacromial space.

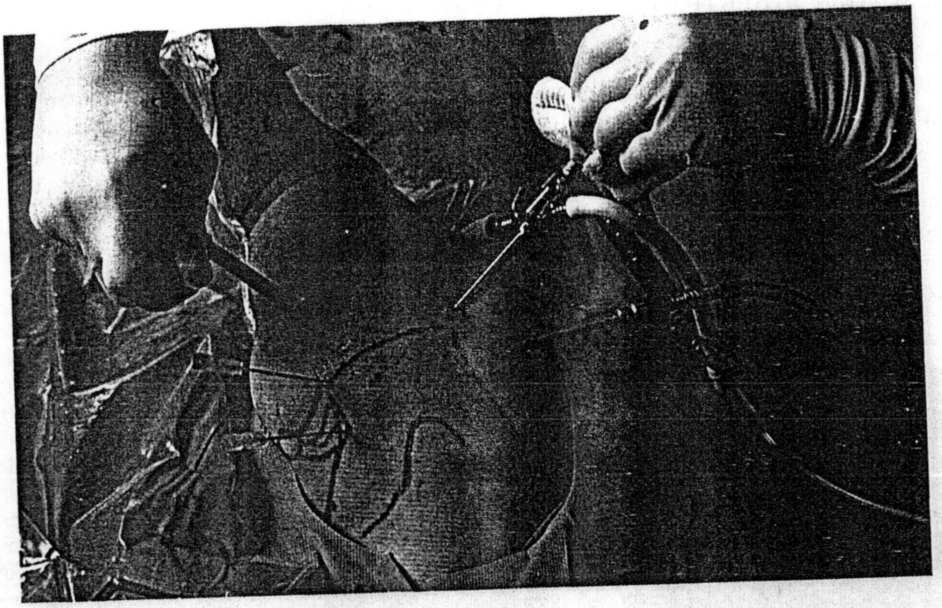

C

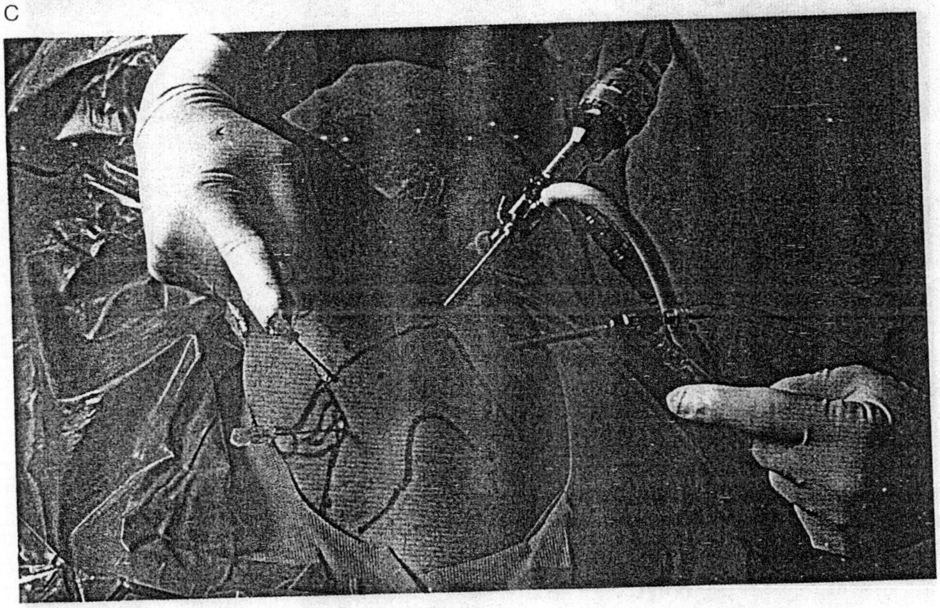

D

must be planned carefully to avoid the need to create additional portals, thereby leaving an opening for fluid to escape into the surrounding tissues. A definite "give" is appreciated as the obturator penetrates the bursal wall. Palpation of both the lateral and the medial pins with the tip of the obturator is possible when placement is correct. All the equipment for surgery in the subacromial space is now in position (Fig. 5–19).

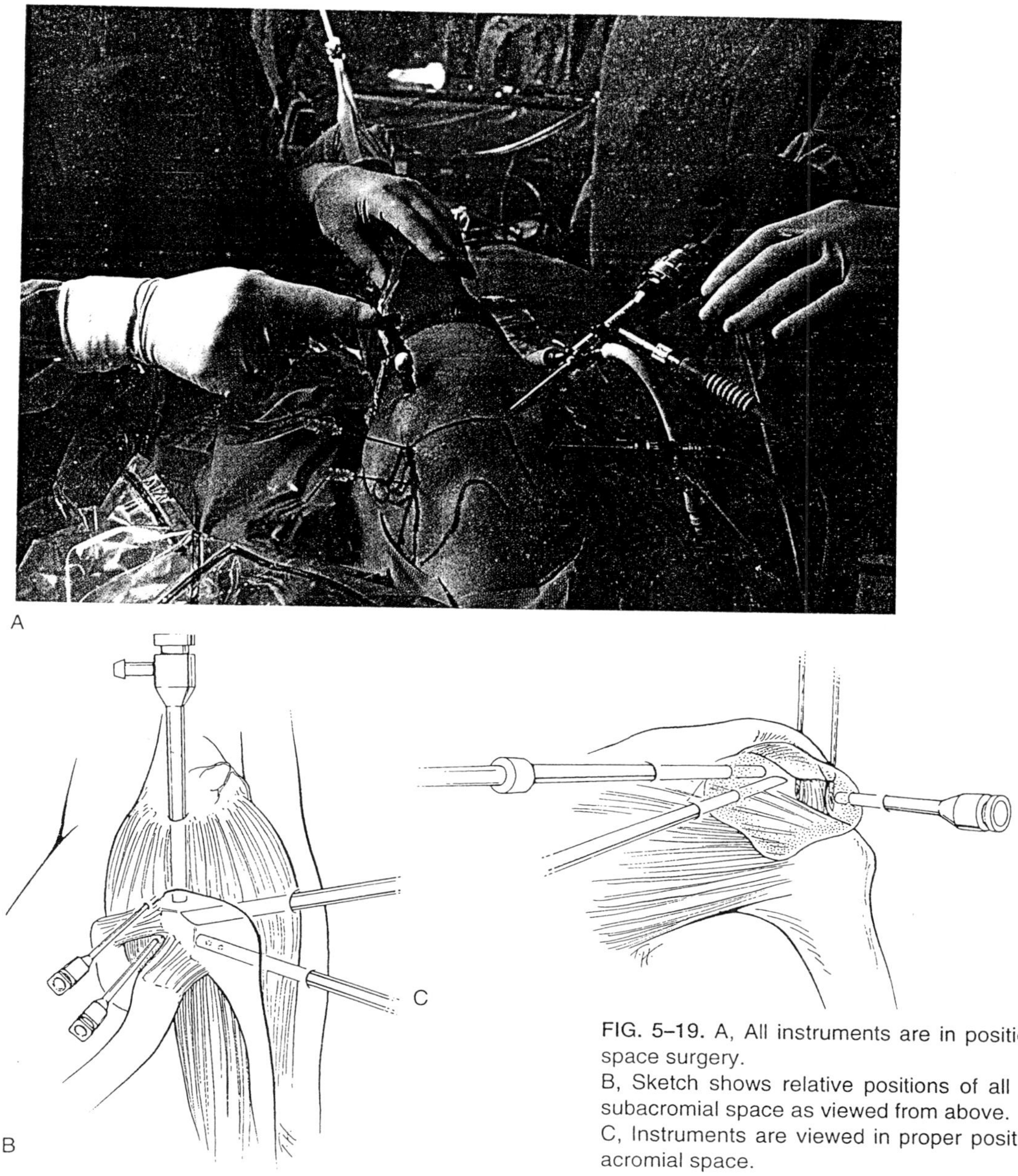

FIG. 5–19. A, All instruments are in position for subacromial space surgery.
B, Sketch shows relative positions of all instruments in the subacromial space as viewed from above.
C, Instruments are viewed in proper position within the subacromial space.

BURSECTOMY

Because the subacromial space usually is obscured by hypertrophic bursa, the next step is a methodical shaving of this tissue to allow identification of the landmarks and completion of the decompression. A synovial shaver is passed through the operating cannula. A synovial resector with either an angled or a serrated tip is preferred. The end of the instrument is positioned below the anterior third of the acromion, and the lens of the arthroscope is advanced to visualize the end of the shaver. At times, the bursa may be so thickened that the examiner can feel the instruments touch each other, but the shaver still cannot be seen. In this instance, the tip of the shaver is rotated so that the cutting surface is away from the lens, and suction shaving is begun. Movement is seen as the shaver begins to clear the area. The tip gradually appears as if it were a butterfly emerging from a cocoon (Fig. 5–20).

One should be careful at this stage to avoid engaging the tip of the lens into the shaver. The lens follows the shaver as the subacromial space is gradually cleared. An effort is made first to clear the bursa in the region of the lateral pin and then to move medially to expose the medial pin. The shaving should not proceed posteriorly much beyond the anterior third of the acromion. The posterior veil in this region must be cleared enough to allow the lens to adequately visualize the anterior acromial structures without impairment. Wiggling of either the medial or lateral pins during the shaving helps to identify them and gradually leads to a comfortable orientation within the subacromial space (Fig. 5–21).

Both the surgeon and the assistant should orient themselves to the position of their instruments by frequently looking away from the video monitor and directly at the patient's shoulder. The tendency to stray both posteriorly and medially into areas of increased vascularity can be avoided by doing so. A glance at the shoulder quickly indicates whether the instruments are working appropriately beneath the anterior acromion. The region of surgery lies directly below the distal phalanx of a thumb placed directly on top of the acromion.

A word of caution is necessary during this phase of the procedure. The stroma in some patients is vascular, and bleeders must be identified and coagulated as they appear. Do not use the shaver too aggressively in the region medial to the

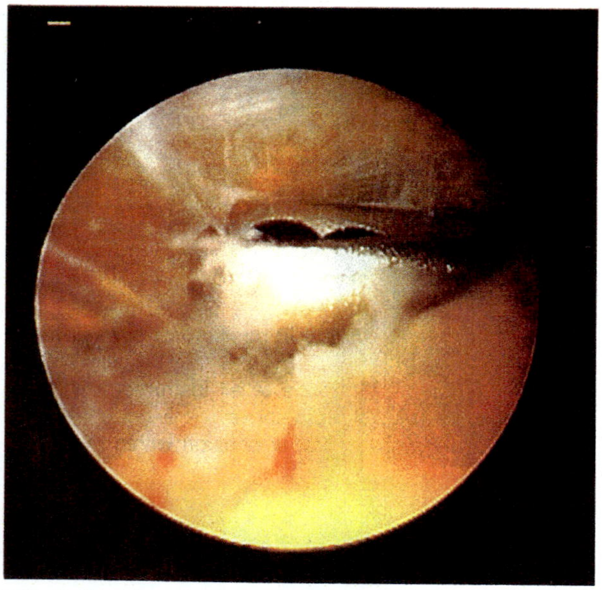

FIG. 5–20. The shaver gradually appears as subacromial bursectomy is performed.

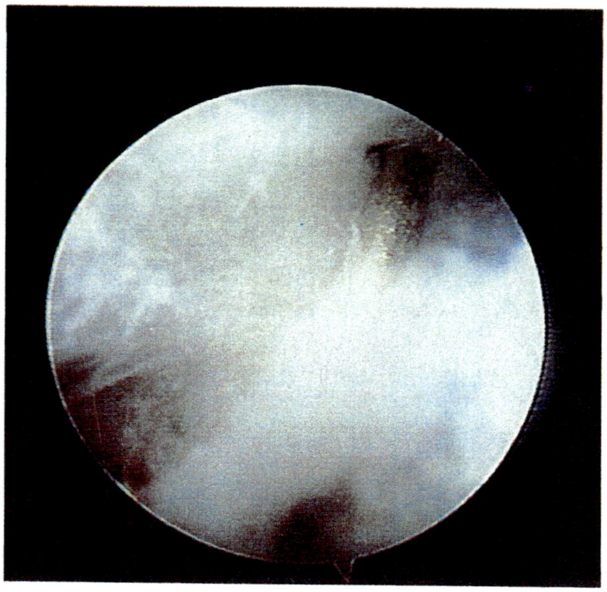

FIG. 5–21. The lateral marker pin is emerging and barely visible as debridement of the hypertorophic bursal stroma progresses.

musculotendinous junction of the cuff; invasion of the muscle may provoke considerable bleeding. Such caution is appropriate also when debriding the subdeltoid region of the bursa. Shaving that is too aggressive not only may clean the bursa, but also may remove some fibers from the undersurface of the deltoid.

SUBACROMIAL SPACE INSPECTION

Once the subacromial space has been thoroughly debrided and bleeding has been controlled, its contents can be explored (Fig. 5–22A). Orient the arthroscopic image so that the two marker pins are vertical. The anterior third of the acromion forms the roof of this small cavern, and the downcurving anterior edge is bounded by the marker pins. The coracoacromial ligament attaches to this anterior margin and, in our arthroscopic view, descends vertically (Fig. 5–22B). The subacromial bursa attaches to the undersurface of the acromion and a portion of the coracoacromial ligament. A thickened bursa obscures the ligament, but in some patients this structure may be seen quite clearly. Inspection of the anterior margin of the acromion may reveal the crabmeat-like fraying of tissue that is the hallmark of mechanical impingement (Fig. 5–22C).

Now, rotate the 30°-angled lens of the arthroscope to look downward on the rotator cuff. Rotate the arm internally and externally while inspecting the cuff. Abduct the arm to identify the insertion of the supraspinatus in the trough between the tuberosity and the humeral head. Introduce a probe through the operating cannula and probe the surface of the cuff to discover any perforations, thinning, or buckling (Fig. 5–22D). If tearing of the bursal surface is revealed, debride the free ends to make them smooth and probe again to determine whether the bursal defect communicates with the glenohumeral joint. The 3-mm bent-arm arthroscopic probe is used to measure and classify the tear. Complete the inspection by exploring into the lateral and medial gutters as far as the limits of the bursa permit (Fig. 5–22E).

RELEASE OF CORACOACROMIAL LIGAMENT

The right-angled plastic-coated meniscectomy electrode is used to release the attachment of the coracoacromial ligament. The plastic coating, which extends almost to the tip of the electrode, permits this electrosurgical instrument to work effectively in a normal saline medium. A specially conductive irrigating fluid is not required. This electrode is inserted into the pencil-like control device. The tip of the electrode extends upward in relation to the buttons that control the coagulation and cutting currents. The control on the electrosurgical generator is set at the minimal level that will permit effective coagulation and cutting. Electrothermal damage to contiguous structures results from improper settings.

The tip of the electrode is placed just medial to the medial pin, and cutting proceeds medial to lateral in a direct line with the anterior margin of the acromion (Fig. 5–23A). The position of the marker pins and the placement of the anterolateral portal in a direct line with the pins facilitate this cut. The attachment of the coracoacromial ligament is outlined by the marker pins, and a cut that connects the distance between the two pins reliably includes the ligament attachment when the pins have been properly placed (Fig. 5–23B). As much as 3 to 6 mm of thickened bursa may have to be cut through before the ligament fibers can be encountered. This layer of thickened bursa should be

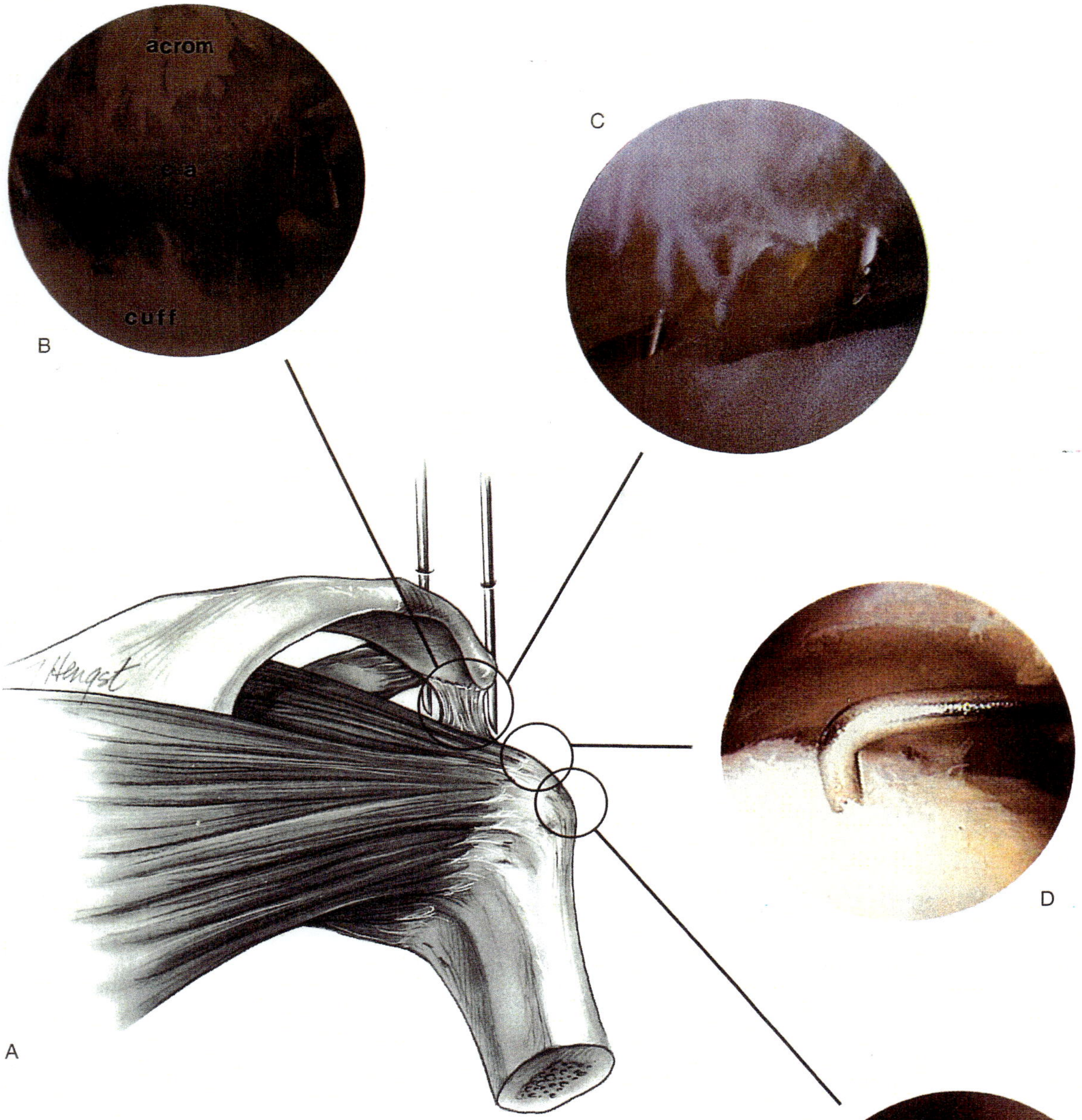

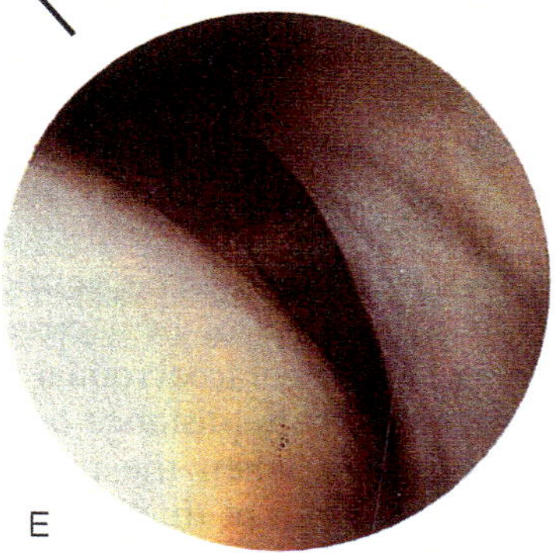

FIG. 5–22. Subacromial space inspection.
A, Orientation sketch.
B, Arthroscopic photograph shows the anterior undersurface of the acromion (acrom) above. The rotator cuff (cuff) is below. The coracoacromial ligament (c-a lig) descends vertically from the anterior edge of the acromion. The lateral marker pin (right) and the medial marker pin (left) are visible.
C, Crabmeat-like fraying of tissue under anterior acromion.
D, A probe has been introduced to palpate the surface of the rotator cuff.
E, The lateral gutter is explored at the limits of the bursa.

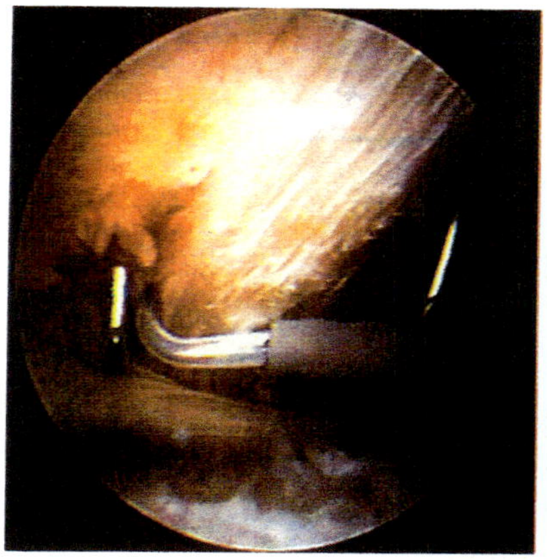

B

C

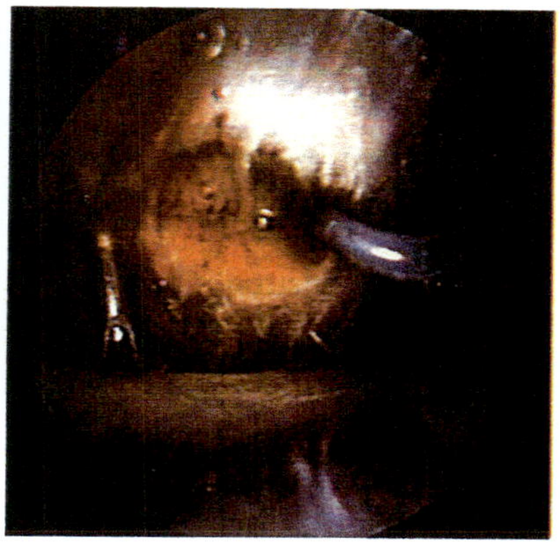

D

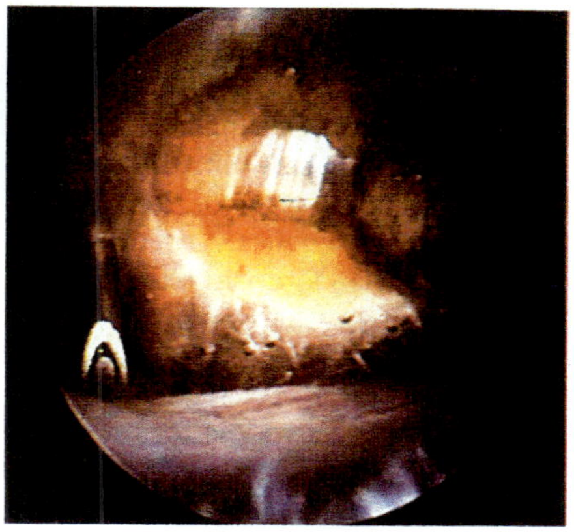

FIG. 5–23. Release of coracoacromial ligament.
A, Orientation sketch with inset shows ligament being cut from medial to lateral pin.
B, Arthroscopic photo with electrode at medial pin.
C, Cut is three-quarters complete.
D, Note shiny, thin, tightly packed fibers of ligament still intact in depths of cut.
E, Ligament completely released. Note exposed broad, reddish deltoid fibers.

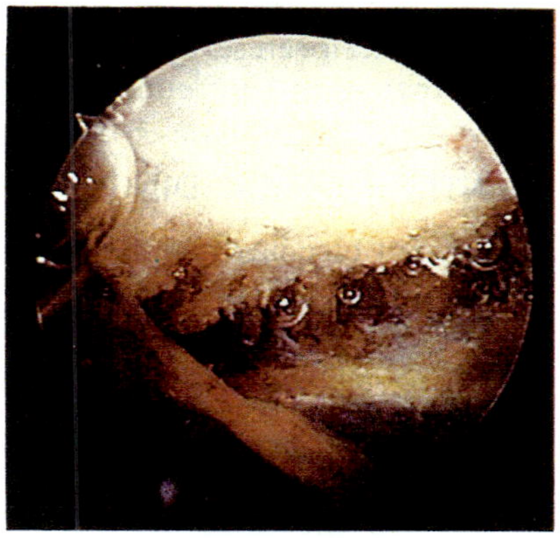

E

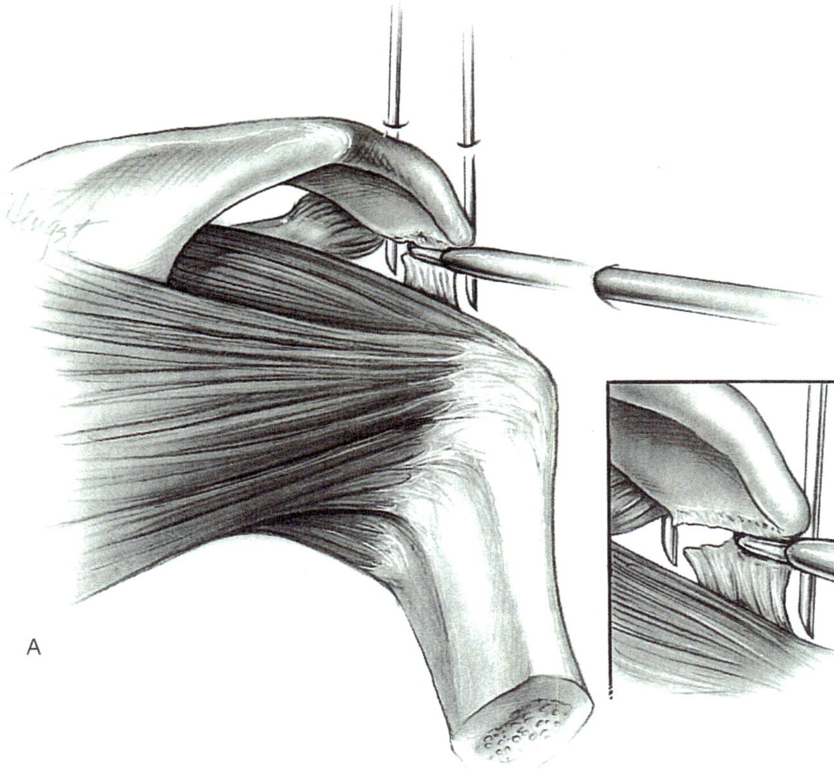

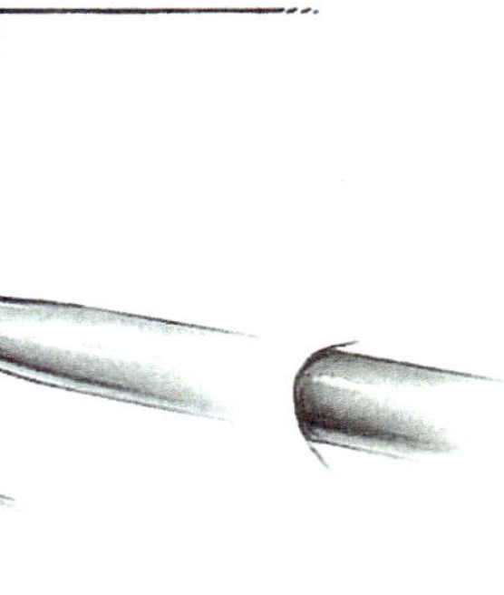

A

incised uniformly across the region of the cut before cutting the actual ligament (Fig. 5–23C). The coracoacromial ligament is approximately as broad and thick as a table knife. The ligament has a silvery-white appearance, and the fibers are quite thin and closely packed (Fig. 5–23D). This appearance contrasts with the deltoid muscle fibers, which appear pink and much broader (Fig. 5–23E).

As the ligament is cut across from below upward, care should be taken to avoid extending the cut into the deltoid attachment. The arthroscope should be brought directly beneath the cutting electrode with the lens positioned upward. The ligament can be cut lightly with short strokes in ever-deepening layers. As the cut is completed, the ligament appears to give way as its acromial insertion is released. The deltoid fibers are exposed, and the electrode can be used somewhat as a probe to palpate the fibers. The ligament may be cut 3 to 5 mm away from its point of attachment, thereby leaving a tiny beard of tissue across the anterior edge of the acromion. This beard of tissue may be easily removed with a basket forceps or an aggressive shaver. The surgeon can resect a portion of this ligament more easily by following this procedure than by attempting to grasp the free-floating edge of the released ligament and resecting it with a basket forceps. The subsequent resection of the anterior edge of the acromion for 8 to 10 mm (described later) further widens the gap between the end of the released ligament and the acromion. This precise surgical release is far superior to any method of detaching the ligament by simply burring away the anterior acromial margin

The acromioclavicular branch of the thoracoacromial artery lies above the ligament within soft tissue. This artery is seldom encountered when the ligament is cut within 5 mm of its attachment to the anterior edge of the acromion. Bleeding most commonly develops during this stage of the procedure if deltoid fibers are cut, an outcome that occurs if the cautery strays too deeply after the ligament has been severed. Should the coracoacromial artery be cut, the hemorrhage may appear torrential.

CONTROL OF BLEEDING

Significant bleeding may impair visualization during any step of this procedure. Various methods are available to control bleeding. Electrocautery should be carried out promptly when bleeding develops. The position of the surgical cannula should be maintained if hemorrhage occurs while the shaver or other instruments are being used. The electrosurgical pencil is introduced promptly into the area where bleeding develops. Rapid, intermittent suction helps to clear this area so that the origin of the bleeding can be identified and cauterized.

Elevation of the fluid bags, or an increase in pump pressure, retards hemorrhage by increasing intrabursal pressure. Approximately 22 mm Hg of increased pressure results from every 1 foot above shoulder level that a fluid bag is elevated. We routinely begin shoulder arthroscopy with the 3M pump set at between 35 to 40 mm Hg. Pressure may be increased to as high as 90 mm Hg for short intervals. Whether gravity or pump systems are used, pressure should be lowered promptly to diminish tissue extravasation.

Hypotensive anesthesia effectively controls bleeding, but must be used cautiously in older patients. The injection of 1 ml of 1:1,000 adrenaline into a 3-L bag of saline irrigation fluid produces an adrenaline concentration of 1:300,000. When instilled, vasoconstriction results. Removal of the traction weights and entrance of air into the joint also may promote coagulation. The operation can resume in 2 to 3 minutes, if feasible. Blunt surfaces of the intraarticular cannula

TABLE 5–1. EIGHT STEPS TO CONTROL BLEEDING

1. Promptly institute electrocoagulation.
2. Maintain cannula position.
3. Apply rapid intermittent suction.
4. Elevate fluid bags or increase pump pressure.
5. Use hypotensive anesthesia.
6. Instill 1:300,000 adrenaline solution in irrigating fluid.
7. Attempt internal/external manual tamponade.
8. Interrupt procedure for 2 to 3 minutes.

or mechanical instruments can be used as extensions of your finger to tamponade bleeding vessels. We would not attempt arthroscopic subacromial decompression without an electrocautery system. The 8 steps followed in an attempt to control bleeding are summarized in Table 5–1.

ACROMIOPLASTY

DENUDING THE AREA

Preparation for the acromioplasty requires removal of the thickened bursa and fibers of ligament and periosteum that invest the undersurface of the anterior acromion. This step is best begun with the electrosurgical instrument. Beginning at the anteromedial pin, the area from which bone will be removed is outlined. This area extends from the anteromedial pin backward along the AC joint for a distance of 2.5 cm and then laterally across the full width of the acromion to return anteriorly along the lateral border of acromion to the anterolateral pin (Fig. 5–24A, A′). The tissue within this area is morseled with electrosurgery and then thoroughly removed with a suction shaver (Fig. 5–24B, B′). An open arthroscopic curette can also be used to denude this area (Fig. 5–24C, C′). Use of the electrocautery minimizes bleeding

EXTENT OF BONE REMOVAL

The digital analogy can demonstrate the extent of the area from which bone is removed in an acromioplasty. Look at your thumb from the lateral aspect with the distal phalanx gently curved. Recall the similarity of the thumb to the length and breadth of the acromion. The area of bone removal in acromioplasty generally extends from front to back for 2.5 cm, about the length of the distal phalanx. The goal is to remove the anterior acromial hook and flatten the undersurface across the full width of the acromion to widen the supraspinatus outlet. The best way to begin removal is to recess the anterior edge 8 to 10 mm. Recessing automatically eliminates the most anterior downcurving portion of a hooked acromion (Fig. 5–25). Anterior recession also establishes the thickness of the acromion. Subsequent thinning and tapering from back to front produces a flattened acromion with the anterior aspect assuming the shape of the trailing edge of an airplane wing (Fig. 5–26).

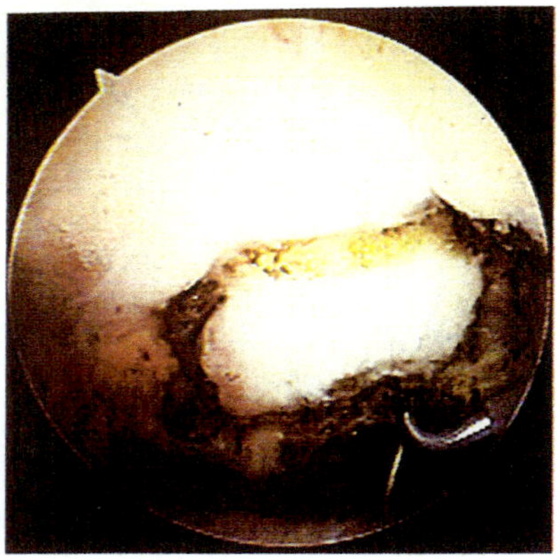

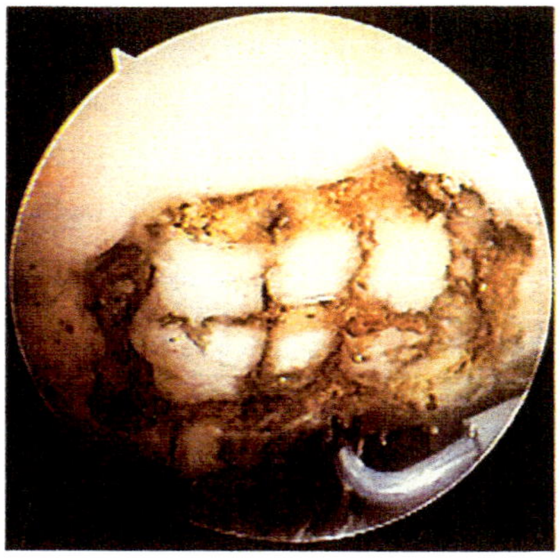

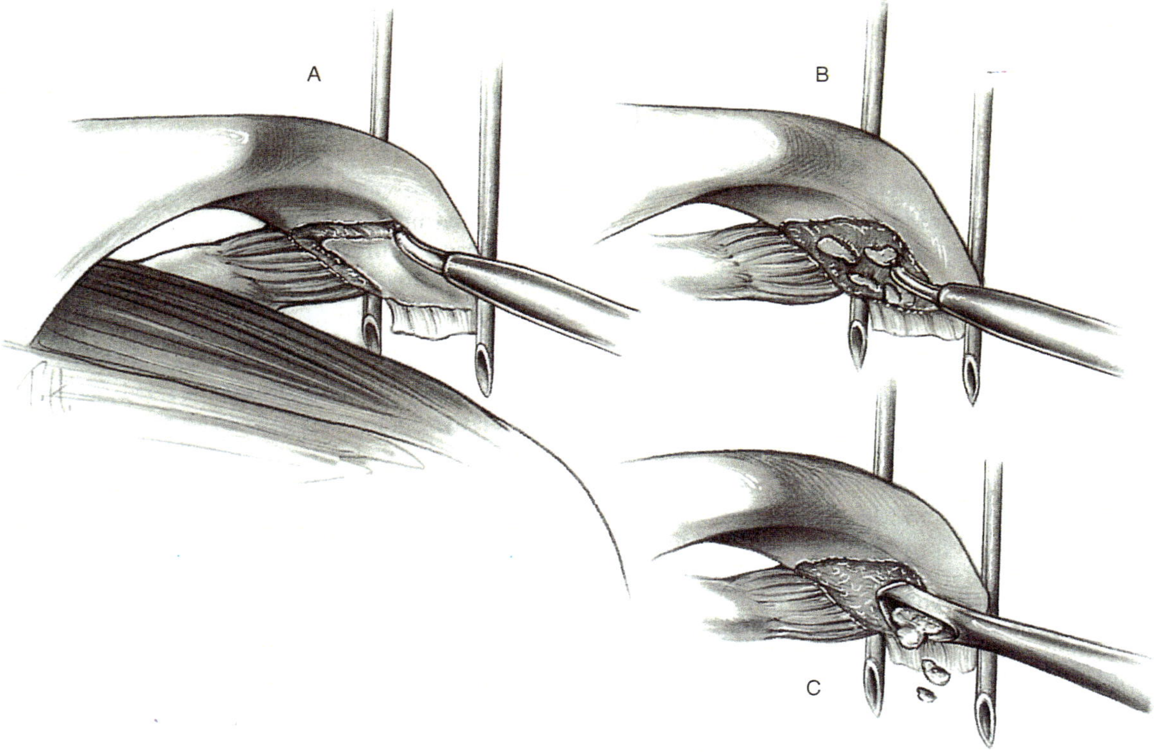

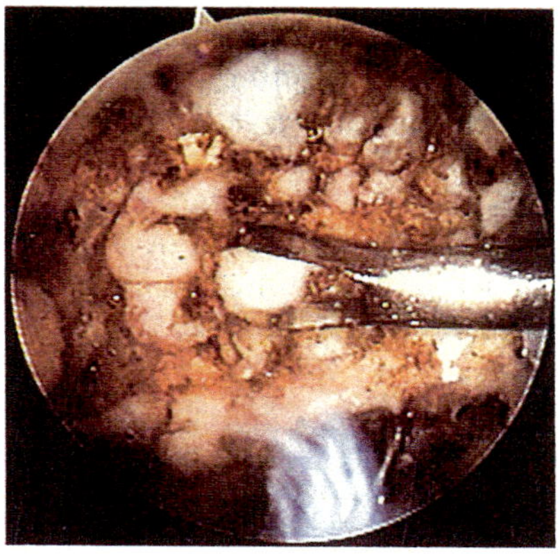

FIG. 5–24. Denuding the area for acromioplasty.
A, A′, The area for bone removal is outlined with the electrode (back 2.5 cm from the front of the acromion and across the full width).
B, B′, Debris within this area morselated.
C, C′, Complete denudation with open curette.

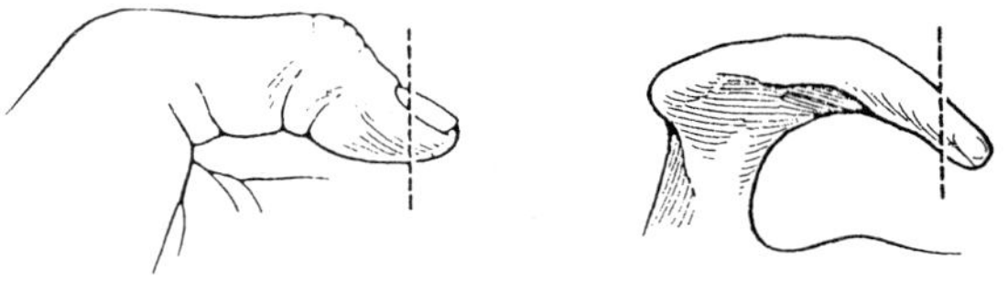

FIG. 5–25. Downcurving portion of hooked acromion is removed by recessing the anterior edge.

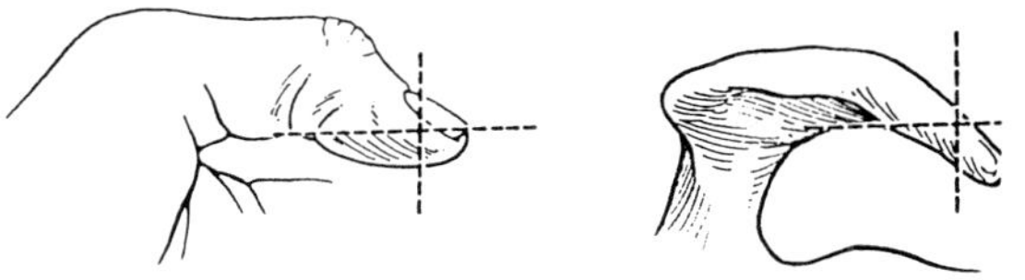

FIG. 5–26. Subsequent thinning and tapering from front to back flattens the acromion.

RECESSING THE ANTERIOR EDGE

The first step in removing the downcurving acromial hook is to recess approximately one-half the thickness of the anterior edge from 8 to 10 mm (Fig. 5–27A, A′). This recessing also begins to establish the thickness of the acromion and helps to flatten the undersurface more easily. The 4.0-mm oval bur is placed directly in front of the medial corner of the acromion and then is drawn from medial to lateral across the full width. This anterior recession should continue until the full thickness of the 8 to 10 mm of bone has been removed. This measurement can be judged by using the known size (4.0 mm) of the sleeve of the bur. The thickness of the acromion is now seen (Fig. 5–27B,B′).

FLATTENING THE UNDERSURFACE

Anteroposterior furrows are then made from the front of the recessed acromion posteriorly for 2 cm. The task is most easily accomplished by beginning the first furrow laterally and tapering from front to back (Fig. 5–28,A,A′). The initial lateral furrow is then advanced medially to produce another furrow of similar depth (Fig. 5–28B,B′). Two or three repetitions with the large oval bur are generally enough to cross the full width of the acromion. The process is then repeated, tapering from front to back, until the anterior edge of the acromion resembles the trailing edge of an airplane wing (Fig. 5–28C,′). The area is polished in a circular fashion to remove any valleys or peaks. The lateral and medial borders should be inspected to ensure that no lateral or medial shelf of bone remains.

REMOVAL OF ACROMIOCLAVICULAR SPURS

The medial border identifies the AC joint. At this point, the undersurface of the clavicle is identified by exerting external downward pressure and watching the acromial end of the clavicle move in relation to the acromion. Any protuberance of this undersurface that exists should be carefully removed. Some additional shaving may be necessary at this anteromedial corner to adequately expose the AC joint (Fig. 5–29A,A′, B,B′, C,C′). A third pin placed at the posterior margin of the AC joint aids orientation during removal of acromioclavicular spurs.

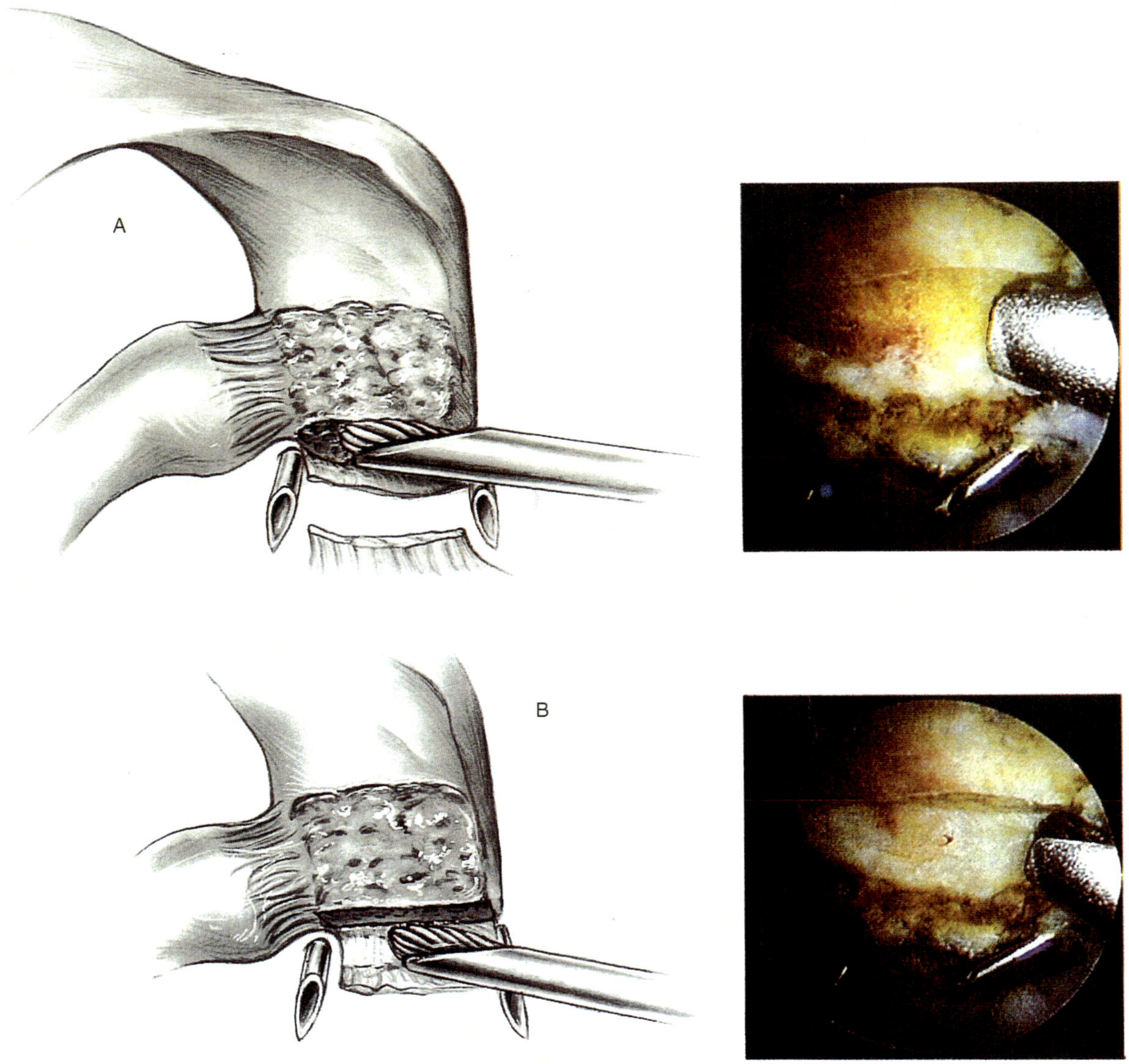

FIG. 5–27. A, A′, One-half thickness of anterior edge has been removed.

B, B′, The full width of the anterior edge has been recessed 8 to 10 mm. Note that the white undersurface of periosteum formerly covering the acromion is exposed, thereby indicating the extent of the recession. The thickness of the acromion is now seen.

FIG. 5–28. Flattening the undersurface of the acromion. ▶
A, A′, The initial furrow is made beneath the lateral border of the acromion. The furrow is deepest at the anterior margin and tapers to remove less bone as it travels posteriorly.

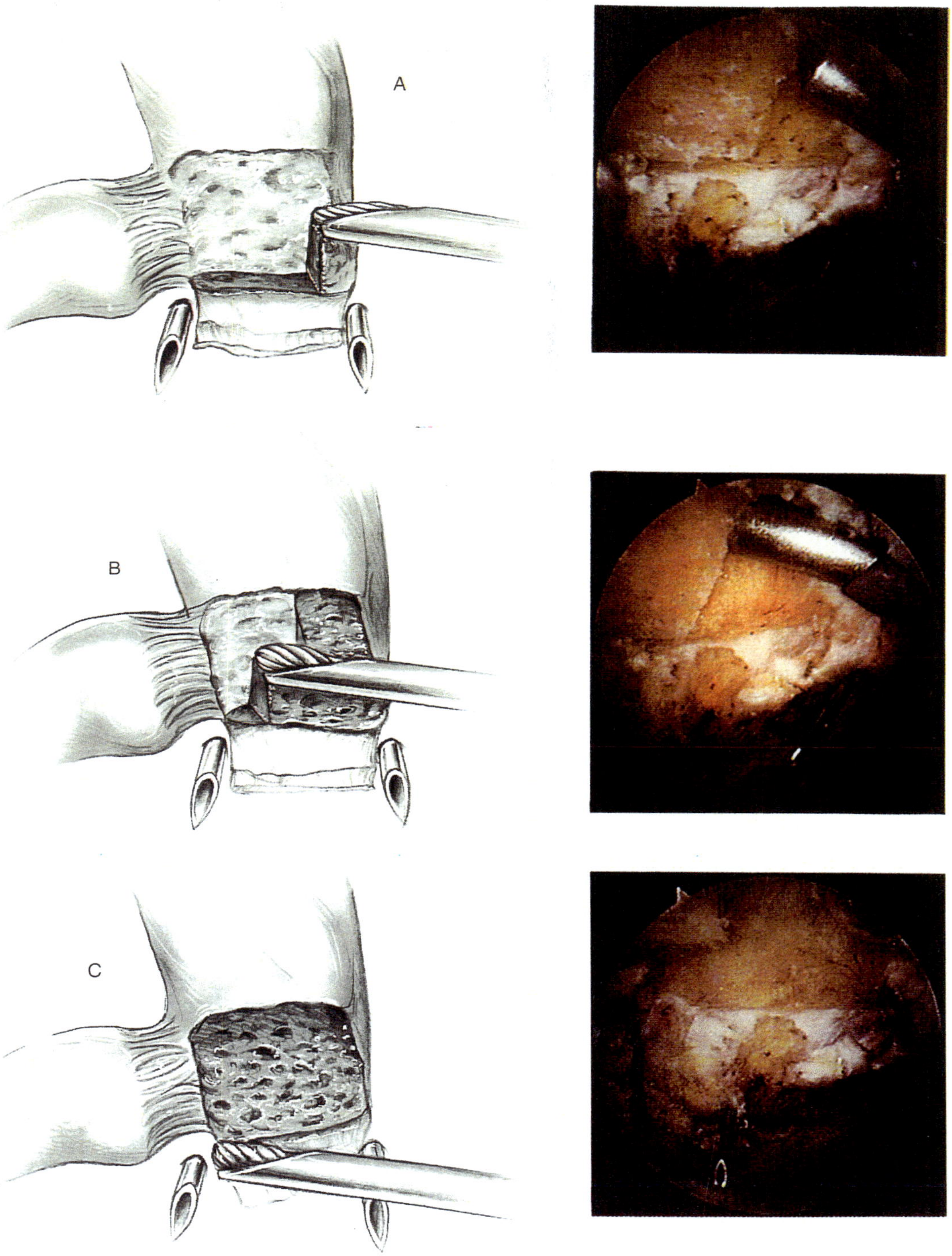

B, B′, Additional furrows are added. The amount of bone removed is readily visualized. C, C′, Deepening process may be repeated until desired amount of bone has been removed. The anterior edge of the acromion resembles the trailing edge of an airplane wing.

THE COMPLETED ACROMIOPLASTY

Prior to concluding the procedure, the flatness of the acromion can be confirmed by using the fluid-ingress cannula to palpate from back to front while viewing with the arthroscope. An alternate method of confirmation is to exchange the arthroscope and anterolateral operating cannula by using switching sticks and to have a lateral view of the acromion while palpating through the posterior portal with a probe. Following completion of the acromioplasty, the undersurface should appear flat across the full width of the acromion and tapered gently from back to front for a distance of nearly 2 cm. The anterior margin of the acromion should appear thin, and an overhang of 8 to 10 mm of superior periosteum should reflect the distance that the anterior edge was recessed prior to flattening. No residual element of coracoacromial ligament should be attached to bone (Fig. 5–29C,C′).

Before closing, traction should be released and the arm abducted and flexed through an arc of elevation while the impingement area is inspected to ensure that the acromioplasty is clinically adequate.

A mixture of 10 ml of bupivacaine with adrenaline is then instilled into the subacromial space, and the portals are closed with interrupted sutures of No. 4 prolene. A compression bandage is applied for 2 or 3 hours following surgery. Prior to discharge from the outpatient center, the compression dressing is removed and small adhesive bandages are applied. Elderly individuals who require postoperative monitoring or those who must travel long distances may be kept overnight. The patient is not fitted with a sling and is encouraged to resume activities of daily living as tolerated.

POSTOPERATIVE COURSE

REHABILITATION

Because no deltoid was removed, the patient may resume activities of daily living as tolerated. Gentle range-of-motion exercises (supine forward elevation, external rotation, and pendulum) are performed every morning and evening to avoid stiffness. Strengthening exercises with rubber tubing are begun at 3 weeks. These initial exercises are performed in the subimpingement range. More strenuous resistance exercises start in the sixth week and continue until the individual goals of rehabilitation are reached. A detailed protocol with illustrated exercises for rehabilitation following arthroscopic subacromial decompression is presented in Chapter 24.

FIG. 5–29. A, A′, Shaving beneath the distal end of the clavicle to expose the acromioclavicular joint. ▶

B, B′, Bur has removed downward-protruding spurs from undersurface of clavicle. Note the exposed acromioclavicular joint as it appears somewhat obliquely between the clavicle and acromion.

C, C′, Completed acromioplasty.

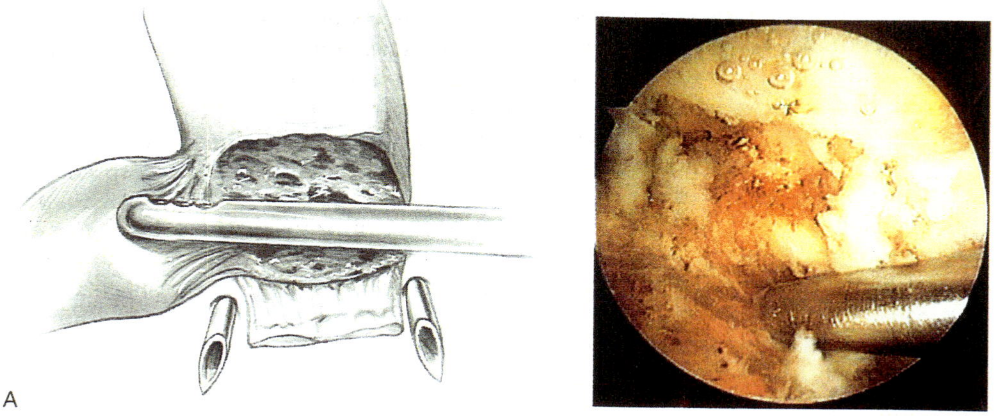

A

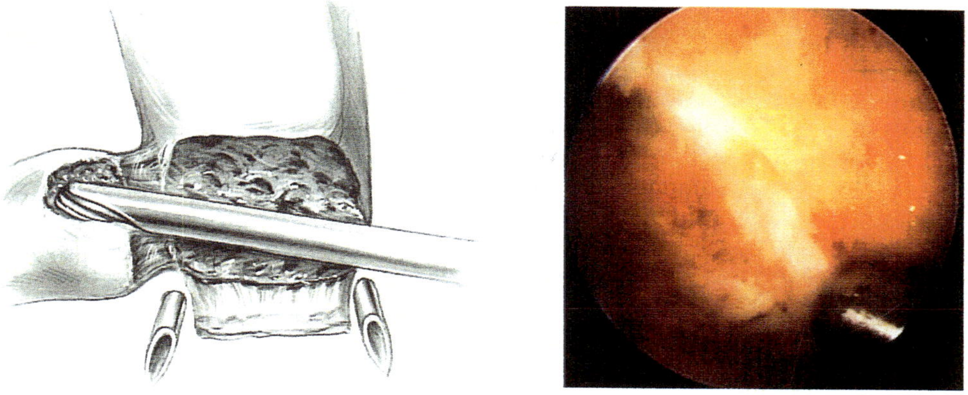

B

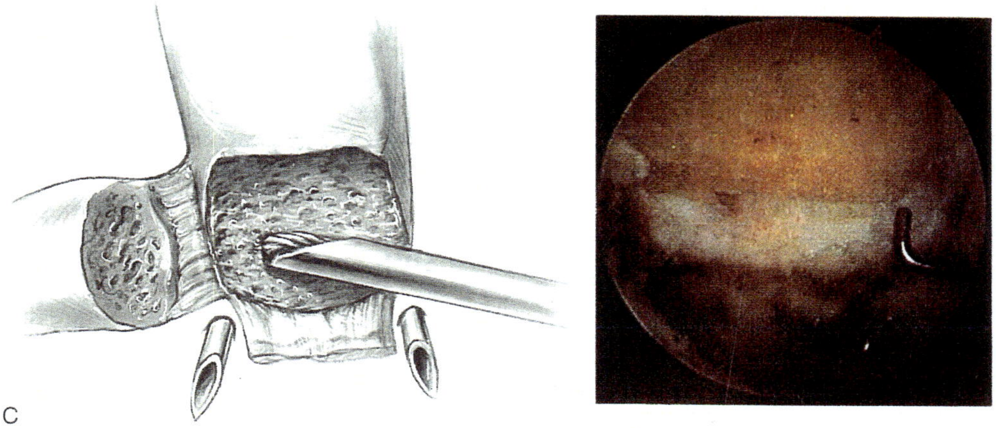

C

FIG. 5–29

RETURN TO WORK OR SPORT

Most patients experience a significant decrease in shoulder discomfort within 2 or 3 weeks following arthroscopic subacromial decompression. An occasional patient reports dramatic relief of pressure and night pain within the first week. The discomfort associated with forward elevation usually disappears by 6 weeks; however, some pain may be provoked by combining pure adduction to 90° with internal rotation for 3 to 6 months following surgery. Restoration of a smooth fibrous undersurface to the acromion following acromioplasty requires at least 3 months. Activities that prematurely stress healing in this area retard convalescence.

Desk work may be resumed within 2 to 3 days following surgery. Light overhead work is allowed in 2 to 4 weeks, but strenuous and repetitive overhead activity should be avoided for 6 to 12 weeks. Sports activities may be gradually resumed at 6 weeks, but should be somewhat restricted for 3 months.

DELAYED RECOVERY

Restricted motion prolongs convalescence following arthroscopic subacromial decompression. Patients with preoperative restriction of motion, as well as those who develop postoperative capsulitis, usually remain symptomatic until motion is restored. Every effort is made during the first few weeks to prevent postoperative adhesion formation by performing gentle active assisted range-of-motion exercises every morning and evening. Patients with capsulitis are monitored closely to prevent any further loss of motion during the immediate postoperative period. After 3 or 4 weeks, a more aggressive program to re-establish external rotation and internal rotation is begun. The patient should be able to externally rotate at least 30° before stretching in forward flexion is initiated. Efforts to mobilize the scapula (shoulder shrugs, shoulder pinches, and manual mobilization) are important in this group of patients. Patients who have impingement with moderate preoperative capsulitis are advised that restoration of motion may take as long as 6 months following surgery.

Patients with *partial-thickness tears* may take longer than patients without tears to achieve a satisfactory result. Patients with partial-thickness tears do not achieve as high a percentage of satisfactory results following arthroscopic subacromial decompression as do patients without evidence of cuff tear. Preliminary studies suggest that tears involving more than one-half thickness of the cuff do not tolerate a return to strenuous activity well in spite of adequate acromioplasty. These facts should be considered in patient selection.

CAUSES OF FAILURE

The final result of arthroscopic subacromial decompression should not be judged until at least 6 months following the procedure. Causes of failure following arthroscopic subacromial decompression (arthroscopic acromioplasty) are similar to the causes of failure following open acromioplasty.

IMPROPER DIAGNOSIS

A painful arc of shoulder elevation may be caused by a myriad of disorders. Most of the conditions simulating impingement syndrome can be excluded by clinical evaluation and appropriate diagnostic imaging. Arthroscopic evaluation of the glenohumeral joint done concurrently with subacromial space surgery at times reveals unexpected disorders.

A significant degree of second- and third-degree *chondromalacia* with cartilaginous loose bodies has been found in more than 7% of our patients. *Bicipital tendon tears* are often found in patients undergoing surgery for impingement lesions. An incomplete tear of the tendon may be so advanced that, in spite of decompression, shoulder pain persists unless bicipital tenodesis is performed. Failure to recognize *acromioclavicular arthritis* or *osteolysis* as a primary cause of shoulder pain is a common reason for the failure of subacromial decompression.

When *impingement* is *secondary to instability,* symptoms are likely to recur in spite of an adequate acromioplasty. The failure to recognize instability as the primary diagnosis is one of the most important causes of failure following acromioplasty, whether the operation is performed with arthroscopic techniques or as an open procedure. Hyperlaxity is evident on arthroscopic evaluation.

The humeral head appears to be displaced anteriorly and inferiorly in relation to the rim of the acromion. The anterior capsule may appear patulous. On occasion, a true Bankart lesion may be found, but in most instances of atraumatic joint laxity, the labrum is simply attenuated, scuffed, or frayed. Intensive rehabilitation following surgery may help to stabilize the joint in many patients, but the symptoms of impingement often recur when strenuous sports or work activities are resumed. The instability should be considered the primary disorder in these patients and should be treated appropriately.

INADEQUATE BONE REMOVAL

One of the most common causes of failure of either open or arthroscopic acromioplasty is inadequate bone removal. Impingement persists when the acromial undersurface is not adequately flattened or the anterior margin is allowed to protrude beyond the line of the clavicle. Failure to thin the lateral margin of the acromion adequately may cause an unsatisfactory acromioplasty. The method of performing arthroscopic acromioplasty described previously in this chapter is designed to eliminate these inadequacies by first recessing the acromion and then beginning to thin the acromion with progressive furrows that remove the lateral margin first to establish the depth of bone removal. The decompression must extend beneath the AC joint to remove any downward protruding spurs. A bulbous enlargement of the lateral clavicle should be flattened to the level of the acromion.

FAILURE TO RELEASE LIGAMENT

A retained coracoacromial ligament attachment may cause decompression to fail. Some fibers of the ligament are attached as far medially as the anterior capsule of the AC joint. Complete detachment of the ligament is best documented by observing the appearance of intact deltoid fibers across the full width of the acromion after the ligament has been completely cut (Fig. 5–30).

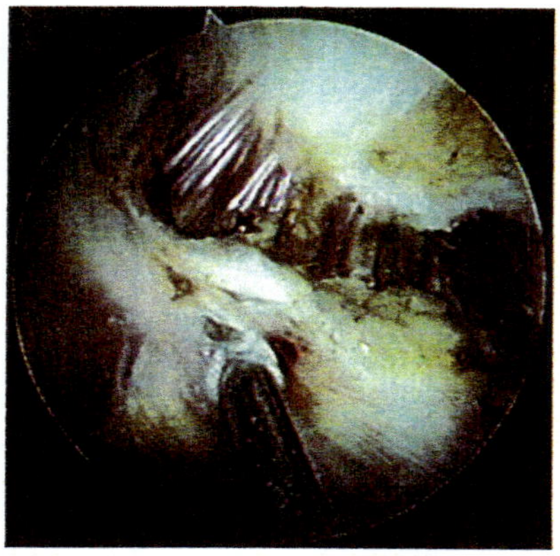

FIG. 5–30. A few silvery fibers of coracoacromial ligament are still intact medially. The broad, pale, reddish fibers of the deltoid have been exposed laterally where the ligament has been completely released. ac = acromion; c-a lig = coracoacromial ligament.

PREMATURE STRENUOUS ACTIVITY

The premature resumption of strenuous sports or overhead vocational activity may discourage the healing process and contribute to an unsatisfactory result. A smooth fibrous undersurface eventually covers the exposed cancellous bone following acromioplasty. Inappropriate activity, however, impairs this healing process. The time for healing simply cannot be rushed. The patient who experiences rapid and gratifying initial relief of pain following the procedure may be quite disappointed a few weeks later if this admonition is ignored.

For this same reason, strengthening exercises should be performed in the subimpingement range for at least 6 weeks. Early efforts at elevation should be carried out in forward flexion with the palm upward to ensure some degree of external rotation. This precaution avoids a collision between the greater tuberosity and the healing subacromial tissue. Pure abduction also should be eliminated until full external rotation is possible to avoid the same problem. Any therapist involved in the rehabilitation process should be quite familiar with these precepts. Overly zealous efforts to restore motion and strength can be counterproductive.

RESULTS

We have independently reported the outcome following arthroscopic subacromial decompression (arthroscopic acromioplasty) in the treatment of rotator cuff disorders. The results of these studies were remarkably similar and, therefore, are combined for this review.

A total of 259 shoulders have been followed for more than 2 years.[39,90,92] Sixty-five had full-thickness rotator cuff tears. The rotator cuff in the remaining 194 shoulders was either intact or partially torn. Results were evaluated on the UCLA or American Shoulder and Elbow Surgeons Shoulder Rating Scale. The patients with intact or only partially torn rotator cuffs achieved an 88.5% satisfactory result. The overall satisfactory result of those with full-thickness rotator cuff tears was 55.4%. A further analysis of the group with a full-thickness tear indicates that the size of the tear had some bearing on the functional outcome. With this in mind, patient selection based on such additional factors as age, handedness, and level of activity becomes important in deciding whether rotator cuff failure is to be treated by arthroscopic or open techniques. Chapter 15, entitled The Scalpel or the Scope? Decision Making in Glenohumeral Instability, is devoted to this subject.

TREATMENT OF PARTIAL-THICKNESS ROTATOR CUFF TEARS: ARTHROSCOPIC AND MINI-OPEN

6

The histopathologic changes involved in progressive failure of the rotator cuff are described in Chapter 4. Simply stated, the rotator cuff insertion shows signs of wear before it tears completely. Codman described these incomplete lesions involving the articular, bursal and interstitial regions of the rotator cuff.[11] On rare occasions, the arthrogram may demonstrate a partial-thickness tear (Fig. 6–1). Ultrasonography may suggest a partial lesion, but it lacks specificity (Fig. 6–2). The MRI is of value for determining partial lesions. The T_2-weighted images are particularly sensitive in disclosing partial lesions (Fig. 6–3). The arthroscope allows confirmation of these lesions under direct vision. With this valuable tool, the location and extent of cuff fiber failure can be determined (Fig. 6–4), thereby enabling the examiner to deal with each lesion in an appropriate fashion and, ultimately, enhancing our understanding of rotator cuff disease and its treatment.

The prevalence of partial-thickness supraspinatus ruptures increases with age. DePalma reported the incidence of partial-thickness tears in 96 shoulders of patients aged 18 to 74 years.[47] Partial ruptures were found in 37%. Lohr and Uhthoff found a comparable incidence of 32% partial tears after examining 306 rotator cuffs at autopsy.[43] The age of these specimens ranged from 26 to 95 years. Nearly 20% of their specimens also had full-thickness tears. A smaller incidence of incomplete tears (13%) was reported by Yamanaka and Fukuda in their study of 249 anatomic specimens.[97] We estimate that, based on previously published studies,[58] partial tears of the articular surface outnumber those of the bursal surface in a ratio of 3:1.

CONSERVATIVE TREATMENT

The prevalence of partial-thickness tears revealed in anatomic studies suggests that such tears are not all symptomatic. On the other hand, a significant number of patients who are treated for stage II impingement ("fibrositis and tendinitis") could have some degree of undisclosed tendon rupture. Most patients with stage II impingement symptoms respond to conservative management, which includes (1) rest and avoidance of an offending activity, (2) nonsteroidal anti-inflammatory drugs, and (3) physical therapy, including methods to control discomfort and strengthening exercises within the subimpingement range designed to restore the balance of the rotator cuff musculature. No more than three steroid

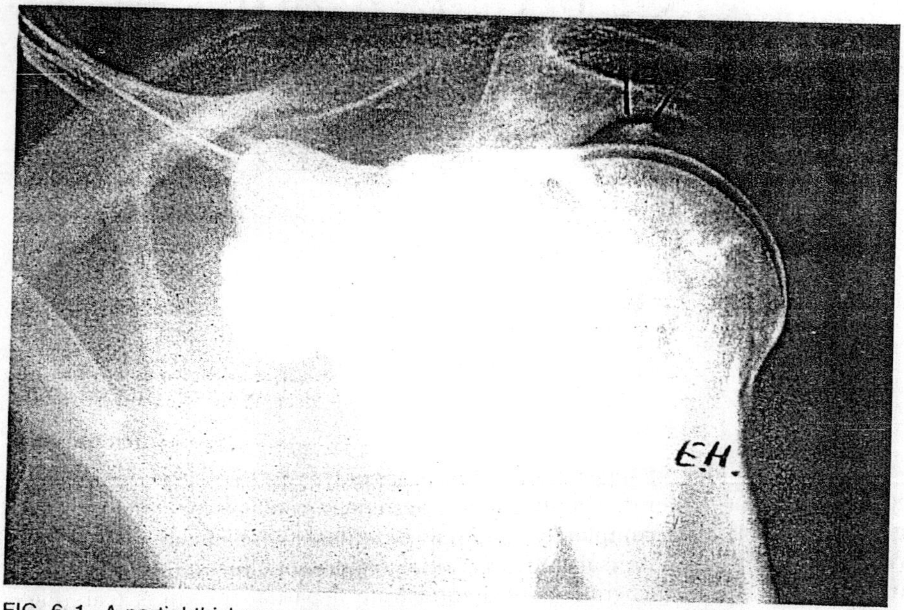

FIG. 6–1. A partial-thickness rotator cuff tear is occasionally demonstrated on a double-contrast arthrogram.

FIG. 6–2. Sonogram shows a band of echogenicity (white arrows) within the rotator cuff, thus suggesting partial-thickness tear.

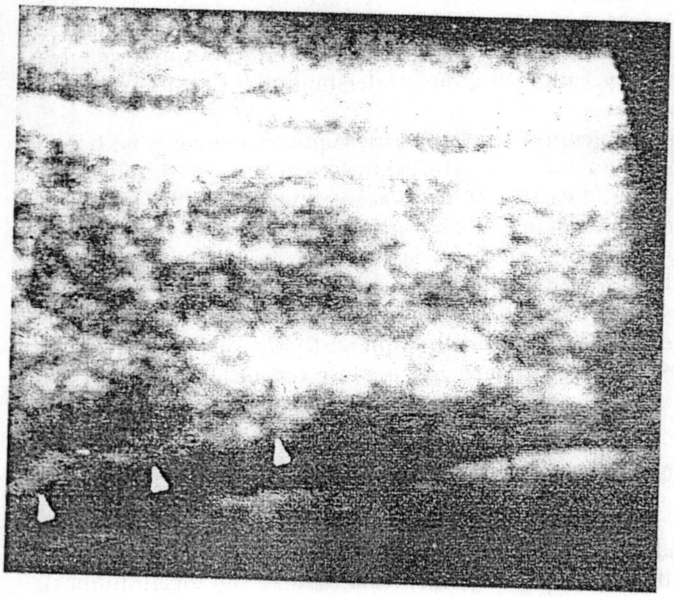

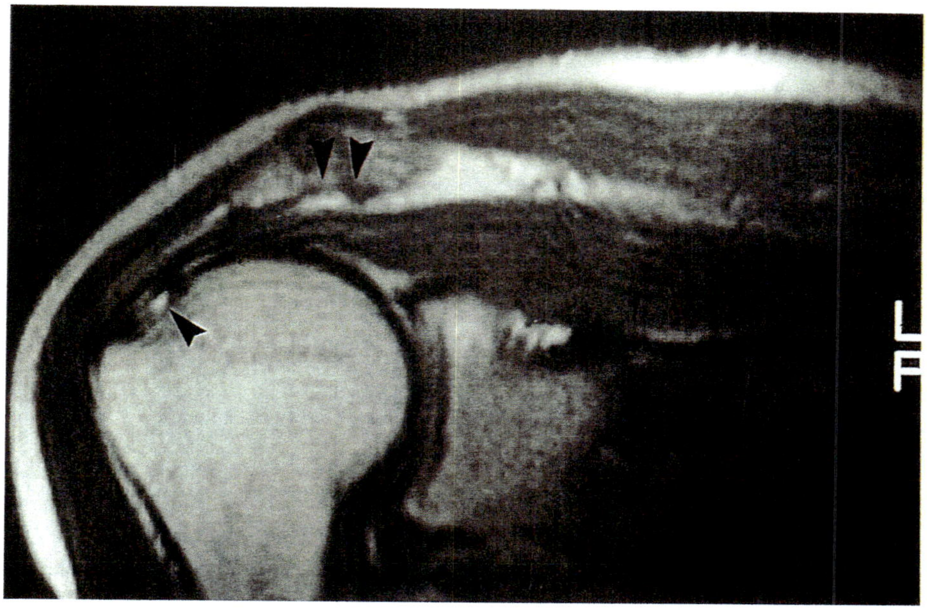

FIG. 6–3. T_2-weighted MRI image: Partial tear (grade 2A) in a 51-year-old tennis player. (From Ellman, H.: Diagnosis and treatment of incomplete rotator cuff tears. Clin. Orthop., *2*:54, 1990.)

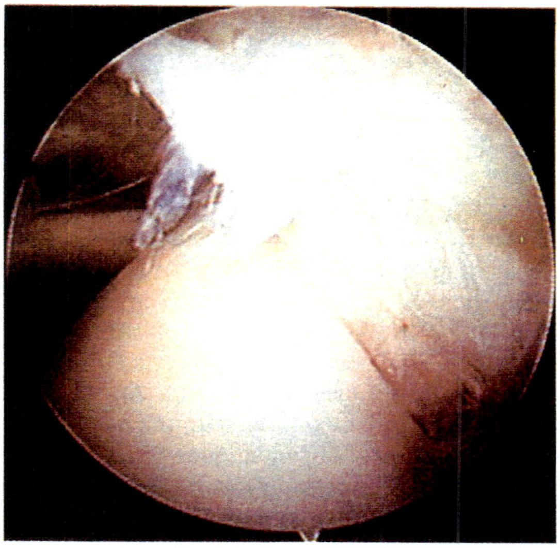

FIG. 6–4. Arthroscopic view of partial-thickness rotator cuff tear.

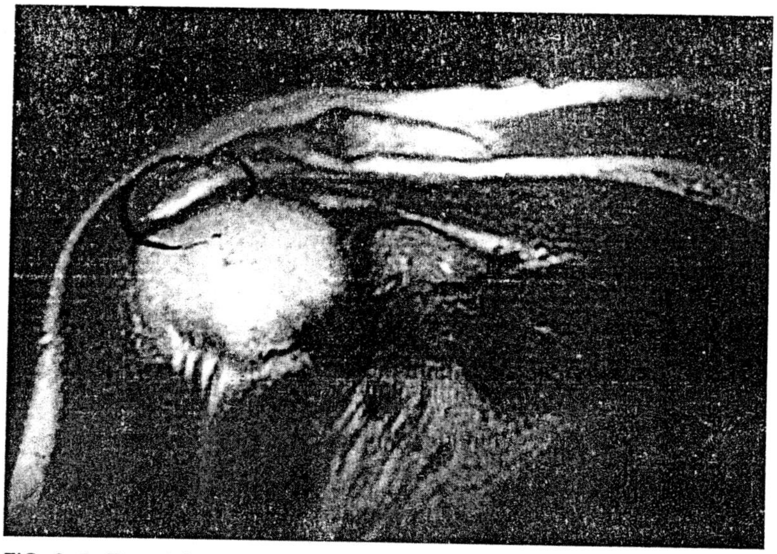

FIG. 6–5. T_2-weighted MRI study: The high-intensity (white) area within the circle demonstrates a full-thickness rotator cuff tear.

FIG. 6–6. Orientation sketch shows normal supraspinatus insertion.

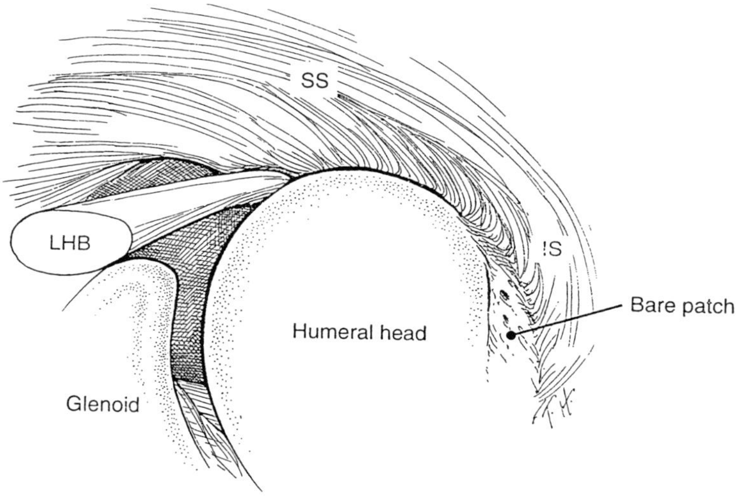

injections should be allowed during the course of treatment. When a full-thickness rotator cuff tear is suspected in individuals over 40 years of age, an arthrogram is recommended if improvement does not occur after 2 or 3 months of conservative management. MRI, particularly the T_2 -weighted studies (Fig. 6–5), can be useful for screening patients who have been treated conservatively for more than 6 months, regardless of age. The previously mentioned caveat should be heeded, however; even the most sophisticated MRI studies report difficulty in imaging partial-thickness or small full-thickness rotator cuff tears.

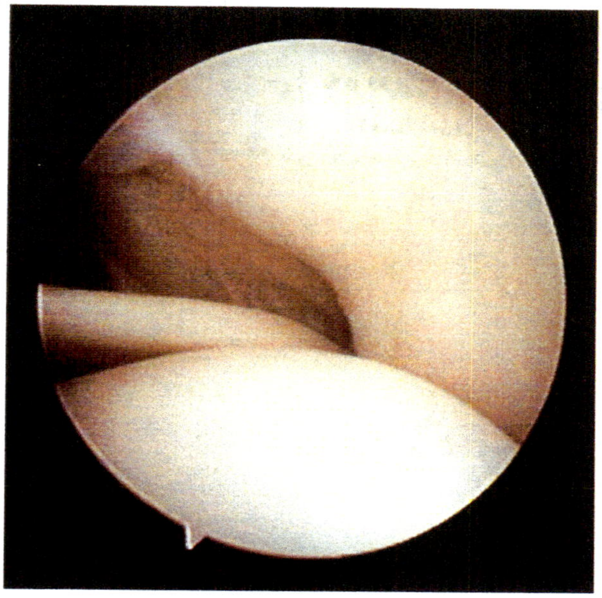

FIG. 6–7. Normal supraspinatus insertion.

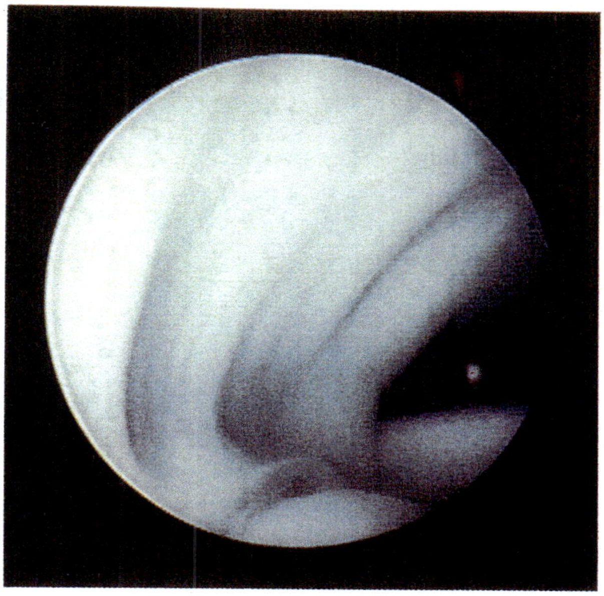

FIG. 6–8. Minute separation of the supraspinatus insertion is seen (left shoulder).

ARTHROSCOPIC MANAGEMENT

The patient with a probable partial-thickness rotator cuff tear who has failed to respond to conservative measures is a candidate for arthroscopic evaluation and treatment. The *articular surface* attachment of the rotator cuff tendons is examined through the posterior portal, as described in Chapter 3.

SUPRASPINATUS INSERTION

The supraspinatus insertion is just posterior to the point where the long head of the biceps tendon exits the glenohumeral joint (Fig. 6–6). The normal supraspinatus tendon hugs the articular cartilage in this region (Fig. 6–7). One of the earliest disruptions of the supraspinatus attachment that we have observed arthroscopically is illustrated in Figure 6–8. A minute separation is observed in the synovium and in tendinous fibers of the supraspinatus attachment into the sulcus adjacent to the articular border of the humeral head. This arthroscopic photograph corresponds to the pathologic section published in Codman's 1934 textbook on supraspinatus ruptures.[11] More commonly, the early articular lesion presents an irregular, frayed appearance (Fig. 6–9). This frayed capsule and strands of ruptured fibers tend to obscure the full extent of the lesion. Superficial debridement with a suction shaver is necessary to determine the extent of the defect.

An anterior portal is established with the Wissinger rod. The shaver is introduced and manipulated into a position superior to the long head of the biceps (Fig. 6–10A). As the shoulder is abducted and externally rotated slightly, the shaver is worked into a position where it can lightly debride the frayed capsule

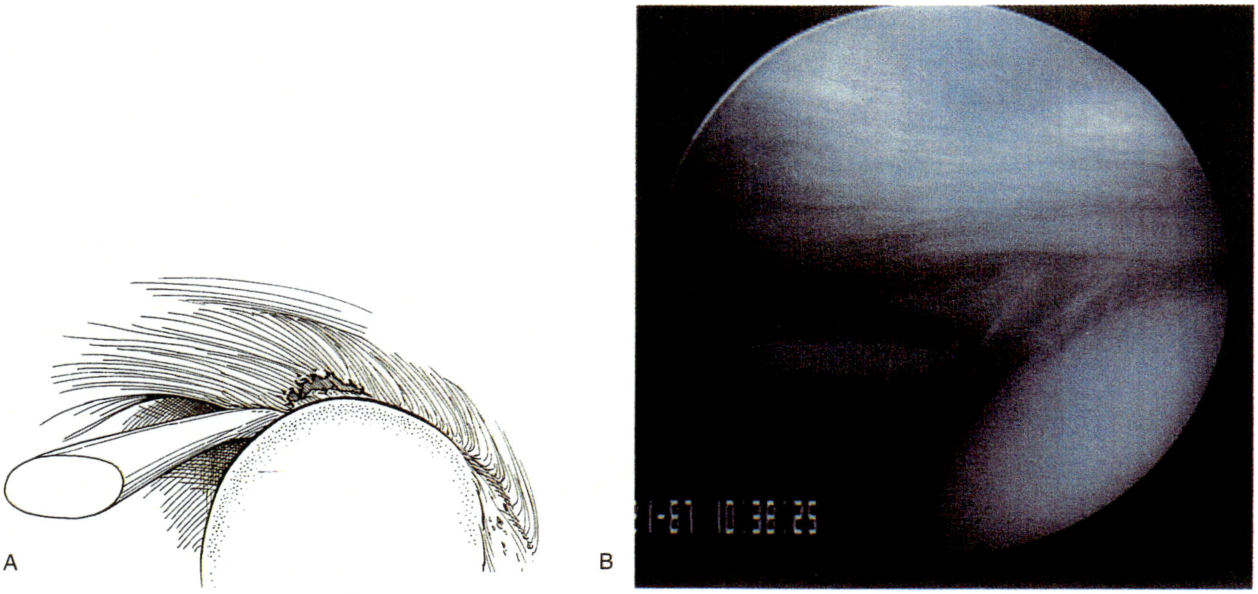

FIG. 6–9. Partial articular-surface tear.
A, Partial tear located in supraspinatus immediately behind the long head of the biceps.
B, Capsule and ruptured strands of fiber obscure full extent of lesion.

and torn cuff fibers (Fig. 6–10B). The shaver should not be so aggressive as to be capable of damaging intact fibers of cuff insertion. After light debridement, a 3-mm bent-arm probe is introduced through the anterior cannula and the defect is inspected (Fig. 6–10C). The probe may be used to measure the depth of the tear, as well as the area of the defect (Fig. 6–10D). The known diameter of the suction shaver is also helpful in estimating the dimensions of the defect.

In larger defects, a perforation of the cuff may be apparent after debridement (Fig. 6–11A). The probe may pass deeply into a laminated interstitial tear or, if the perforation is complete, may pass completely through the substance of the tear into the subacromial space. The deep partial tear can also be probed from the superficial surface. The lateral subacromial portal is established, and the plastic operating cannula with its blunt obturator is inserted. The obturator is used to palpate the subacromial surface and may enter the glenohumeral joint if a full-thickness defect is present (Fig. 6–11B).

Chronic, progressive rupture of insertional fibers produces a large articular defect with the osseous changes of insertional tendinopathy. As the cuff fibers separate from the articular attachment, they no longer hug the articular surface (Fig. 6–12). The exposed osseous surface of the trough between the humeral head and the tuberosity assumes the appearance of "craters and volcanoes" as described by Codman.[11] The process has been termed enthesopathy by Lohr and Uhthoff.[43] These cystic caverns or sclerotic osseous protuberances are easily seen on plain roentgenograms. The findings are often a reliable indicator of chronic cuff disease.

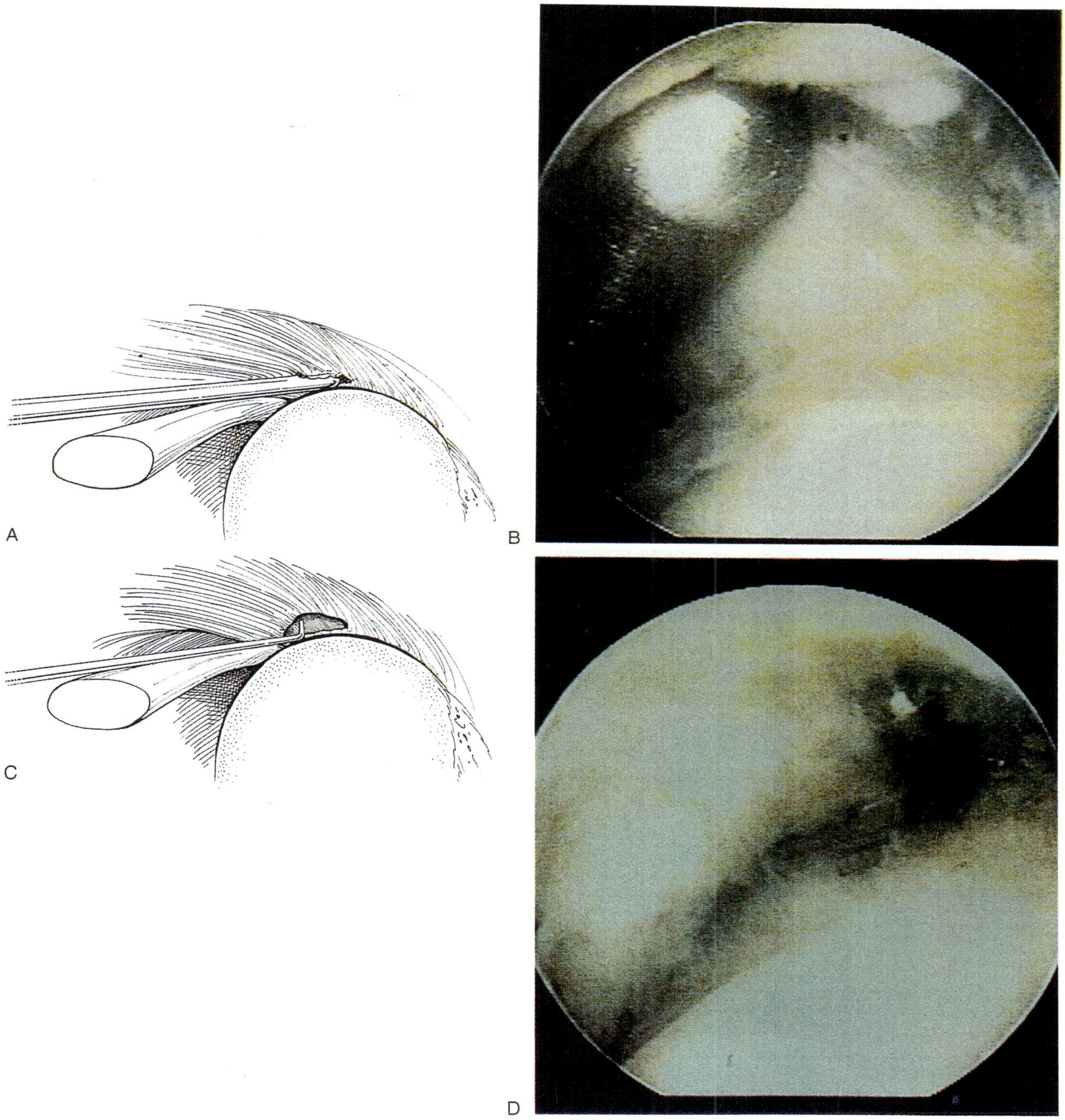

FIG. 6–10. Debridement and measurement of partial tear.
A, A suction shaver is introduced through the anterior portal and is positioned to begin debridement.
B, Debridement completed. Depth of defect is less than 3 mm, judging from known diameter of shaver.
C, A 3-mm bent-arm probe is introduced to inspect the defect.
D, A probe is used to measure depth and area of defect.

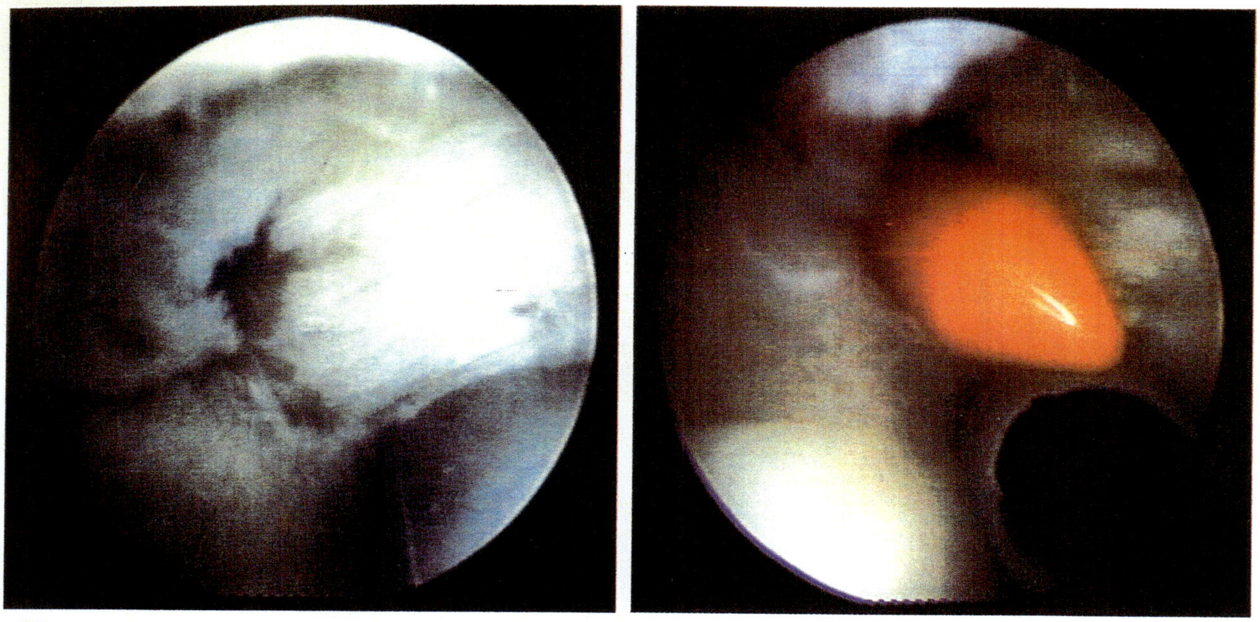

A B

FIG. 6–11. Full-thickness perforation.
A, Following debridement, a perforation is apparent.
B, A blunt probe, palpating from the superior surface, passes through the perforation.

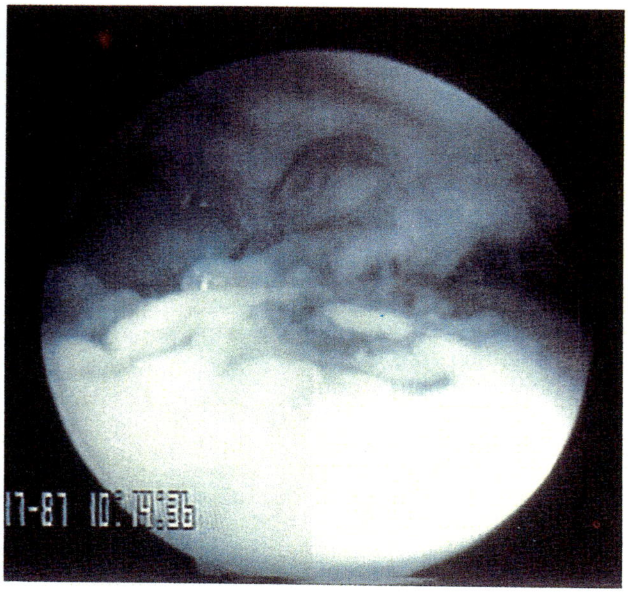

FIG. 6–12. With progressive failure, the tendon no longer hugs the articular surface, and "craters and volcanoes" are seen in the trough between the articular surface and tuberosity. The cuff is above, and the humeral head is below. (From Ellman, H.: Diagnosis and treatment of incomplete rotator cuff tear. Clin. Orthop., *2*:54 1990.)

INFRASPINATUS AND TERES MINOR INSERTIONS

The insertions of the infraspinatus and teres minor are inferior and somewhat lateral to the supraspinatus insertion (Fig. 6–13A and B). The more lateral insertion of the infraspinatus and teres minor exposes a portion of the intracapsular neck of the humerus that has been referred to as the "anatomic bare patch." The region is characterized by the appearance of several small, pitted openings, which presumably are the point of entrance for nutrient arteries (Fig. 6–13C, D,

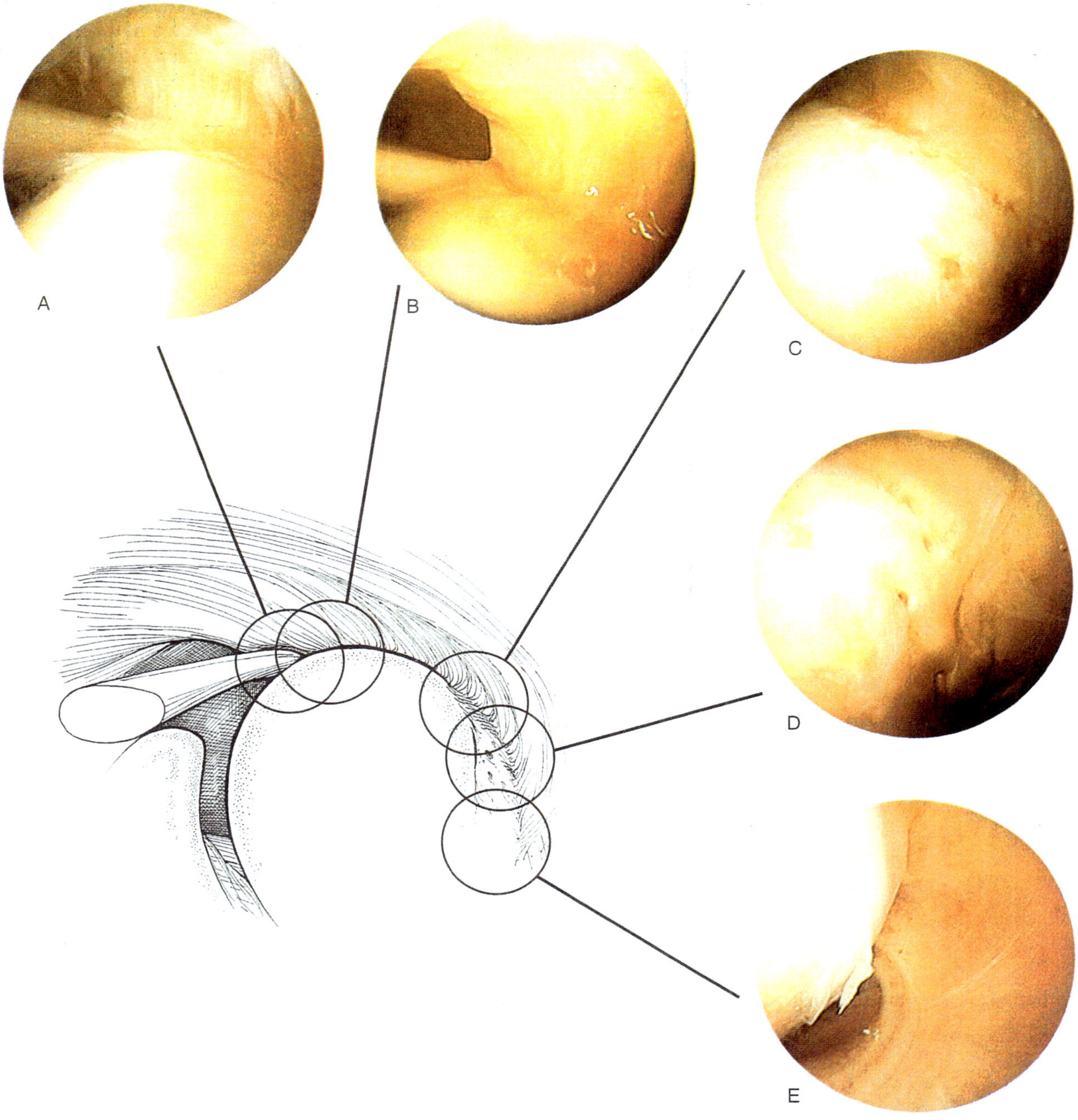

FIG. 6–13. Infraspinatus and teres minor insertions.
A, Supraspinatus insertion has been lightly debrided to show shallow partial tear in 68-year-old woman.
B, The beginning of the infraspinatus insertion is seen as a small portion of the intracapsular neck of the humerus is exposed.
C, The infraspinatus insertion is well lateral to the articular margin. Note small pits for nutrient arteries that characterize the "anatomic bare patch."
D, Still lower, the fibers of the teres minor are observed.
E, The inferior recess is coming into view at the posterior-inferior aspect of the joint.

and E). This anatomic area devoid of cartilage should not be confused with the Hill-Sachs' lesion. In most instances, involvement of the infraspinatus tendon insertion accompanies a lesion of the supraspinatus. On occasion, isolated ruptures of the infraspinatus and teres minor have been observed.

MARKER SUTURE INSERTION

Before leaving the glenohumeral joint, the location of a partial-thickness articular surface tear is tagged by placing an absorbable suture through the lesion. The location of the lesion thus is marked when bursal surface inspection is carried out. The technique for insertion is quite simple. With the arm in 20° of abduction and neutral rotation, a 20-gauge spinal puncture needle is introduced close to the anterolateral margin of the acromion. The tip of the needle can usually be directed into the area of the tear from this position (Fig. 6–14A and B). A No. 1 PDS suture is then passed through the needle into the joint. Enough suture is threaded intra-articularly to allow withdrawal of the lumbar puncture needle without extracting the suture as well (Fig. 6–14C). The point of exit through the cuff is seen on subacromial inspection once visibility has been established (Fig. 6–14D and E).

BURSAL SURFACE EVALUATION

Inspection for bursal surface tears of the rotator cuff requires the establishment of subacromial space portals (see Chap. 5). Chronic impingement provokes considerable bursal hypertrophy. An extensive bursectomy is necessary before the superficial aspect of the rotator cuff can be adequately inspected (Fig. 6–15A). Codman described the classic impingement lesion as "a deep red, more or less vascular zone of turgid membrane lying on the base of the bursa in the region of the supraspinatus facet."[11] We have noted that this lesion does not extend into the substance of the tendon; however, a whitish, anemic center has been observed (Fig. 6–15B and C). In more advanced cases, the tendon fibers in this area are damaged. Codman also described thin straps of supraspinatus tendon fibers separated from the tendon that "seemed to be worn as if from friction" (Fig. 6–15D).[11] Following bursectomy, the bursal surface of the cuff should be carefully probed through the operating cannula. The marker suture should be located and the contiguous area carefully probed for thinning, buckling, or perforation. Figure 6–15E shows an extensive incomplete bursal surface tear lying directly below the anterior hook of the acromion.

INTRATENDINOUS TEARS

Intratendinous tears may be present in many patients with "chronic tendinitis." Arthroscopic examination cannot identify these intratendinous disruptions until a tear has developed in either the articular or the bursal surface. Codman was ". . . convinced that some of the central fibers of the tendon may wear without those which are superficial to it on the bursal side, or beneath it on the joint side, being ruptured" (Fig. 6–16).[11] Yamanaka and Fukuda found that more than one half of the 33 partial-thickness supraspinatus tears found in 249 anatomic specimens were intratendinous.[97]

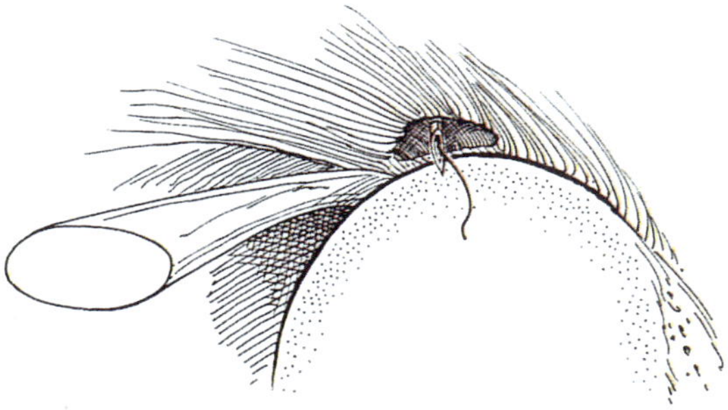

A

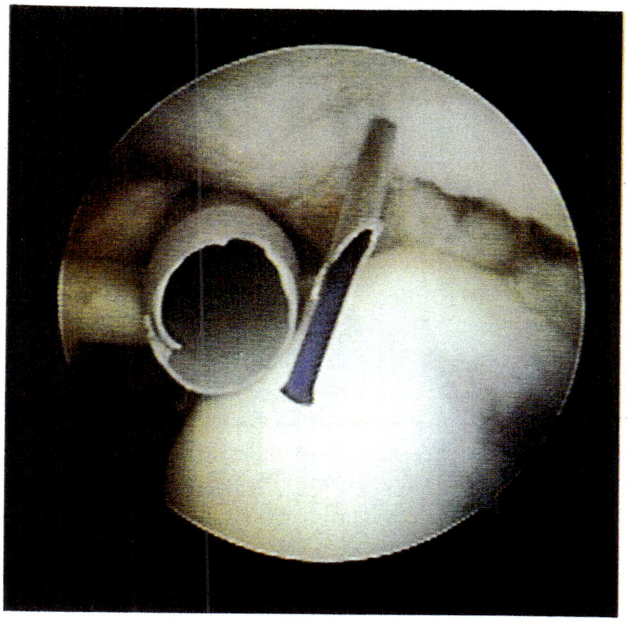

B

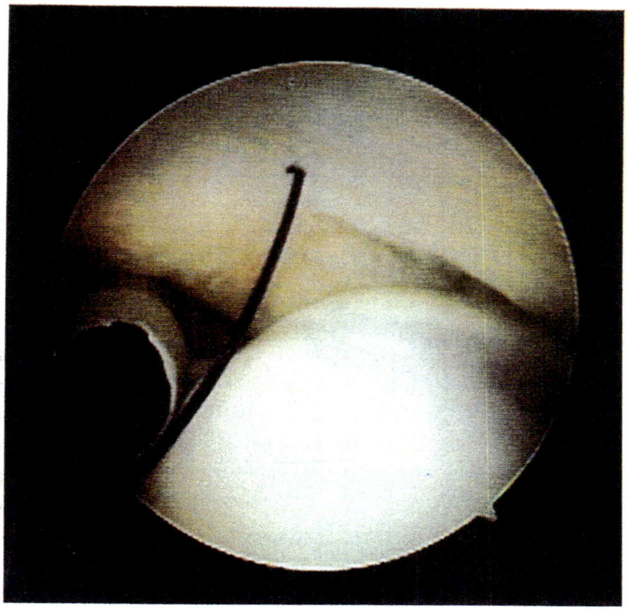

C

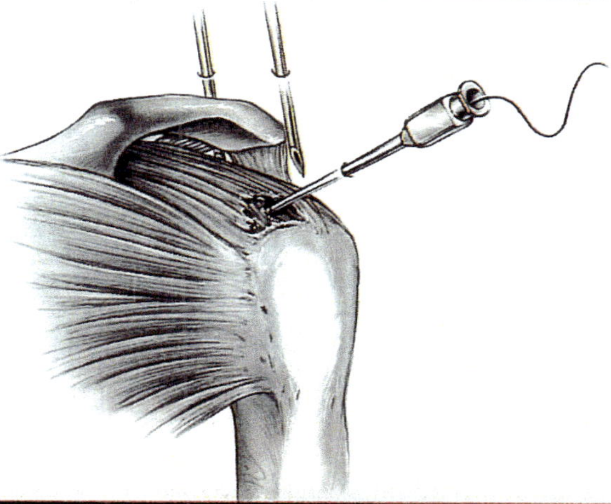

D

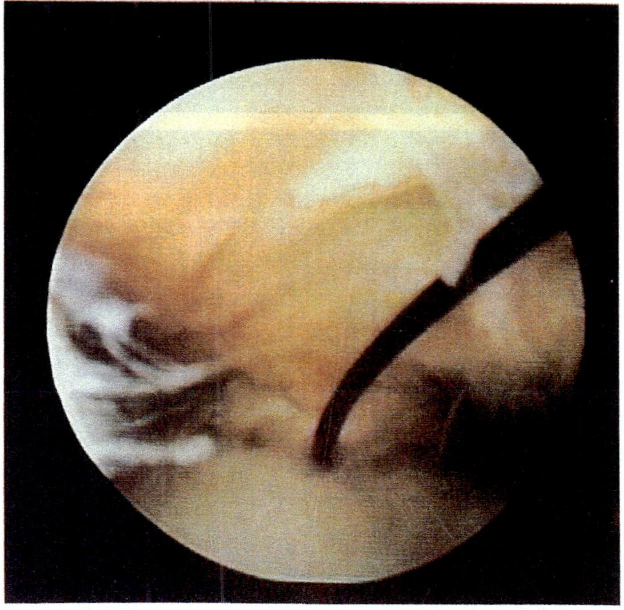

E

FIG. 6–14. Marker suture insertion.

A, A 20-gauge spinal puncture needle is introduced from above into the area of the tear.

B, The needle is in position, and a No. 1 PDS suture is being passed through the needle.

C, The needle is withdrawn carefully, and the PDS suture remains in place.

D, Position of LP needle used for insertion of marker suture is seen from the bursal aspect.

E, Spinal needle has been removed, and suture is seen from the bursal surface as it emerges through the cuff, thereby indicating the area of defect.

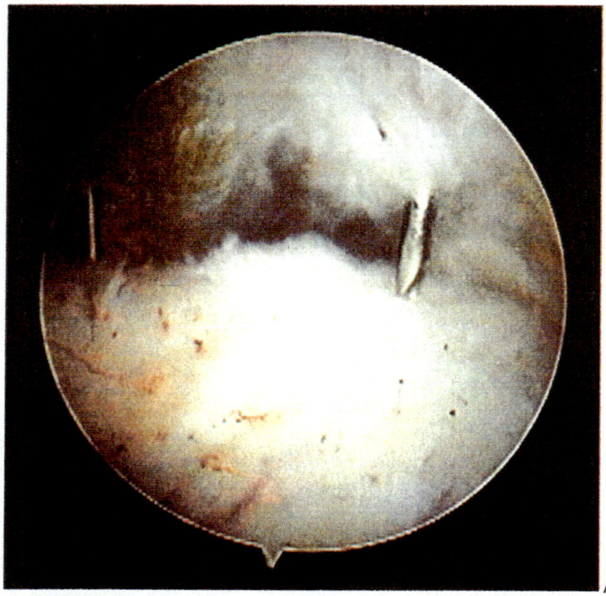

A

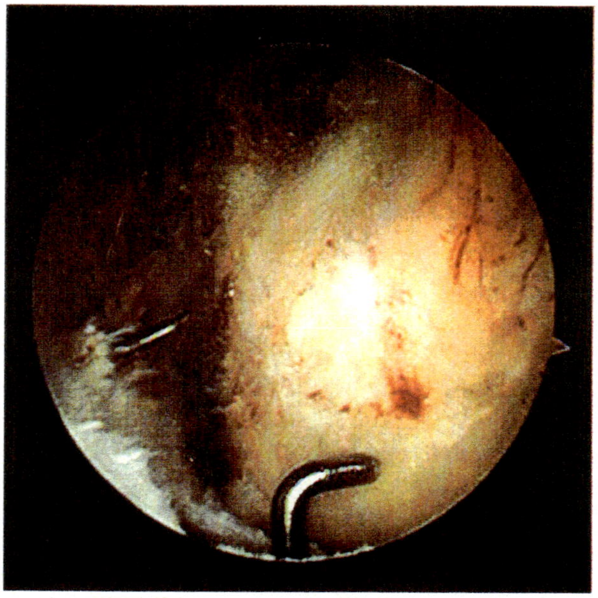

B

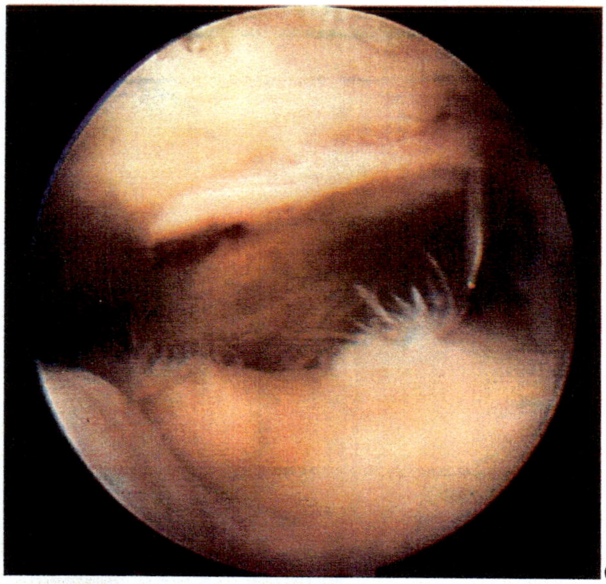

C

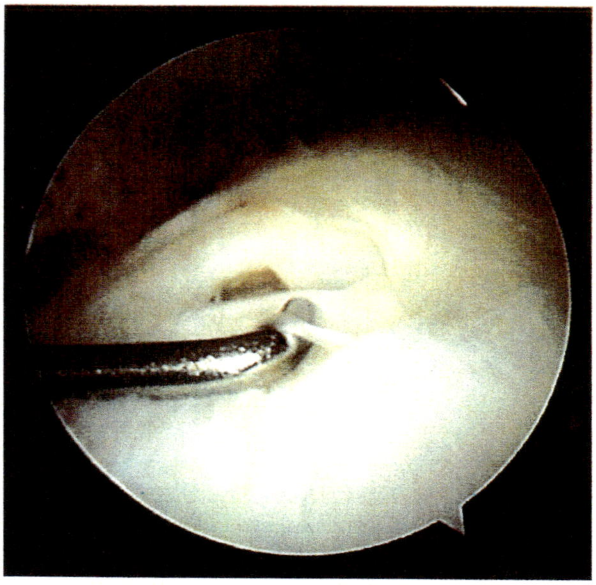

D

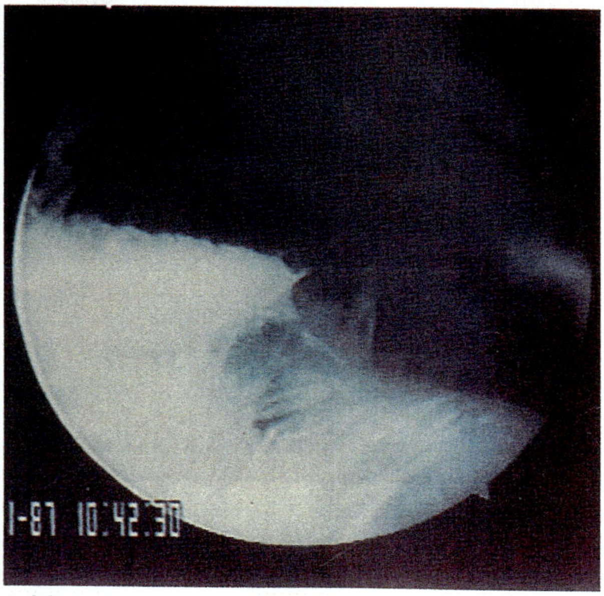

E

FIG. 6–15. A, Extensive bursectomy has been completed to begin inspection of the rotator cuff.
B, The superficial aspect of the cuff is eroded in the impingement area.
C, Bursal fraying is seen beneath the anterolateral corner of the acromion and is indicative of chronic impingement.
D, Small "straps" of worn tendon are seen at the periphery of a small full-thickness tear.
E, Extensive bursal-surface incomplete tear (grade 3B). (From Ellman, H.: Diagnosis and treatment of incomplete rotator cuff tear. Clin. Orthop., *2*:54, 1990.)

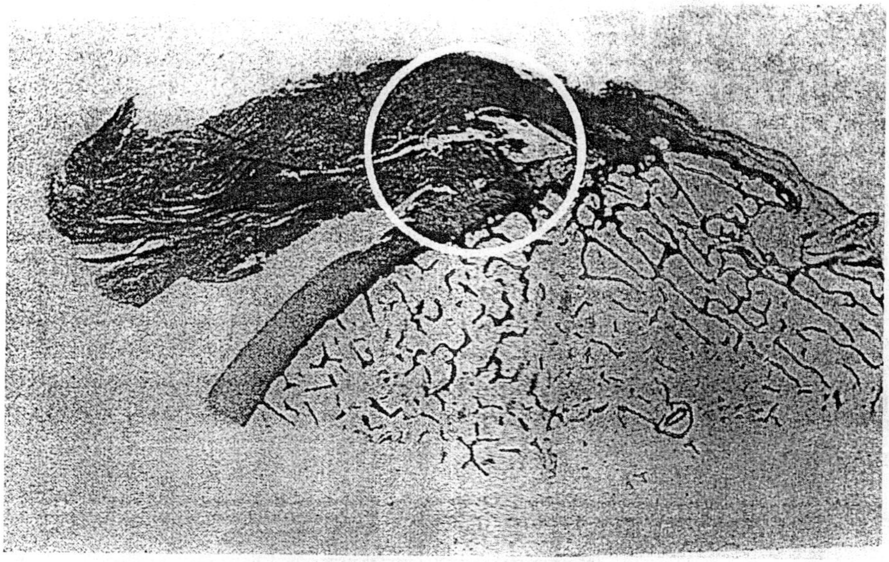

FIG. 6–16. Microphotograph of intratendinous tear. (From Codman, E.A.: The Shoulder. Boston, Thomas Todd, 1934.)

ARTHROSCOPIC TECHNIQUE

The arthroscopic treatment of partial-thickness tears is based on debridement of frayed and fibrotic cuff margins. Debridement is followed in most patients by arthroscopic subacromial decompression (see Chap. 5). Neer has described the rationale for anterior acromioplasty as follows: "The value of anterior acromioplasty is . . . that it retards the wear caused by persistent impingement and may prevent rupture of the supraspinatus."[1] An arthroscopic subacromial decompression is indicated in nearly every patient in whom mechanical impingement is the primary cause of a significant full-thickness tear.

PARTIAL TEARS SECONDARY TO INSTABILITY

In patients with partial tears associated with instability, the instability should be addressed primarily. These patients are commonly young competitive athletes who participate in sports that use racquets or require throwing. Whether the articular surface tear results from tension overload, external compression, or a combination of both, we recommend that *the primary treatment should be directed toward correcting the instability.* The goal is to compensate for the loss of overstretched capsular restraints by strengthening the more dynamic muscular restraints. If surgery becomes necessary, the instability should be corrected and significant rotator cuff tears repaired. Subacromial decompression fails when the instability has not been overcome.

CLASSIFICATION OF PARTIAL TEARS

Direct arthroscopic visualization allows classification of partial-thickness tears involving the articular or bursal surface according to the extent to which the cuff insertion has been disrupted. The classification indicates the location of the tear and grades the depth of the tear in relation to the full thickness of the tendon (Fig. 6–17) (see Chap. 4). A grade 1 partial tear is a relatively minor but definite disruption of tendinous insertion. The depth is less than 3 mm as measured by a small arthroscopic probe with a 3-mm bent arm or by the known diameter of a suction shaver (Fig. 6–18). A grade 2 lesion extends well into the substance of the cuff but does not exceed approximately one half of the thickness of the tendon. This lesion is generally between 3 and 6 mm deep (Fig. 6–19). Grade 3 represents a significant disruption that extends through more than one half of the tendon (greater than 6 mm) (Figs. 6–20 and 6–21). In this grade 3 lesion, some cuff fibers, either articular or bursal surface, are intact, but continuity appears tenuous (Fig. 6–22).

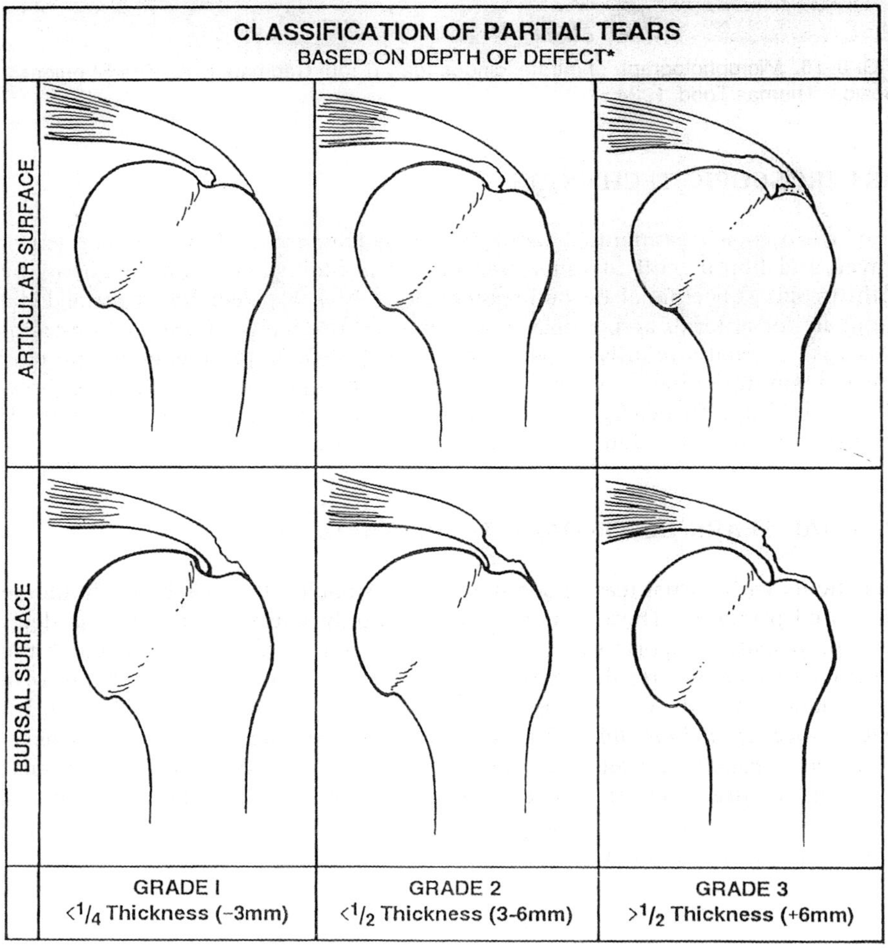

*Indicate AREA OF DEFECT: Base of tear × maximum retraction = mm^2

FIG. 6–17. Ellman classification of partial-thickness tears.

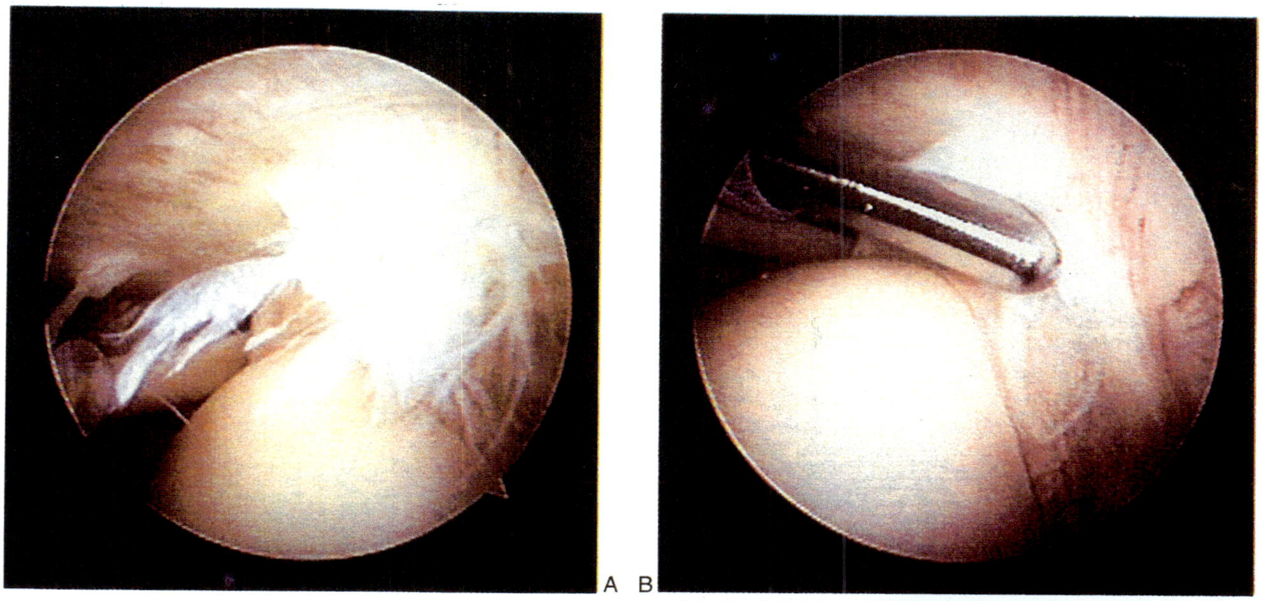

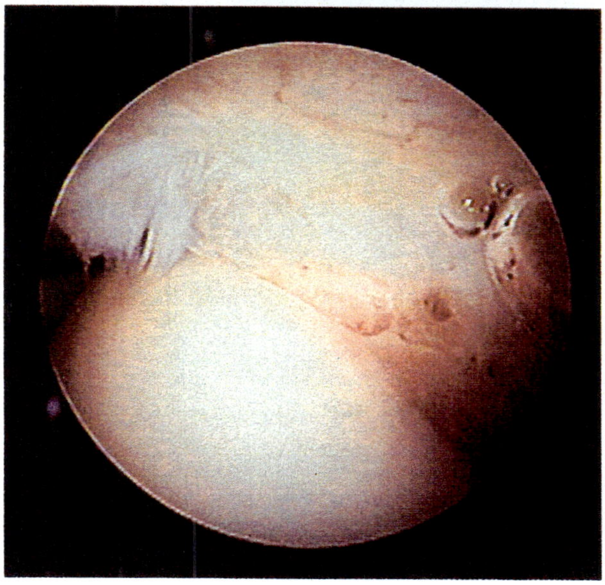

FIG. 6–18. Grade 1 articular tear.
A, Initial appearance of tear involving supraspinatus.
B, Debridement in progress with shaver 5 mm in diameter.
C, Final inspection shows that rotator cuff defect is quite superficial (less than 3 mm). Area of defect is estimated at 6 × 12 mm.

The description of a partial tear is completed by including the *area of defect*. This area is expressed in mm^2 by multiplying the length of the base of the tear by the width of maximum retraction (see Table 6–1). This comprehensive description of the cuff defect has considerable clinical relevance in deciding the method of treatment for an individual patient. In addition, an orderly classification standardizes the observations of future investigators into the study of incomplete tears.

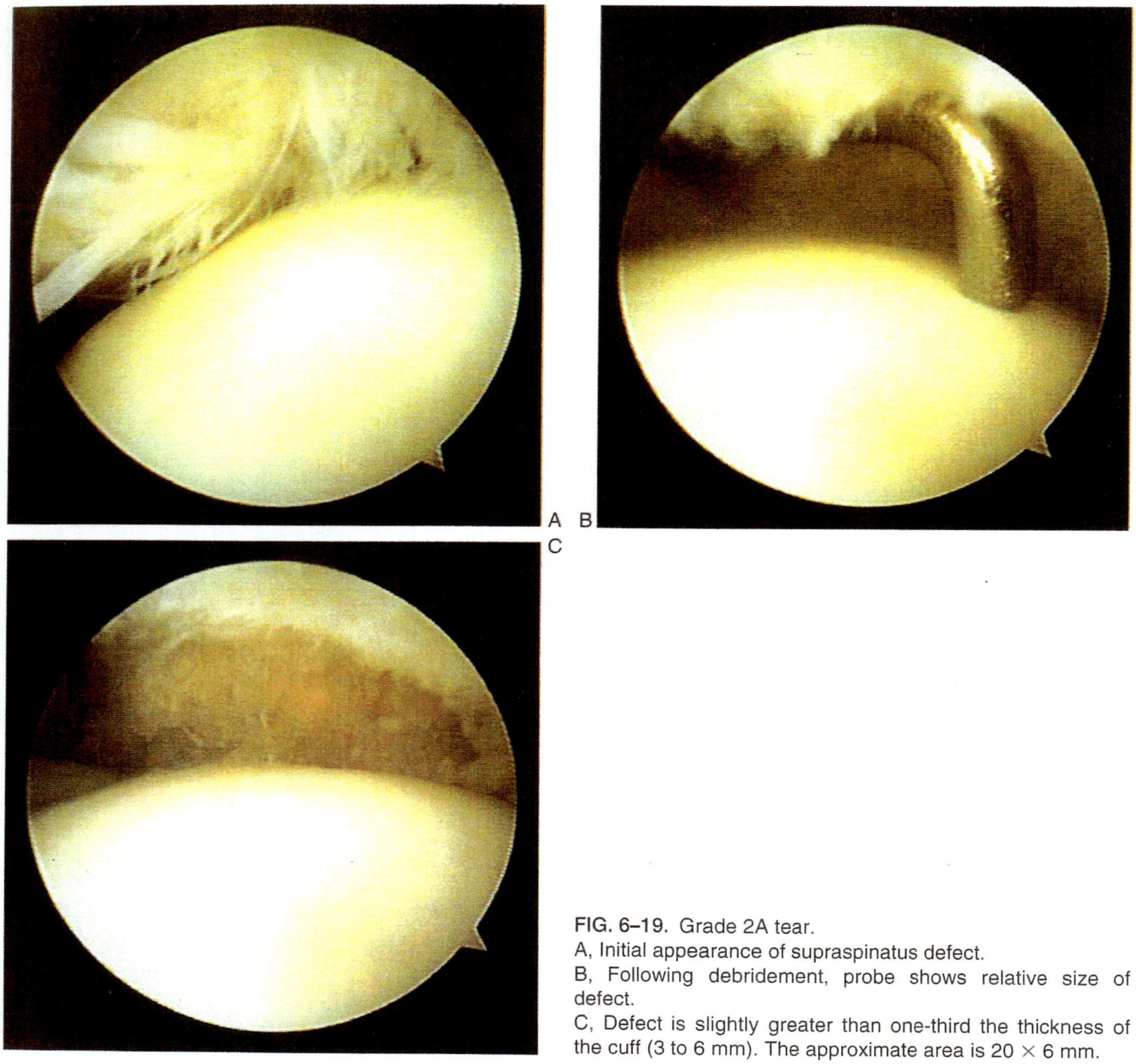

A B
C

FIG. 6–19. Grade 2A tear.
A, Initial appearance of supraspinatus defect.
B, Following debridement, probe shows relative size of defect.
C, Defect is slightly greater than one-third the thickness of the cuff (3 to 6 mm). The approximate area is 20 × 6 mm.

CLINICAL APPLICATION OF ARTHROSCOPIC TECHNIQUE

Our rationale for the arthroscopic treatment of partial-thickness rotator cuff tears is based on the extent of the defect, as well as on the activity level, arm dominance, and age of the patient. One cannot discuss the arthroscopic management of partial-thickness tears without considering the importance of acromioplasty in the treatment of these disorders. Although the cause of cuff failure is multifactorial, few shoulder surgeons would consider repairing a rotator cuff tear

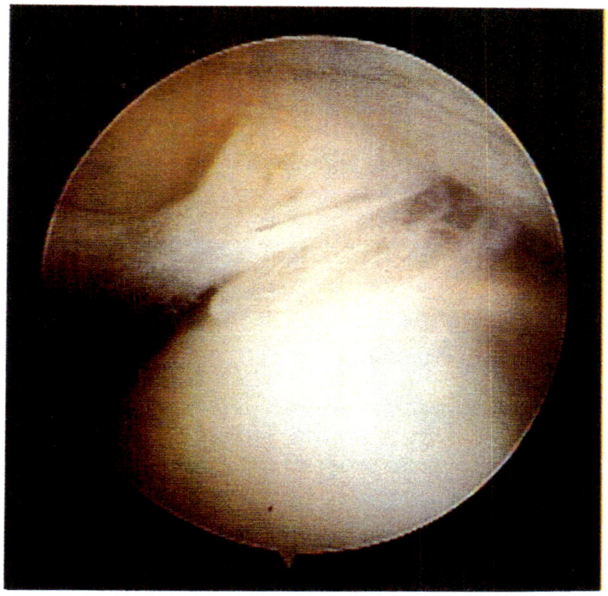

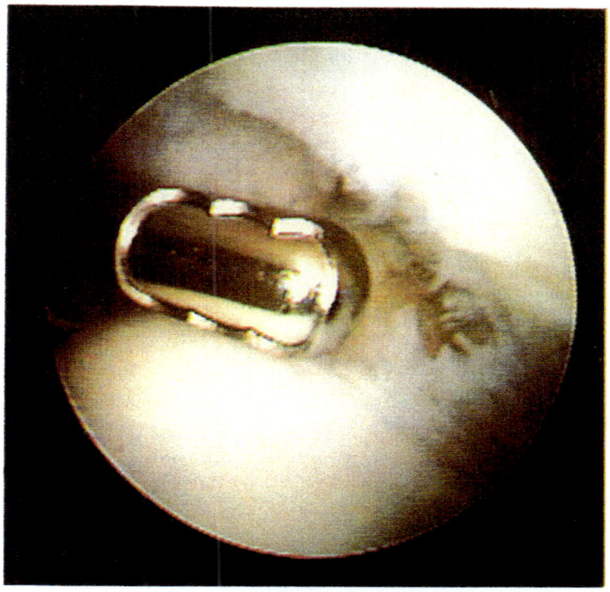

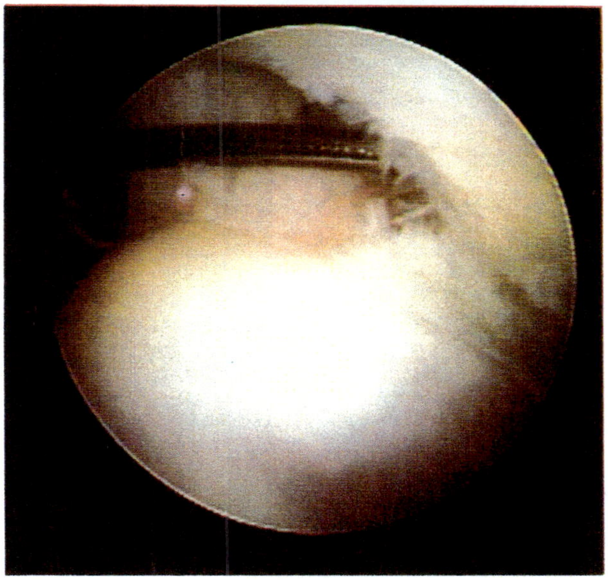

FIG. 6–20. Grade 3A partial-thickness tear.
A, Initial appearance of tear involving supraspinatus.
B, Debridement with 5-mm suction shaver. A portion of the tear extends deeper than one-half the thickness of the cuff.
C, A probe has been inserted in the region of the grade 3 defect.

without also performing an anterior acromioplasty. The relief of the symptoms following arthroscopic acromioplasty in patients with advanced stage II impingement syndrome without evidence of rotator cuff tear has been well documented. The results of arthroscopic acromioplasty reported by various authors have been less favorable when partial-thickness tears were present.[41,58,98,99] Although various factors influence the result, we believe that a vigorously active individual with a *sizable* partial defect requires not only acromioplasty but excision and repair of that partial defect to sustain the level of activity. Therefore, surgical decisions are divided into two categories, initially based on whether the tear involves less than or more than one-half the thickness of the cuff.

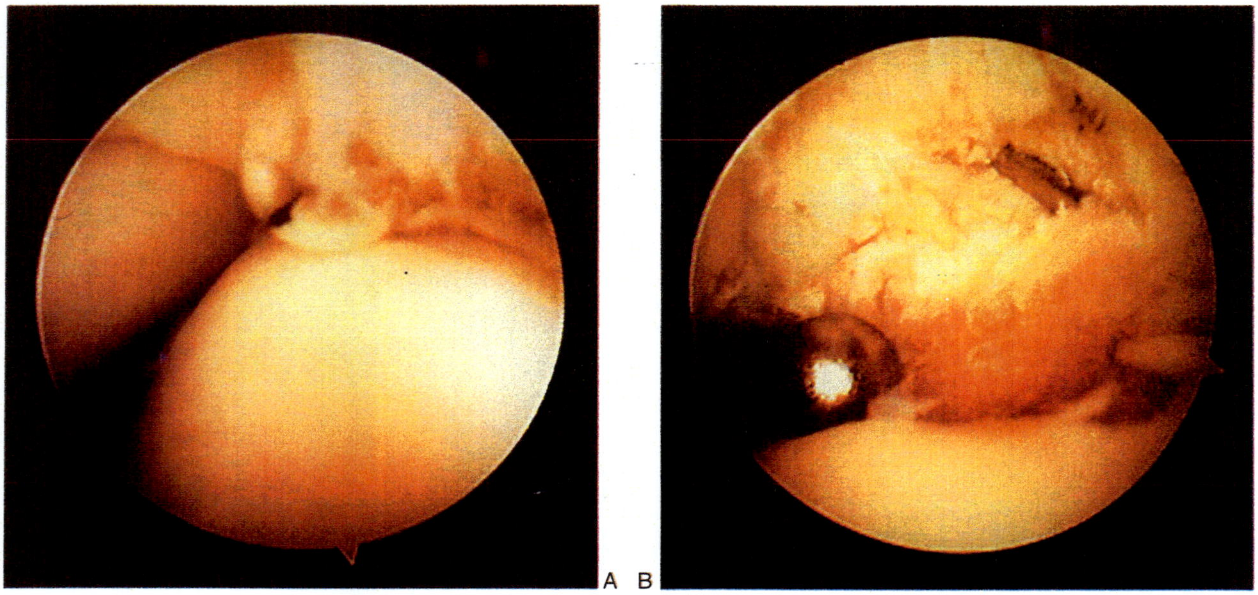

A B

FIG. 6–21. A more extensive grade 3 defect.
A, Initial appearance.
B, Extensive area of fiber failure with small full-thickness perforation.

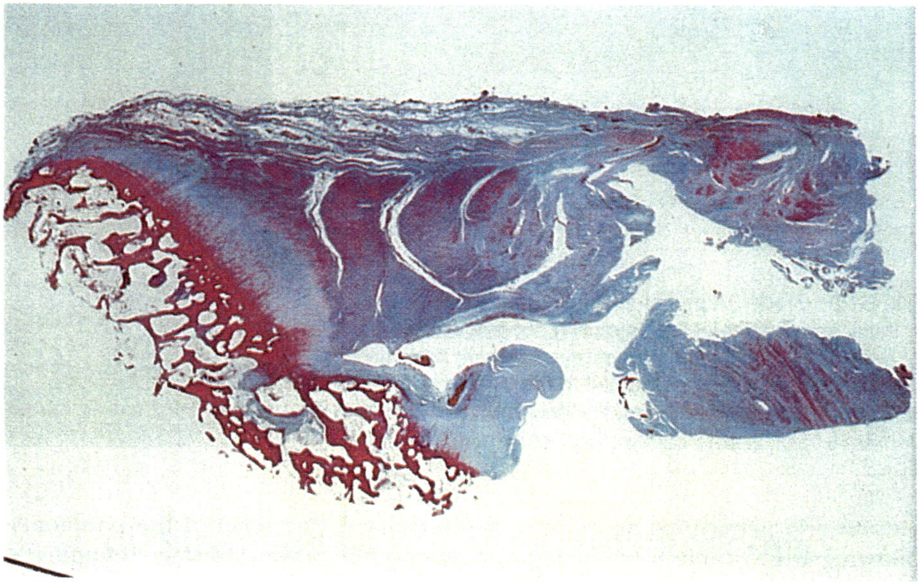

FIG. 6–22. Histologic section of extensive grade 3 articular-surface defect. The tuberosity insertion is on the right, the bursal surface is seen superiorly. The articular defect extends widely through the cuff substance and leaves only a thin superior bursal covering intact. (Slide courtesy of Hiro Fukuda, M.D.)

LESS THAN ONE-HALF THICKNESS

Tears that involve less than one-half the substance of the tendon thickness (grades 1 and 2) are debrided and decompressed, except in the young athlete who must throw and who still has an unfused acromial epiphysis. The coracoacromial ligament is released in these patients.

MORE THAN ONE-HALF THICKNESS

When the partial tear involves more than one-half the thickness of the tendon (grade 3), the surgical decision depends on whether the patient intends to return to a high level of strenuous repetitive activity with this shoulder. We have observed that when the supraspinatus insertion is torn more than halfway through, the competitive athlete involved in throwing, racquet sports, volleyball, and weight-lifting is much more likely to be dissatisfied with the result when a sizable partial-thickness tear is treated only by arthroscopic acromioplasty. The same, of course, is true for persons who must return to strenuous overhead occupations as well. On the other hand, less active individuals seem to get along rather well with debridement and decompression of a partial tear. Handedness is also a factor; the minor arm is less critical than the major. The reader should understand that these recommendations are based on the authors' clinical impressions gained from their experience. Ongoing end-result studies of these concepts are in progress. Another 15 to 20 years may be required to conclude a meaningful study.

TABLE 6–1. ELLMAN CLASSIFICATION OF PARTIAL-THICKNESS ROTATOR CUFF TEARS (STAGE P)

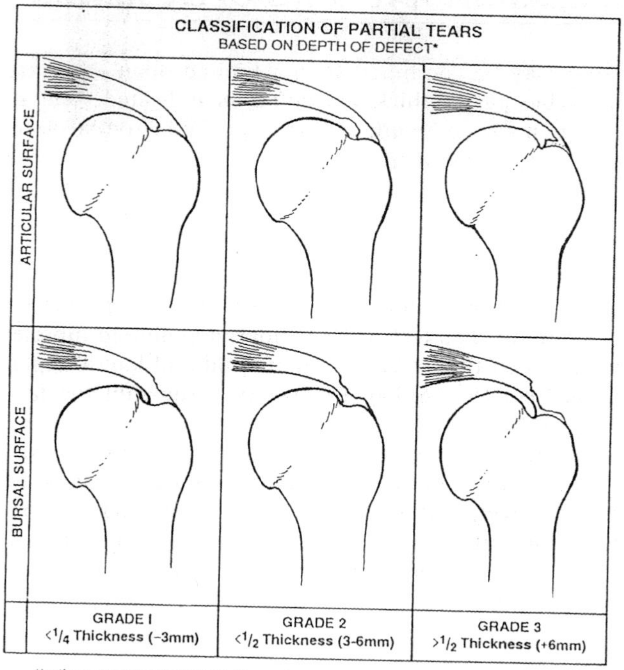

*Indicate AREA OF DEFECT: Base of tear × maximum retraction = mm²

THE PREOPERATIVE CONFERENCE

Increasingly sophisticated methods of diagnostic imaging, particularly MRI and ultrasonography, have demonstrated that specificity, sensitivity, and accuracy of interpretation decrease as the size of the defect decreases. Even the most experienced radiologist has difficulty determining the difference between "tendinitis," partial-thickness tears, and small (less than 2 cm) full-thickness cuff ruptures. This imprecision should be called to the patient's attention during preoperative discussions.

The patient and clinician together decide in advance on the course of action to be followed once the degree of fiber failure has been confirmed by arthroscopic inspection. The individual who anticipates full return to strenuous overhead activity, either vocational or athletic, is advised to undergo a mini-open repair following arthroscopic subacromial decompression if a significant defect is found. The patient is also informed that the mini-open procedure requires at least an overnight hospitalization and the same postoperative protocol for rehabilitation suggested for the open repair procedure. The patient participates in the decision, and the surgeon is advised to have this "what do I do if I find. . . ?" conversation preoperatively with every patient undergoing arthroscopic surgery for rotator cuff disease. The active patient undergoing arthroscopic subacromial decompression for advanced impingement syndrome is encouraged to consent to "possible mini-open repair" in the event that arthroscopic evaluation discloses a more significant cuff defect than was anticipated following clinical evaluation and diagnostic imaging.

COMBINED APPROACH: ARTHROSCOPIC DECOMPRESSION AND MINI-OPEN REPAIR

Arthroscopic technique may be combined with a limited open exposure when reconstruction of a sizable partial-thickness defect is indicated. The so-called "mini-open" approach is made following arthroscopic subacromial decompression and debridement of the partial tear.

EXPOSURE

The skin incision extends from the anterolateral portal proximally for 3 to 4 cm to the corner of the acromion (Fig. 6–23). The underlying deltoid muscle is then split along the raphe between the anterior longitudinal and lateral bipenniform fibers for a distance of 3 cm (Fig. 6–24). Extension of the split too far distally jeopardizes the axillary nerve.

The muscle is retracted, and the underlying bursa is split to expose the supraspinatus insertion. Bursal surface and small full-thickness tears are easily visualized (Fig. 6–25); however, partial articular surface tears may not be readily apparent through the intact superficial fibers of the cuff. Palpation may demonstrate buckling of the thinned tendon, but as noted earlier, the defect can be marked precisely during arthroscopy.

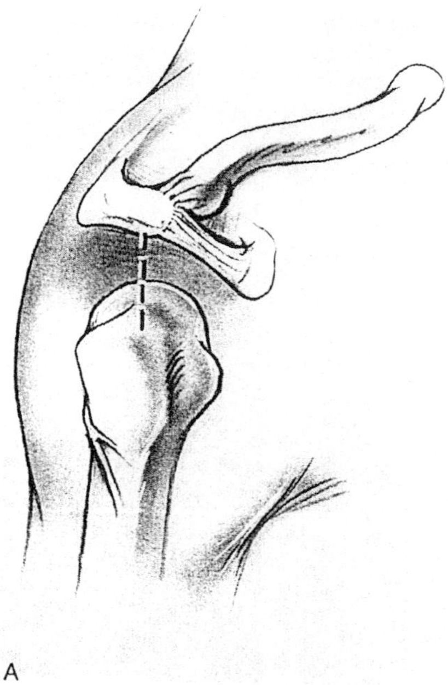

A

FIG. 6–23. Mini-open approach: Skin incision.
A, The anterior lateral portal is extended proximally to the corner of the acromion.
B, Scalpel at upper margin of anterior portal.
C, Incision completed.

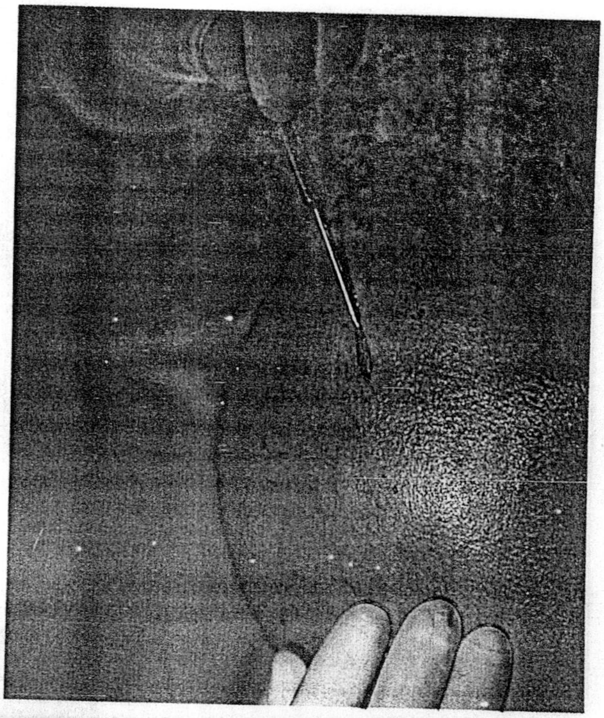

B

C

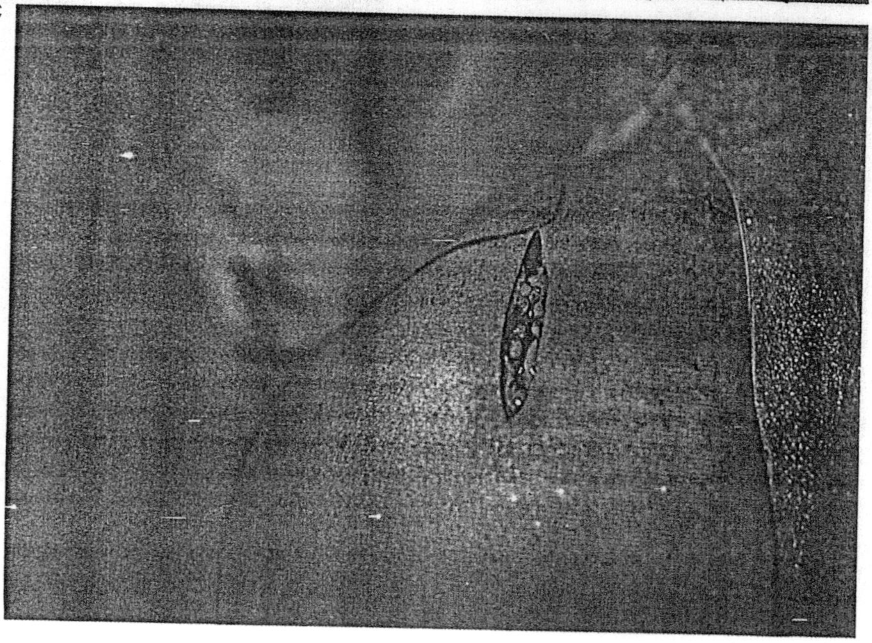

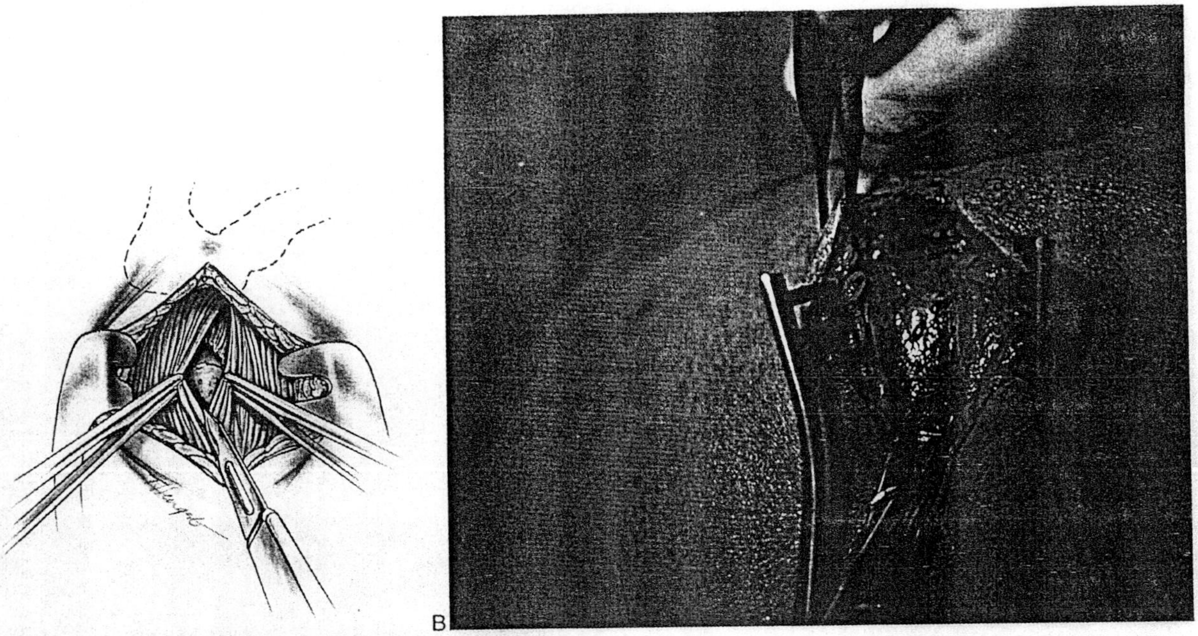

A B

FIG. 6–24. A, Deltoid split along raphe between the anterior longitudinal and lateral bipenniform fibers.
B, Extension of the split too distally jeopardizes the axillary nerve.

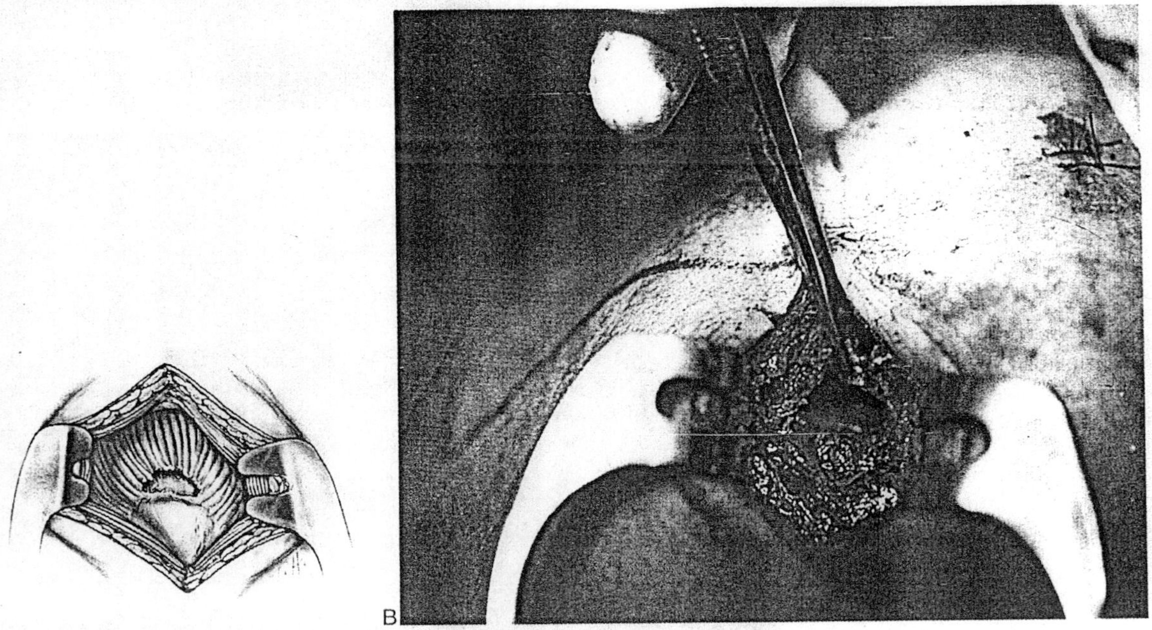

A B

FIG. 6–25. Mini-open approach: Tear exposed.
A, Muscle retracted to expose cuff tear.
B, Margin of tear is elevated to show extent of defect.

LOCALIZING A PARTIAL TEAR

Following debridement of an articular surface tear, an absorbable suture is threaded through a spinal needle as described earlier and is left in place to localize the area for subsequent viewing from the bursal surface (see Fig. 6–14). An alternate method of localizing an articular tear is to introduce a needle into the torn tendon and inject a dilute solution of sterile methylene blue.[100] The degenerated tendon becomes stained, and the discoloration usually can be seen from the bursal surface.

RESECTION AND REPAIR

Following identification of the area of partial rupture through the mini-incision, the overlying cuff is incised in the line of fibers for about 12 mm. This opening is widened as the degenerated margins of the torn tendon are progressively debrided back to normal tendon. A surprising amount of interstitial lamination may be encountered. Following resection of the degenerated cuff tissue, two patterns of defect are encountered: elliptic and crescent shaped.

ELLIPTIC DEFECT

An elliptic defect requires side-to-side closure (Fig. 6–26). Repair is made by apposing one side to the other with No. 1 nonabsorbable suture. Degenerated tendon should be adequately excised so that closure involves the approximation of normal tendon on either side of the ellipse.

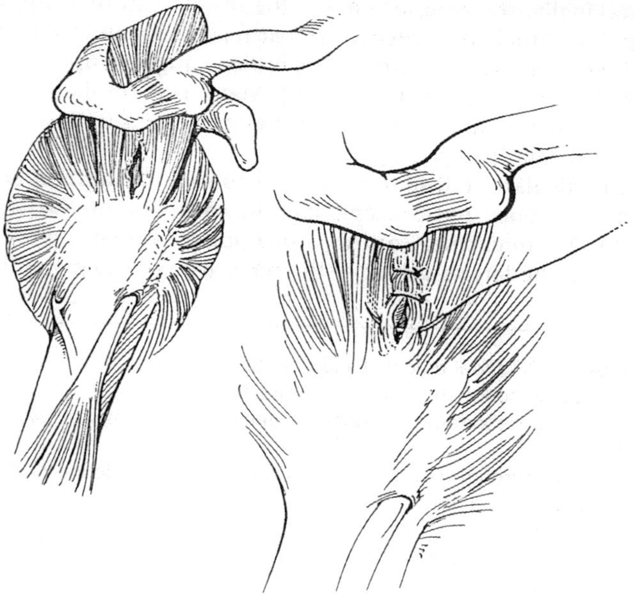

FIG. 6–26. Rare elliptic defect: Following excision of degenerated margins, defect is repaired from side to side with No. 1 nonabsorbable suture.

CRESCENT DEFECT

A crescent defect requires tendon-to-bone closure. In most instances, the resection of a partial tear leaves a crescent-shaped defect less than 2 × 2 cm in area (Fig. 6–27A). After thorough debridement, a horizontal mattress suture (No. 1 or No. 2 nonabsorbable) is placed into strong cuff tissue within 1 cm of the resected margin (Fig. 6–27B). The suture begins on the articular surface, penetrates to the bursal surface of the tendon, and then returns back through the tendon to exit the articular aspect.

The crescentic margin of the torn tendon should be returned directly into bone to restore normal tendon function. A shallow trough is prepared with a mechanized bur just lateral to the articular surface of the humeral head (Fig. 6–27C). Lightly bleeding cancellous bone must be exposed. An intraosseous suture is required for fixation. Every effort is made to create the origin of these osseous tunnels 2 to 2.5 cm distal to the tip of the greater tuberosity. The cortical bone may be quite thin proximally; consequently, more distally placed tunnels afford a stronger bony bridge for suture fixation. Abduction of the shoulder facilitates the preparation of the tunnels with a straight drill (Fig. 6–27D_1). Three tunnels are usually made for a small defect. The bony bridge between cortical holes should optimally be at least 1.5 cm.

A malleable suture passer with a nylon loop on the end (Richards) can be used to pass the suture through the osseous tunnel. The passer is bent into a gentle curve and threads through the most posterior hole first from below to exit in the groove adjacent to the humeral head (Fig. 6–27D_2). One end of the suture is captured by the nylon loop and pulled through the tunnel (Fig. 6–27D_3). The passer is then placed through the middle tunnel. The remaining strand of the first suture is combined with the more posterior strand of the second, and these are combined and pulled through the middle tunnel. The ends are sorted and paired appropriately. Different-colored sutures may be used for easy identification. Finally, the anterior limb of the second suture is brought through the most anterior tunnel and matched. The arm is then abducted to relieve tension on the cuff while the two sutures are each tied snugly to approximate the cuff margins into the bony groove (Fig. 6–27E). Tension is checked with the arm at the side as well as in rotation and flexion to ensure that undue stress will not be placed on the repair during rehabilitation.

A particularly efficient method of tunnel preparation and suture passing has been developed by Concept, Inc., in collaboration with S. Snyder, M.D. (Fig. 6–28). A semicircular cortical gouge punch is used to prepare a curvilinear tunnel from the lateral cortex to the bony trough. A circular bone rasp widens and

FIG. 6–27. Crescent defect: Tendon-to-bone closure. ▶
A, A small crescent-shaped defect is illustrated.
B, Following debridement, horizontal mattress sutures are placed through the cuff margins.
C, A shallow trough is prepared just lateral to the articular surface of the humeral head with a mechanized bur.
D, Preparation of bony trough: 1, Drill prepares intraosseous tunnel. 2, Malleable suture passer is used to capture suture. 3, Suture through osseous tunnel pulls margin of tendon into bony trough.
E, Cuff closure: Osseous tunnels are approximately 1.5 cm apart and 2 cm distal to the tuberosity. The middle tunnel shares a strand from each of the mattress sutures. The arm should be gently abducted to relieve tension while sutures are tied.

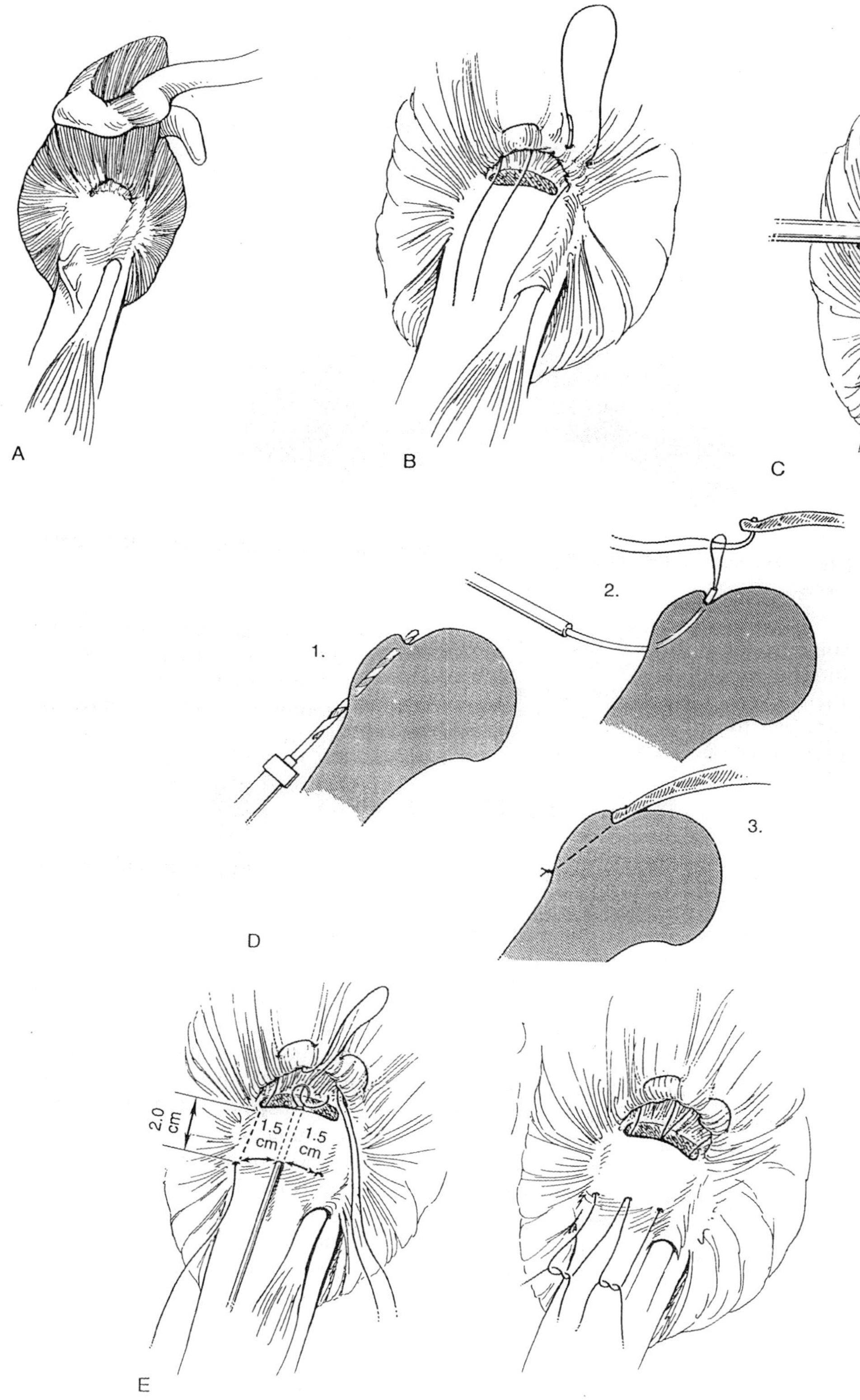
A
B
C
1.
2.
3.
D
2.0 cm
1.5 cm
1.5 cm
E

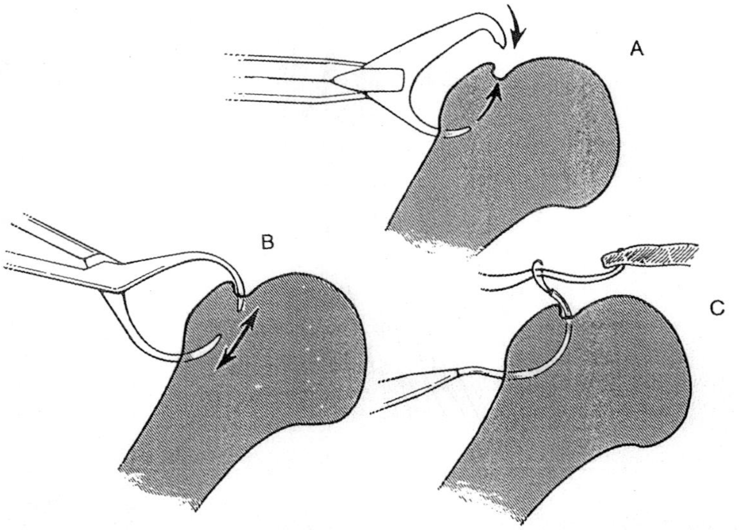

FIG. 6–28. Special instruments facilitate the development of osseous tunnel and suture passer.

smooths the tunnel. A disposable suture retriever of similar curvature is then introduced through the lateral cortex to retrieve the suture and pull it through the tunnel. The instruments are made in three sizes to vary the distance between the tuberosity and the lateral cortical osteotomy, as well as between each of the openings.

REHABILITATION

When the partial-thickness tear has been treated by debridement and decompression only, the rehabilitation is identical to that for patients without cuff tears who have undergone arthroscopic subacromial decompression. Passive range of motion is resumed as tolerated. No sling is required.

When mini-open repair has been performed for a large partial tear, the rehabilitation program is rather similar to the protocol followed by patients who have undergone open reconstruction for a full-thickness tear. A sling is worn for 3 to 6 weeks, depending on the size of the defect and the quality of the repair. Passive range of motion is begun on the initial postoperative day to minimize adhesion formation. The mini-open repair that was closed by side-to-side suture or the small crescent tear that was closed without undue tension is allowed antigravity motion at 3 to 4 weeks, but resistance exercises or lifting is avoided for a full 6 weeks. Morbidity following mini-open repair is much reduced in comparison to that following full open exposure. Because deltoid function is not impaired with the mini-open procedure, the patient regains shoulder control rapidly. Although length of postoperative hospitalization and amount of analgesic relief required are lesser for the minimally invasive procedure than for the open procedure, ample time must be allowed in either situation for the cuff to heal properly before the shoulder is subjected to stressful activity.

OPEN REPAIR OF FULL-THICKNESS ROTATOR CUFF TEARS

7

A successful open reconstruction of a full-thickness rotator cuff tear produces optimal functional results when compared to the results from any other method of treatment. Open reconstruction is routinely accompanied by anterior acromioplasty, release of the coracoacromial ligament, and removal of any downward protruding spurs arising from the acromioclavicular (AC) joint.

This chapter is devoted to the technique of open reconstruction of full-thickness rotator cuff tears. The technical difficulty involved in repair, as well as the eventual results, are influenced by the size of the defect and the quality of the tissue being repaired.

PATTERNS OF TEAR

The progressive failure of cuff fiber insertion produces several types of commonly encountered defects. Once the tendon separates from its insertion, the torn margin is retracted by the unopposed pull of the torn muscle and its neighbors. An understanding of these patterns of tear facilitates reconstruction. The musculotendinous rotator cuff is illustrated in Figure 7–1.

CRESCENT TEARS

With few exceptions, a full-thickness tear initially involves the supraspinatus muscle. Medial retraction presents a crescent-shaped defect beginning near the long head of the biceps tendon and arching medially and posteriorly for 2 to 3 cm (Fig. 7–2). Extension of the tear gradually (and at times acutely) involves the origin of the infraspinatus, beginning at its most anterior aspect and extending posteriorly and inferiorly as its insertion arches around the tuberosity. Involvement of the infraspinatus not only widens the defect, but tends to pull the apex somewhat posteriorly. Isolated tears of the supraspinatus (Matsen stage 1) are relatively small, often 2 cm or less. Extension of the tear into a second muscle, the infraspinatus, progressively widens the base of the crescent and allows a greater degree of retraction by the combined forces of both the supra- and the infraspinatus (Matsen stage 2).

FIG. 7–1. Rotator cuff musculature.

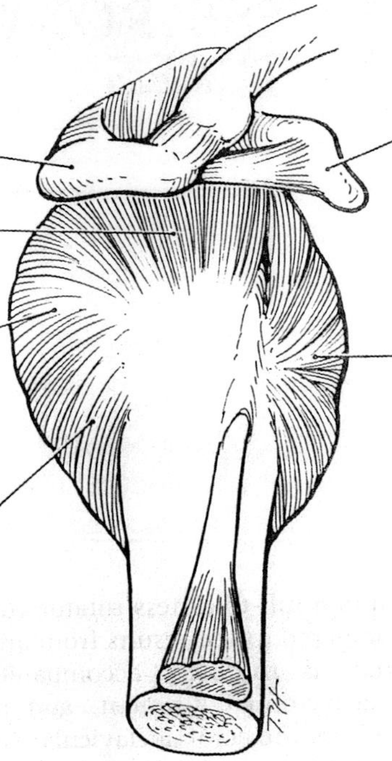

TRIANGULAR DEFECT (REVERSE-L OR L-SHAPED TEAR)

A moderate-sized triangular defect is most commonly produced when a supraspinatus tear extends medially along its anterior border in a line with the long head of the biceps tendon (Fig. 7–3A). This limb of the tear is located through the relatively thin fibrocapsular area between the subscapularis and supraspinatus. The long head of the biceps tendon travels below the interval, whereas the coracohumeral ligament joins this interval from above as it courses toward its insertion. The torn surfaces outline a reverse L. The cuff margin retracted medially and posteriorly forms the hypotenuse of the triangular defect.

A less commonly observed variation involves a tear of the supraspinatus with extension of the tear medially between the junction of the supra- and the infraspinatus fibers (Fig. 7–3B). In this *L-shaped* tear, the torn end of the infraspinatus has retracted medially and somewhat anteriorly. The pattern of retraction must be appreciated to identify the retracted edge and return it to its origin. Larger L-shaped tears are created as increasing portions of the infraspinatus become involved.

TRAPEZOIDAL TEARS

The trapezoidal tear generally develops when both the supraspinatus and the infraspinatus are torn (Matsen stage 2) and the tear extends anteriorly along the rotator interval and posteriorly into the interval between the infraspinatus and teres minor (Fig. 7–4). The torn edges of the supra- and infraspinatus may be retracted medially to the level of the glenoid. In some instances, portions of the tendon and its musculotendinous junction may be literally ground away

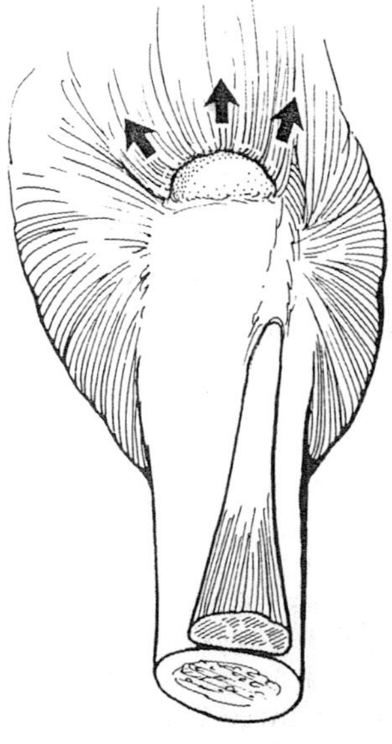

CRESCENT

FIG. 7–2

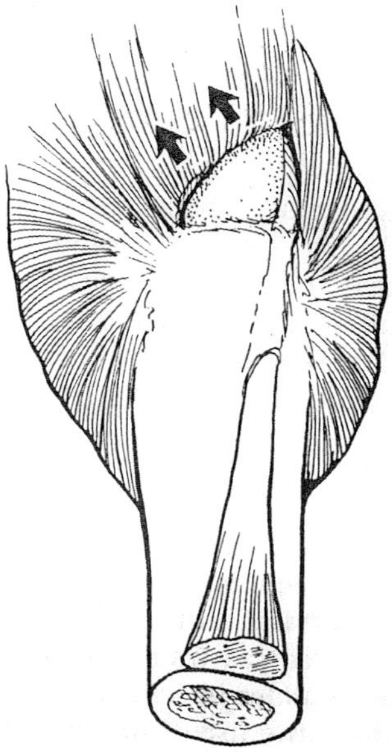

REVERSE "L"

FIG. 7–3A

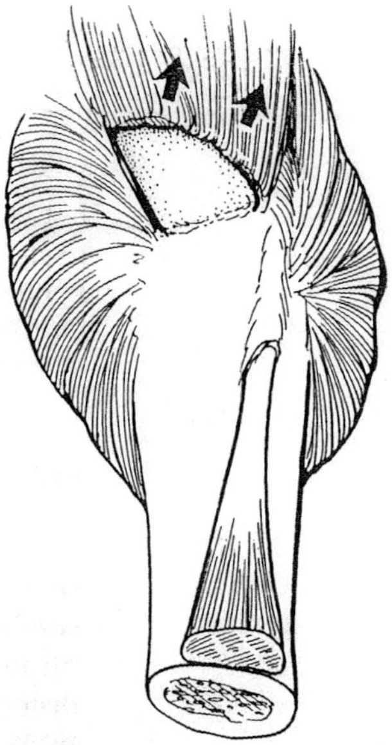

L-SHAPED

FIG. 7–3B

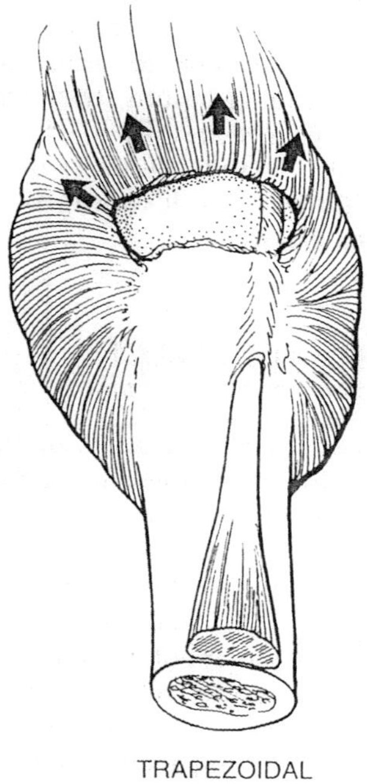

TRAPEZOIDAL

FIG. 7–4

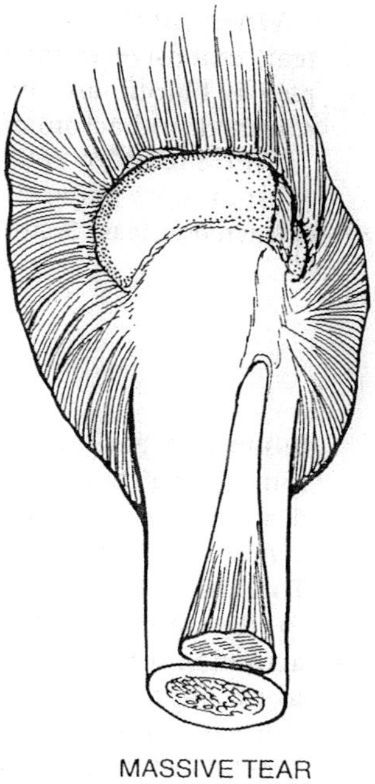

MASSIVE TEAR

FIG. 7–5

FIG. 7–2. Crescent tear: Tear involves supraspinatus tendon. Note direction of muscle pull (arrows).

FIG. 7–3. Triangular defect (reverse L or L-shaped tear). Arrows show direction of muscle pull.
A, Reverse L: Supraspinatus tear extends medially through rotator cuff interval in line with long head of biceps tendon.
B, L-shaped tear: Supraspinatus tear has extended through junction with infraspinatus, thereby producing an anteromedial displacement.

FIG. 7–4. Trapezoidal tear: This tear results when both supraspinatus and infraspinatus are torn. As more of the infraspinatus insertion fails, the trapezoid enlarges. Arrows show direction of muscle pull.

FIG. 7–5. Massive tear: When three muscles are involved, the tear is usually massive. Two-muscle tears should be retracted at least 5 cm to be designated massive.

between the undersurface of the acromion and the humeral head as the head rises superiorly during overhead elevation of the arm. A pebbled and irregular appearance of the humeral head suggests the lengthy presence of the cuff defect. On the other hand, a relatively smooth, glistening dome suggests that the extensive two-muscle tear may be more recent in origin and more likely repairable.

MASSIVE TEAR

The pattern of a massive tear is somewhat unpredictable (Fig. 7–5). The Matsen staging system for degenerative tears describes a stage 3 tear as including the supraspinatus and infraspinatus, as well as the subscapularis. Tears of this magnitude commonly occur as traumatic avulsions associated with acute anterior dislocation of the shoulder in individuals older than 40 years of age. Few objections can be made to the use of the term "massive tear" in these circumstances. Although some degree of cuff degeneration may have pre-existed the acute trauma, extensive areas show evidence of recent avulsion. The long head of the biceps is often displaced in these circumstances.

When chronic progression of cuff degeneration has caused all three muscles to tear, extensive retraction is present, and the retracted musculotendinous complex is fibrotic and inelastic. In long-standing lesions, the greater tuberosity is rounded, and acromiohumeral arthritis is present.

The literature reflects some diversity in the definition of a "massive tear." Most authors agree that a tear should involve at least 2 muscles and should be retracted at least 5 cm to be designated massive.

SURGICAL APPROACH

Surgery is performed under endotracheal anesthesia with the patient in the semi-sitting (beach chair) position. Following sterile preparation of the skin and draping, the bony landmarks are outlined. The anterosuperior skin incision is centered over the acromion and placed along lines of skin cleavage (Fig. 7–6A). The total length of the incision is approximately 8 cm, beginning 3 cm posterior to the anterior edge of the acromion and extending distally beyond the acromion for no more than 5 cm. The subcutaneous tissue is dissected medially to expose the AC joint and laterally beyond the lateral margin of the acromion. Curved Adson cerebellar retractors are placed to maintain exposure. The deltoid is detached from the anterior acromion by using a surgical electrode. The dissection begins on the superior surface of the acromion, about 0.5 cm posterior to its anterior edge. A thick osteoperiosteal flap is developed, beginning just lateral to the AC joint and extending to the anterolateral margin of the acromion. From this point, the deltoid is split distally between the longitudinal fibers of the anterior deltoid border and the thicker bipenniform fibers of the lateral deltoid. The deltoid should not be split distally for more than 4 cm in the average-sized person. In small individuals a split beyond 3 cm may endanger the nerve. A suture is placed at the distal most point of deltoid split to serve as a reminder against extending the split more distally and thereby placing the axillary nerve in jeopardy. The anterior deltoid is carefully peeled from the margin of the acromion without yet releasing the coracoacromial ligament attachment (Fig. 7–6B). The deltoid split is facilitated by splitting the fibers with a Kelly forceps directed downward until the whitish dome of subacromial bursa is exposed. A sharp periosteal elevator is then used to complete the deltoid detachment while exposing the superior surface of the coracoacromial ligament. An acromioclavicular branch of the thoracoacromial artery courses superior to the ligament and must be identified and cauterized. The deltoid then can be peeled away from the underlying ligament, as well as from the bursa. The ligament should be exposed most of the way to its coracoid insertion. The bursa is incised to expose the greater tuberosity and visualize the cuff rupture. Abduction and rotation of the arm demonstrate the impingement phenomenon in most instances.

ANTERIOR ACROMIOPLASTY[1] (OPEN SUBACROMIAL DECOMPRESSION)

The subacromial space is decompressed to facilitate exposure, eliminate encroachment after repair, and reduce postoperative pain. The decompression begins by releasing the coracoacromial ligament from the anteroinferior margin of the acromion with the surgical electrode (Fig. 7–6C). The released margin of the ligament is grasped with a Kocher's forceps, and when a large tear is present, a sizable portion of the ligament is resected and preserved for possible use as an autologous graft. The technique of open acromioplasty is the same whether the operation is done in conjunction with repair of a full- thickness tear or simply for the relief of chronic impingement syndrome. The acromioplasty diminishes the impingement process and retards progression of the disease process.

The anterior portion of the acromion is exposed across the full width by peeling back the superior periosteal structures for 1 cm. A rongeur is then used to recess the anterior edge for a distance of 1 cm (Fig. 7–6D_1). This recession automatically eliminates the most anterior downcurving portion of the acromion and associated spurs. The thickness of the acromion is revealed after this anterior resection has been completed. A broad Key elevator is placed beneath the acromion with the tip located well posteriorly to wedge the subacromial space wide open. Distal traction on the extremity is also helpful at this point.

A wedge of bone approximately 8 mm in thickness and extending posteriorly for nearly 2 cm is then removed from the anterior undersurface of the acromion (Fig. 7–6D_2). A sharp, thin osteotome, 2.5 cm in width, is used to accomplish the acromioplasty. The wedge of bone removed should extend from the anterolateral corner to the anteromedial corner of the acromion. The risk of fracturing the acromion is significant at this stage; great care should be taken to lever the osteotome distally as the wedge is separated from the undersurface of the acromion. If the handle of the osteotome is levered superiorly, an acromial fracture could occur. Sharp dissection is usually necessary to free the resected wedge of bone from soft tissues. The lateral deltoid attachment should not be violated while doing so. After the wedge of bone has been removed, the osteotome is placed against the undersurface of the full length of the acromion to determine whether the undersurface has been completely flattened. The thickness of the residual anterior acromion is also determined. A large oval bur is used to flatten the undersurface if any additional resection is required and also to remove any protuberances (Fig. 7–6D_3).

Next, a finger is placed beneath the AC joint, and the area is palpated for any downward protruding spurs. The rounded prominence of the lateral clavicular

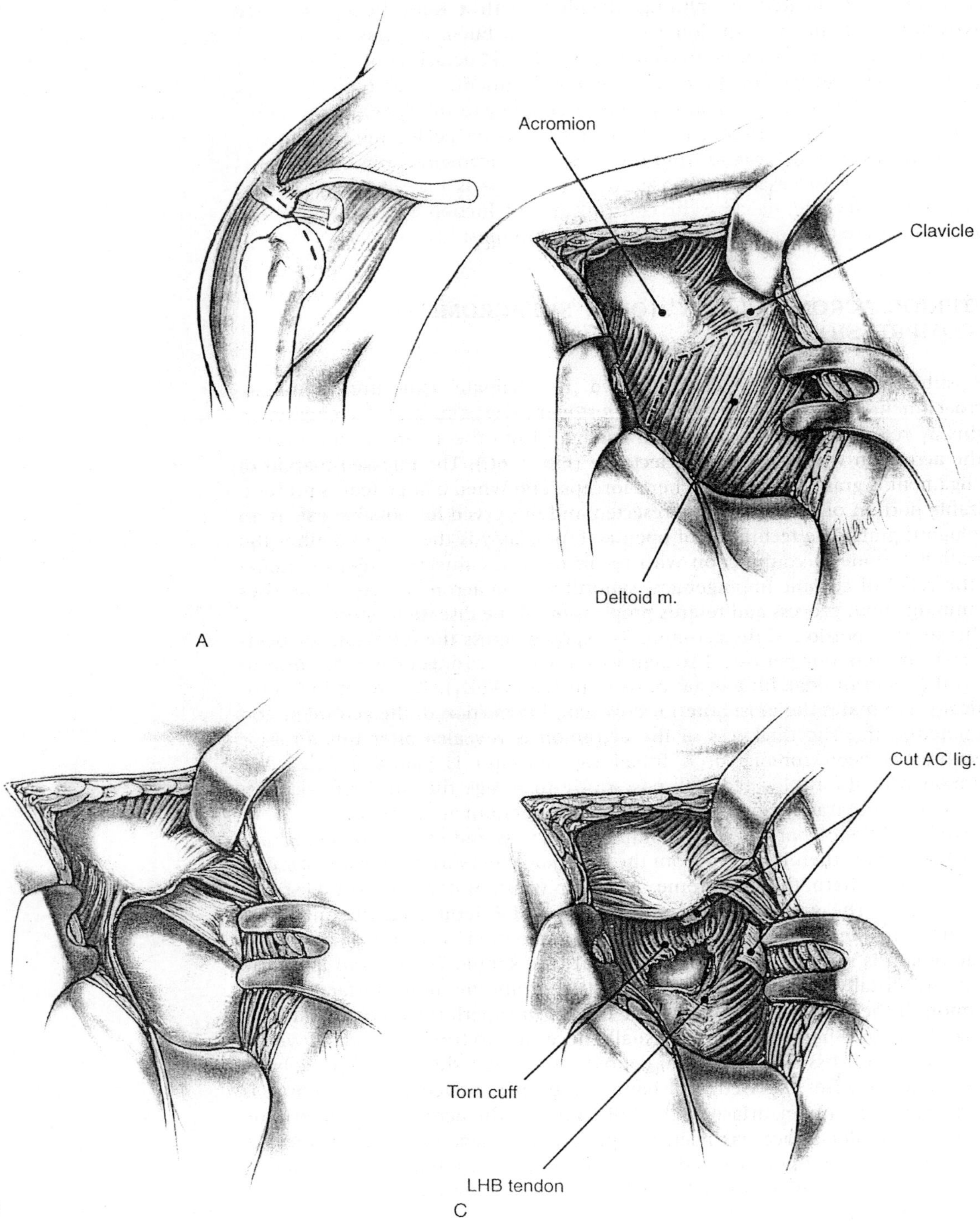

Acromion
Clavicle
Deltoid m.
A
Cut AC lig.
Torn cuff
LHB tendon
B
C

FIG. 7–6.

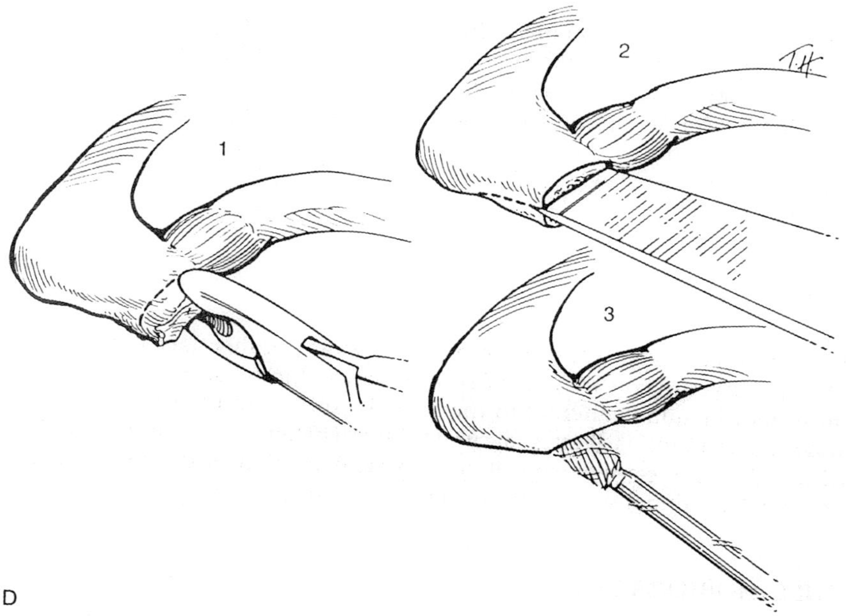

D

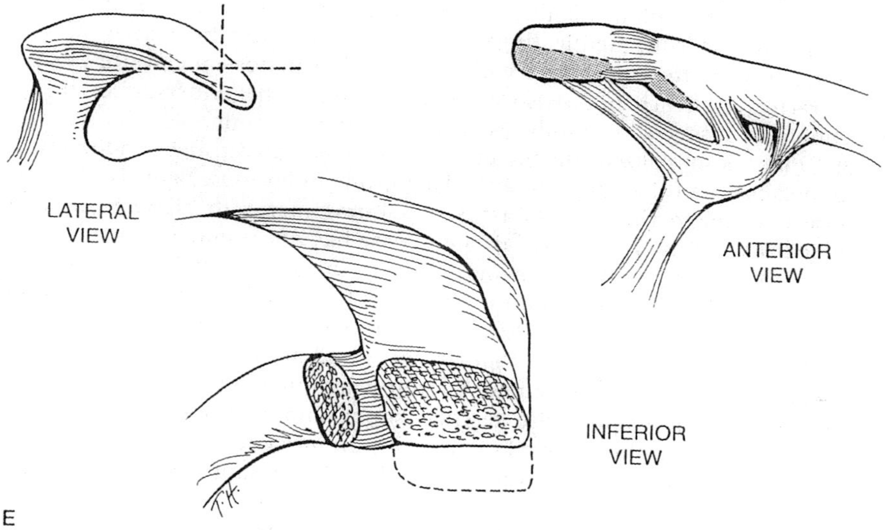

E

FIG. 7–6. (continued) Surgical approach, including acromioplasty.

A, Line of skin incision indicated in inset. With subcutaneous tissue retracted, the deltoid release is shown by dotted line.
B, Deltoid has been released from anterior acromion and split distally for 3 cm. The coracoacromial ligament is exposed.
C, Coracoacromial ligament released and a portion excised. Bursa has been removed to expose torn cuff.
D, (1) Rongeur resects anterior 1 cm of acromion. (2) Osteotome removes a wedge of bone to flatten undersurface of acromion. (3) Large oval bur removes any remaining protuberances from beneath acromion, as well as from below outer edge of clavicle.
E, The amount of bone removed during acromioplasty as viewed from the lateral, anterior, and inferior direction.

undersurface may compromise the supraspinatus outlet as well. This prominence and any spurs should be removed with an oval bur to provide a spacious tunnel for the supraspinatus muscle. A full resection arthroplasty of the AC joint is seldom performed in primary repairs. AC joint resection is occasionally necessary to gain exposure of a retracted supraspinatus muscle or in the event of *symptomatic* acromioclavicular arthritis. Figure 7–6E depicts the extent of bone removed during acromioplasty.

BURSECTOMY

We perform an extensive subacromial bursectomy at this stage of the procedure. The unwary surgeon may mistake a hypertrophic bursa for cuff margin. The bursa may be quite adherent to the superior surface of the retracted cuff, and a wide bursectomy facilitates accurate identification, as well as mobilization. Although the bursa may contribute to vascularization of the torn tendon, bursectomy has not negatively affected clinical results.

CUFF MOBILIZATION

A series of horizontal mattress sutures is placed in the exposed cuff margins to facilitate mobilization. Clamps are avoided, as they invariably damage the substance of the cuff. Gentle finger dissection separates the cuff from adherent bursa or from the undersurface of the deltoid. A periosteal elevator or Chandler retractor can reach otherwise inaccessible areas. The undersurface of the cuff should be inspected carefully. Tears are frequently laminated, and separate layers must be mobilized independently. The articular capsule is adherent to the undersurface of the cuff. The articular capsule often must be incised at its labral insertion below the supraspinatus and infraspinatus to allow maximum cuff mobilization (Fig. 7–7). This capsule release has not resulted in instability; however, care must be taken to avoid injury to the supraglenoid attachment of the long head of the biceps when the capsule is freed in this area. Attempts to mobilize the supraspinatus along the neck of the glenoid must be carefully carried out to avoid injury to the suprascapular nerve and artery as they wind around the spinoglenoid notch and extend inferiorly to innervate the infraspinatus. The coracohumeral ligament also restricts supraspinatus mobilization and must be released either at the coracoid origin or by an incision through the rotator interval adjacent to the anterosuperior border of the supraspinatus. This incision must be closed later.

When mobilization has been completed, the irregular, avascular fibrotic margins of the torn cuff are resected. This resection should be kept to the minimum required to establish a firm, viable margin. Laminated tissue should be freshened and incorporated into the repair. Only after mobilization has been completed and the degenerated edges excised can the full extent of the defect be defined. The method of reconstruction varies with the pattern and size of the defect. Closure occasionally may be accomplished by tendon-to-tendon repair, but in most patients, closure involves suture of the torn edge of tendon directly into the bony trough or, at times, a combination of side-to-side approximation of tendon to tendon in combination with tendon-to-bone fixation.

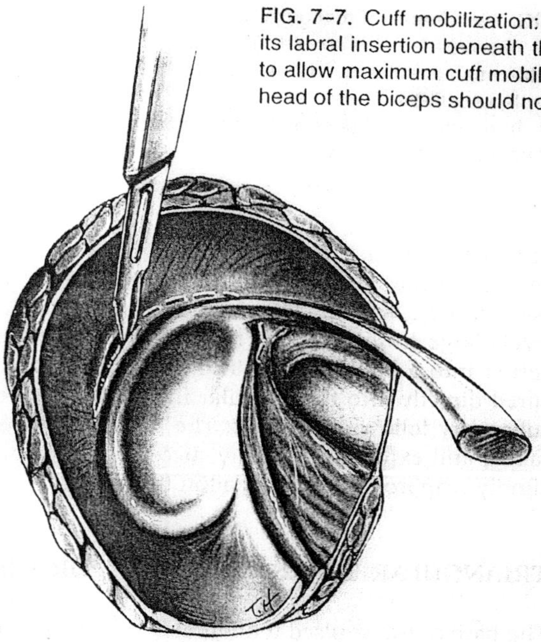

FIG. 7-7. Cuff mobilization: The articular capsule is incised at its labral insertion beneath the supraspinatus and infraspinatus to allow maximum cuff mobilization. The attachment of the long head of the biceps should not be disturbed.

CLOSURE OF DEFECTS

The optimal goal following cuff mobilization is to close the defect and re-establish the insertion of the torn tendon into a bony trough that lies between the articular surface of the humeral head and the greater tuberosity. This procedure should be accomplished without undue tension in most closures while the arm is resting at the side. The closing techniques of various patterns of tear are described individually.

VERTICAL TEARS

Vertical tears extending along the line of cuff fibers are relatively rare and comprised only 4% of our series of full-thickness cuff repairs.[28] A somewhat elliptic full-thickness tear may result following the excision of a sizable partial-thickness tear. This type of tear may be treated with excision of the degenerated cuff margins and side-to-side suture of the torn tendon margins with interrupted nonabsorbable sutures. The technique for closure of vertical tears was detailed in the preceding chapter.

CRESCENT TEARS

Small to moderate crescent tears may be mobilized readily and inserted into a bony trough. They are held by intraosseous sutures, as described in the prior chapter. The larger crescent tears, generally involving the entire supraspinatus

FIG. 7–8. Repair of triangular tears.
A, Reverse-L tear should be mobilized and reapproximated to the tuberosity with intraosseous sutures. The vertical limb is approximated to the rotator interval with interrupted sutures.
B, In repair of L-shaped tear, the vertical defect between infraspinatus or teres minor is repaired by side-by-side apposition.

and a portion of the infraspinatus, may be converted into an inverted-Y shape by closing the more medial portion with a shoelace suture and then fixing the base to bone, as illustrated in repair of trapezoidal defects (see Fig. 7–9). A relatively large crescent tear of recent origin often may be easily mobilized and reinserted into a bony trough. The torn edge of the tendon should never be resutured directly into the irregular fragments of tendon that remain on the greater tuberosity following rupture. The rotator cuff insertion in this area has already failed, and expectation of any success is unreasonable if the ends of the tear are simply reapproximated as tendon to tendon.

TRIANGULAR TEARS (REVERSE-L OR L-SHAPED)

The base of the avulsed tendon(s) should be identified, mobilized, and reinserted into a bony trough. The resulting vertical limb of the tear, in the case of the commonly encountered reverse-L configuration, should be reapproximated to the rotator interval of subscapularis (Fig. 7–8A). The L-shaped pattern requires similar efforts at mobilization of the retracted tendon, followed by side-to-side closure of the resulting vertical defect between the infraspinatus or teres minor (Fig. 7–8B), depending on the size of the tear.

TRAPEZOIDAL DEFECTS

A trapezoid-shaped defect is generally associated with a large cuff tear involving both the supraspinatus and the infraspinatus muscles with considerable medial retraction. Both the base of the tear and the extent of retraction equal 4 cm. This 4 × 4 cm tear outlines an area of defect measuring 16 cm^2. Long-standing tears of this type may be quite challenging to repair, particularly if the remaining musculotendinous structures are atrophic and fibrotic. The inverted-Y closure advocated by McLaughlin may be effective here (Fig. 7–9). In some instances, a few millimeters of encroachment into the articular surface of the humeral head may be necessary for placement of the bony trough so that the defect can be reconstructed without undue tension.

MASSIVE TEARS

A truly massive tear involves rupture of the supraspinatus, infraspinatus, and subscapularis. The term *global* tear also describes a tear of this magnitude. This three-muscle tear frequently accompanies anteroinferior dislocation of the shoulder in older individuals. The biceps tendon is usually dislocated from its groove as well. A prompt reconstruction generally allows the return of the avulsed tendons to their bony origin with transosseous sutures. Chronic degen-

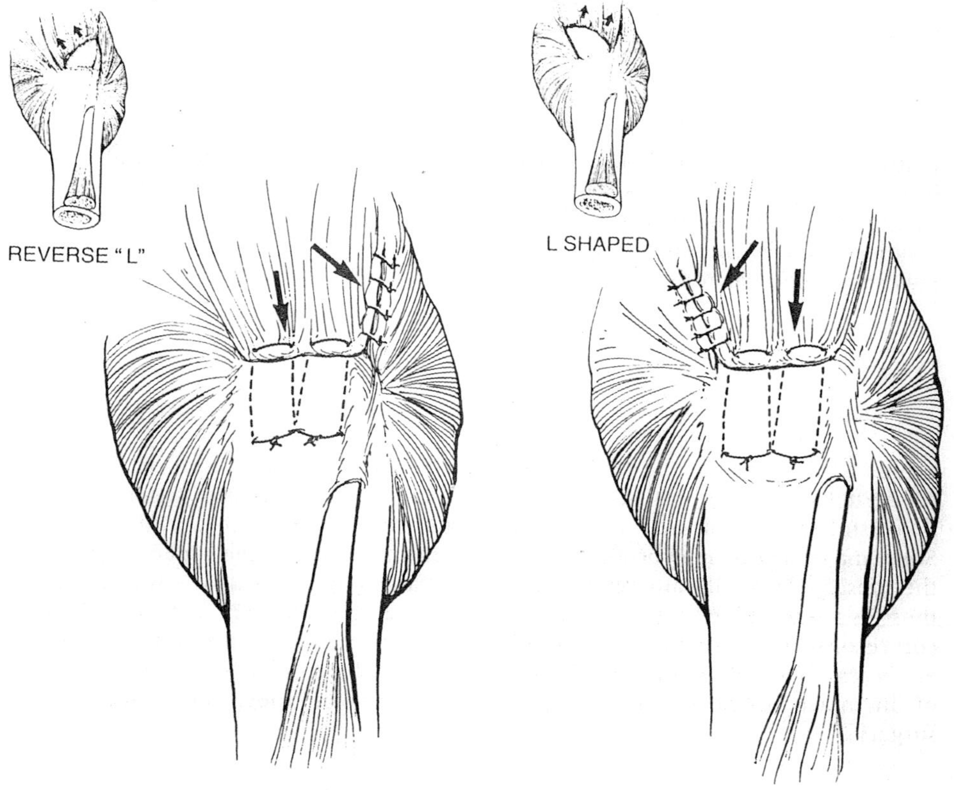

FIG. 7–8.

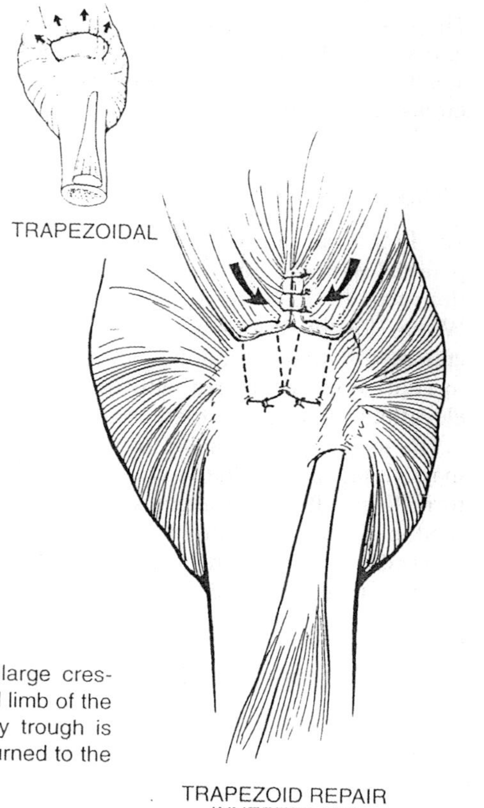

FIG. 7–9. Inverted-Y closure of trapezoidal or large crescent defect. After mobilization, the medial vertical limb of the Y is sutured with a "shoelace stitch." The bony trough is fashioned in a V shape, and the tendons are returned to the bony trough.

erative tears involving only the supraspinatus and infraspinatus may deservedly be considered *massive* tears when substance of the tendon has been ground away by the mortar-and-pestle action caused by a high-riding humeral head and the residual retracted musculotendinous complex is fibrotic and inelastic. Such tears may require heroic measures to restore cuff function.

TENDON TRANSPOSITION

Transposition of the superior half of the subscapularis muscle has been advocated by Neer.[31] The underlying capsule containing the glenohumeral ligaments should be left intact as the superior portion of the subscapularis is detached and reinserted superiorly. Cofield[29] and Neviaser and Neviaser[30] have reported the successful transfer of the entire subscapularis while leaving the capsule intact. Some major defects may be closed by combining a transfer of the superior half of the subscapularis with any remaining infraspinatus (Fig. 7–10A). The transposed muscles are combined superiorly and reattached in the bone (Fig. 7–10B). When cuff reconstruction requires transposition techniques, the overall results are generally less favorable than when a direct repair can be performed. Transposition of an intact muscle could make patients weaker than they were before the surgery.

CORACOACROMIAL LIGAMENT PATCH

The entire coracoacromial ligament can be harvested during the acromioplasty and used subsequently as an autologous graft in difficult tears. This relatively small patch graft is used primarily to achieve a watertight repair rather than to enhance strength.

BICEPS TENODESIS

The long head of the biceps may hypertrophy to several times its normal size in patients with chronic cuff rupture. This hypertrophied tendon appears to function actively as a head depressor, and its insertion should not be disturbed. When closure cannot be completed in any other fashion, the broadened and generally flattened tendon can be incorporated into the repair by being attached to contiguous structures with interrupted nonabsorbable sutures. Some loss of elevation range seems to accompany this tenodesis.

The long head of the biceps may dislocate from the intertubercular groove in massive tears, particularly when the superior portion of the subscapularis is also torn. If an effective transverse humeral ligament cannot be reconstructed, the tendon should be sutured to the adjacent cuff musculature. This tenodesis is preferable to sacrificing the head depressor/flexor function of an intact long head of the biceps tendon.

BICEPS TENDON GRAFTS

The long head of the biceps tendon is commonly ruptured in advanced cuff tears. The rupture generally occurs in the superior aspect of the intertubercular sulcus. The tendon may retract completely to create a characteristic bulge in the distal portion of the upper arm. Occasionally, the torn tendon becomes adherent

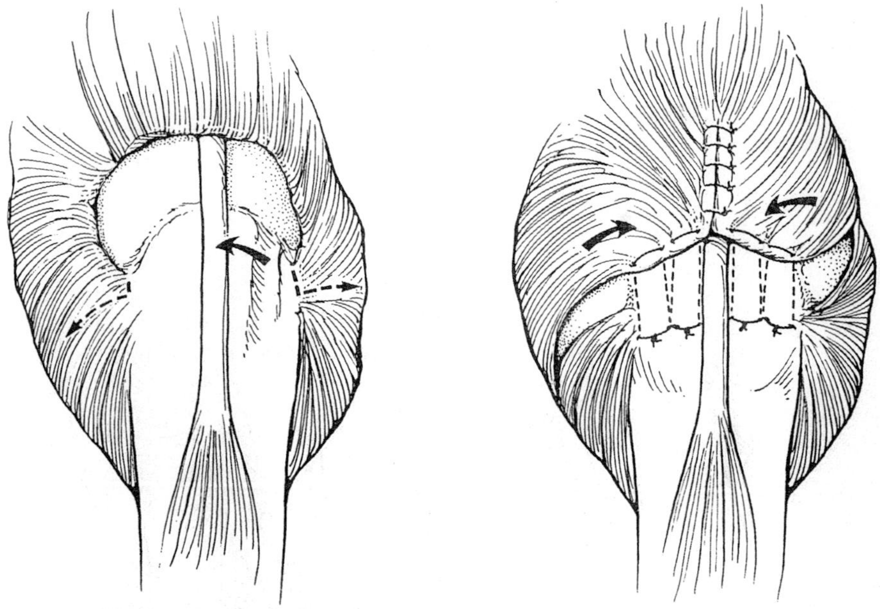

FIG. 7–10. Tendon transposition for massive tear.
A, Releasing incisions are made in the upper half of the supscapularis and remaining infraspinatus prior to transfer. If intact, the long head of the biceps tendon is moved more laterally from its groove to the center of the tuberosity, where a new groove is created.
B, The transposed tendons are individually reattached with transosseous sutures into a bony trough. The long head of the biceps tendon undergoes tenodesis in the vertical closure with interrupted sutures.

within the intertubercular groove, a form of self-tenodesis. In either instance, a sizable stump of proximal biceps tendon may be encountered during the repair. This stump of tendon can be detached and used as a graft in difficult reconstructions.[22] The tendon is sliced down the middle and opened like a book. The shiny side of this split tendon should face the articular surface of the joint when it is incorporated as a graft.

FASCIA LATA GRAFTS

The use of fascia lata grafts for reinforcement and bridging of major defects was described by McLaughlin.[15] Bateman reports the use of fascia lata in 323 patients, with a satisfactory result in 80.5%.[101] Most shoulder surgeons employ mobilization techniques and occasional muscle transposition at this time rather than utilize fascial grafts.

HOMOLOGOUS OR SYNTHETIC GRAFTS

Cadaver grafts or synthetic materials are infrequently used. In our opinion, the value of these materials in comparison to other techniques has not been established.

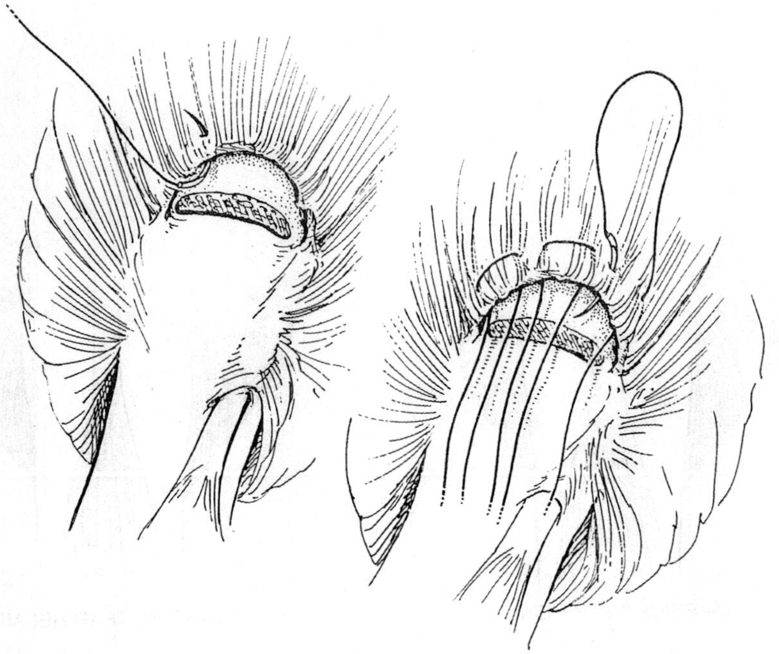

FIG. 7–11. Horizontal mattress sutures: After mobilization and excision of the degenerated margins, a series of horizontal mattress sutures is placed near the cuff margin. Three sutures are used for this large crescent tear.

TENDON-TO-BONE FIXATION: INTRAOSSEOUS SUTURE TECHNIQUE

Most repairs are successful only when the torn tendon is returned to its bony origin. The technique of osseous fixation involves placing sutures in the tendon and then preparing a bony trough and intraosseous tunnel.

TENDON SUTURE PLACEMENT

Cuff repair fails when the suture pulls out of the tendon or cuts through the bony bridge that secures it. Braided polyester (nonabsorbable) No. 1 or No. 2 sutures are used. A variety of methods have been advocated to capture the freshened tendon margin and lead it securely into a bony trough. A horizontal mattress suture is commonly used (Fig. 7–11). The horizontal limb of the mattress suture usually lies along the bursal surface of the tendon but may be placed in a reverse fashion if doing so improves tendon-to-trough approximation.

When the tendon margin is atrophic or friable, a new, modified Mason-Allen technique described by Gerber has been shown to improve tensile strength.[32] The suture is placed within 5 to 10 mm of the tendon margin (Fig. 7–12). Beginning on the articular surface, the suture is passed obliquely through the tendon to emerge on the bursal aspect. The suture is then brought back horizontally to a point where vertical penetration of the tendon causes the suture to emerge near the initial point of insertion. The suture is then brought horizontally along the articular surface for a distance corresponding to the bursal hori-

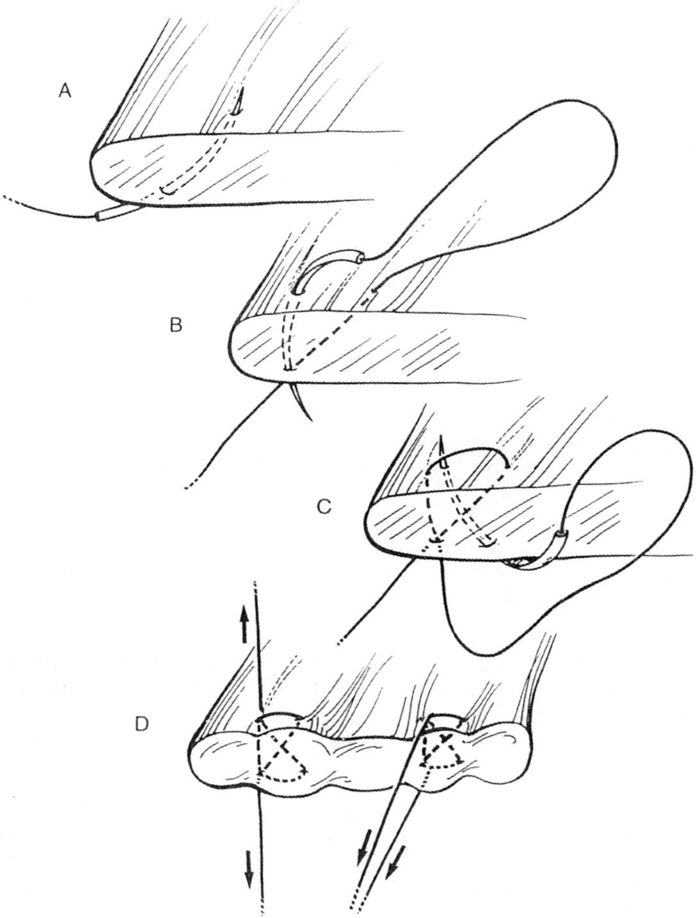

FIG. 7–12. Modified Mason-Allen suture is used to improve tensile strength when tendon margin is atrophic or friable. *A*, The suture initially passes obliquely from articular to bursal surface. *B*, The suture returns to the articular surface vertically to emerge near the site of initial penetration. *C*, The suture reenters the articular surface and crosses the previous oblique limb in the opposite direction. *D*, The modified figure-of-eight suture is tightened by pulling the ends in opposite directions.

zontal limb of the suture. The articular surface is again penetrated in an oblique direction to cross the previous oblique limb in the opposite direction and emerge from the bursal surface, as illustrated. The suture is tightened by pulling in the opposite direction on both ends. This modified vertical figure-of-eight suture grasps tendon bundles as it tightens and improves tensile strength by a factor of 2. The superoinferior placement guides the tendon nicely into the bony trough.

BONY TROUGH PREPARATION

A sharp osteotome is used to prepare a shallow bony trough just lateral to the articular surface of the humeral head for reinsertion of the supraspinatus (Fig. 7–13). As the trough is prepared more posteriorly to reconstruct the infraspinatus, it moves incrementally away from the articular border to conform to the anatomic insertion. The trough should be relatively shallow but deep enough to

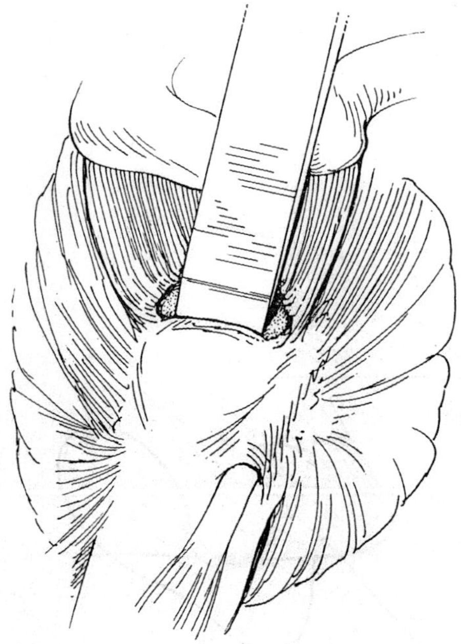

FIG. 7–13. Bony trough preparation: A sharp osteotome prepares a shallow trough lateral to the articular surface of the humeral head. An oval bur may be used to widen and deepen the trough as required.

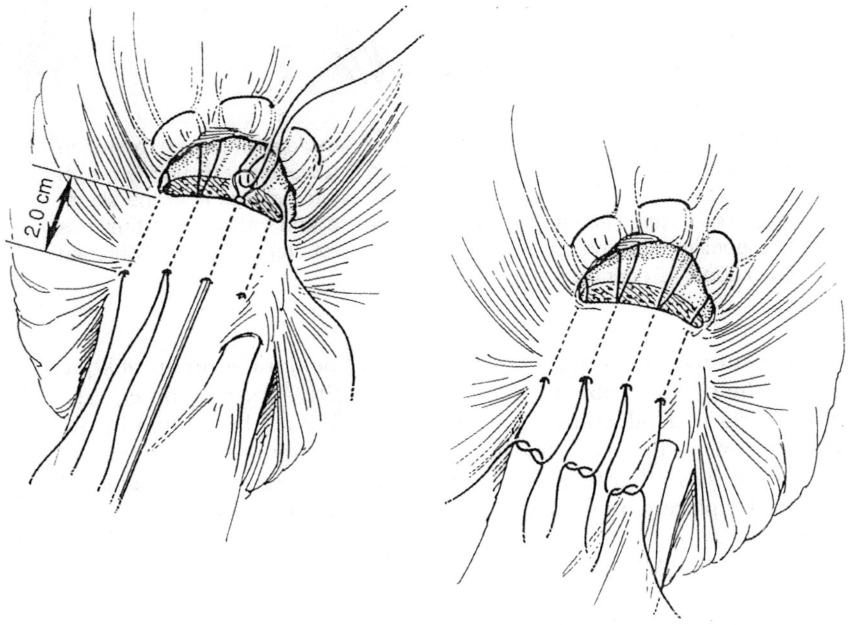

FIG. 7–14. Intraosseous tunnels are made as illustrated in Chapter 6 (Figs. 6–27D and 6–28). The arm is abducted while sutures are tied.

expose cancellous bleeding bone. The trough begins just posterior to the intertubercular sulcus, behind the long head of the biceps when it is intact in the groove. An oval bur is used to widen and deepen the trough as required. This region may have become quite sclerotic in long-standing cuff tears, and a freely bleeding cancellous surface must be exposed to ensure subsequent healing. The frayed stump of torn tendon in the region should be removed with a rongeur. A prominent tuberosity is flattened and smoothed with the bur to eliminate postoperative impingement by this structure.

INTRAOSSEOUS TUNNEL PREPARATION

This technique is illustrated in Chapter 6. The osseous tunnel should originate between 2 and 2.5 cm distal to the tip of the greater tuberosity (Fig. 6–27D). The cortical bone may be quite thin proximally; therefore, more distally placed tunnels afford a stronger bony bridge for suture fixation. Abduction of the shoulder facilitates the preparation of the tunnel with a straight drill. Traction on the split deltoid must not damage the axillary nerve. From 2 to 5 tunnels may be made, depending on the size of the tear. The bony bridge between cortical holes should be at least 1 cm.

A malleable suture passer with a nylon loop on the end (Richards) may be used to pass a suture through the osseous tunnel. The passer is bent into a gentle curve and is threaded through the most posterior hole first from below to exit in the groove adjacent to the humeral head. One end of the suture is captured by the nylon loop and pulled through the tunnel. The passer is then placed through the next tunnel. The remaining strand of the first suture is combined with the more posterior strand of the second, and these are combined and pulled through the next tunnel. The ends are sorted and paired appropriately. Different-colored sutures may be used for easy identification. This process is repeated until the appropriate number of tunnels has been made (Fig. 7–14). The arm is then abducted to relieve tension on the cuff while the sutures are individually tied snugly to approximate the cuff margins into the bony groove. Tension is checked with the arm at the side as well as in rotation and flexion to ensure that undue stress will not be placed on the repair during rehabilitation.

Special instruments designed for tunnel preparation and suture passing are described in Chapter 6 (Fig. 6–28).

CLOSURE OF DELTOID

The deltoid must be meticulously restored to its origin at the conclusion of the cuff repair. Failure of deltoid repair results in a serious and disabling complication. The deltoid should be resutured through osseous tunnels to the anterosuperior margin of the acromion (Fig. 7–15). When an adequate acromioplasty has been performed, osseous sutures often can be placed through the acromion from below upward. Alternatively, drill holes may be made at least 1 cm posterior to the tip of the acromion. Nonabsorbable figure-of-eight sutures are placed through these holes in the anterior acromion to ensure firm muscle-to-bone contact. These sutures may be reinforced with additional fascial-periosteal sutures between the trapezius insertion and the deltoid. If the AC joint has been

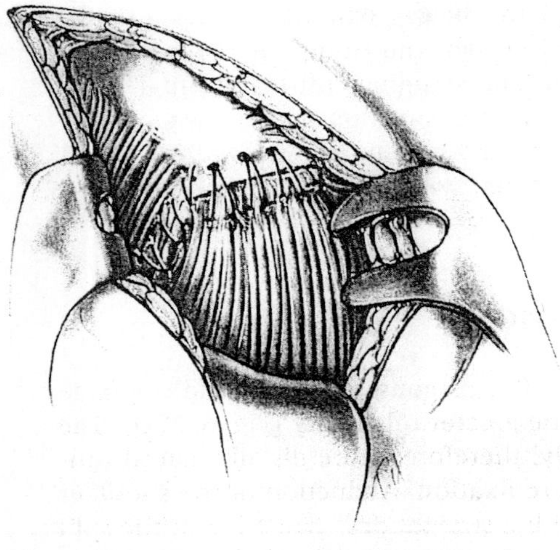

FIG. 7–15. Closure of deltoid: The deltoid is reattached securely to the anterior acromion and acromioclavicular region with interrupted nonabsorbable figure-of-eight sutures. The deltoid split is also sutured securely.

resected, sutures between the trapezius and deltoid are essential. The deltoid repair must be protected throughout the initial 4 to 6 weeks of rehabilitation.

ALTERNATE EXPOSURES

DELTOID DETACHMENT

An alternate method of detaching the deltoid from the anterior acromion is available. The routine anterosuperior skin incision is made as previously described. The fascial extension of the deltoid and periosteum overlying the anterior acromion is split in the same parasagittal direction of the skin incision by utilizing either electrocautery or sharp dissection. The flaps are dissected cleanly off the acromion medially to the AC joint and laterally to the lateral margin of the acromion. Fibers of the deltoid are split along this same line for 3 to 4 cm distally while avoiding injury to the axillary nerve. The anterior acromion is literally "shelled out" of this fascial-periosteal sheath. The acromioplasty and open cuff repair then can be performed. The medial and lateral flaps are reapproximated during closure with interrupted nonabsorbable sutures. Advocates of this method of exposure indicate that a more secure restoration of deltoid continuity is accomplished by this method and that, in fact, the fibers of insertion remain in continuity with the fascial extensions shared by the deltoid and trapezius on the top of the acromion.

In practice, we have found two problems with this exposure. First, the fascial-periosteal sheath in older patients may be quite thin over the more lateral aspect of the acromion; in some individuals, the thickness is less than 2 mm. Consequently, reconstruction is tenuous. Second, we have encountered problems involving the anterior deltoid fibers that have been peeled away. The transition between the thick deltoid and the thin fascial-periosteal sheath is abrupt when the dissection has been completed, particularly in muscular individuals.

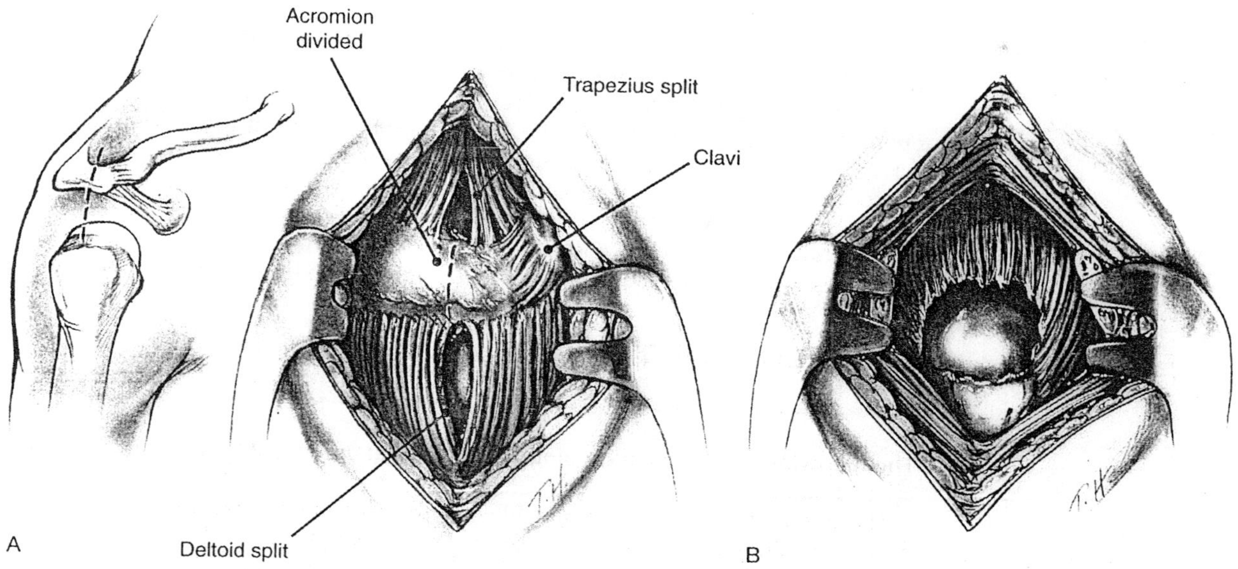

FIG. 7–16. Kessel modification of Debeyre incision.
A, Acromion split in the coronal plane along a line drawn from the posterior border of the clavicle.
B, Deltoid split along line of fibers for 3 to 4 cm. Acromion retracted to expose tear.

Most patients in whom we have used this exposure have required the placement of figure-of-eight sutures through the anterior 1 cm of acromion to reinsert the anterior deltoid securely. This situation occurred so often during our trials of this exposure that we returned to the more traditional method of deltoid detachment and reinsertion previously described.

DEBEYRE APPROACH

Debeyre and associates originally described an acromial-splitting technique for performing a supraspinatus slide in patients with massive defects.[18] The exposure was modified by Kessel and Watson, who shortened the incision and essentially used only the lateral half.[102] Exposure is based on splitting the acromion in the coronal plane along a line drawn from the posterior border of the clavicle, extending laterally (Fig. 7–16A). This route actually bisects the intermuscular attachment of the deltoid and trapezius. The split acromion is spread with a self-retaining retractor, and the deltoid is split along the lines of its fibers laterally for 3 to 4 cm. The lateral portion of the supraspinous fossa is exposed (Fig. 7–16B). This exposure may facilitate mobilization of a torn and retracted supraspinatus tendon.

Debeyre extended this incision medially along the full length of the supraspinatus. The trapezius was released from the scapular spine, and the entire supraspinatus was mobilized from its fossa. The dissected muscle, tethered only by the suprascapular nerve and artery, was translated laterally to cover the defect. The suprascapular nerve is in some jeopardy during this procedure, and significant postoperative weakness has been encountered. The procedure is not widely used.

Kessel believed that the acromial split gained wider access to a retracted cuff than did more conventional exposures limiting the incision to the more lateral aspect. We have observed some difficulties and do not use this acromial-splitting approach. At times, spreading of the acromion widely after it is split is quite difficult. In some patients, a fibrous union has resulted from the acromial split. An anterior acromioplasty is more difficult to perform with the split acromion procedure than with the more conventional anterior exposure.

Currently, most surgeons perform a wide excision of the AC joint to achieve a greater exposure of the supraspinatus as it emerges from the fossa.

USEFUL INSTRUMENTS FOR OPEN SHOULDER SURGERY

The following is a compilation of instruments that are valuable when performing open shoulder surgery.

The operating room shelves are filled with instruments that are designed for other disciplines but are valuable also in shoulder surgery.

1. Curved Adson cerebellar retractor (Fig. 7–17A): The curvature of this instrument adapts nicely to the contours of the shoulder. It is superior to the straight Langenbeck retractors. We use a pair to spread the skin.
2. Baby Balfour retractor (Fig. 7–17B): This retractor is widely used in abdominal surgery on children. The three-piece design works well to retract the deltoid.
3. Goulet retractor (Fig. 7–17C): A pair of these gently curved blades (larger at one end than at the other) may be used to retract the deltoid atraumatically for long periods.
4. Special shoulder retractors: Numerous self-retaining retractors designed exclusively for use in the shoulder are commercially available. We routinely use a medium-sized retractor with two small curved blades in smaller patients (Fig. 7–17D).

   Equally valuable is a larger self-retaining retractor that has interchangeable blades conforming somewhat to the design of a Goulet retractor. One set of blades is deeper than the other (Fig. 7–17E).
5. Weighted vaginal speculum (Fig. 7–17F): This unlikely instrument is attached to a simple loop in the region of the wrist and effectively holds the patient's arm across the chest in an internally rotated position. This instrument comes in handy during subcutaneous and skin closure.
6. Shoulder holder (Fig. 7–17G): During rotator cuff repair, the surgeon or assistant usually must hold the arm in one position or another throughout the procedure. The reader might scour the operating room for attachments that provide some support. This homemade gutter splint works well.
7. Chandler retractor (Fig. 7–17H): These flat, blunt, semi-curved instruments are available in four sizes. Originally designed as periosteal retractors, they provide an easy, safe method of reaching entirely around the proximal humerus in the subdeltoid region to release adhesions. This instrument saves wear and tear on the fingers.

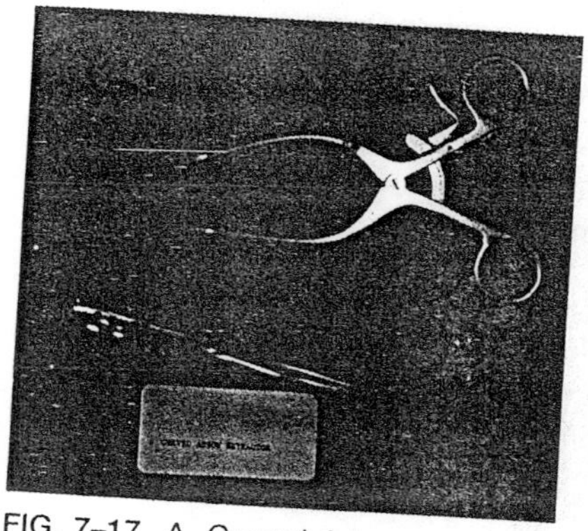

FIG. 7–17. A, Curved Adson cerebellar retractor.

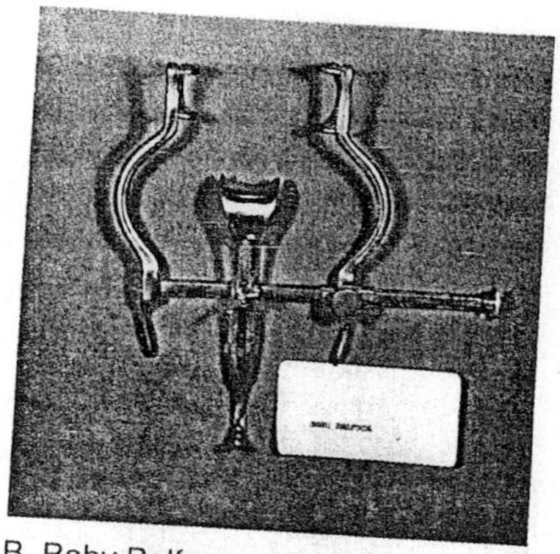

B, Baby Balfour retractor.

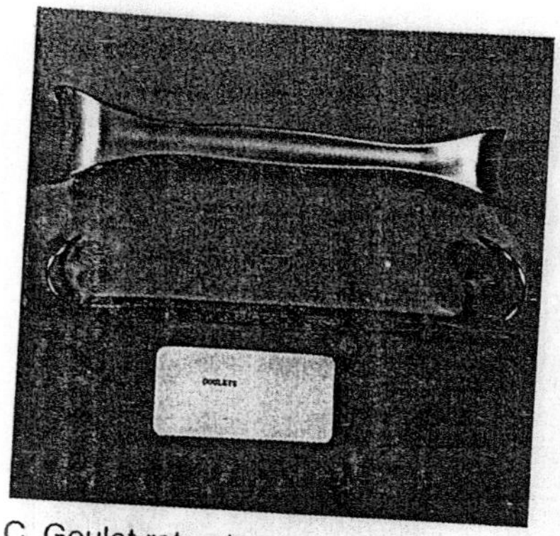

C, Goulet retractor.

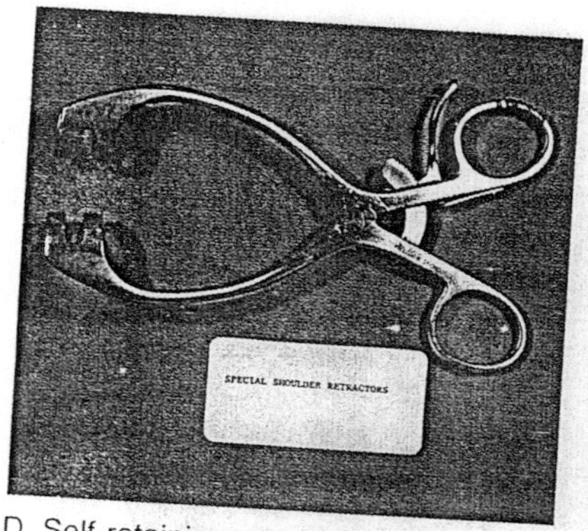

D, Self-retaining retractor with two small curved blades.

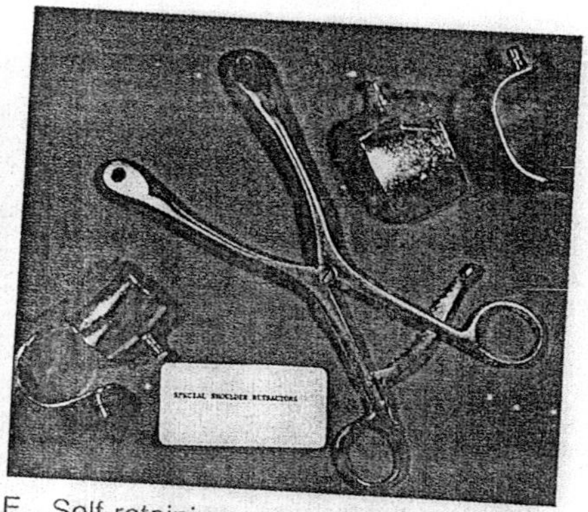

E, Self-retaining retractor with interchangeable blades (one long, one short).

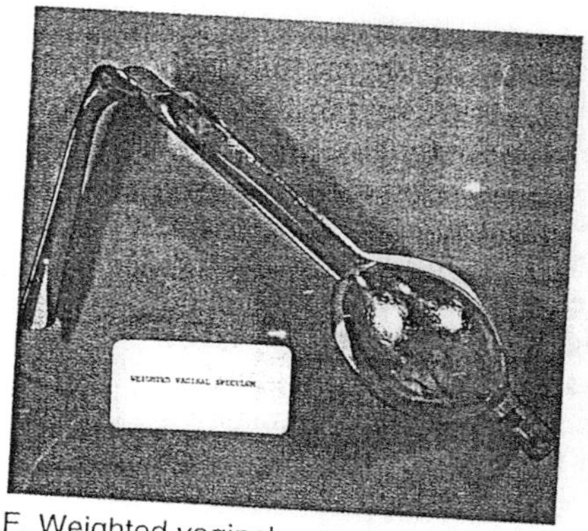

F, Weighted vaginal speculum.

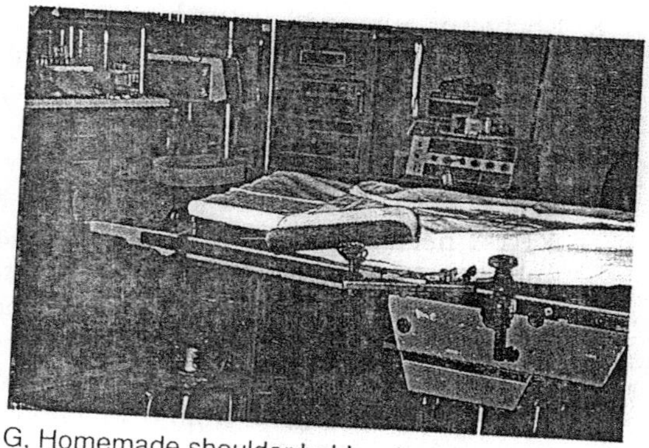

G, Homemade shoulder holder. (continued)

FIG. 7–17 (continued)

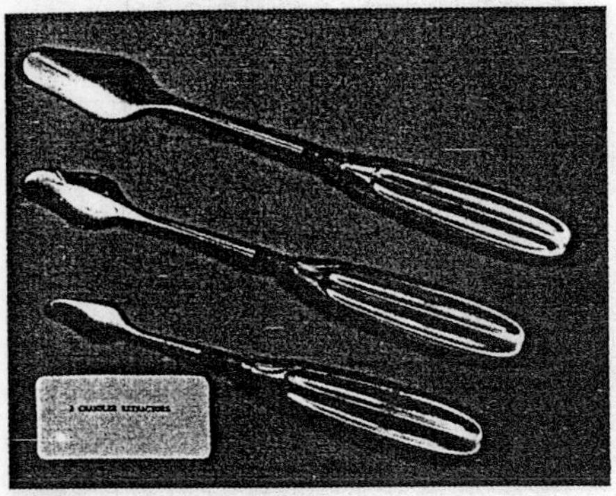

H, Chandler retractor.

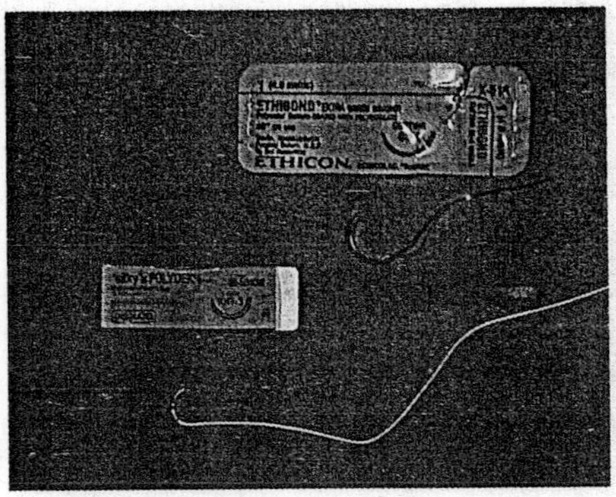

I, Suture material.

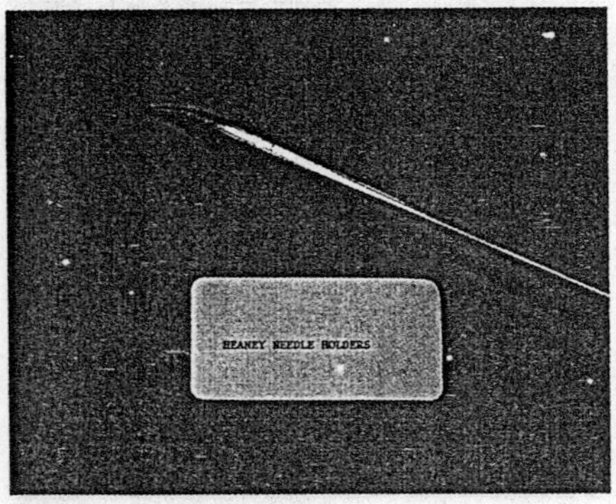

J, Heaney suture driver.

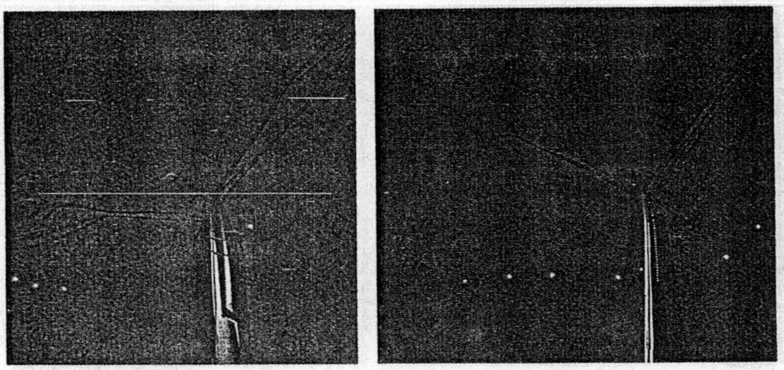

K, Slip knot to secure sutures.

8. Kocher or other types of clamps are never placed on the margins of the cuff during mobilization. They destroy tissue. Horizontal mattress sutures, placed through firm cuff tissue, should be used when all the tugging and pulling are going on.
9. We use nonabsorbable No. 1 sutures (occasionally No. 2) in our repair (Fig. 7–17I). The suture is swaged on 2 sizes of cutting needles. The KHT-3 needle (Polydek-Deknatel) is small enough to work with in the subacromial space, yet is stout and serviceable. A somewhat larger OM-3 needle (Ethibond-Ethicon) is a good size for thicker cuffs and for deltoid reattachment. Our criterion for an adequate acromioplasty is that the acromion must be thinned enough to permit the OM-3 needle to be passed through it from below upward with reasonable force.
10. Heaney suture driver (Fig. 7–17J): This gynecologic instrument has a curved rather than a straight nose to hold the suture. The instrument is helpful when trying to pass a suture through cuff margin retracted deeply into the narrow confines of the shoulder.
11. We have a special twist for holding the free ends of the suture in a Kelly clamp to keep the suture from pulling out while tugging (Fig. 7–17K1, K2). Throw a simple slip knot over the tip of the clamp before grasping the ends of the suture, and then tug away.

MANAGEMENT OF THE IRREPARABLE ROTATOR CUFF AND CUFF ARTHROPATHY

The progressive nature of degenerative rotator cuff disease dictates that some defects will be more difficult to repair than others. In some patients, tissue destruction and chronic contracture produce an irreparable cuff. The ability to repair any cuff defect may vary with the skill and experience of the surgeon. The primary repair of reattaching a torn tendon to bone in or near the region of anatomic insertion produces the best result in regard to restoration of motion and strength. When muscle transposition or grafts are required in a primary repair, function suffers, but reasonable motion and the restoration of adequate strength can be achieved. More heroic measures designed to substitute for the deficient cuff include latissimus transfer,[32,103] trapezius transfer,[104] or the construction of a deltoid flap to attach to the retracted cuff margin.[105] The functional goal in any of these procedures is limited, and they are designed to salvage as much function as possible. The results of any method of treatment are often disappointing when lesions such as those demonstrated in Figure 8–1 are encountered.

THE IRREPARABLE CUFF

The irreparable cuff is the enigma of the shoulder surgeon. Occasionally, a patient appears with the classic findings of advanced cuff failure, including severe atrophy of the supra- and infraspinatus, and yet is able to elevate the arm overhead with little or no discomfort. These patients have achieved a functional pseudoarticulation. A radiograph reveals that the humeral head has risen upward from the glenoid and migrated somewhat medially to nestle beneath the bony coracoclavicular-acromial arch (Fig. 8–2A). The acromiohumeral distance is reduced to 2 or 3 mm. The undersurface of the acromion appears sclerotic and curved and seems to articulate with the humeral head. Adaptive changes have eroded the greater tuberosity, and the entire proximal humerus appears rounded.

The biomechanics of cuffless abduction in this situation are relatively straightforward. During normal elevation, an intact cuff stabilizes the humeral head centrally in the glenoid (Fig. 8–2B and C). The absence of rotator cuff function

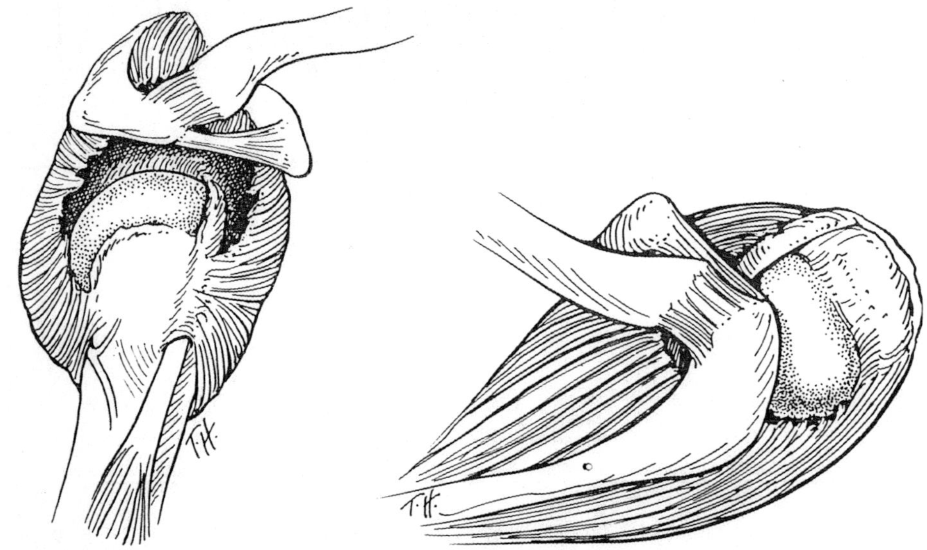

A LATERAL VIEW B SUPERIOR VIEW

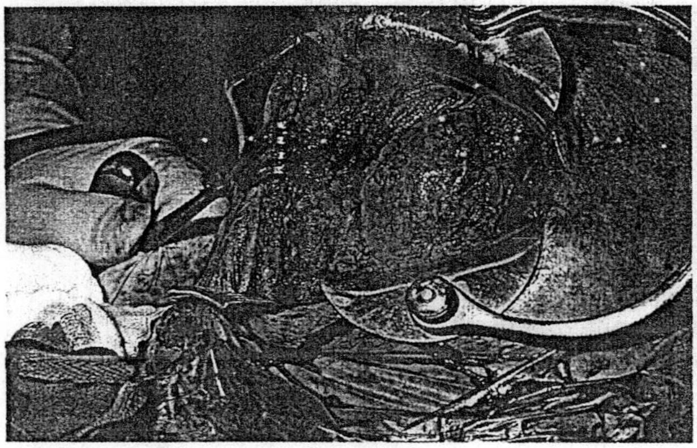

C

FIG. 8–1. Massive rotator cuff defects.
A, Massive defect seen from lateral view.
B, Massive defect seen from superior view.
C, Photograph of massive, irreparable cuff tear. All cuff tissue superior to the dome of the humeral head has been ground away. The head has a pebbled, irregular appearance from articulating directly with the undersurface of the acromion.

allows the head to migrate superiorly when the deltoid is contracted. Once the head is stabilized beneath the coracoacromial arch, combined deltoid contraction and scapular rotation permit elevation in the plane of the scapula (Fig. 8–3). Anterior and posterior stability are necessary for the pseudoarticulation to function. Anterior displacement is stabilized by a relatively intact subscapularis, and remnants of the infraspinatus and teres minor support the joint posteriorly. When either anterior or posterior stabilization is absent, the head displaces anteriorly or posteriorly (Fig. 8–4). In such a circumstance, overhead elevation cannot be achieved.

The muscles that rotate the scapula are important in shoulder elevation. The

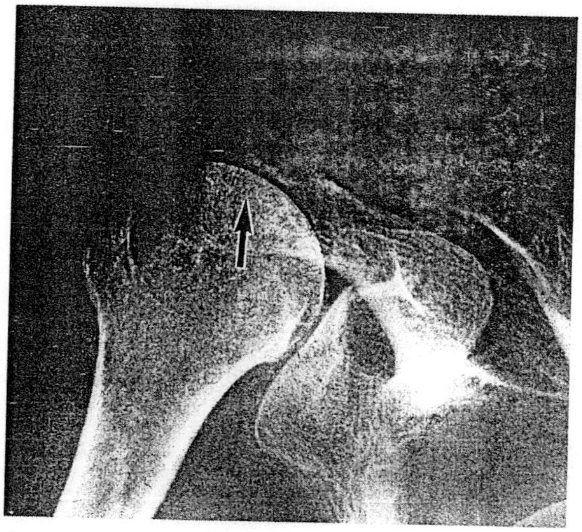

A

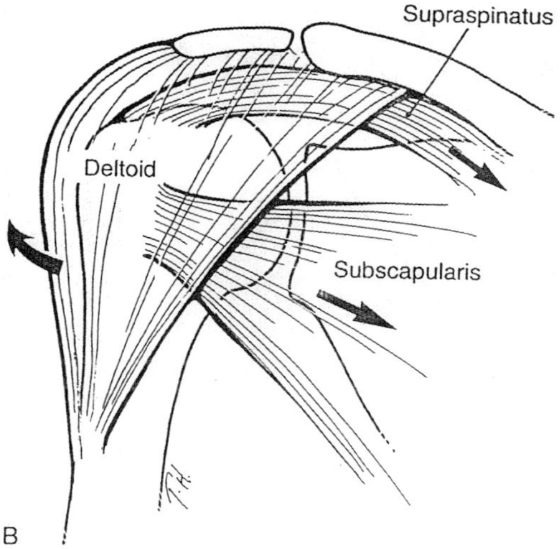

B

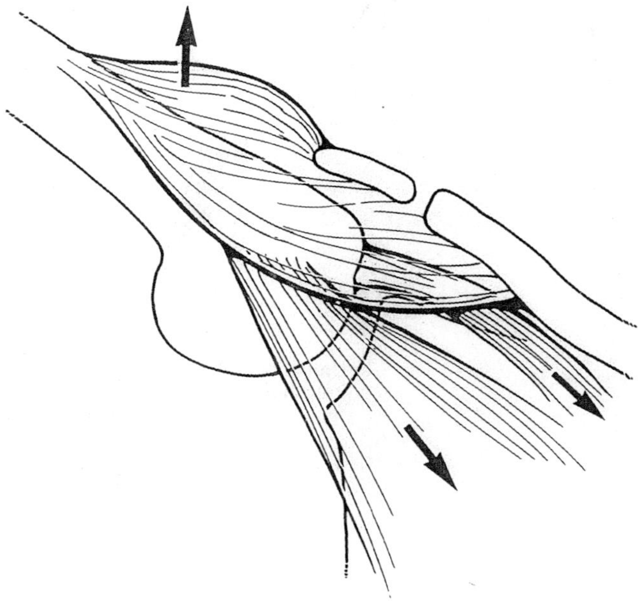

C

FIG. 8–2. A, Pseudoarticulation: The humeral head has migrated superiorly and medially to articulate with the coracoacromial arch (arrow).
B, The deltoid works as a force-couple with the stabilized humeral head to elevate the extremity.
C, Intact rotator cuff musculature stabilizes the humeral head against the glenoid.

serratus and levator form a force-couple, which works synergistically with the upper and lower trapezius fibers to rotate the scapula during elevation. A surprising degree of elevation can be achieved in spite of cuff deficiency when the deltoid and scapular musculature are strengthened by rehabilitation. The extremity nevertheless remains weak through the midrange of abduction in the scapular plane.

The pseudoarticulation cannot function well when the joint is painful. A surprising amount of pain can be relieved in a patient with an irreparable tear by debridement of the torn, floppy, fibrotic margins of the torn cuff, glenohumeral synovectomy, and subacromial decompression. As pain is relieved, strengthening exercises gradually restore functional overhead elevation in many patients. The decompression and debridement may be done as an open procedure or with arthroscopic techniques.

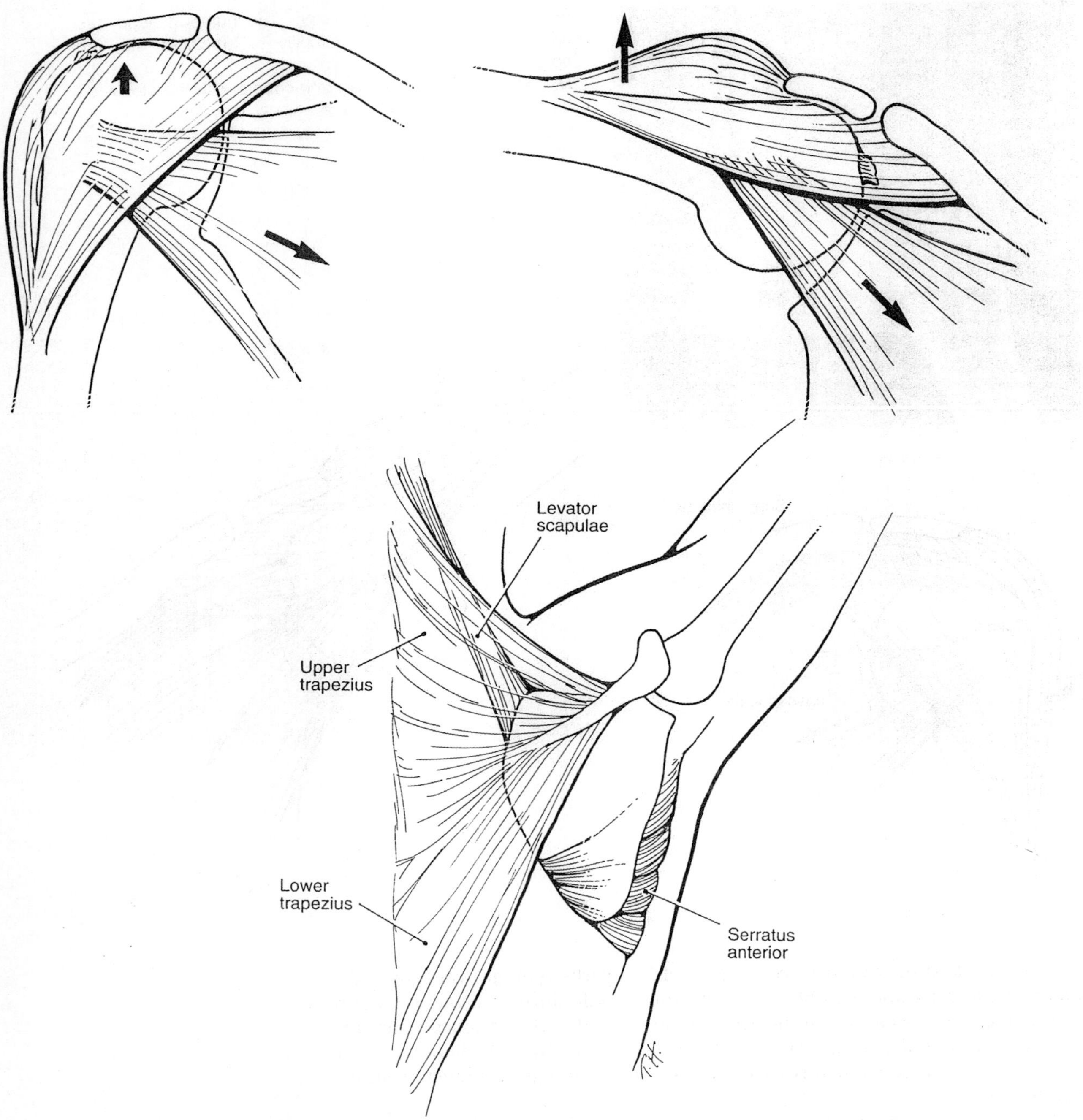

FIG. 8–3. Cuff-deficient pseudoarticulation.
A, Absence of the superior cuff permits the humeral head to ride upward with deltoid contraction.
B, Once the cuff stabilizes superiorly, limited elevation can be accompanied by deltoid contraction in combination with scapular rotation.
C, The principal scapular rotators that are helpful in cuff-deficient elevation.

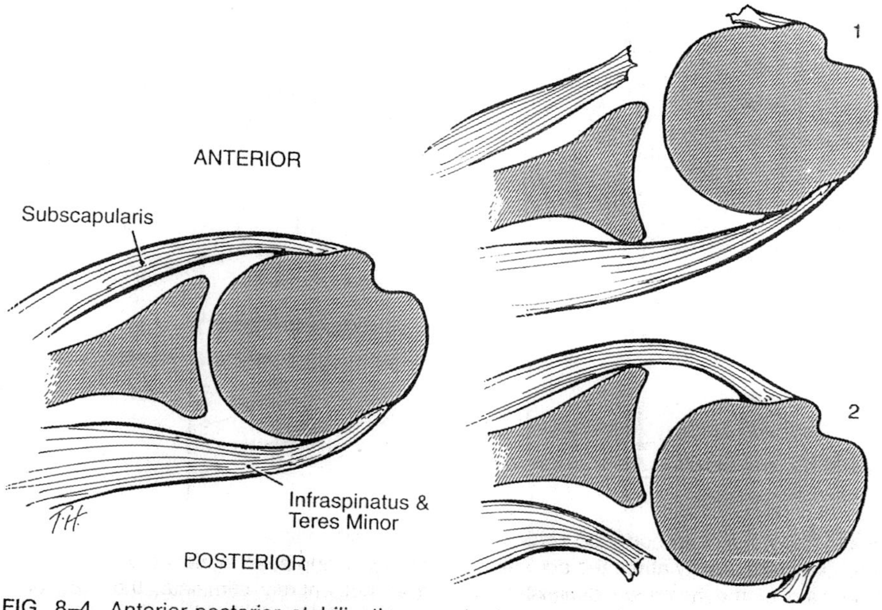

FIG. 8–4. Anterior-posterior stabilization required for the pseudoarticulation to function. (1) Absent subscapularis permits anterior displacement. (2) When infraspinatus and teres minor support is lost, the shoulder displaces posteriorly.

OPEN DEBRIDEMENT AND DECOMPRESSION

Rockwood and Burkhead reported the results of open debridement and subacromial decompression in a series of 15 patients followed for 7.2 years.[38] Through a conventional anterosuperior approach to the joint, a thorough acromioplasty was performed, including release of the coracoacromial ligament and extensive bursectomy. The cuff was inspected, and an effort was made to mobilize the retracted margins. When a massive defect could not be repaired without relatively heroic measures, the torn, fibrotic, and irregular margins of the retracted cuff were debrided extensively and the deltoid securely repaired. Rehabilitation started on the first postoperative day. Strengthening exercises were continued until the patient had obtained the maximum function achievable. They reported the relief of pain, with satisfactory strength and function, in all of the patients.

Burkhart has substantiated these results.[106] His biomechanical analysis suggests that patients with a shortened acromion (as a result of the acromioplasty) achieve greater elevation (Fig. 8–5). Rounding off the tuberosity also improves range of motion. These observations are valid provided the joint has adequate anterior and posterior stabilization.

ARTHROSCOPIC DEBRIDEMENT AND DECOMPRESSION

The principles of treatment by arthroscopic methods are comparable to those of the open procedure. The cuff defect is carefully inspected arthroscopically to determine the size of the defect and the quality of residual tissue. Retraction of

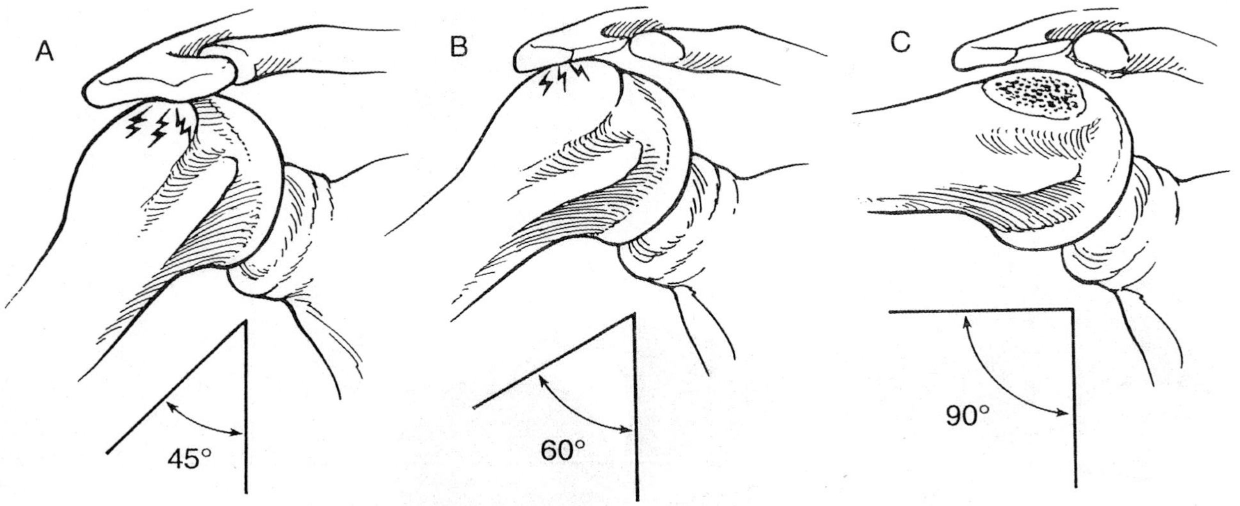

FIG. 8–5. The value of a shortened acromion and tuberosity-plasty.
A, A prominent tuberosity abuts the acromion as the high-riding head is elevated.
B, Shortening of the acromion diminishes, but does not entirely eliminate, the area of abutment.
C, Rounding off the tuberosity (tuberosity-plasty) improves the range of elevation.

the massively torn cuff is so extensive that both the articular and bursal surfaces of the cuff can be inspected from the posterolateral subacromial portal (Fig. 8–6). A grasping forceps is introduced to ascertain cuff mobility (Fig. 8–7). Irreparable defects generally involve rupture and retraction of both the supraspinatus and the infraspinatus. The retracted cuff tissue may be fibrotic and irregular or appear thin and inelastic. The superior articular surface of the humeral head may be worn or pebbled by repeated contact with the undersurface of the acromion. A surprising amount of reactive synovial changes may be found in the interstices of the glenohumeral joint or in the recesses of the subacromial space (Fig. 8–8). These grape-like clusters of synovial tissue can be quite vascular.

DEBRIDEMENT

Debridement begins with an extensive synovectomy. Portals for the arthroscope and shaver are reversed during the synovectomy to gain maximum access to the glenohumeral recesses. Hypertrophic bursal tissue is removed from the subacromial space. The irregular, fibrotic margins of the cuff are then debrided (Fig. 8–9). A relatively smooth, stable margin should result. Irregularities of the biceps tendon are also smoothed when the tendon is intact. If rupture has occurred, any remaining stub of tendon is removed.

TUBEROSITY-PLASTY

The greater tuberosity is usually worn and irregular in these patients (Fig. 8–10). Any remaining prominence is superfluous and should be removed with a mechanical bur. The proximal humerus should present a congruous roundness for the pseudoarticulation to function well.

FIG. 8–6. Orientation view and photograph of an extensive cuff defect.

A, Rotator cuff defect in a right shoulder as viewed through the posterior portal. The bursal structures are exposed, and the undersurface of the acromion, the coracoacromial ligament, and marker pins are seen.
B, Arthroscopic photograph of a comparable view to that in A. The articular surface of the tuberosity and the long head of the biceps appear worn, and crab-like, frayed, fibrous tissue hangs downward from the acromion.

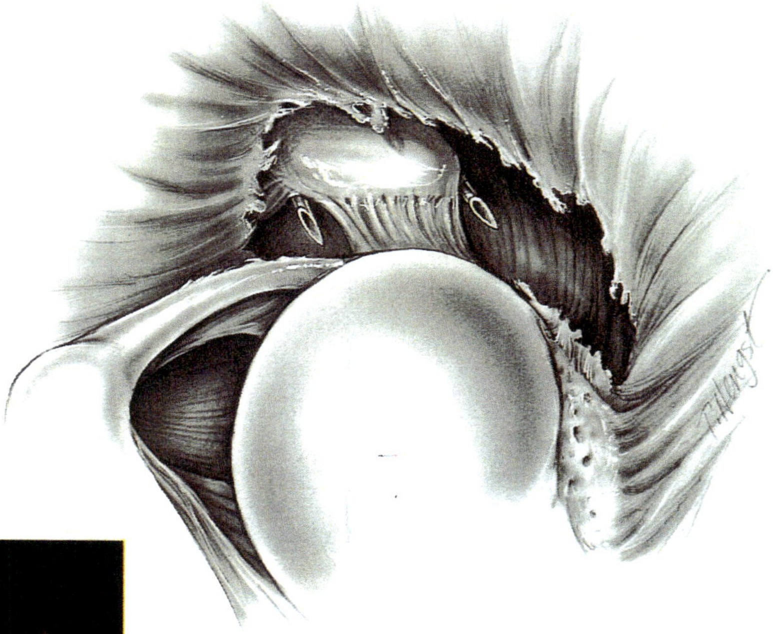

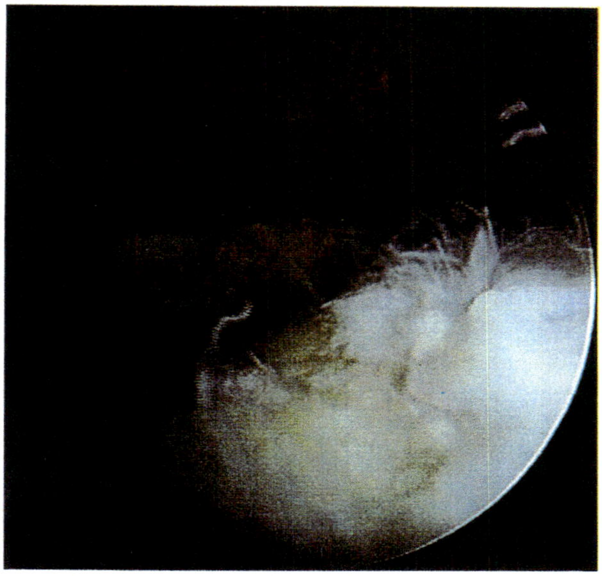

A
B

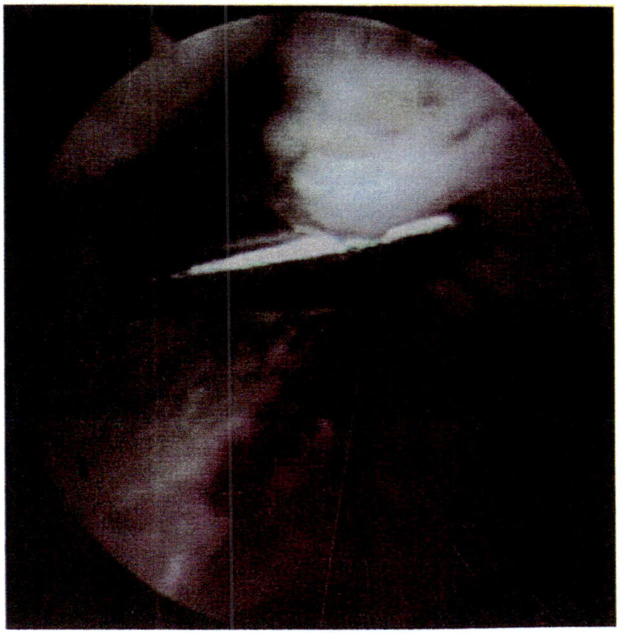

FIG. 8–7. A grasping forceps is introduced to ascertain cuff mobility.

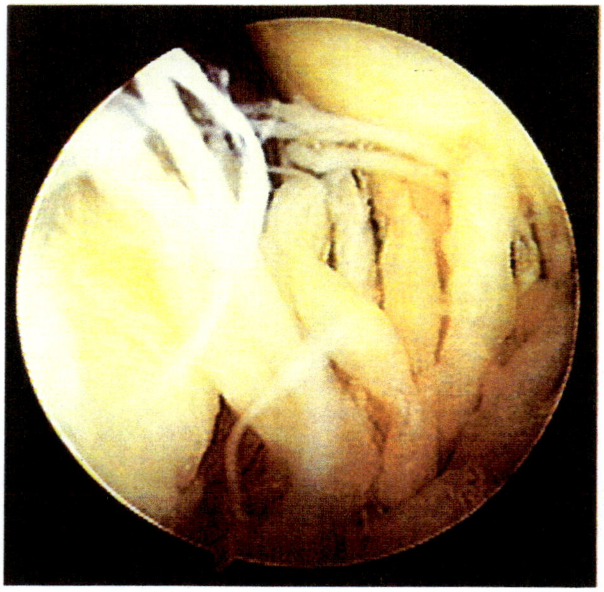

A

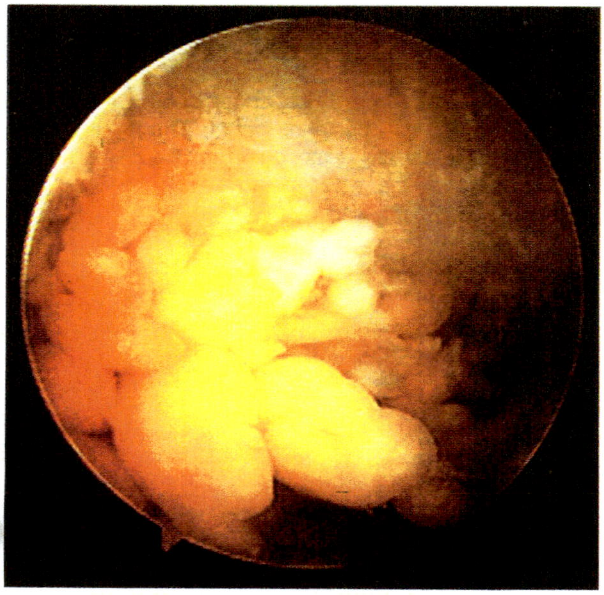

B

FIG. 8–8. Chronic synovitis associated with massive cuff tears. A, Long strands of synovial tissue found in inferior recess. B, Grape-like clusters of synovitis in subacromial space.

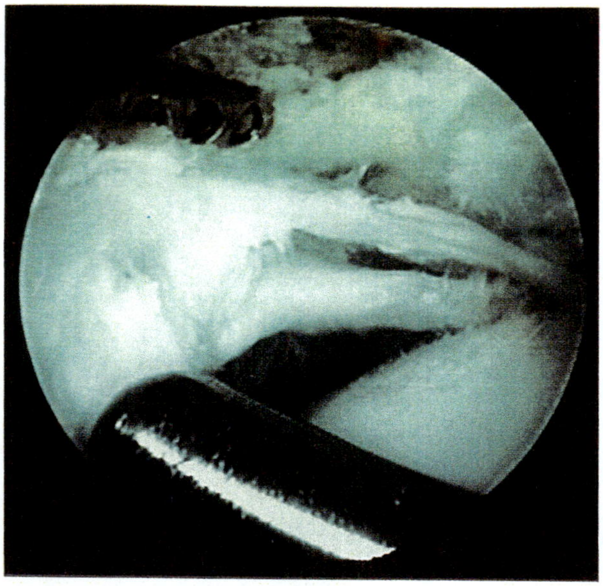

FIG. 8–9. Fibrotic margins of the cuff are debrided.

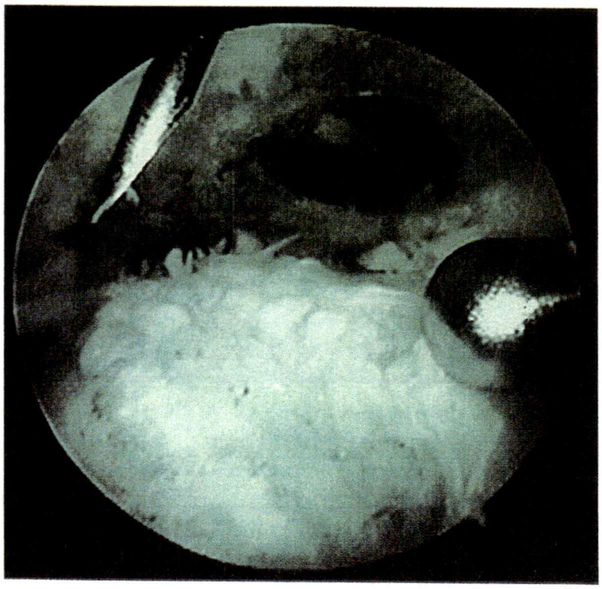

FIG. 8–10. Tuberosity-plasty: The irregular surface of the tuberosity is debrided and then rounded with a bur.

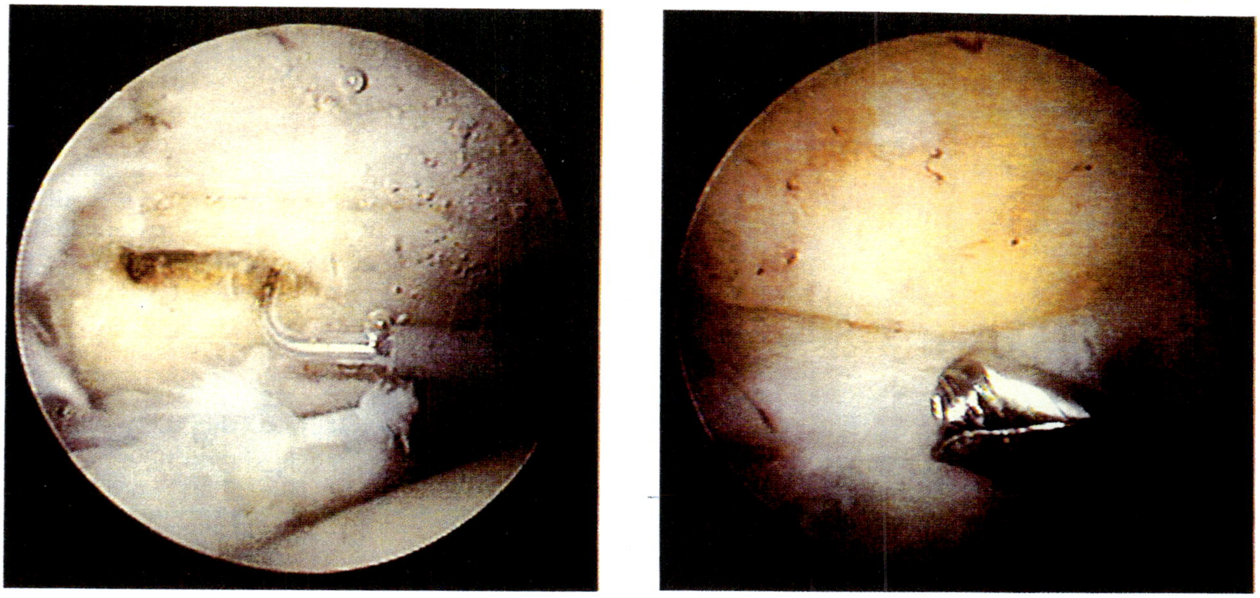

A B

FIG. 8–11. Acromioplasty.
A, Release of coracoacromial ligament.
B, The completed acromioplasty. Bur has recessed 1 cm from the anterior edge of the acromion.

ACROMIOPLASTY

Arthroscopic release of the coracoacromial ligament and acromioplasty are carried out as the final step of this procedure (Fig. 8–11). Following release of the ligament, the anterior acromion is recessed at least 1 cm and then is tapered to flatten the undersurface and eliminate spurs. As mentioned earlier, the shortened acromion appears to allow greater elevation in these patients. The decompression is considered essential in the treatment of these irreparable lesions. Synovectomy and debridement without decompression do not yield comparable results.[107]

REHABILITATION

The key to establishing a functional pseudoarticulation following arthroscopic subacromial decompression and cuff debridement lies in strengthening the deltoid and scapular rotators. For the first 2 postoperative weeks, the patient is simply encouraged to use the arm as much as possible for the activities of daily living. Passive assisted forward elevation, external rotation, and pendulum exercises are performed 2 times daily to avoid adhesion formation. As postoperative discomfort diminishes, isometric and then minimally stressful resistance exercises are introduced. Dental dam or rubber tubing is used to strengthen the external rotators and the anterior, posterior, and medial fibers of the deltoid in the subimpingement range (ABC exercises, see Chap. 25). Efforts to lift the extremity against the resistance of gravity are encouraged after the third week.

By the sixth week, the patient should be able to begin the limited phase III resistance protocol (see Chapter 25). Even a 1-pound weight may be difficult to lift at first. Improvement of strength is gradual over the next few months. Pain diminishes slowly. If the weight-training program is initially too aggressive, the patient may become discouraged by pain associated with the therapy sessions. The rate of weight resistance advancement must be monitored carefully by a skillful therapist. Reasonable goals must be set. In time, pain relief is gratifying. Residual weakness in elevation is inevitable when both the supraspinatus and the infraspinatus have been irreparably torn. The ability to use the arm overhead effectively for light activities usually returns within 3 to 6 months.

CLINICAL TIP

Patients with irreparable cuff deficiency are usually elderly. The preoperative conference should establish realistic goals. The patient should understand that normal strength cannot be restored and that the primary objective is to reduce pain. As long as 6 months may be needed for significant improvement to occur.

CUFF TEAR ARTHROPATHY

The end stage of rotator cuff disease has been termed "cuff arthropathy" (Fig. 8–12).[45] This entity has been estimated to develop in fewer than 4% of individuals with long-standing massive rotator cuff tears. The diagnosis is established by a triad of findings: collapse of the humeral head, chronic synovitis (often hemorrhagic), and instability. Crystalline deposits within the synovium have been observed. Cuff arthropathy appears to be quite similar to the entity known as "Milwaukee shoulder."[46]

This condition must be differentiated from various other causes of glenohumeral arthritis. The radiographic collapse of the humeral head may appear similar to that seen in avascular necrosis (Fig. 8–13); however, the rotator cuff is usually intact with avascular necrosis. Osteoarthritis is readily differentiated from cuff arthropathy by its characteristic marginal osteophytes, osseous eburnation at the point of joint reactive forces, and a usually intact cuff. Rheumatoid arthritis of the shoulder, in contrast to cuff arthropathy, is associated with distinctive involvement in multiple joints, as well as with corroborating laboratory data. The cuff in a rheumatoid patient may be thinned but is usually intact until the later stages of the disease. Pyogenic arthritis produces cartilage destruction and eventual osteolysis. The infected joint is distinguished by local heat, leukocytic response in the synovial fluid, and a positive culture. Neuropathic joint destruction, such as that seen with Charcot's joint or syringomyelia, is more disorganized in appearance than is cuff arthropathy.

TREATMENT

The treatment of cuff arthropathy is directed primarily toward relief of pain. Although nonconstrained shoulder arthroplasty is generally considered the treatment of choice, arthroscopic surgery offers an alternative method.

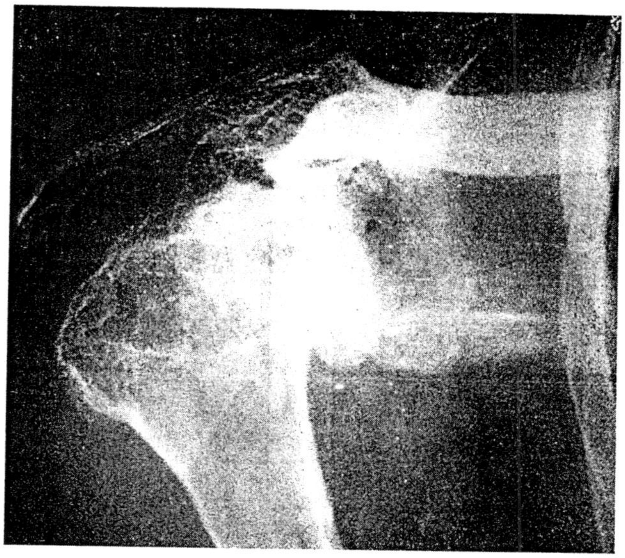

FIG. 8–12. Cuff arthropathy: The radiograph shows extensive bone destruction and collapse of the humeral head in this 83-year-old patient with end-stage rotator cuff dis ease.

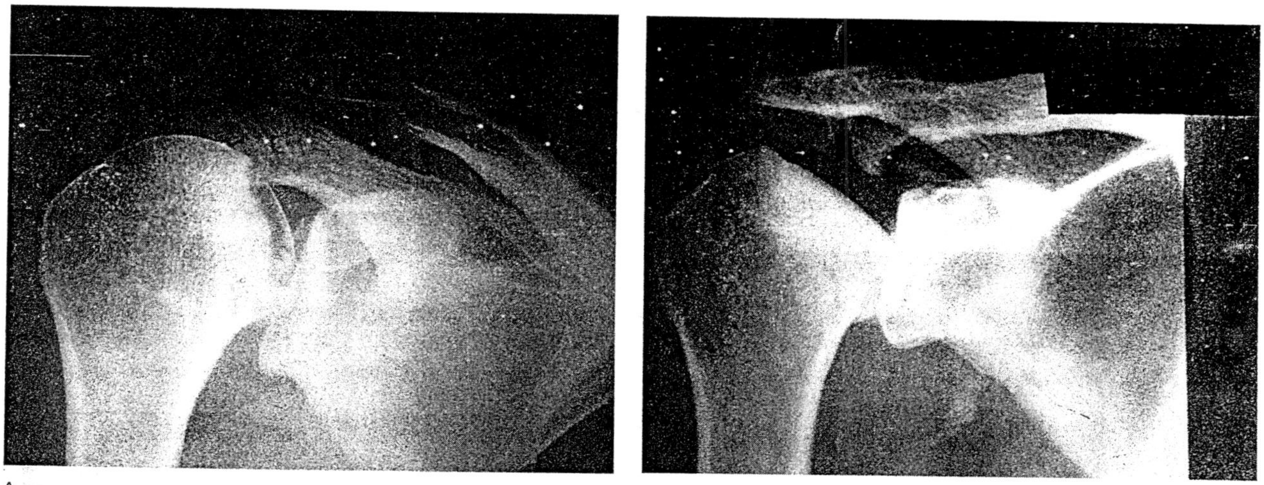

A B

FIG. 8–13. Differential diagnosis between avascular necrosis and cuff arthropathy.
A, Avascular necrosis with collapse of humeral head. The rotator cuff is intact.
B, Cuff arthropathy associated with chronic massive rotator cuff tear. Note spurs projecting downward from anterior acromion and lateral aspect of clavicle.

OPEN SURGERY

Most authors recommend hemiarthroplasty rather than total joint replacement. Franklin and associates[108] and Arntz and colleagues[109] have shown that a persistent high-riding humeral head produces a "rocking-horse" force against the glenoid that eventually causes it to dislodge. For this reason, a glenoid component is avoided and a relatively large humeral component is used in these

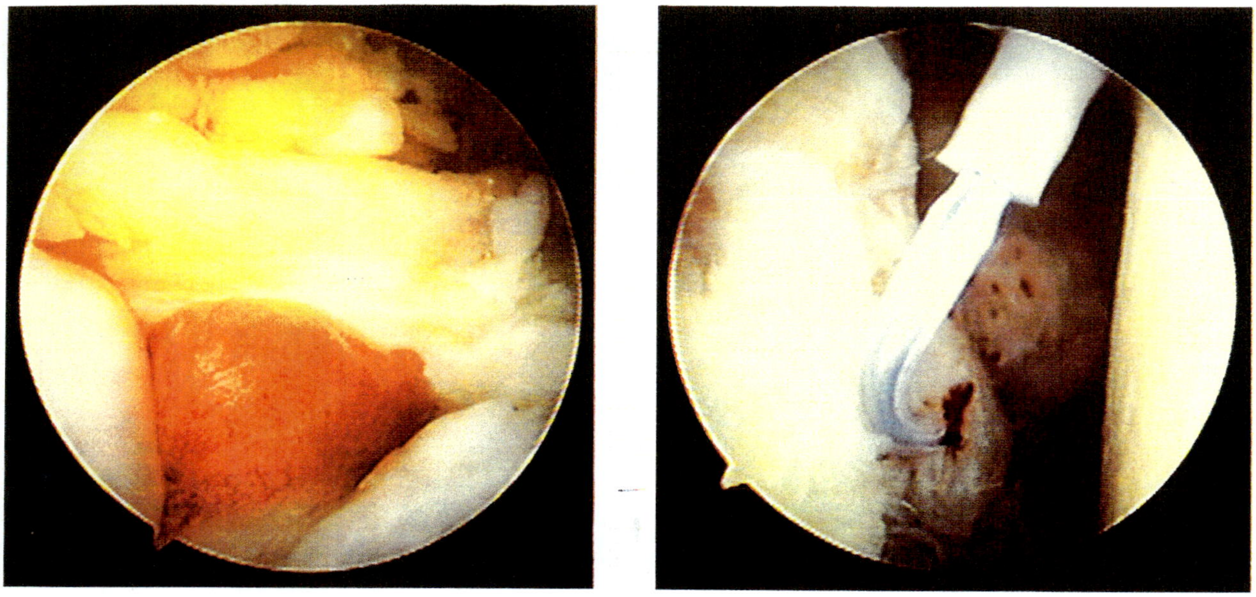

A B

FIG. 8–14. Debridement of hemorrhagic synovium.
A, Hemorrhagic synovial pod responsible for commonly seen hemorrhagic synovitis in this condition.
B, Following synovectomy, electrocautery is essential to control bleeding.

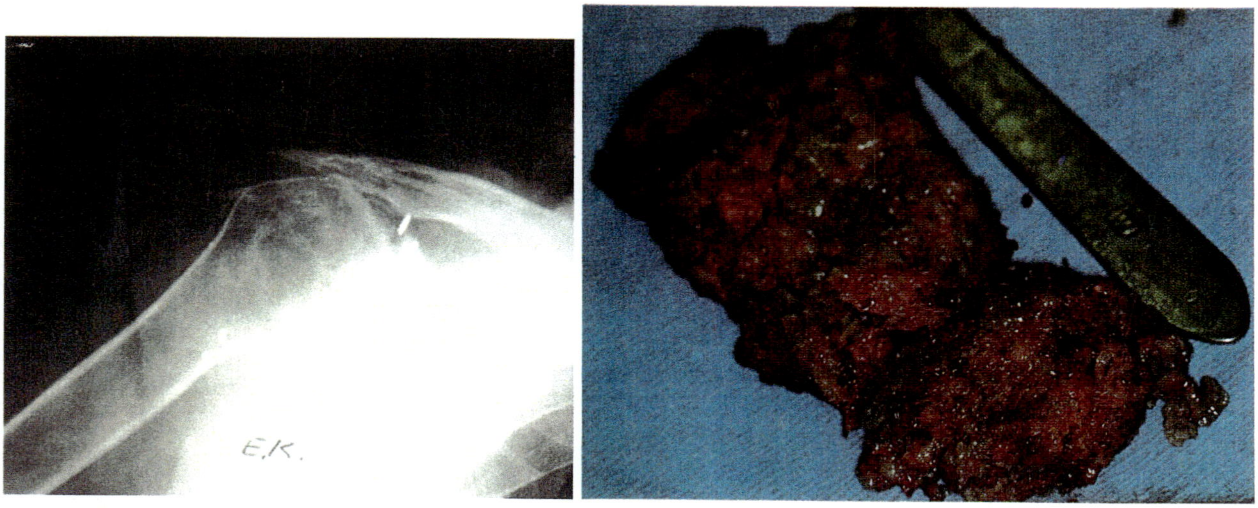

A B

FIG. 8–15. Material removed during debridement, synovectomy, and decompression.
A, Preoperative radiograph of 82-year-old patient with cuff arthropathy.
B, Amount of material removed during debridement, synovectomy, and decompression is massive when shown in comparison to the size of a scalpel handle.

patients. When repair of the remnants of rotator cuff seems possible, a relatively small amount of deformed humeral head is removed and replaced by a smaller, short head. This short head may permit transposition of the subscapularis superiorly in an effort to cover the head.

The goals of rehabilitation following open surgery are quite limited in these unfortunate patients. Instability is difficult to overcome. The synovectomy that accompanies joint replacement diminishes or eliminates the effusion. Pain is usually diminished but not entirely relieved. Unfortunately, the cuff cannot be repaired in most patients with cuff arthropathy, and functional impairment is profound in the cuffless arthroplasty.

ARTHROSCOPIC SURGERY

Arthroscopic treatment has achieved a limited-goals result in a few patients with advanced cuff arthropathy.[40] The procedure consists primarily of an extensive synovectomy and joint debridement. The shaggy edges of any cuff that remains are removed, and downward-protruding acromial or acromioclavicular spurs are eliminated. The grape-like clusters of hypertrophic synovium that develop in this condition may be quite vascular (Fig. 8–14A). Adequate joint distention must be maintained to tamponade bleeding. The equipment for intra-articular electrocautery is essential during the procedure (Fig. 8–14B). Chronic synovitis, including the recurrent hemorrhagic synovitis that often occurs, can be markedly diminished or eliminated by a thorough synovectomy (Fig. 8–15). Reasonable pain relief has been documented in most of these patients for as long as a 5-year follow-up period. Although a modest improvement in function accompanies pain relief, these patients should clearly understand that an arthroscopic procedure cannot materially improve their range of motion or strength. The instability found in a patient with cuff arthropathy is accompanied by a loss of anterior stabilization (subscapularis) and/or posterior stabilization (supraspinatus, teres minor). As a result, the pseudoarticulation required by the deltoid force-couple to elevate the arm is unlikely to develop. Pain relief is the primary goal of the operation.

RESULTS

A group of 20 shoulders with massive, irreparable tears was selected for arthroscopic treatment and followed for 2 to 6 years.[40] Of the shoulders in this study, 5 had cuff arthropathy. Based on the UCLA Shoulder Rating Scale, 10 good, 6 fair, and 4 poor results were achieved. Not one excellent result was achieved. Given the limited-goals aspect of this group of patients, the shoulders with good and fair ratings were considered to represent favorable outcomes. The UCLA score gives a total of 10 points each for pain and function, 5 points each for range of motion and strength, and 5 points for patient satisfaction with the result. The maximum score is 35 points. The average preoperative score of the shoulders studied was 13; the average postoperative score was 27.6, an increase of more than 100%. Most patients who considered this operation successful were able to lift their arms up to or above shoulder level against gravity; however, they were unable to perform this movement repetitively when more than 1

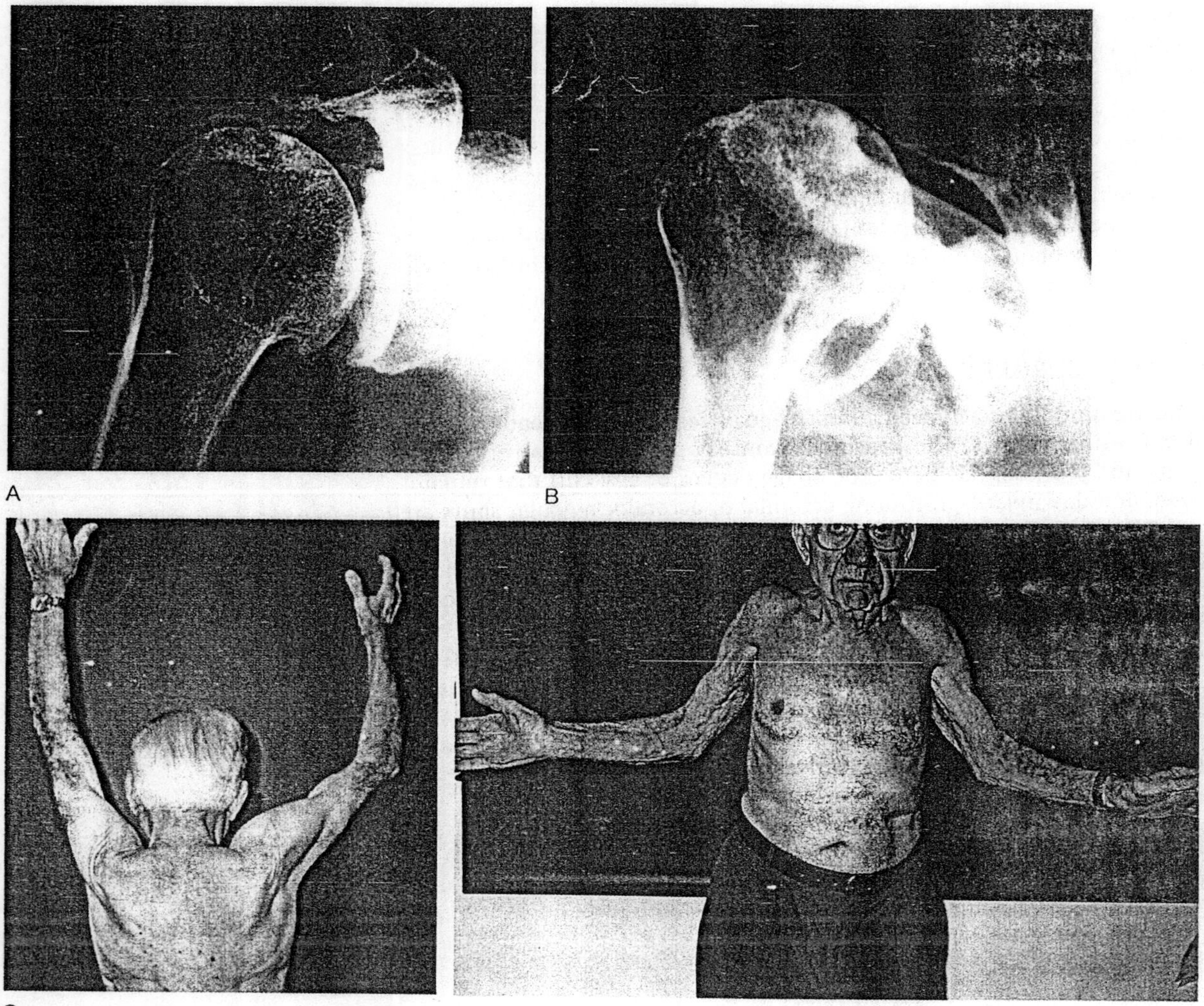

A B C D

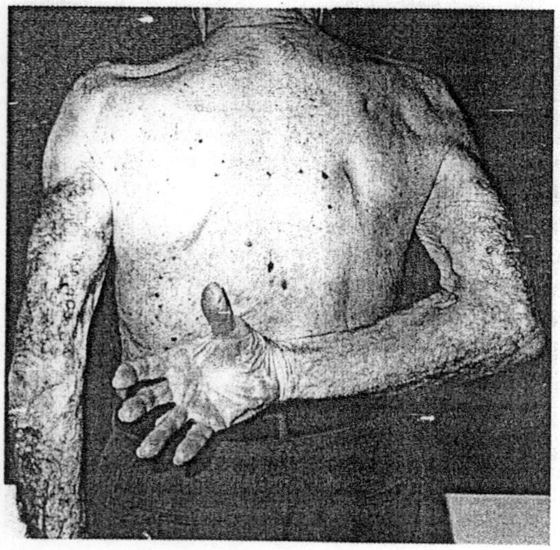

E

FIG. 8–16. Follow-up study: Good result following arthroscopic decompression and cuff debridement.

A, Preoperative radiograph of 80-year-old man shows nearly complete obliteration of acromiohumeral distance. He had undergone repeated aspirations for hemorrhagic synovitis and disabling pain.

B, Six-year follow-up radiograph. The head has risen upward in relation to the glenoid and moved medially to develop pseudoarticulation.

C, Six-year follow-up examination of patient aged 86 years. The patient is pain free and able to achieve functional elevation in the plane of the scapula. Note deltoid hypertrophy.

D, Comparison of external rotation of both extremities.

E, Internal rotation. Thumb touches dorsal 10. Patient is free of pain.

or 2 pounds of weight were added. Five patients could lift up to 5 pounds, and only one patient could manage 10 pounds.

We believe that the arthroscopic debridement and decompression procedure is a reasonable method of treatment for irreparable cuff tears and cuff arthropathy. The functional results are similar to, and at times better than, more heroic salvage procedures in selected patients with massive, irreparable cuff tears (Fig. 8–16).

CALCIFIC TENDINITIS

Calcific tendinitis is a unique lesion among the disorders that produce impingement symptoms in the shoulder. The precise stimulus that provokes calcium deposition is uncertain. Codman described the condition in detail.[11] McLaughlin believed that the pathogenesis involved the degeneration of collagen tissue and, therefore, that the condition was a degenerative disease.[110] Uhthoff and associates disagree and have pointed out that this condition is different from the relatively small flakes of dystrophic calcification seen in degenerative tendinitis.[111] The average age of the patient with acute or chronic calcific tendinitis is younger than that of the patient with degenerative cuff disease. The condition is rarely seen in heavy laborers. As many as 65% of patients who have calcific deposits in the shoulder also have calcific deposits elsewhere in the body. Involvement in repetitive overhead activities of a strenuous nature is not a significant factor in patients with calcific tendinitis.

CAUSES OF CALCIFICATION

Numerous factors influencing the deposition of calcium, such as an increase in the calcium/phosphorus saturation or the existence of a substance that could create nucleating sites or remove them, have been proposed as the causative agent. The question regarding precisely which agent induces calcification to occur biomechanically is still unanswered. A decrease in pO_2 has been confirmed.

The theory proposed by Uhthoff has become a unifying concept in our management of this condition and has enhanced our understanding of this unique lesion.[111] Uhthoff theorizes that calcific tendinitis is a "self-healing tendinopathy" and describes a *formative/resorptive cycle* (Fig. 9–1). He postulates a precalcifying phase in which a reduction in oxygen tension transforms a portion of the tendon into fibrocartilage, where chondrocytes mediate the deposition of calcium at multiple foci. Following this formative phase, the calcium may exist for an indefinite period of time. Eventually, phagocytic cells accumulate around individual foci, and concomitant vascular proliferation occurs. The resorptive phase begins when these new vascular channels provide a pathway for resorption and restore normal perfusion and oxygen tension to the tissues. After the calcification is resorbed, the tendon is capable of returning to normal function, presum-

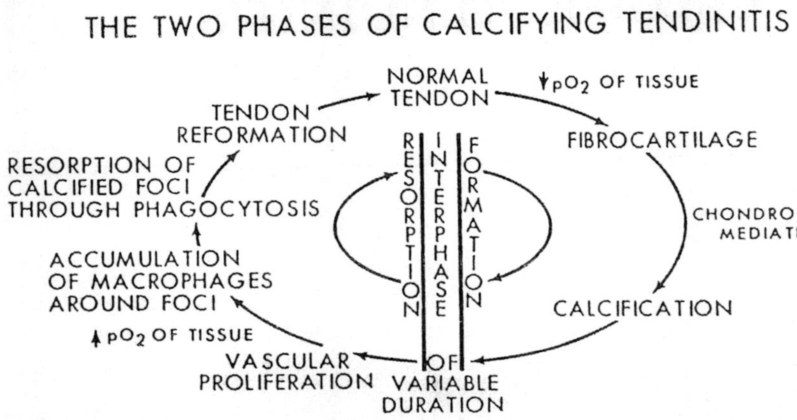

FIG. 9–1. Formative/resorptive cycle of calcification. (From Uhthoff, H.K., Sarkar, K., and Maynard, J.A.: Calcifying tendinitis: A new concept of its pathogenesis. Clin. Orthop., *118*:164, 1976.)

ably by new matrix formation. Symptoms intensify during this resorptive phase. Both phases may exist concurrently.

RADIOGRAPHIC APPEARANCE

Based on roentgenographic appearance, DePalma and Kruper divided calcific deposits into type I, "fluffy, amorphous lesions" that were usually associated with acute symptoms (Fig. 9–2A), and type II, "defined, homogenous lesions" with subacute or chronic clinical symptoms (Fig. 9–2B).[112] Uhthoff and associates agreed that fluffy calcific deposits are often associated with acute symptoms and noted that a patient with chronic calcification may develop acute symptoms when the process of resolution is occurring.[111] Pinals and Short have also noted that disintegration of calcific deposits occurred concurrently with acute attacks of pain.[113] Attempts to control pain and assess the calcification serially for evidence of resorption are prudent steps to take prior to considering surgical intervention, even in the case of chronic deposits.

Conversely, McKendry and colleagues have also noted that 50% of patients with an acute onset of symptoms failed to develop resorptive features.[114] They also noted that "fully 30% of patients continued to have pain and shoulder dysfunction for more than 12 weeks" following open removal of calcium.

LOCALIZATION OF DEPOSITS

Calcific deposits in the shoulder may be uni- or multiloculated. The deposits may occur in more than one tendon in the same shoulder. The location of the deposit(s) must be identified to initiate appropriate treatment.

Radiographs taken in the anteroposterior projection in both internal and external rotation, as well as an axillary view, help the surgeon to localize the deposit. Calcifications involving the supraspinatus tendon maintain a position superior to the humeral head in both internal and external rotation. When the

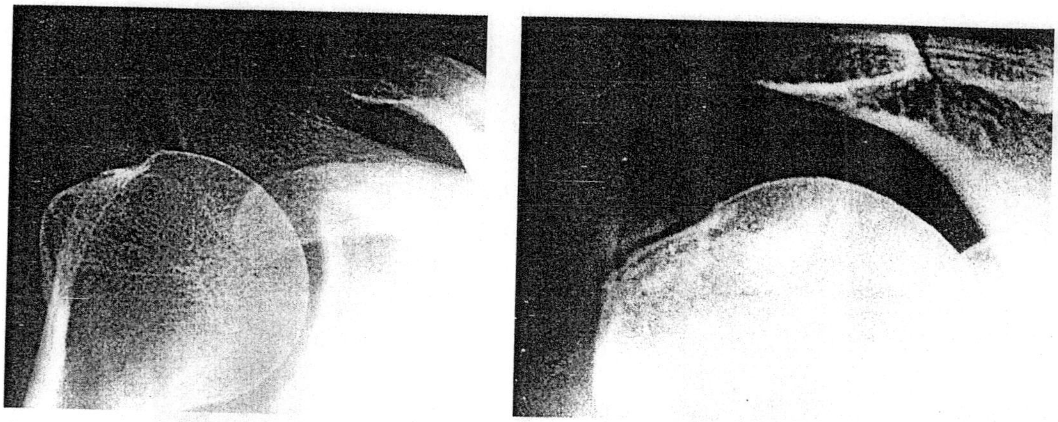

A B

FIG. 9–2. Types of calcification.
A, Type I: Fluffy, amorphous lesion.
B, Type II: Defined, homogenous lesion.

calcification is located more posteriorly (within the tendon of the infraspinatus, for example), the greater tuberosity may obscure the calcification in the externally rotated anteroposterior view (Fig. 9–3A). The calcification may only appear in a somewhat lateral and inferior position to the tip of the tuberosity as the arm is internally rotated (Fig. 9–3B). The axillary view is most helpful in identifying calcifications in the subscapularis anteriorly, as well as in the infraspinatus or teres minor posteriorly (Fig. 9–3C). The supraspinatus outlet view (arch view) can also be helpful (Fig. 9–3D).

CONSERVATIVE MANAGEMENT

Conservative management is based on the recognition and localization of the calcific deposit as a source of shoulder pain. The clinical presentation most often is that of the impingement syndrome. The intratendinous calcification produces an "intrinsic tendinopathy" that compromises the supraspinatus outlet by both tendinous enlargement and reactive subacromial bursitis. On occasion, a patient with a known chronic deposit or a previously unknown lesion experiences an acute onset of excruciating shoulder pain. This acute phase appears to be associated with the resorption of some aspects of the chronic deposit or with a potential rupture of the calcification into the subacromial space. In either instance, the patient may appear in need of emergency relief following a sleepless night during which all measures of pain relief had failed (Fig. 9–4A). The introduction of a local anesthetic (bupivacaine, 0.25%) into the subacromial space (Fig. 9–4B), in conjunction with needling of the calcification, can produce dramatic pain relief (Fig. 9–4C). The addition of a soluble steroid reduces the bursal reactive changes and diminishes pain after the anesthetic wears off.

An amorphous deposit of calcific granules occasionally can be aspirated in the process of local anesthetic infiltration. If a second needle with a somewhat larger bore can be introduced into the calcific deposit, a considerable amount of calcium can be removed by barbotage (Fig. 9–5). More often, the calcium is too

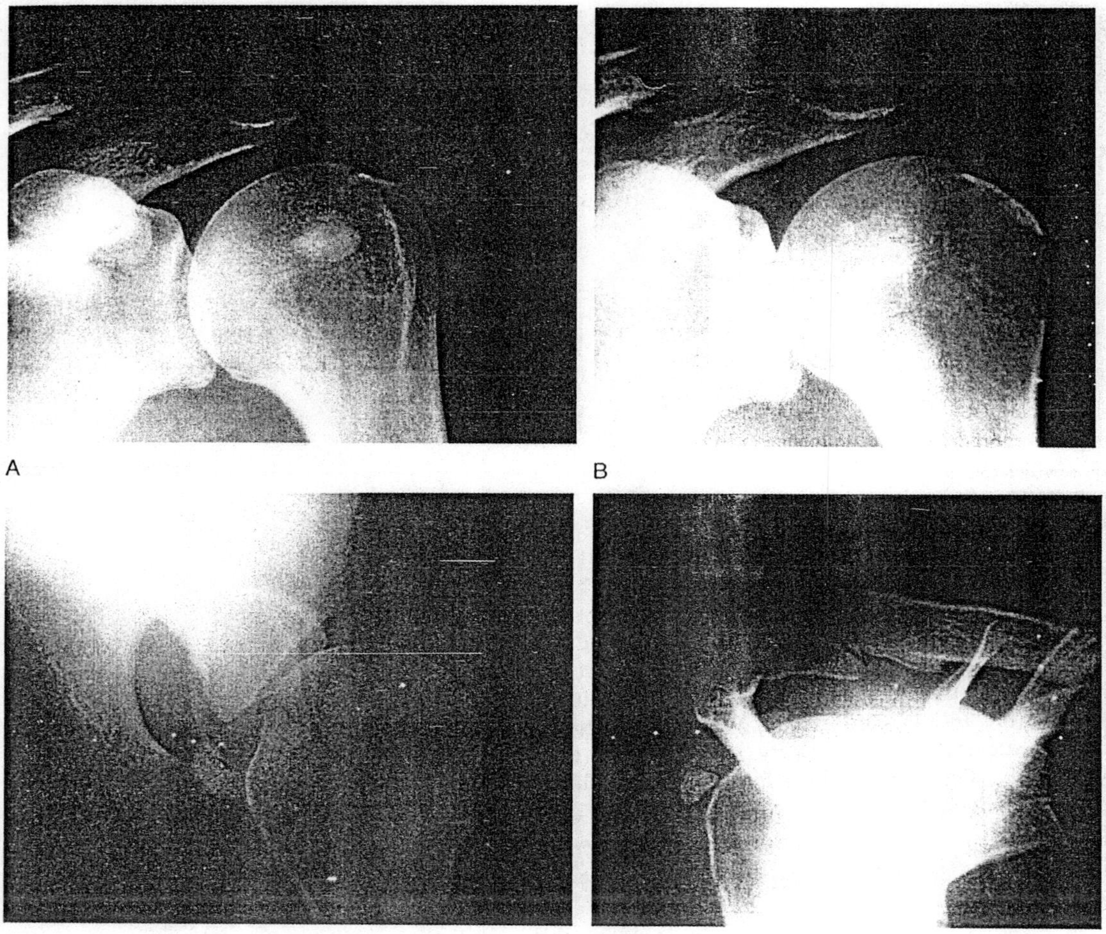

A B C D

FIG. 9–3. Radiographic localization of calcific deposit.
A, Anteroposterior view in external rotation reveals single deposit obscured by humeral head.
B, Internal rotation view reveals two separate areas of calcification in the supraspinatus.
C, Axillary view shows both deposits in the infraspinatus; one is more anterior than the other.
D, Supraspinatus outlet (arch) view helps further to localize deposits.

inspissated to permit aspiration. The gritty sensation of a chronic deposit can be appreciated as the needle is introduced. In theory, needling the region of a chronic calcareous deposit introduces a channel for vascular ingrowth and thereby stimulates the process of resorption.

The patient suffering from calcareous tendinitis should be encouraged to perform range-of-motion exercises to tolerance to avoid the development of capsulitis. After barbotage and/or needling, the patient is advised to apply ice packs to the shoulder and is given analgesic medication to relieve the pain that will develop after the local anesthetic wears off.

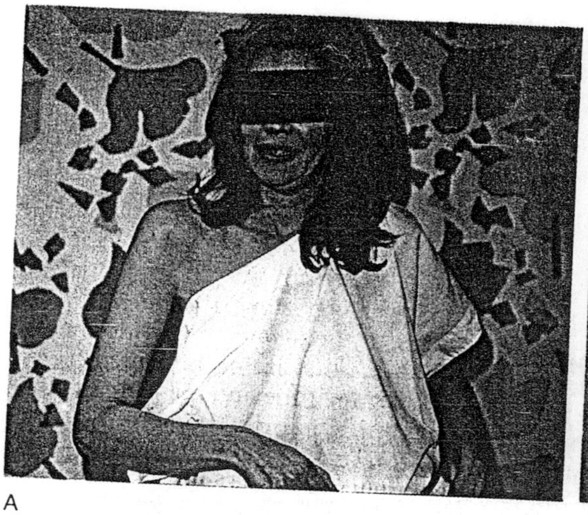

A

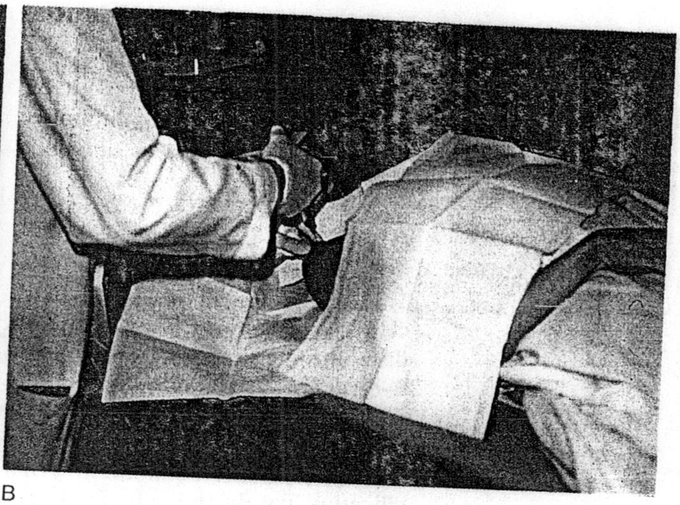

B

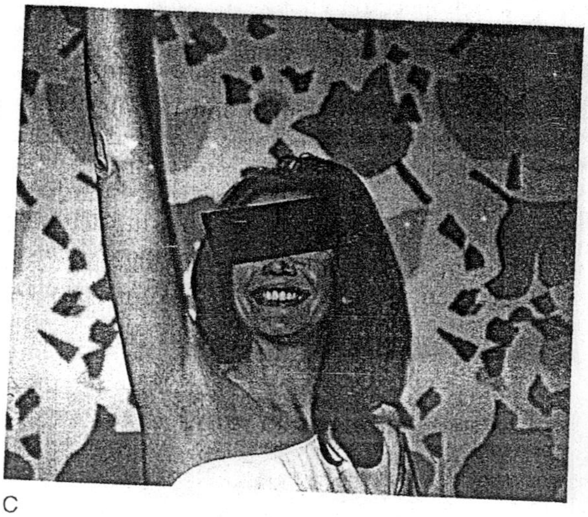

C

FIG. 9–4. Conservative treatment.
A, Woman, 42 years of age, had experienced 24 hours of intractable pain. She was unable to abduct.
B, Injection of local anesthetic with steroid. Calcium is needled.
C, Dramatic relief. Patient was advised regarding post-anesthetic use of ice and analgesics.

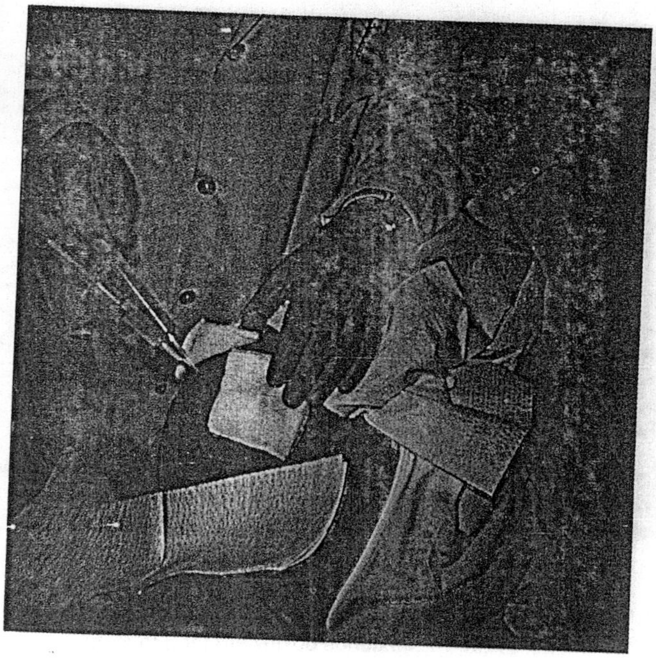

FIG. 9–5. Barbotage: On occasion, amorphous calcium can be removed by irrigation with two syringes of local anesthetic.

SURGICAL MANAGEMENT

Prior to the development of arthroscopic techniques, patients with refractory cases of calcareous tendinitis who had endured recurrent symptoms for more than 2 years were treated by arthrotomy and surgical removal of the deposit.

OPEN TECHNIQUE

The shoulder is approached through a short incision along the lines of skin cleavage, beginning at the anterolateral aspect of the acromion and extending distally for no more than 3 to 4 cm depending on the size of the patient (Fig. 9–6A). The deltoid is split along the junction between the anterior longitudinal fibers and the more lateral bipenniform fibers of the muscle. Following incision of the bursa, the shoulder is internally and externally rotated to visualize the intratendinous calcification in either the supraspinatus or the infraspinatus (calcification within the subscapularis requires a deltopectoral approach). Regional swelling, whitish discoloration, or injection often localize the site of a significant deposit. When the deposit can be readily identified, a small incision is made along the line of cuff fibers, and a curette is introduced to remove calcification (Fig. 9–6B). In some patients, the calcification is interstitial and not apparent from the bursal surface. In this circumstance, the suspected area is probed with a 20-gauge lumbar puncture (LP) needle. The obturator of the LP needle is removed, and following each penetration, the lumen is inspected to see if it has encountered any calcium. An exploratory incision is then made after the deposit has been located. A single absorbable suture is occasionally used to approximate the cuff defect after a sizable deposit has been removed.

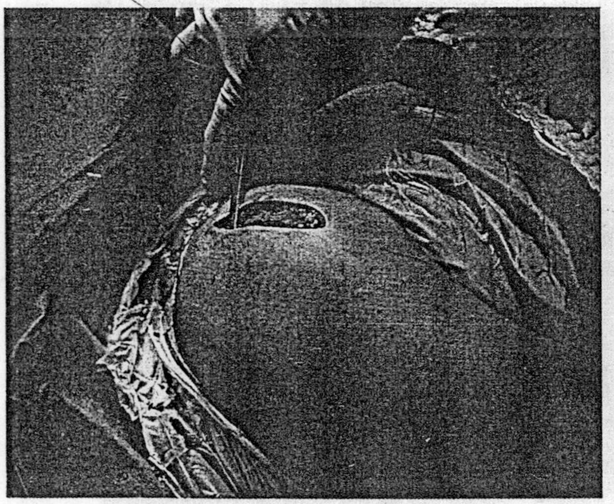

A

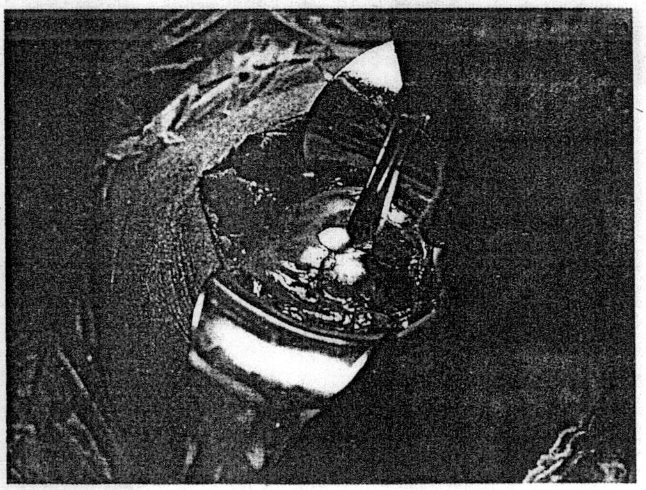

B

FIG. 9–6. Open surgical removal.
A, Short deltoid-splitting exposure begins at the anterolateral corner of the acromion and extends downward for 3 to 4 cm.
B, Cuff incised in line of fibers to release a copious amount of amorphous calcium.

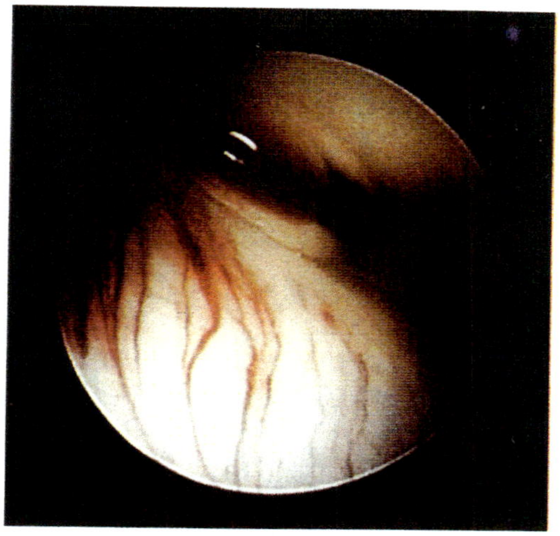

A

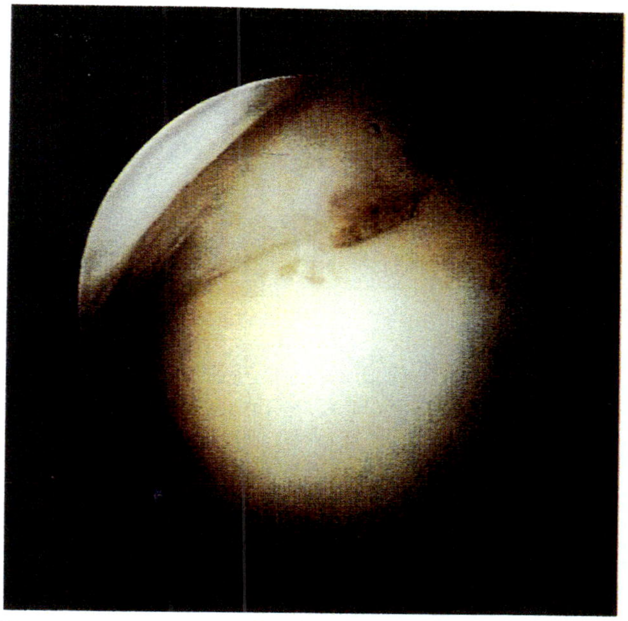

B

FIG. 9–7. Arthroscopic treatment: Glenohumeral inspection.
A, Hyperemic capsule below calcium deposit.
B, Small chondral lesion invading articular surface of humeral head directly below calcific deposit.

ARTHROSCOPIC TECHNIQUE

The patient is prepared for shoulder arthroscopy as described in Chapter 3. The posterior soft-spot portal is established and diagnostic glenohumeral arthroscopy is performed. Particular attention is directed to the capsule in the region where calcium is considered to be present. Although visualization of calcific deposits from the articular surface is highly unusual, the synovium may appear locally hyperemic (Fig. 9–7A). Isolated chondral defects near the margins of the humeral head have been noted occasionally directly below a calcific deposit (Fig. 9–7B). Introduction of a "marker suture" into the joint is helpful (see Chap. 6, Fig. 6–14). A 20-gauge LP needle is introduced vertically from a point adjacent to the anterolateral border of the acromion directly into the joint under arthroscopic surveillance. The obturator of the needle is removed prior to insertion, and if the needle passes through a deposit in the supraspinatus, flakes of calcium will be seen as the joint is penetrated. A No. 1 absorbable (PDS) suture is passed through the lumen, and the needle is withdrawn carefully to leave the suture in situ (Fig. 9–8). The location of this suture becomes a reference point when the bursal surface of the cuff is inspected. The location in which the marker suture is introduced may be varied if preoperative assessment suggests a more posterior (infraspinatus) location of the deposit.

Routine portals for subacromial space arthroscopy are then established (see Chap. 5). Visualization generally is difficult until a mechanical shaver is introduced and a subtotal bursectomy performed. The bursa may be inflamed and hypertrophic; however, at times this structure appears quite pristine except for some local hyperemia. Control of bleeding is maintained by electrocautery.

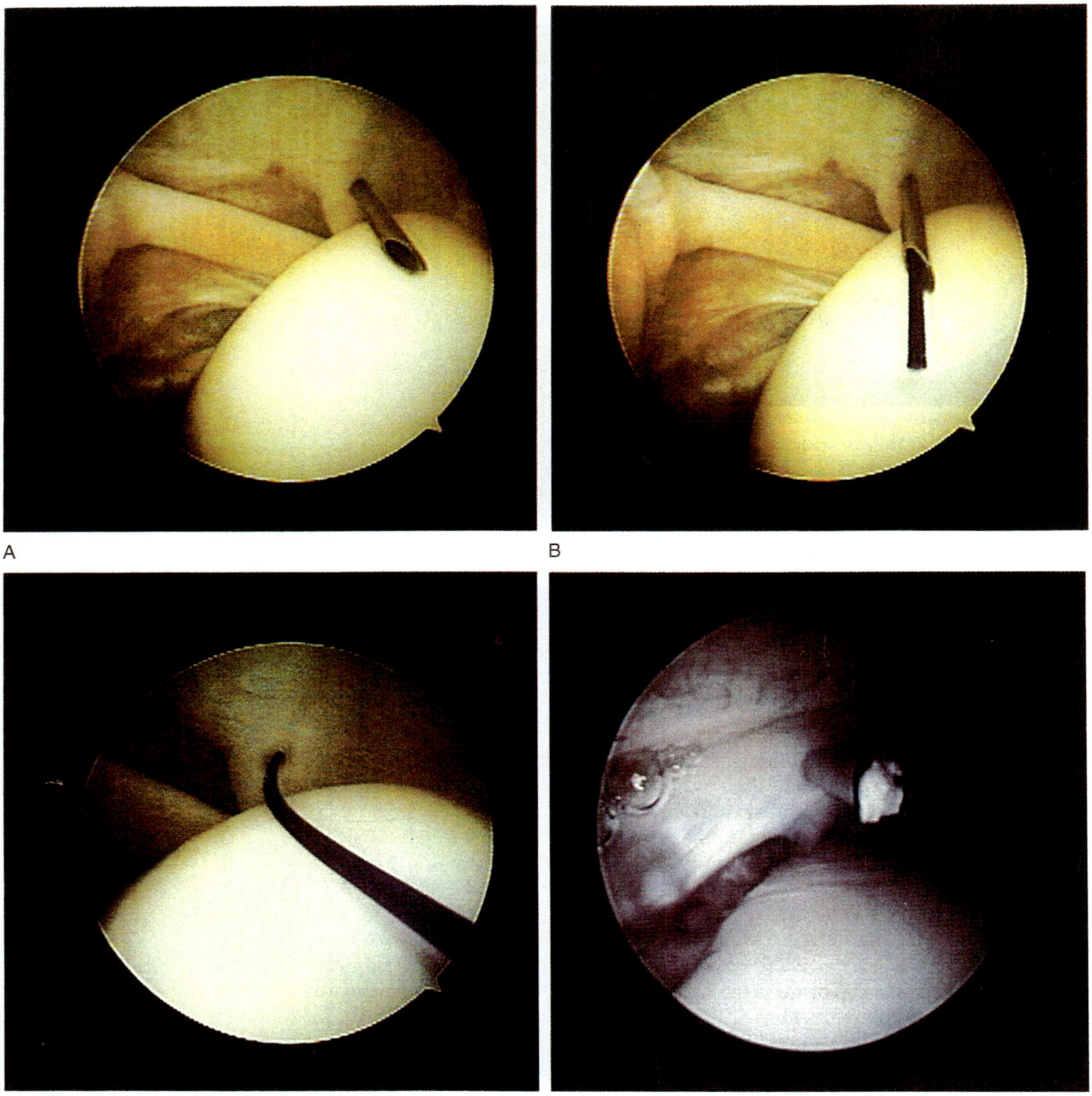

A B C D

FIG. 9–8. Introduction of marker suture to aid localization.
A, A 20-gauge lumbar puncture needle is introduced through anterior margin of subscapularis tendon.
B, Absorbable (PDS) suture introduced through needle.
C, Needle is removed, leaving marker suture in position.
D, In this instance, the needle has been passed directly through the calcific deposit. Note the plug of calcium in the lumen.

After a thorough bursectomy, the superior surface of the rotator cuff is inspected to locate the calcific deposit. The dome of larger deposits may be visualized; however, in many instances, the calcification is interstitial and cannot be seen through the superior intact tendon fibers. After reviewing the preoperative radiographs to establish the likely location of the calcification(s), a 20-gauge LP needle is used to explore the cuff. The presence of a marker suture exiting the bursal surface of the cuff through a predetermined area is most helpful for orientation at this point.

Multiple punctures with the LP needle placed in the area of suspected calcification usually liberate a few snowflake-like flecks when calcium is encountered. Multiple penetrations, as well as wiggling the needle within the foci, liberate a great deal of calcium. An opening large enough to admit a 3-mm arthroscopic curette can be made in this fashion. On occasion, after the needle has located a deposit, the 3-mm arthroscopy knife may be used to make a small incision in the cuff in line with the fibers. The curette then can be introduced through this opening. When the calcification is multiloculated, the additional areas should be searched for diligently.

Because of the cyclic nature of this disorder, some areas of calcification may be quite inspissated and granular, whereas others may be more fluffy and amorphous. The fluffy, amorphous type oozes freely through the needle penetrations and is easiest to eradicate. A synovial shaver may be used to trim the frayed tendinous margins of the calcareous deposit. Copious irrigation in combination with the suction shaver should be used to remove the many calcific granules that have been liberated within the subacromial space. Even after an extensive deposit has been debulked, small granules of calcium can be noted in an interstitial position. The amount of calcium that may be removed without causing injury to the cuff is limited. Needling of the periphery of larger deposits creates new vascular channels and facilitates resorption of the remaining material. Figure 9–9 illustrates the techniques just described.

On occasion the foci of calcification may be difficult to locate. Consequently, the equipment needed to secure an intraoperative radiograph should be available to aid in the search. An intraoperative radiograph also helps to assess the amount of calcium that has been removed. We generally place an x-ray cassette beneath the shoulder before beginning the procedure.

ROLE OF ACROMIOPLASTY

In most patients, we have performed subacromial decompression in conjunction with the removal of calcific deposits. Based on our recent findings, however, this procedure may be necessary for only certain patients. Calcific tendinitis produces impingement symptoms by virtue of the intrinsic reaction that causes the tendon to swell. When calcification reaches the bursal surface, a significant bursal reaction is also provoked. We believe that the postoperative course is benefitted by decompression. DePalma advised release of the coracoacromial ligament following removal of calcium to ensure free excursion of the humeral head under the coracoacromial arch.[112] We believe acromioplasty is definitely indicated in two situations. The first is in any shoulder with a type III down-curving acromion that shows arthroscopic evidence of mechanical impingement. The second is in the rare case when a small intrinsic calcification cannot be identified even after extensive needling.

At the conclusion of the procedure, 10 ml of 0.25% bupivacaine are instilled within the subacromial space, and the portals are closed with 3-0 nylon sutures.

(text continues on p. 230)

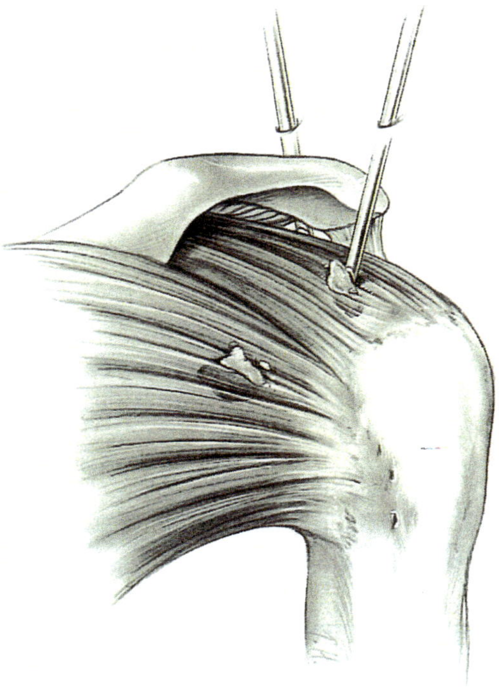

FIG. 9–9. Arthroscopic localization and removal of multifocal calcific deposits.
A, Marker suture is emerging from the joint below through inflamed bursal surface. Suture is adjacent to white, round calcific deposit.
B, The deposit is penetrated with an LP needle from above, thereby liberating flakes of calcium.
C, A curet is used to liberate large amounts of calcium.
D, A 3-mm rosette knife incises the cuff in line of fibers over a second deposit.
E, The opening liberates an oval-shaped solid mass of inspissated calcium.
F, The lump of calcium is removed from the joint. Note superficial round defect through which calcium emerged.
G, A shaver debrides the area. Considerable suction lavage is carried out to cleanse the subacromial space of calcific fragments. The coracoacromial ligament is released, and an anterior acromioplasty is performed to decompress the subacromial space.
H, This final picture shows the flattened acromion above and the cuff surface below.

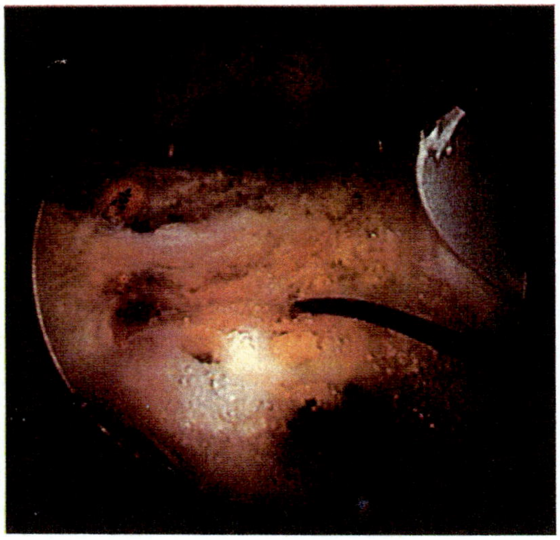

A

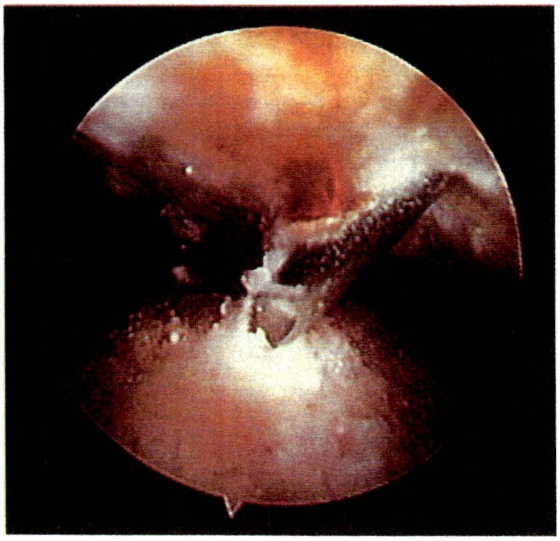

B

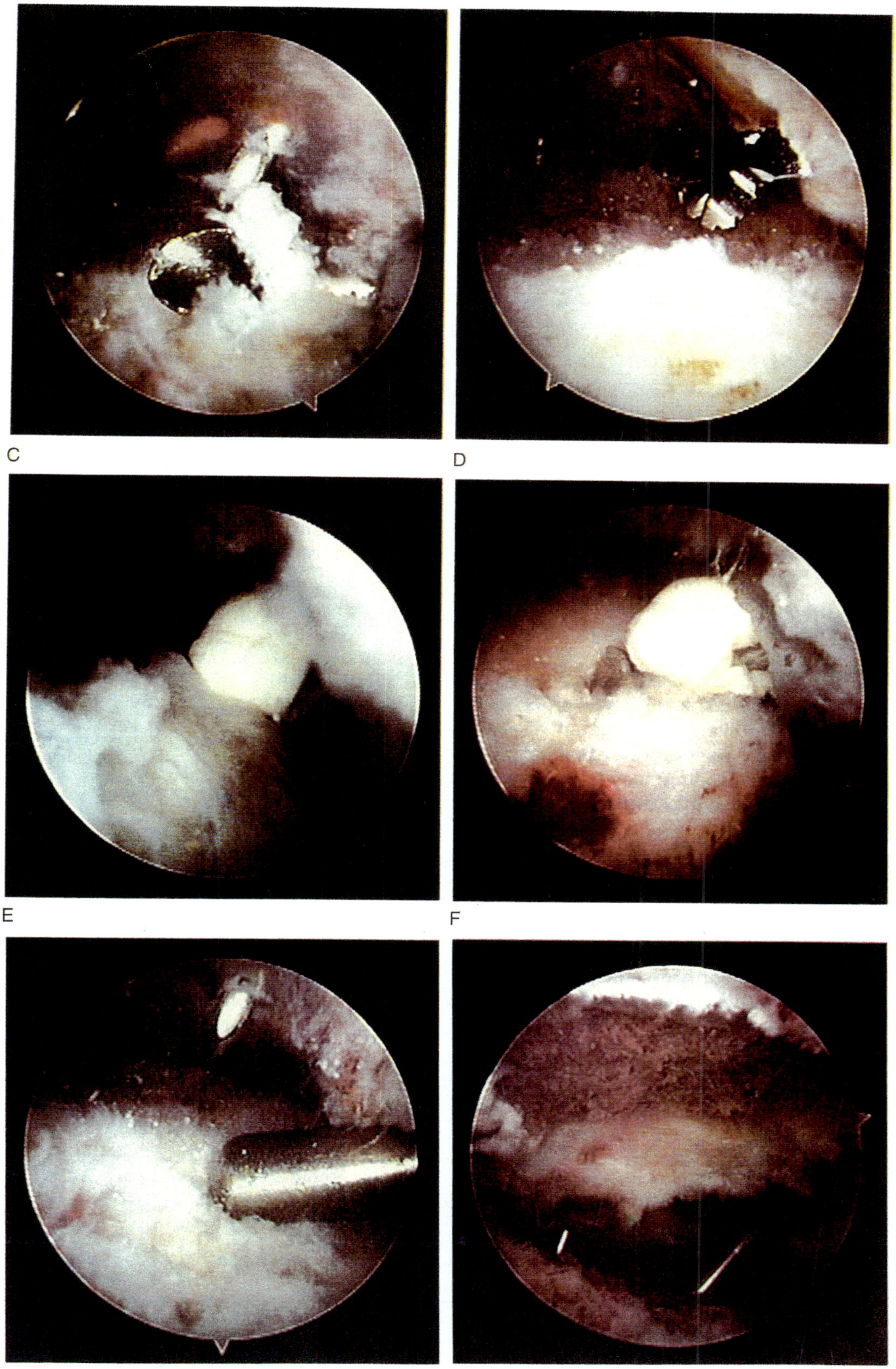

C D E F G H

FIG. 9-9 (continued)

POSTOPERATIVE MANAGEMENT

Patients are encouraged to perform active and active-assisted range of motion in forward flexion and external rotation in the supine position beginning on the day of surgery. Circumduction is added the next day. These exercises are performed twice daily for only 3 to 5 repetitions. The goal is simply to avoid adhesion formation. A sling is not necessary, and the patient may resume activities of daily living as tolerated. Isometrics are instructed at 3 weeks, and muscle-strengthening exercises with surgical tubing are initiated after 6 weeks.

FATE OF CALCIFICATION

Operative radiographs were taken during or immediately following the arthroscopic procedure for removal of calcification.[115] In some patients, particularly those with a large unilocular deposit, all the calcium appeared to have been removed (Fig. 9–10). In other patients, the postoperative radiograph showed that the calcification had been "debulked" but not eliminated (Fig. 9–11). Serial follow-up radiographs in these patients showed the gradual resolution of calcium over a variable period of time, anywhere from 2 weeks to 6 months. In some patients, especially when multiloculated deposits were present, the immediate postoperative film showed that some areas of calcification remained intact. In each instance, however, an attempt had been made to locate and needle these deposits. The eventual disappearance of calcific foci in all but one of these patients was rewarding but not surprising in view of current theory. The extensive needling may have brought vascular channels to the region and undoubtedly aided in stimulating resorption.

RESULTS

Ellman studied 16 patients who had endured the symptoms of calcific tendinitis for an average of 2.4 years prior to surgical intervention to evaluate the efficacy of the arthroscopic procedure described above.[115] The average number of preoperative corticosteroid injections was 4.4, with a range of from 1 to 20 injections.

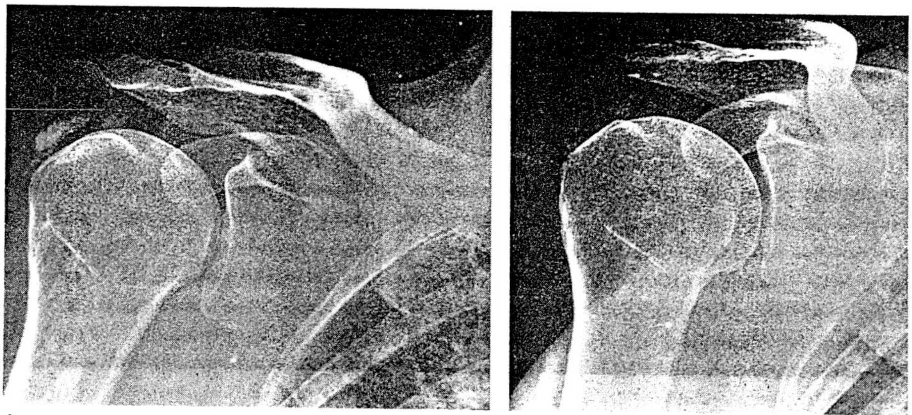

A B

FIG. 9–10. Fate of calcification.
A, Preoperative radiograph.
B, Postoperative film taken 1 week later.

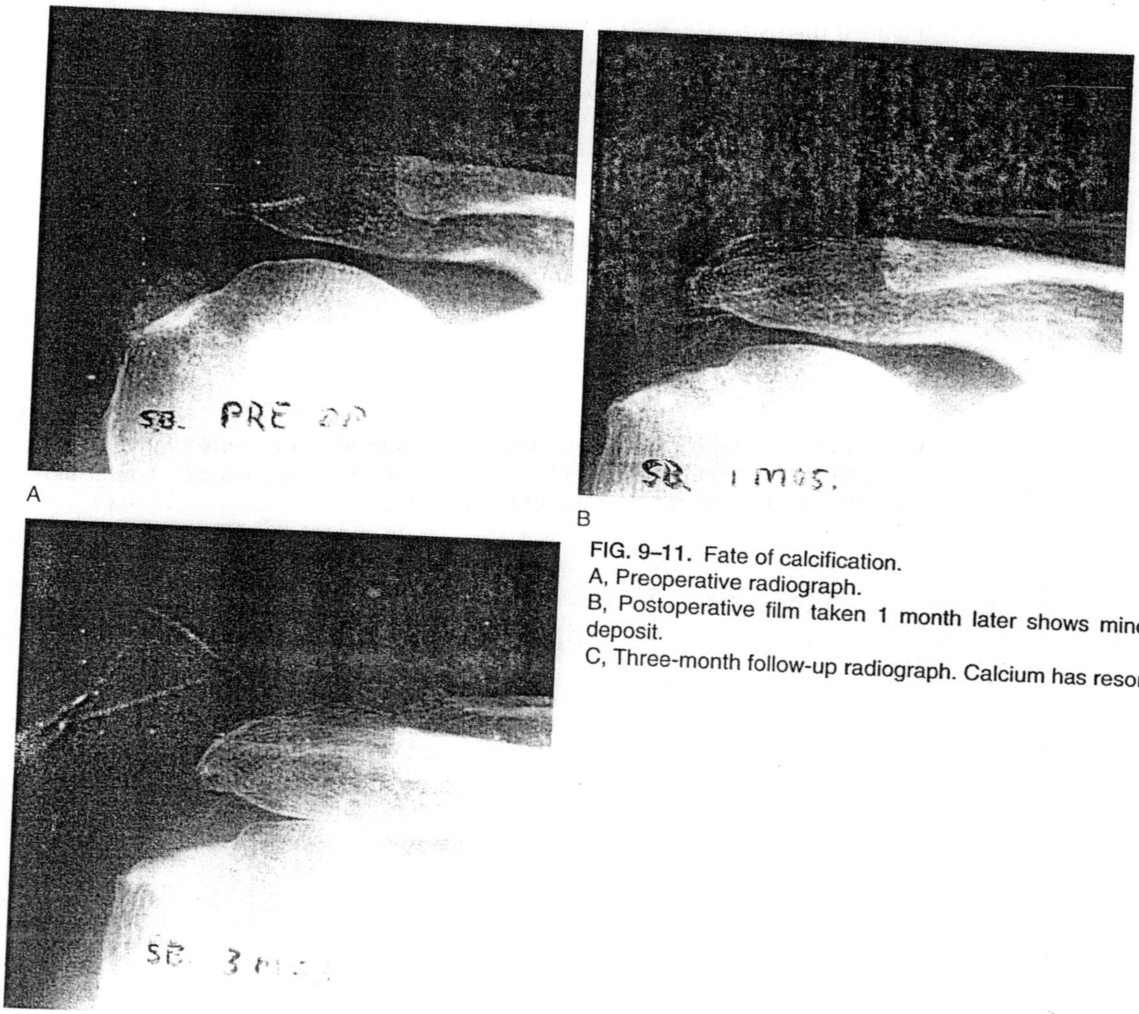

A B C

FIG. 9–11. Fate of calcification.
A, Preoperative radiograph.
B, Postoperative film taken 1 month later shows minor residual deposit.
C, Three-month follow-up radiograph. Calcium has resorbed.

The average calcification was nearly 2 cm in size. The minimum 1-year follow-up results, measured on the UCLA Shoulder Rating Scale, were 94% satisfactory and 6% unsatisfactory.

Ark and colleagues reported the results of 33 patients treated arthroscopically with an average follow-up of 26 months.[116] Satisfactory results were reported by 91%. Techniques used among the patients were similar; however, only 9 of their patients had a coracoacromial release, and only 3 of the patients initially had undergone an arthroscopic acromioplasty. Of the 20 patients who did not have acromioplasty, 2 had persistent pain and required a second operation. These patients were the only 2 patients who reported unsatisfactory results. Ark and colleagues believed that an impingement lesion had been overlooked. An arthroscopic acromioplasty was performed in a second operation on both of these patients, and they eventually achieved a satisfactory result.

A recent American multicenter study on arthroscopic treatment was reported at the Vth International Conference on Surgery of the Shoulder.[117] The study included the patients from the aforementioned reports plus the patients of three additional practitioners. Of the 131 patients studied, 93 had acromioplasties and 37 did not. One case was undocumented. No significant correlation existed between the global results of the patients who had acromioplasty and those who did not. Satisfactory relief of pain and restoration of range of motion and function were uniformly achieved by more than 90% of the patients reported by the participants.

An extended period of conservative management had been carried out in these patients. The average duration of symptoms prior to surgery was 29.4 months.

SUMMARY

Most patients with calcifying tendinitis respond to conservative care. Arthroscopic intervention should be reserved until it has been clearly established that spontaneous resorption is not likely to occur.

10

LONG HEAD OF BICEPS TENDON LESIONS

The long head of the biceps (LHB) tendon arises from the supraglenoid tubercle and travels across the anterosuperior aspect of the humeral head within the glenohumeral joint. It then enters the bicipital sulcus (intertubercular groove), where it is held in place superiorly by the transverse humeral ligament and inferiorly by the broad tendon of the pectoralis major insertion. Synovial membrane from the joint accompanies the tendon into the sulcus. Below the sulcus, the LHB merges with the short head to form the body of the biceps brachii. This muscle acts as a powerful supinator and flexor of the forearm. The LHB helps to hold the humeral head in its socket, especially during external rotation of the humerus. The tendon of the LHB also serves to depress the humeral head during elevation of the arm. The hypertrophy of the tendon that occurs when the rotator cuff has been torn attests to this function.

ARTHROSCOPIC INSPECTION

During arthroscopic inspection of the glenohumeral joint, the intact tendon has a round cord-like appearance. The surface is smooth and white (Fig. 10–1A). The tendon marks the interval between the supraspinatus and subscapularis muscles. When viewed through the posterior portal, the tendon is seen exiting into the sulcus adjacent to the most anterior fibers of the supraspinatus insertion (Fig. 10–1B). With the arm in neutral rotation, a spinal needle placed vertically down from the anterolateral corner of the acromion into the joint penetrates the supraspinatus just posterior to the LHB tendon. A second needle passed vertically downward in front of the acromioclavicular joint is seen just anterior to the tendon (Fig. 10–1C). The tendon lies directly beneath the anterior acromion at this point and is vulnerable to the same mechanical factors of impingement produced by a downcurving acromion[1] or by distally pointing osteophytes[57] as are the cuff tendons, depending on rotation during elevation.

TYPES OF LESIONS

Bicipital tendinitis, rupture, subluxation, and dislocation are the most commonly encountered lesions involving the LHB. The pathologic changes that occur within the sulcus cannot be visualized arthroscopically, but the *effects* of chronic inflammation, degeneration, or displacement are readily seen.

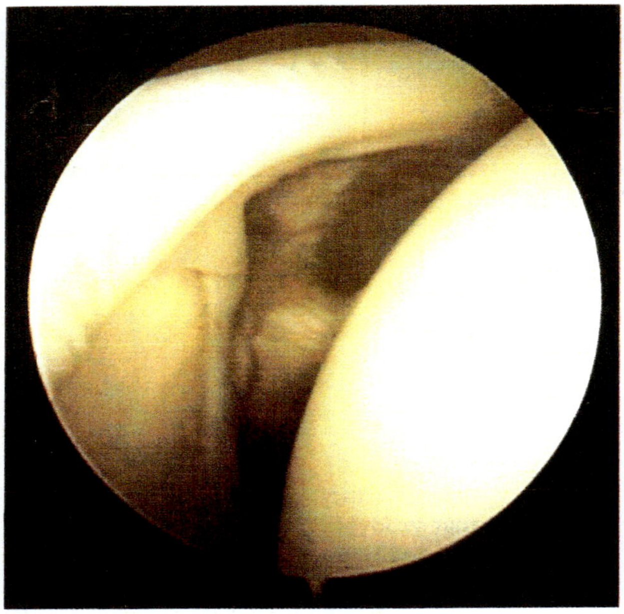

A

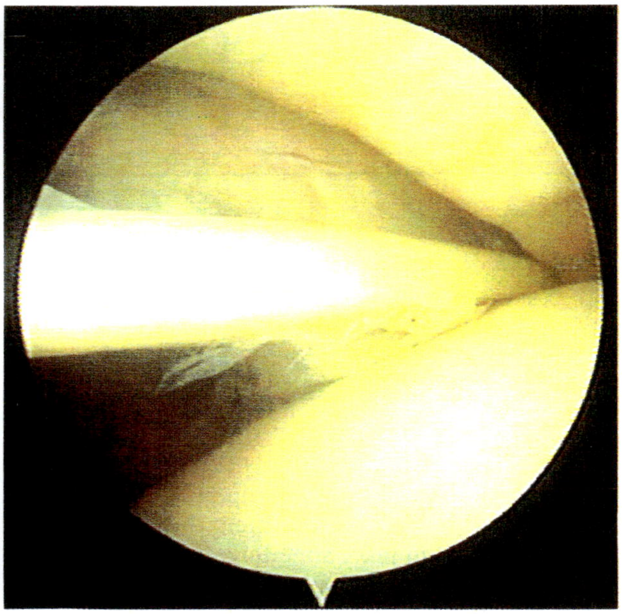

B

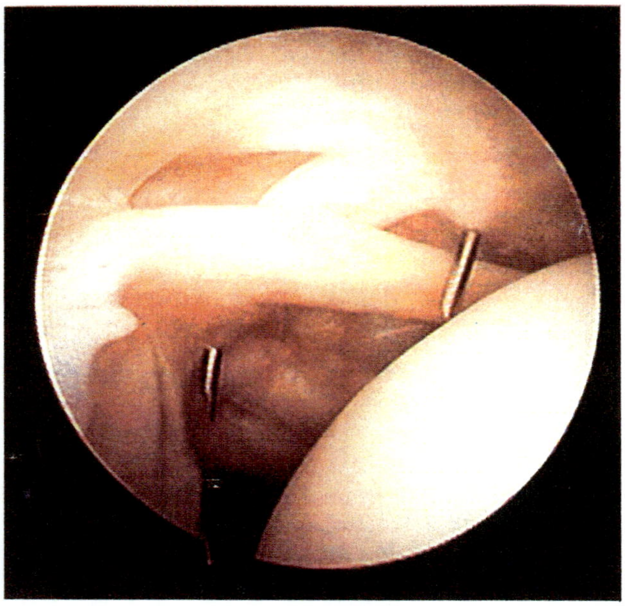

C

FIG. 10–1. A, The round, cord-like long head of the biceps tendon arises from the top of the glenoid.
B, The long head of the biceps exits into the sulcus immediately adjacent to the anterior margin of the supraspinatus.
C, Marker needles have been introduced at the anterolateral and anteromedial aspects of the acromion. Note how the long head of the biceps lies directly under the anterior acromion as it passes between the two needles.

BICIPITAL TENDINITIS

The LHB tendon does not move within the groove when the muscle is contracted. Rather, the groove moves around the relatively fixed tendon when the shoulder is elevated or rotated.[118] In the acute phase of bicipital tendinitis (commonly provoked by excessive activity), capillary dilatation, edema of the tendon and synovium, and cellular inflammation have been demonstrated.[119] The clini-

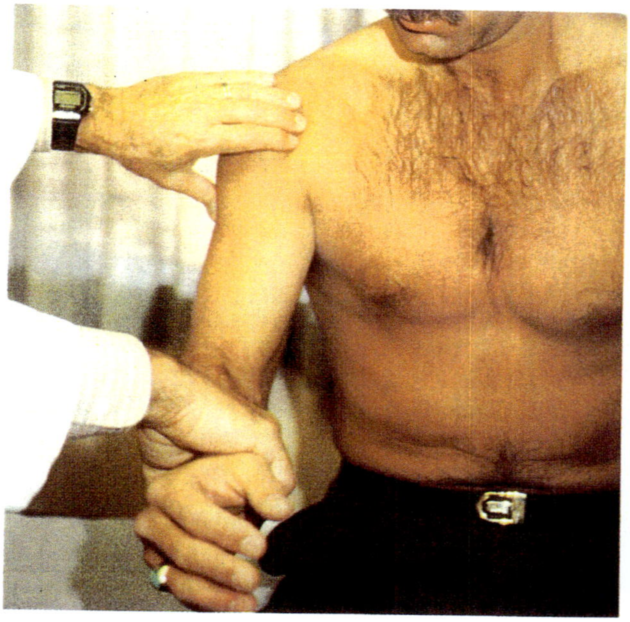

A

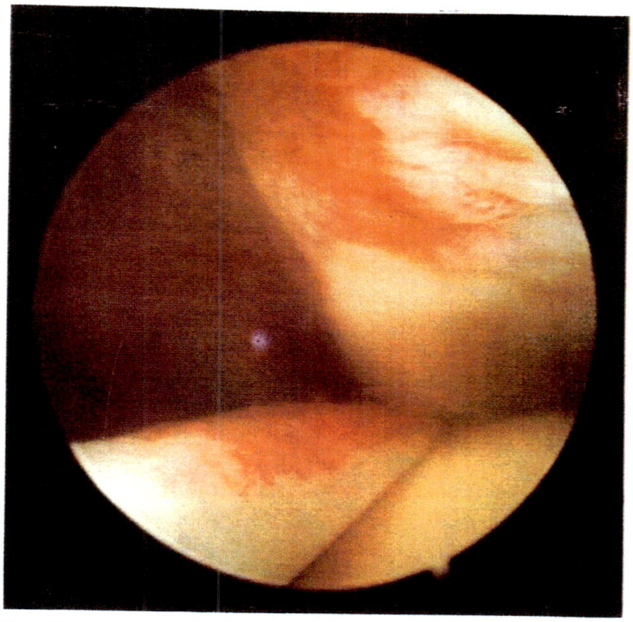

B

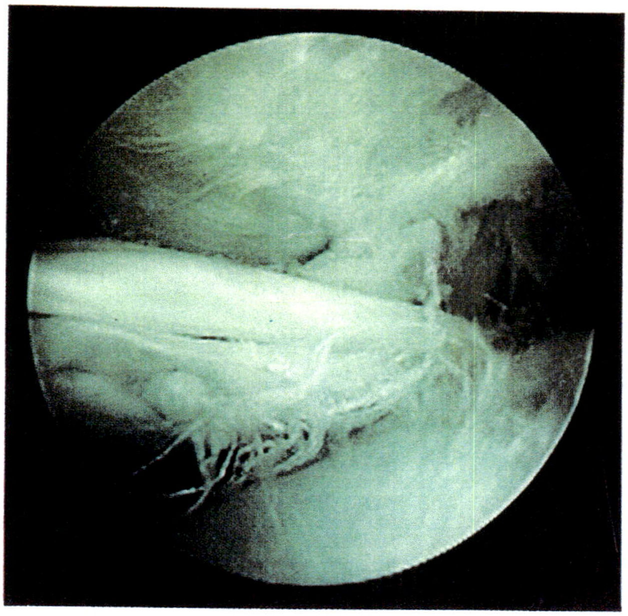

C

FIG. 10–2. A, Yergason test: With the elbow flexed, forced supination is resisted. Pain is referred to the bicipital sulcus in the presence of an injured long head of the biceps (LHB).
B, Capillary dilatation on the superior surface of the LHB as it enters the sulcus.
C, Extensive fraying is noted in the tendon at its point of exit into the sulcus.

cal consequences of these changes are localized tenderness and painful motion. The Yergason test (resisted supination with the elbow flexed) refers pain to the sulcus (Fig. 10–2A). When bicipital tendinitis becomes chronic, the tendon becomes frayed, narrowed, and fibrosed, thereby causing dense adhesions between the tendon and its sheath.[120]

During the acute phase, capillary dilatation may be seen through the arthroscope on the surface of the tendon as it enters the sulcus (Fig. 10–2B). The fraying associated with chronic tendinitis is seen in the same location (Fig. 10–2C).

PARTIAL AND COMPLETE RUPTURES

Progressive attrition and fraying of both the intra-articular and the intertubercular portions of the LHB were observed by Meyer in 1928.[121] He called attention to the supratubercular ridge on the lesser tuberosity as a factor in producing widening, flattening, and fibrillation of the articular portion of the LHB tendon. These changes in the tendon are seen arthroscopically in various stages that progress from partial tears to complete rupture (Fig. 10–3). Most tears are located in the lateral intra-articular portion of the tendon and extend into the sulcus, where they disappear from view.

Following complete rupture, the stump of tendon retained in the joint varies in length. When rupture of the LHB is associated with chronic massive rotator cuff tears, the stump is invariably quite short. Most ruptures occur in the proximal portion of the sulcus, thereby suggesting that the intra-articular portion of the tendon had been ground away between the superiorly migrated humeral head and the acromion. Smaller cuff tears associated with LHB rupture may disclose a longer stump of tendon. On occasion, a complete rupture of the LHB may be observed in the absence of a clinically apparent "bunching up" of the retracted muscle into the distal portion of the arm. Chronic adhesions within the intertubercular sulcus can prevent distal retraction of the degenerated tendon.

SUBLUXATION AND DISLOCATION

Arthroscopic examination is a definitive method of confirming the presence or absence of a subluxing biceps tendon. Hitchcock and Bechtol believed that a shallow bicipital groove contributed to displacement of the tendon, with resultant clinical symptoms.[122] We rarely observe either subluxation or dislocation of this tendon *unless* the adjacent subscapularis tendon is ruptured at its superior insertion. In most of these instances, the supraspinatus tendon is also torn. The LHB loses its proximal tether as the relatively weak transverse humeral ligament gives way, and the tendon migrates medially over the degenerated subscapularis.

When traumatic anterior dislocation of the shoulder occurs in a patient over the age of 40, a major rupture of the rotator cuff may be present. Avulsion of the subscapularis insertion permits the LHB to dislocate acutely. The displacement may be so severe that reduction is blocked by the posteriorly displaced tendon.

MANAGEMENT OF LESIONS

The origin of LHB lesions is multifactorial and activity related. Two groups of patients are encountered from a clinical point of view. The first group is comprised of younger individuals engaged in strenuous lifting (either vocational or avocational), or in throwing and racquet sports. This group, particularly the dedicated weight-lifters, develop primary bicipital tendinitis and, with persistent overuse, may progress to tendon rupture (Fig. 10–4). The second group is older, and the bicipital lesions are associated with the impingement mechanism. Changes in the supraspinatus tendon develop concurrent with biceps tendon degeneration. The two groups tend to merge in middle age, but the individual

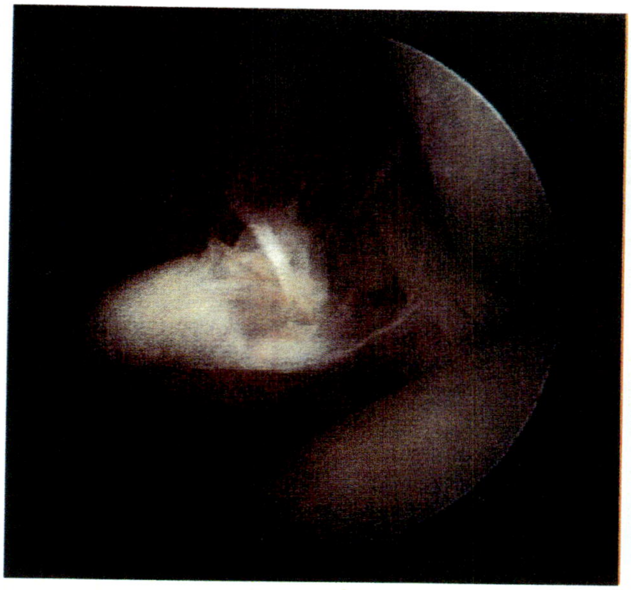

A

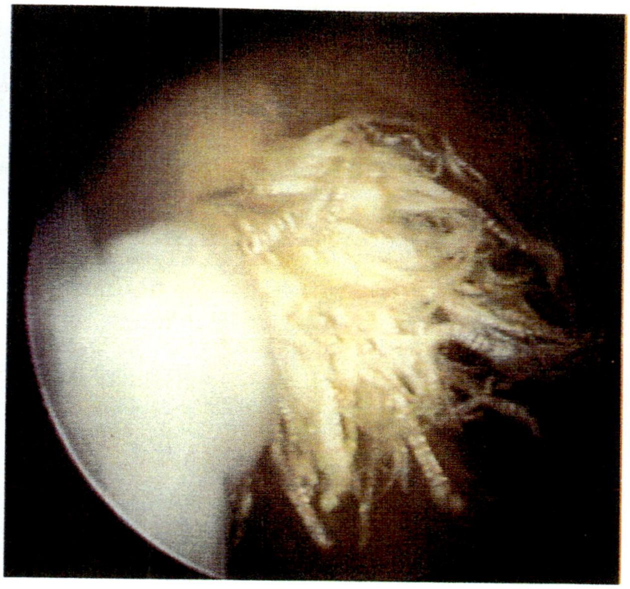

B

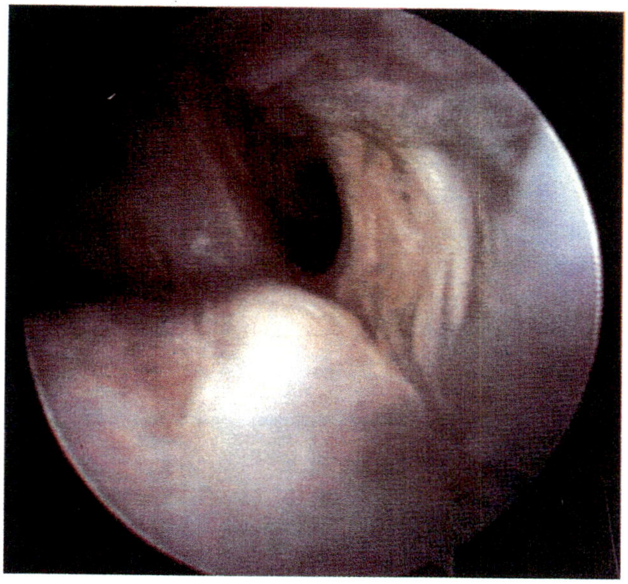

C

FIG. 10–3. Partial and complete ruptures of the long head of the biceps (LHB).

A, Partial rupture of the LHB occurring just proximal to its exit from the glenohumeral joint. Margin of supraspinatus tendon is above and humeral head is below.

B, Complete rupture of LHB at insertion into supraglenoid tubercle.

C, Same patient as in Figure 10–3B. Note the empty oval sulcus through which the LHB has retracted.

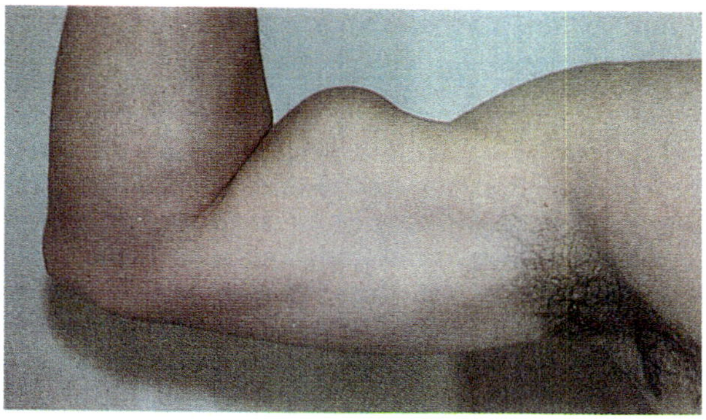

FIG. 10–4. Deformity caused by acute ruptured long head of the biceps tendon in a young, muscular patient.

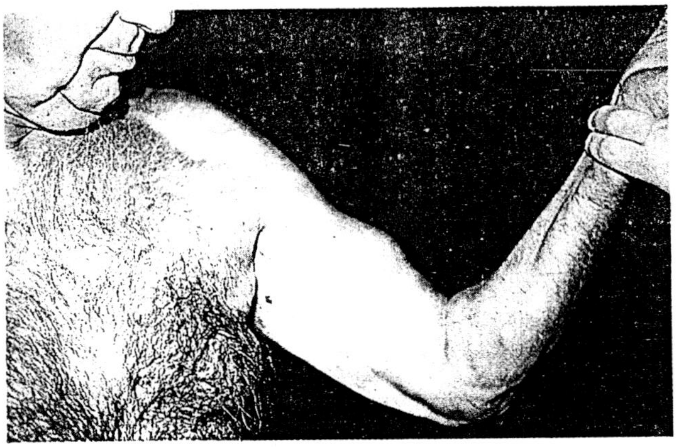

FIG. 10–5. Deformity in an older patient with associated rotator cuff tear.

who has been strenuously active is more likely to have more degenerative changes than is a sedentary counterpart (Fig. 10–5). Neer has advised that every patient over 40 years of age with a ruptured LHB should have an arthrogram to rule out rotator cuff tear.[60]

CONSERVATIVE TREATMENT

The basis of conservative treatment is rest and avoidance of offending activities. A sling is advised when symptoms are acute. Nonsteroidal anti-inflammatory drugs are helpful. Steroid injections into the tendon or its synovial sheath are avoided. Any attendant relief afforded by local steroids is often overcome by the patient's propensity to return prematurely to the offending activity. This propensity, combined with the deleterious effect of steroid on collagen, illustrates why tendon rupture often occurs following a series of injections. The relief of persistent disabling symptoms may require surgical intervention.

ARTHROSCOPIC TREATMENT

Glenohumeral joint inspection readily discloses bicipital tears or instability. Partial-thickness tears are debrided lightly; care must be taken to avoid disruption of intact fibers (Fig. 10–6). If the tear exceeds one-half the thickness of the tendon, subsequent rupture is likely in an active individual. When this patient fits the profile for primary tendinitis rather than for impingement and has no acromial abnormalities, an arthroscopically assisted transposition of the LHB is performed.

When a partial LHB tear is seen in older patients with a profile suggesting chronic impingement, the treatment is directed primarily to relieve the impingement. Following debridement of the partial tear, cuff inspection usually discloses at least a partial lesion in the supraspinatus tendon as well (Fig. 10–7). An arthroscopic subacromial decompression (see Chap. 5) is performed in these patients. The decompression generally relieves symptoms and retards the progression of both LHB and cuff tendon failure. The patient is warned that subsequent rupture of the LHB may occur. A prophylactic tenodesis is not warranted in this older group, except in individuals who plan to return to strenuous activi-

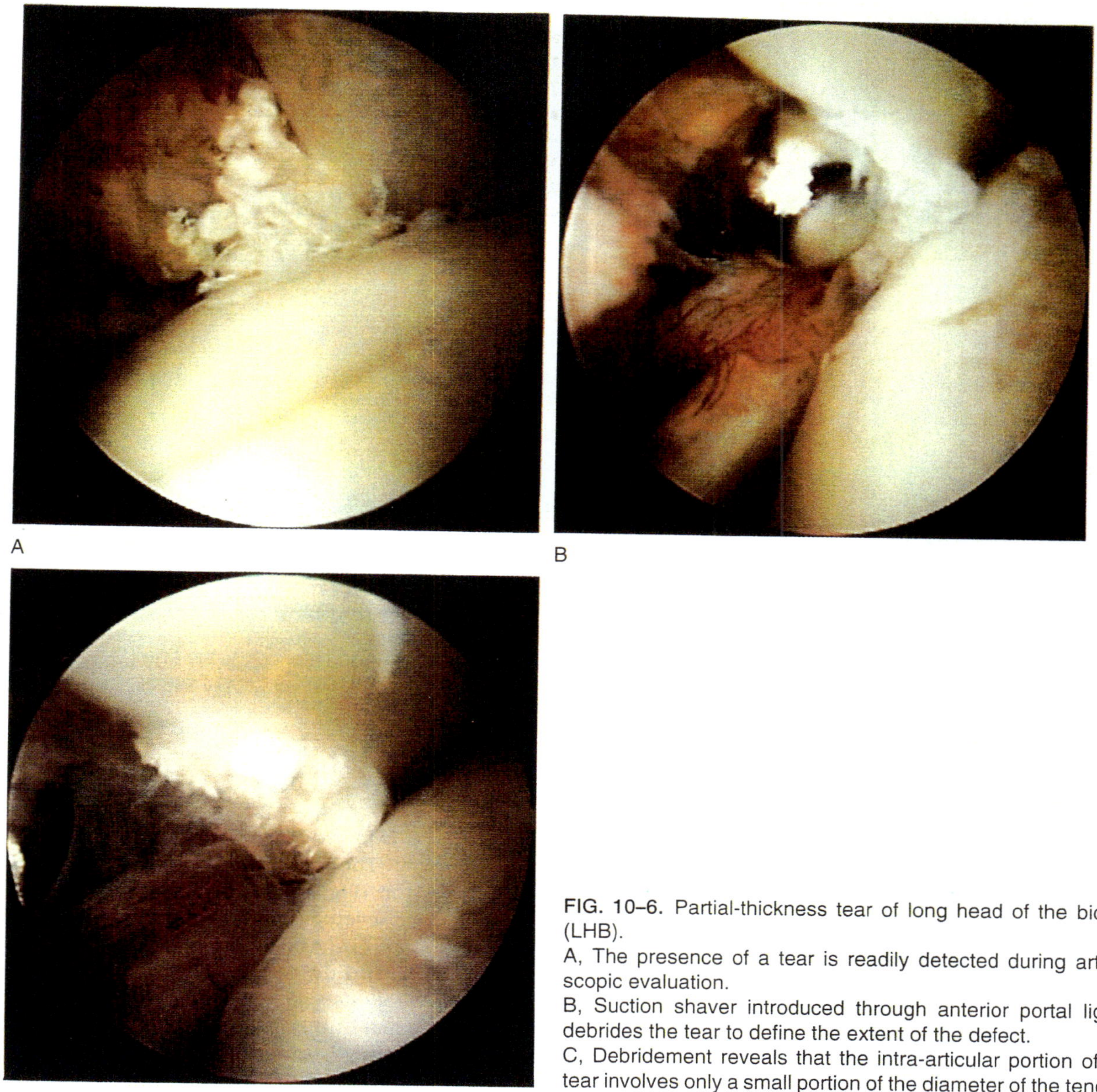

A

B

C

FIG. 10–6. Partial-thickness tear of long head of the biceps (LHB).
A, The presence of a tear is readily detected during arthroscopic evaluation.
B, Suction shaver introduced through anterior portal lightly debrides the tear to define the extent of the defect.
C, Debridement reveals that the intra-articular portion of the tear involves only a small portion of the diameter of the tendon.

ty. These older patients are advised that LHB rupture is not likely to create a significant functional impairment. A large stump of tendon following rupture is often encountered in patients with rotator cuff tears. The stump is shaved or resected if it appears large enough to be symptomatic (Fig. 10–8).

TECHNIQUE OF ARTHROSCOPICALLY ASSISTED LHB TENODESIS

Posterior and anterior glenohumeral portals are established as previously described. The insertion of the torn LHB tendon is identified through the posterior arthroscopic portal. A loop of PDS suture is passed through the tendon 1 cm

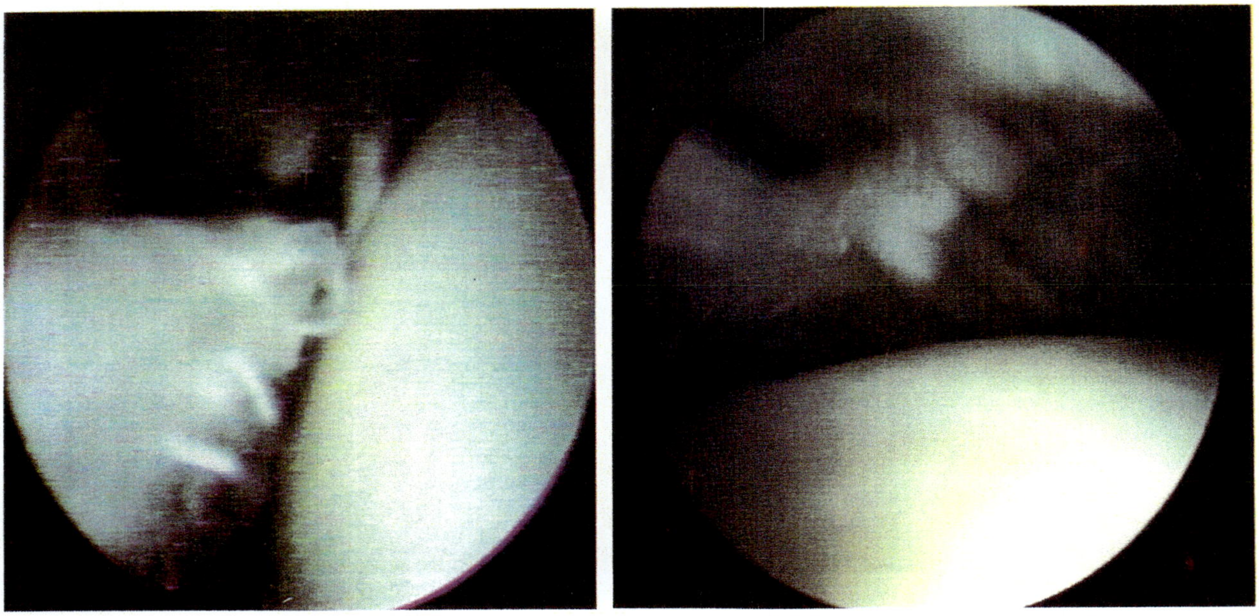

A B

FIG. 10–7. Partial tear of the long head of the biceps (LHB) and rotator cuff secondary to impingement.
A, Appearance of a partial tear near the approach of the tendon to the sulcus.
B, Partial tear of the supraspinatus is seen adjacent to the LHB. Treatment consisted of debridement followed by arthroscopic subacromial decompression.

distal to its attachment via the anterior portal. Both ends of the suture are brought out through the anterior canulla and held securely with a Kelly snap. An arthroscopic scissors or basket forceps is introduced through the anterior portal and brought to the base of the tendon. The tendon is severed from its insertion without disturbing the glenoid labrum (Fig. 10–9A). The suture exiting the anterior canulla prevents retraction of the severed tendon. Any roughened edges of the LHB stump are trimmed with a shaver. Arthroscopic detachment eliminates the extended deltopectoral incision and dissection necessary to enter the joint for release of the tendon prior to tenodesis.

The intertubercular sulcus of the proximal humerus is exposed through a limited deltopectoral incision. The cephalic vein is identified in the deltopectoral groove and is retracted laterally. The sulcus is palpated as the proximal humerus is rotated. The synovial sheath of the LHB is incised vertically to expose the tendon. The clamp controlling the severed end of the tendon is loosened and the tendon is pulled out of the groove and inspected (Fig. 10–9B). The point where appropriate resting tension can be re-established should be marked with methylene blue on the midportion of the sulcus. The proximal end of the tendon may be knotted or rolled to reinforce the area of partial defect and create a bulbous end. Several sutures are placed to reinforce the end. A keyhole-shaped osteotomy is made at the previously determined isometric point in the sulcus. The rounded proximal opening should admit the bulbous end, and the thinner inferior slot captures the tendon. The walls of the sulcus distally are roughened to encourage fixation. After stuffing the proximal end into the intramedullary

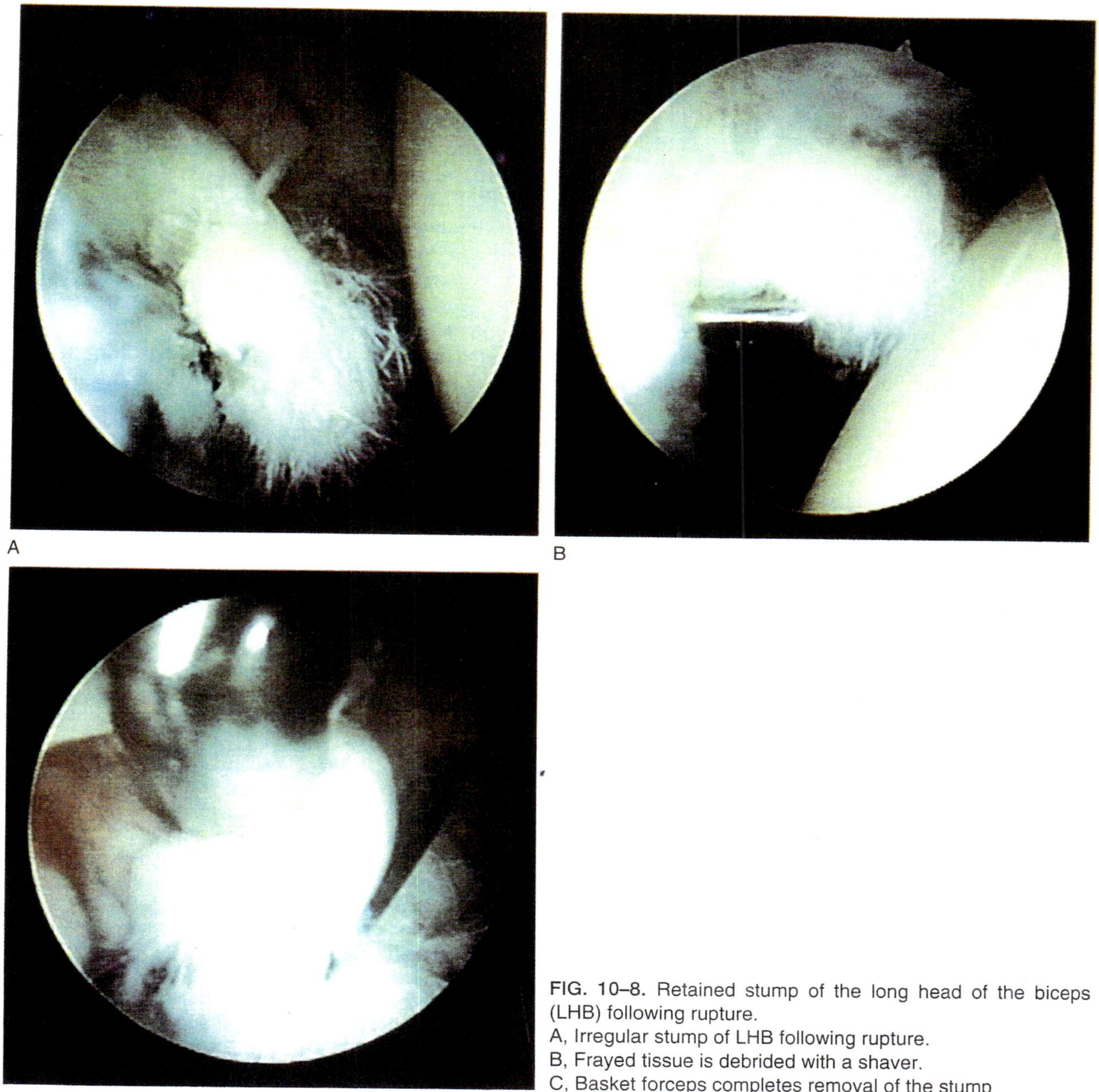

A

B

C

FIG. 10–8. Retained stump of the long head of the biceps (LHB) following rupture.
A, Irregular stump of LHB following rupture.
B, Frayed tissue is debrided with a shaver.
C, Basket forceps completes removal of the stump

canal, the transposed tendon is reinforced by additional sutures to the medial and lateral soft tissues (Fig. 10–9C).

An alternate method of fixation is to roughen the walls of the sulcus with a gouge and then fix the tendon with multiple transosseous sutures placed in the medial or lateral wall of the sulcus. Repair with metal staples or screws is not usually done, based on our principle of avoiding metal implants in the vicinity of

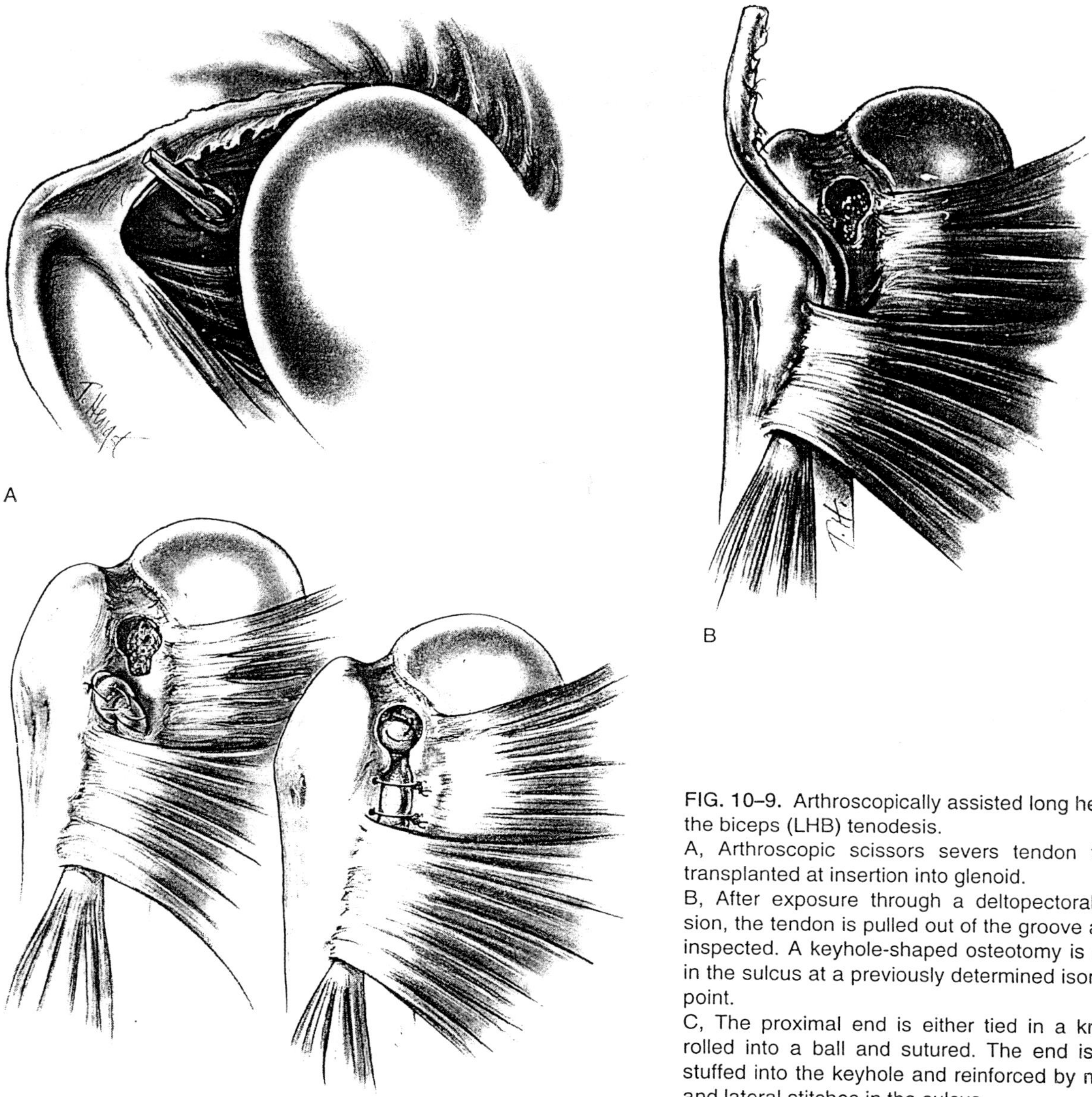

A B C

FIG. 10–9. Arthroscopically assisted long head of the biceps (LHB) tenodesis.
A, Arthroscopic scissors severs tendon to be transplanted at insertion into glenoid.
B, After exposure through a deltopectoral incision, the tendon is pulled out of the groove and is inspected. A keyhole-shaped osteotomy is made in the sulcus at a previously determined isometric point.
C, The proximal end is either tied in a knot or rolled into a ball and sutured. The end is then stuffed into the keyhole and reinforced by medial and lateral stitches in the sulcus.

a joint. Another alternative method of fixation is to suture the proximal end of the tendon to the short head of the biceps tendon near its insertion at the coracoid process.

OPEN SURGICAL TREATMENT

Open surgical treatment is traditionally undertaken either to relieve chronic, incapacitating bicipital tendinitis or to repair an acute rupture of the LHB. Whether the intra-articular portion of the tendon is partially torn cannot be determined in an open procedure until the joint has been opened.

When open tenodesis of an intact but intractably painful tendon is contemplated, the surgeon should carefully assess whether impingement or primary bicipital tendinitis is a factor. Although the impingement sign may be positive in both circumstances, a positive Yergason test implicates the LHB. A radiograph taken in the supraspinatus outlet view (arch view) demonstrates whether acromial structure suggests mechanical impingement. The final decision may require a preoperative magnetic resonance imaging study to determine whether the supraspinatus shows evidence of chronic tendinitis or partial tear. If the study is positive, anterior acromioplasty should accompany tenodesis.

When complete rupture of the tendon occurs, the decision as to whether to reconstruct or to neglect may be difficult. Younger, physically active patients are encouraged to undergo repair of a rupture. Conversely, older, less active patients are advised that acceptance of a deformity need not mean a sacrifice of adequate function. The patient is encouraged to participate in the decision immediately following acute LHB rupture, because reconstruction is more difficult after a delay of more than 3 or 4 weeks.

OPEN TECHNIQUE

The technique of open tenodesis of the LHB is similar to that of the arthroscopically assisted method described earlier in this chapter, except that the deltopectoral skin incision must extend all the way to the clavicle and an arthrotomy of the glenohumeral joint is necessary. After exposing the proximal humerus through a full deltopectoral approach, the synovial sheath of the tendon is incised over the sulcus and extended proximally just anterior to the anterior border of the supraspinatus. This incision travels along the rotator interval that demarcates the supraspinatus and subscapularis. The LHB tendon should lie directly below this interval. When still intact, the diseased tendon should be followed to the origin and detached. If an acute rupture has occurred, the intra-articular stump should be resected through this arthrotomy prior to performing the tenodesis. When indicated, open acromioplasty is performed in conjunction with the tenodesis.

REHABILITATION

The elbow is splinted in 90° flexion for 3 weeks. A sling is worn for an additional 3 weeks while gentle mobilization exercises are carried out to gradually regain full elbow extension.

When arthroscopic acromioplasty is combined with tenodesis, active shoulder mobilization may begin within a few days. If the acromioplasty is performed with the open technique, shoulder motion should be passive at least for the first 3 weeks to protect the deltoid repair. Immobilization is followed by progressive resistance exercises of the shoulder and elbow until function is restored.

[illegible]

[illegible] dependent on the density [illegible] approximately [illegible] adsorption is [illegible] of an adsorbent [illegible]

[illegible]

[illegible] technique [illegible] is similar to that [illegible] discussed [illegible] and desorption [illegible] except that the [illegible] to the [illegible] dependence of [illegible] expression [illegible] is [illegible] adsorption [illegible] along the [illegible] and that [illegible] similar [illegible] dependence [illegible] the first [illegible] a [illegible]

[illegible]

[illegible] advantages [illegible] experimental [illegible] pressure [illegible]

THE SCALPEL OR THE SCOPE? DECISION-MAKING IN THE TREATMENT OF ROTATOR CUFF DISEASE

11

The use of the arthroscope in shoulder surgery has increased the understanding of rotator cuff disorders and modified methods of treatment in many ways. The true value of shoulder arthroscopy lies in the hands of the surgeon who has achieved equal skill in both arthroscopic and open surgical techniques. The preceding chapters on rotator cuff disease have dealt with the pathogenesis and evaluation of cuff failure and described the arthroscopic treatment of stage II impingement and partial-thickness tears. Open methods of rotator cuff reconstruction have also been covered. Arthroscopic treatment of rotator cuff disease involves arthroscopic subacromial decompression and debridement of the torn rotator cuff, for purposes of this discussion. The use of metallic or biodegradable fixation devices to restore a torn cuff into a bony trough is evolving. Repair of smaller mobile tears without open augmentation undoubtedly will be possible in the future. The decision as to whether to perform an open repair of a torn cuff or simply to decompress the subacromial space and debride the defect is the subject of this chapter.

Proper application of arthroscopic techniques requires an understanding of the progressive nature of rotator cuff failure, as well as an ability to assess the degree of fiber failure. The goal is to select the appropriate treatment—open repair, arthroscopic treatment, or a combined approach. The combined approach involves arthroscopic subacromial decompression with a "mini-open" reconstruction of the torn cuff. Performing the decompression arthroscopically should allow the surgeon to repair a relatively small, mobile tear through a small deltoid-splitting incision without detaching any fibers of deltoid insertion.

CLINICAL EVALUATION

The clinical evaluation should include the following pertinent factors.

PERTINENT HISTORY

Physiologic age and hand dominance are important factors. The patient's functional requirements, both occupational and avocational, should be considered. The level of activity should be classified as light, moderate, or strenuous. The duration of symptoms has a bearing on the chronicity of degenerative complaints. The degree of trauma that may have provoked a sudden rupture is pertinent. Although a relatively normal cuff may rupture in the presence of severe injury, most cuff tears occur through an area of prior degeneration as a result of trivial trauma.

PHYSICAL EXAMINATION

The physical examination should include a careful assessment of the patient's *range of motion*, as well as *strength*, after pain ablation. The inability to achieve overhead motion in combination with a classic "shoulder shrug" is clear evidence of a sizable tear. Significant weakness in both abduction and external rotation indicates a tear involving both the supraspinatus and the infraspinatus. Such a tear undoubtedly is large. When pain is ablated by a generous subacromial injection of local anesthetic, the patient with a small tear may display little or no weakness. As the size of the tear increases from moderate to large, the degree of weakness also increases. The massive tear may demonstrate the "drop-arm sign," which indicates that the patient simply cannot maintain his arm against gravity after it has been passively elevated into position overhead.

DIAGNOSTIC IMAGING

A simple radiograph taken in the anteroposterior plane of the glenohumeral joint may suggest, and at times confirm, the presence of rotator cuff disease. Areas of sclerosis and subchondral cyst formation in the trough between the greater tuberosity and humeral head (enthesopathy) often accompany cuff failure (Fig. 11–1).[43] Superior migration of the humeral head occurs in larger tears. The acromiohumeral distance is measured from below the anterior margin of the acromion to the superior aspect of the humeral head. This measurement is most reliable when the film is taken with the arm actively abducted a few degrees. When the acromiohumeral distance measures less than 7 mm, a cuff tear is likely (Fig. 11–2).[66] When the humerus rises upward to within 2 or 3 mm of a concave, sclerotic acromion, the tear not only is massive, but is likely to be irreparable (Fig. 11–3).

Single-contrast arthrography has been the gold standard for determining the presence or absence of a full-thickness rotator cuff tear for many years. *Double-contrast arthrography* (3 ml of radiopaque dye and 10 ml of room air) has the further advantage of assessing both the size of the tear and, in many instances, the quality of the tissue (Fig. 11–4).

Magnetic resonance imaging is emerging as the most valuable method of assessing cuff integrity. Moderate and large tears can be reliably imaged. When the body of the supraspinatus muscle is shown to be atrophic and fibrotic in the presence of a large retracted tear, the prognosis for successful reconstruction is quite poor (Fig. 11–5). Discrimination between "tendinitis" and small full-thickness rotator cuff tears is less reliable with magnetic resonance imaging. T_2-weighted studies help to determine degenerative changes within the tendon. The surgeon should be aware that both false-positive and false-negative readings increase when small lesions are being evaluated.

Arthroscopic examination helps to evaluate the extent of cuff disorders. A par-

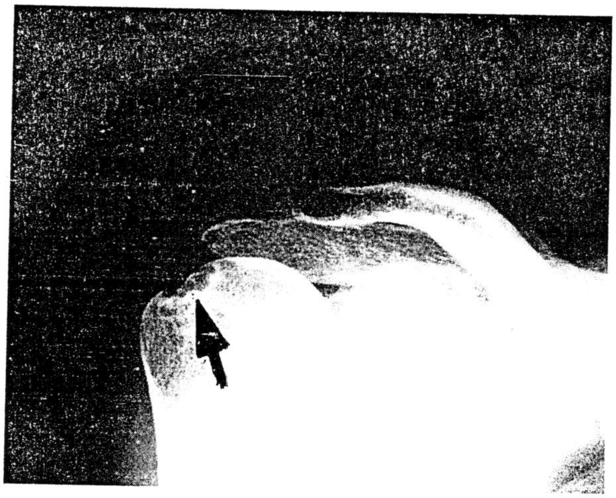

FIG. 11–1. An extensive area of subchondral cyst degeneration (arrow) in combination with marginal sclerosis (enthesopathy) is a sign of significant cuff failure.

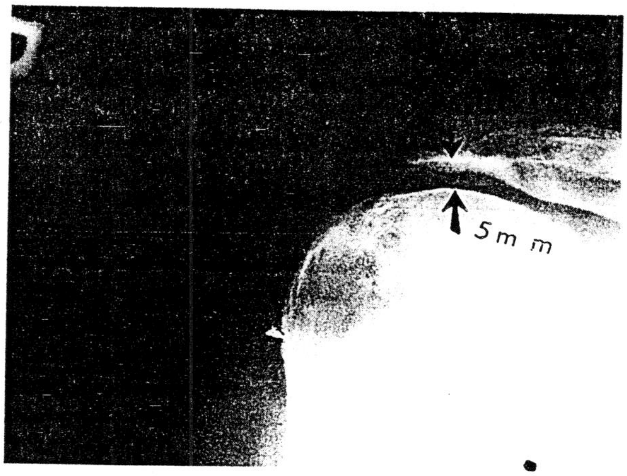

FIG. 11–2. Reduction of the acromiohumeral distance to less than 7 mm suggests a likely cuff tear.

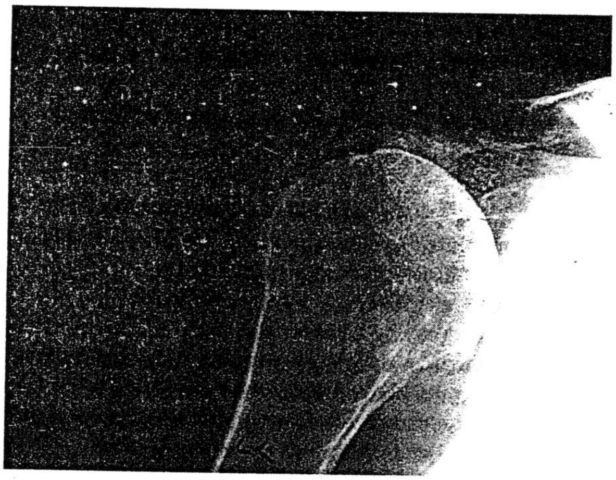

FIG. 11–3. When the humeral head rises upward in relation to the glenoid and within 2 or 3 mm of the undersurface of the acromion, repair is likely to be challenging.

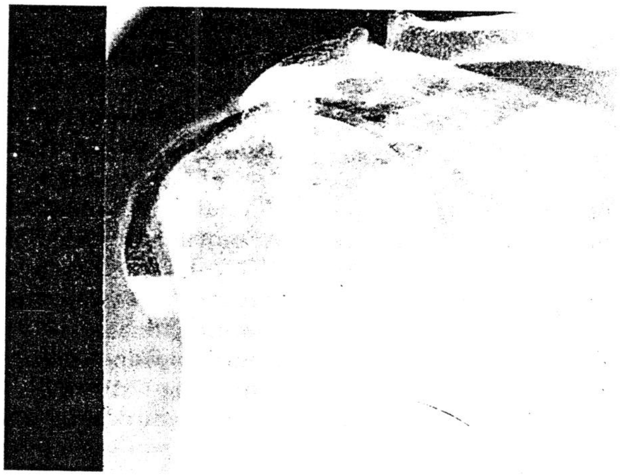

FIG. 11–4. Double-contrast arthrography: This film confirms a massive tear. Cuff tissue between the elevated humeral head and the undersurface of the acromion is absent. Tears of this magnitude are potentially irreparable.

tial-thickness articular surface tear may be debrided to determine the full extent of the lesion. The identification of bursal surface tears requires a thorough bursectomy to visualize the defect thoroughly.

When a massive tear is present, the arthroscope may be used to determine its repairability (Fig. 11–6). A grasping forceps may be introduced through the anterolateral portal and the residual elasticity of the cuff can be determined. Diagnostic use of the arthroscope to confirm a mid-sized full-thickness tear is rarely justified because other accurate and less invasive techniques are available.

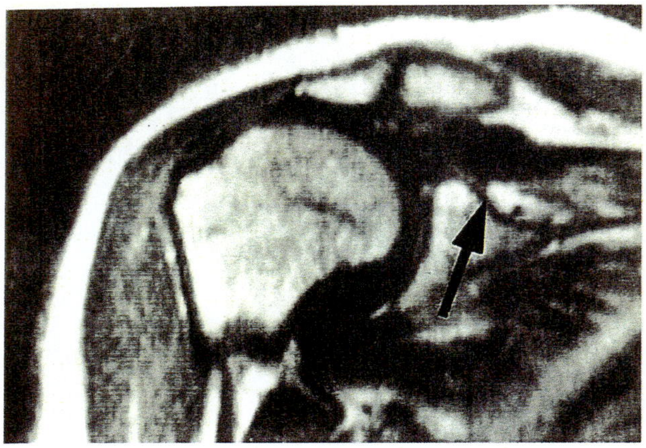

FIG. 11–5. MRI of massive tear: The torn supraspinatus is retracted medial to the glenoid, and the muscle body appears quite fibrotic.

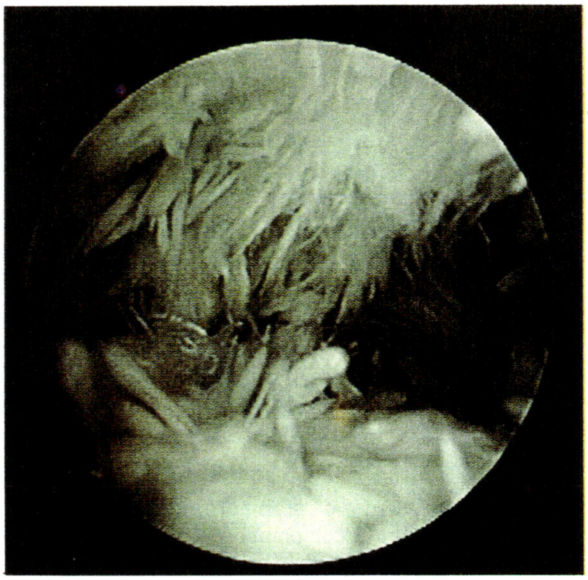

FIG. 11–6. Arthroscopic evaluation of a long-standing massive rotator cuff tear: The cuff has retracted medially, and the shaggy acromial undersurface is seen above while the irregular humeral head is exposed below.

PREOPERATIVE PATIENT CONFERENCE

When clinical assessment has been completed, the patient and the surgeon can decide on the recommended treatment. The anticipated results concerning strength, activity level, and possible future surgery should be discussed, along with the rehabilitation program. The surgeon should also determine and review with the patient *in advance* any alternate method of treatment that should be carried out if the magnetic resonance imaging study or arthrogram is wrong.

CURRENT PROTOCOL

When comprehensive clinical evaluation leads to a recommendation for surgical intervention, the arthroscope is utilized in a variety of circumstances. The current protocol follows:

ADVANCED STAGE II IMPINGEMENT

Arthroscopic subacromial decompression (see Chap. 5) is performed for patients with advanced stage II impingement and no evidence of rotator cuff tear in whom conservative management has failed for a period of 6 to 12 months. Patients in this category, particularly younger athletes, should be carefully evaluated for instability to exclude the possibility that the impingement is secondary to capsular laxity. The supraspinatus outlet view of the acromial arch should reflect a type II (curved) or type III (hooked) acromion. A patient with a flat

RESULTS: ARTHROSCOPIC	
ELLMAN, KAY	89%
GARTSMAN	90%
ALTCHEK, WARREN	83%
MENDOZA	95%
ESCH, et. al.	82%
WASILEWSKI, FRANKL	87%
AVERAGE	87.6%

RESULTS: OPEN	
NEER	94%
RAGGIO, WARREN, et. al.	89%
POST and COHEN	89%
TIBONE, JOBE, et. al.	89%
STUART, AZEVEDO, COFIELD	78%
BIGLIANI, et. al. (under age 40)	81%
AVERAGE	86.6%

FIG. 11–7. Reported results of arthroscopic versus open acromioplasty for stage II impingement were essentially the same.

STAGE II TENDINITIS AND PARTIAL THICKNESS TEARS

ARTHROSCOPIC RX	Stage II	Partial Tear
ELLMAN + KAY	89%	75%
GARTSMAN	90%	82%
ESCH et. al.	82%	76%
ALTCHEK, WARREN	83%	66%
MENDOZA	95%	
SNYDER et. al.		84%

FIG. 11–8. Comparison of results of arthroscopic treatment in patients with and without partial-thickness tear.

(type I) acromion rarely undergoes arthroscopic subacromial decompression. Our overall results following a 2- to 5-year study of patients in this category yielded 89% satisfactory results.[39] Satisfactory results in 4 other studies ranged from 80 to 95%.[41,91-93]

The principal advantage of arthroscopic subacromial decompression is that no deltoid fibers are detached. The published results of arthroscopic acromioplasty compare favorably with the results following open acromioplasty (Fig. 11–7).[84-87,123] The duration of hospitalization, requirements for analgesia, and resumption of activities of daily living all favor arthroscopic over open decompression. The nosocomial infection rate is less following arthroscopic subacromial decompression. The difference in the economic consequences between open and arthroscopic techniques is only minor, because the high cost of instrumentation for shoulder arthroscopy may outweigh the total expenses for an open procedure that requires an additional 1 or 2 days of postoperative hospitalization. The learning curve required to gain proficiency is much steeper for the arthroscopic procedure than for open acromioplasty. Assessment of the amount of bone removed is made more easily during open surgery than during the arthroscopic procedure.

PARTIAL-THICKNESS TEARS

The published results following arthroscopic treatment of partial-thickness tears reflect a less satisfactory outcome following arthroscopic subacromial decompression when the cuff is partially torn (Fig. 11–8).[40,41,92,93] Our experience suggests that both patient selection and extent of the partial tear contribute to these results. The partial-thickness tear involving either the articular or the bursal surface should be carefully debrided and measured as to both the depth and the area of fiber failure.

LESS THAN ONE-HALF THICKNESS PARTIAL TEAR (GRADES 1 AND 2)

Partial tears of either the articular or the bursal surface that involve less than one-half the thickness of the cuff (grades 1 and 2) are debrided and decompressed. An exception is made for the young athlete involved in sports that require throwing who still has an unfused acromial epiphysis. In this situation, only the coracoacromial ligament is released and a bursectomy is performed.

MORE THAN ONE-HALF THICKNESS PARTIAL TEAR (GRADE 3)

When the partial tear involves more than one-half the thickness of the tendon, the surgical decision depends on whether the patient intends to return to a high level of strenuous activity. When the supraspinatus insertion is torn more than halfway through, the competitive athlete involved in throwing, racquet sports, volleyball, and weight-lifting is much more likely to be dissatisfied with the results of arthroscopic acromioplasty. The same is true when the patient is obliged to return to a strenuous occupation that requires overhead movement. On the other hand, less active individuals often are quite satisfied with arthroscopic treatment of a grade 3 tear. Handedness is also a factor, because a grade 3 tear is less critical in a minor arm than in a major arm. Individuals who anticipate a full return to strenuous overhead activity, either vocational or athletic, are advised to have a "mini-open" excision and repair (preferably tendon to bony groove) following arthroscopic subacromial decompression. The patient is also informed that the "mini-open" procedure requires at least an overnight hospitalization and the postoperative open cuff repair protocol for rehabilitation. The patient participates in the decision, and the surgeon is well-advised to have this "What do I do if I find . . . ?" conversation preoperatively with every patient undergoing arthroscopic surgery for rotator cuff disease.

FULL-THICKNESS TEARS

SMALL TEARS (LESS THAN 2 CM)

These relatively small rotator cuff tears, which generally involve only a portion of the supraspinatus, can be treated effectively with arthroscopic subacromial decompression followed by a "mini-open" repair in most patients (Chap. 6). The combined procedure reduces postoperative morbidity by avoiding deltoid release. Postoperative hospitalization is seldom longer than 1 or 2 days.

Occasionally, a small full-thickness tear is treated by arthroscopic decompression and debridement without repair of the tear. This treatment is offered to older (greater than 65 years of age), inactive individuals. The early results following decompression and debridement of small tears have been favorable in a carefully selected group of patients, particularly when the minor arm is involved and adequate strength (4+ or better) is present.

LARGE TEARS (2 TO 5 CM)

Most patients with repairable rotator cuff tears between 2 to 5 cm are treated by open surgical reconstruction. Exceptions include an elderly (older than 72 to 75 years), inactive individual whose primary complaint is pain rather than functional impairment. Performing arthroscopic decompression and debridement on a patient with a repairable rotator cuff tear is a decided comprise.

In 1986, Ellman and associates published an end-results study of 50 full-thickness rotator cuff tears that had been treated by open reconstruction.[28] Satisfactory results were reported in 84%. In 1991, Ellman and colleagues studied the mid-term follow-up results of 40 cases of full-thickness tears that had been treated arthroscopically.[40] The overall results were 55% satisfactory and 45% unsatisfactory. The results in both studies were then divided into 3 categories according to the size of the tear and were compared to determine the efficacy of each type of treatment. Small tears (less than 2 cm) in both groups had a 90% satisfactory result. Note, however, that the arthroscopic patients were selected, in general, because their activity level was less than strenuous and the minor arm was usually the arm involved. In the tears ranging from 2 to 4 cm in size, the group treated with open surgery achieved 83% satisfaction, with nearly half of those considered excellent results. Only a 50% satisfactory result was achieved in the 2- to 4-cm tears that were treated arthroscopically. None of the repairs in this group achieved an excellent rating.

Thus, although some carefully selected small tears can be successfully treated arthroscopically, the best results for larger tears are achieved with an open repair. Any exception is considered a compromise.

MASSIVE, IRREPARABLE TEARS

The patient with a massive, irreparable tear of the rotator cuff is the greatest enigma to the shoulder surgeon. In this category, 20 patients were treated over a 5-year period between 1983 and 1988, with a minimum follow-up of 2 years.[40] Of these patients, 5 had cuff arthropathy. The arthroscopic procedure consisted of an extensive joint debridement and synovectomy, as well as a modified acromioplasty and tuberosity-plasty designed to make the pseudoarticulation between a high-riding humeral head and the coracoacromial arch more congruous. Significant pain reduction was achieved in 18 to 20 patients. Only 3 patients in the group of 20 who were selected for arthroscopic treatment were dissatisfied with the results. Over half of the patients were able to increase their range of motion modestly (12° average) by strengthening the deltoid. The results of arthroscopic treatment of irreparable rotator cuff tears appear to compare favorably to those obtained by the open technique reported by Rockwood and Burkhead.[38]

DECISION-MAKING ALGORITHM

An algorithm designed to summarize important factors considered when making the decision to treat a partial-thickness (Fig. 11–9) or a full-thickness (Fig. 11–10) rotator cuff tear by open (O) or arthroscopic (A) methods is presented. The size of the tear is considered in relation to the age of the patient (under/over age 65), arm dominance (nondominant/dominant), and level of activity (minimal/moderate/strenuous). Preference is indicated by either A (arthroscopic) or O (open). When either method of treatment may be appropriate, a small-case type is used; the slightly preferred technique is indicated by placing its letter designation (either the o or the a) first. All the categories for each size of tear are important in the final decision.

DECISIONS: PARTIAL THICKNESS

SIZE of TEAR	<65	>65	NON-DOMINANT ARM
LESS THAN ½ THICKNESS	A	A	A
MORE THAN ½ THICKNESS	A/O	A	A

ROTATOR CUFF TEARS

DOMINANT ARM	LEVEL OF ACTIVITY		
	MINIMAL	MODERTE	STRENUOUS
A	A	A	A
A/O	A	O/A	O

A = Arthroscopic Rx
O = Open Repair

FIG. 11–9. Factors considered important in the choice of treatment for partial-thickness tears.

DECISIONS: FULL THICKNESS

SIZE of TEAR	<65	>65	NON-DOMINANT ARM
<2cm	O	A	A
2–4cm	O	O/A	O
>4 (5)cm	O	O/A	A/O
IRREPARABLE	A	A	A

ROTATOR CUFF TEARS

DOMINANT ARM	LEVEL OF ACTIVITY		
	MINIMAL	MODERATE	STRENUOUS
O/A	A/O	O/A	O
O	O/A	O	O
O	A/O	O/A	O
A	A	A	A

FIG. 11–10. Factors considered important in the choice of treatment for full-thickness tears.

SUMMARY

Arthroscopic decompression and debridement of small full-thickness rotator cuff tears offer gratifying pain relief and reasonable options for the elderly patient with adequate strength. These patients should be aware that usually 2 to 3 months are required for significant pain relief to occur. Popping and clicking continue indefinitely, and weakness persists. On the other hand, active individuals, regardless of age, can anticipate a favorable result when the cuff rupture is repaired surgically. Arthroscopic treatment may be a reasonable compromise when the rigors of rehabilitation are compared to the functional requirements of the patients. Although acromioplasty appears to retard the progression of many rotator cuff tears, no long-term studies have been concluded. The jury is still out. Patient selection is the *sine qua non* of success when deciding whether to use the scalpel or the scope.

III

SECTION

INSTABILITY

PATHOGENESIS AND CLINICAL EVALUATION OF GLENOHUMERAL INSTABILITY

12

This chapter deals mainly with anteroinferior glenohumeral instability. Posterior instability may be diagnosed, but is rarely treated arthroscopically because the altered anatomy that allows such translation is generally not responsive to arthroscopic treatment. Our knowledge of the structures that maintain glenohumeral stability has been gained from inspection of the damaged tissue during open surgical reconstruction and during anatomic dissection in the laboratory. Arthroscopic anatomy differs in several important ways. Arthroscopic observation of the glenohumeral ligaments is performed in both the injured and the noninjured individual. Many patients with rotator cuff disease and abnormalities confined to the subacromial space undergo arthroscopic surgery, thereby also affording the surgeon a view of undamaged glenohumeral structures. The view obtained during such a procedure does not involve any dissection that could distort the findings. The anatomy is viewed from "inside-out" and close-up. The findings are commonly recorded on videotape for later review. A stress examination for translation can be performed while maintaining the important structures directly within the surgeon's visual field. Thus, any changes in these structures can be noted. Our appreciation of both the abnormal and the normal anatomy critical for joint stability and function is improving.[124,125]

FINDINGS CONSISTENT WITH GLENOHUMERAL INSTABILITY

SUPERIOR GLENOHUMERAL LIGAMENT

Superior glenohumeral ligament (SGHL) injuries include midsubstance and humeral insertion site tears. The SGHL is the most likely of the three anterior glenohumeral ligaments to vary in size, but it is present in 90% of shoulders examined arthroscopically. SGHL attenuation, best judged by probe palpation with inferior distraction to the arm, seems to be most common in individuals with multidirectional instability and recurrent subluxation. An actual tear of the SGHL is most often seen in individuals who sustain a single isolated trauma, often of the distraction type (Fig. 12–1). The tear is often associated with lesions of the rotator interval and, when combined with direct observation of excessive inferoanterior translation, is consistent with symptomatic instability.

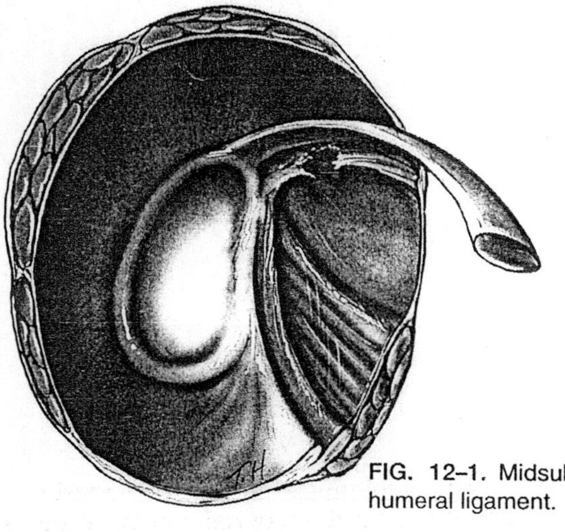

FIG. 12–1. Midsubstance tear of the superior glenohumeral ligament.

MIDDLE GLENOHUMERAL LIGAMENT

The middle glenohumeral ligament (MGHL) may be torn, absent, attenuated, or split. It may be separated from its labrum or glenoid insertion. The MGHL is poorly defined or absent in 25% of patients. Tears of the MGHL are noted more commonly on the glenoid insertion site than on the humeral insertion site. The MGHL occasionally may be absent, perhaps because the ligament had been traumatized and absorbed or was congenitally deficient. The cause of this occasional absence is still unclear. An atrophic MGHL is most often seen with multiaxial subluxation. Often this type of MGHL can be appreciated by direct observation of the thin, atrophic ligament. Occasionally, the ligament looks normal, but when a probe is placed into the glenohumeral joint from an anterior portal (a step that should *always* be performed), a decreased tone in the MGHL can be appreciated. When the humeral head is stressed in an inferior direction or when the arm is taken into abduction and external rotation, the normal tightening of the MGHL does not occur.

Another abnormality is a split in the glenohumeral ligament. A split seems to be most often associated with instability resulting from an isolated trauma rather than from repetitive microtrauma. The MGHL can also be inserted more medially on the glenoid. This abnormality may be the result of a tear that had healed in an inferomedial direction, thereby rendering the shoulder less stable, or it may simply be anatomic. The separation in the ligament insertion site that occurs with the anteroinferior glenohumeral ligament can also occur with the MGHL/labrum complex.

ANTEROINFERIOR GLENOHUMERAL LIGAMENT

Anteroinferior glenohumeral ligament (AIGHL) findings are similar to those described for the MGHL. The AIGHL may be torn, absent, attenuated, recessed, or separated, but is rarely split. The weak link appears to be the glenoid insertion site. Disruption of the humeral head insertion site is rare. Midsubstance tears may occur but are difficult to recognize in patients with chronic instability.

These tears are seen more commonly in acute dislocation.[126] A poorly defined, absent, or attenuated AIGHL is less common than a SGHL or a MGHL with similar characteristics. Often, the anteroinferior ligament complex is lax and poorly defined when the patient is in the decubitus position and the arm is internally rotated. External rotation of the arm makes the superior band more prominent. Separation of the AIGHL, the classic Bankart lesion, is consistent with recurrent instability. A probe should be placed at the AIGHL insertion site when clinical suspicion of instability is high and obvious separation cannot be detected. Often, an apparently well-attached AIGHL can be peeled off the glenoid with minimal pressure. Mild degrees of labral fraying at the 4 to 6 o'clock position are suggestive of instability and may exist with ligament laxity or ligament insertion injuries.

POSTEROINFERIOR GLENOHUMERAL LIGAMENT

The posteroinferior glenohumeral ligament (PIGHL) can be most easily seen with the arm rotated internally. Although our experience in the arthroscopic management of posterior instability is limited, we can easily visualize with the arthroscope the posterior Bankart lesion in the posterior portal. If the ligament insertion site appears normal but clinical suspicion of a defect is high, the arthroscope should be inserted through the anterior portal and a probe should be placed posteriorly to attempt to palpate any defect within the ligament substance or insertion site.

CLASSIFICATION OF GLENOHUMERAL INSTABILITY

Translation is defined as the amount of humeral head movement on the glenoid surface. *Instability* is defined as the symptomatic expression of excessive glenohumeral translation. Conventional classifications of glenohumeral instability generally follow certain accepted criteria. The instability is classified according to its chronicity (acute, chronic), degree (subluxation, dislocation), direction (anterior, posterior, inferior, multidirectional), origin (traumatic, atraumatic), and patient control (voluntary, involuntary). This classification helps the orthopedic surgeon to diagnose the type of instability and, therefore, to perform the appropriate treatment. If the treatment is operative, the classification system helps the surgeon to determine the appropriate operation. For example, a patient with a nontraumatic multidirectional instability may be treated nonoperatively with an exercise program. On the other hand, a recurrent dislocation of traumatic origin usually requires surgical treatment at some point.

This classification is useful, but is limited because it is indirect. The direction, origin, and chronicity are determined by the patient's history, an indirect method. Observations at the time of open surgery are limited because the surgical approach does not give a complete view of the glenohumeral joint without division of the ligaments and capsule.

An arthroscopic classification, however, is based on direct observation of the glenohumeral capsule/ligament complex from the inside of the glenohumeral joint. Incision of the structures is not necessary. The arthroscopic classification is not meant to replace the classic classification system just described, but serves as a parallel or complementary system.

The arthroscopic classification seeks to determine the integrity of the glenohumeral ligament complex. Instability is classified as insertional, ligament substance, functional, or combination (Fig. 12–2A through C). Insertional ligament instability implies that the ligament substance is intact, but its insertion site has been disrupted. The ligament may be disrupted from the labrum, or the ligament may be firmly attached to the labrum, but the labrum is detached from the glenoid. Alternatively, the ligament may be detached from the humeral head.

A ligament substance instability is the result of a midsubstance ligament tear or attenuation (Fig. 12–2D).

Functional instability is rare and implies a mechanical abnormality within the glenohumeral joint. This abnormality, usually a torn labrum or cartilaginous loose body, prevents "seating" of the humeral head. The patient consequently falsely perceives the shoulder as "coming out of joint." Judgment is required to determine whether the mechanical abnormality is truly the cause of the instability or is a result of instability (Fig. 12–2E).

Because three glenohumeral ligaments exist (superior, middle, and inferior), a combination of injuries can occur. Such combination injuries have been better appreciated arthroscopically. One common injury combination is a midsubstance tear of the SGHL and attenuation of the MGHL. Another common pattern is a ligament insertion detachment of the AIGHL combined with a midsubstance tear of the MGHL.

The arthroscopic classification system, which is more anatomically precise than the classic system, is valuable in determining whether surgical treatment is appropriate and, if so, whether that surgical treatment can be accomplished arthroscopically.

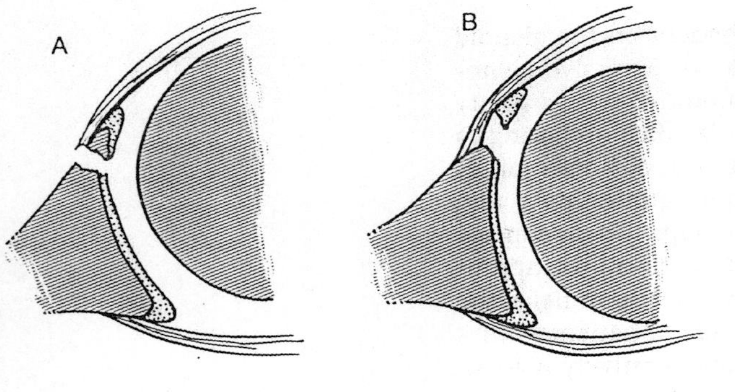

FIG. 12–2. A, Ligament-bone avulsion from the glenoid. B, Ligament avulsion can include a portion of the labrum. C, Ligament avulsion from the humerus. D, Ligament substance lesion resulting from a tear or attenuation of the midcapsule-ligament complex. E, A torn labrum can be interposed between the humeral head and the glenoid, thereby preventing proper "seating" of the humeral head. Such positioning can be perceived by the patient as "instability."

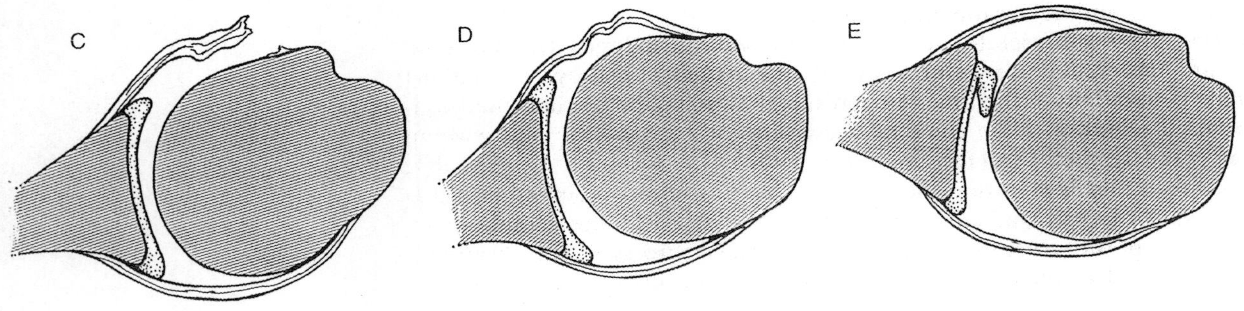

STABILITY FACTORS

The early literature on glenohumeral instability is dominated by the search for a "single essential lesion." Perthes, Broca, and Bankart are all credited with identifying the ligament detachment at the glenoid in patients with recurrent dislocation.[127] Certainly many patients with recurrent dislocation had this lesion, but as more shoulders were treated operatively, individuals with glenohumeral instability without ligament detachment were identified. Various other mechanisms were explored based on glenoid or humeral head version, capsular laxity, or subscapularis muscle strength. Today, we realize that no single essential lesion exists and that stability of the glenohumeral joint is the result of numerous factors that each contribute to some degree.

PASSIVE STABILIZERS

Five factors that contribute as passive stabilizers of the glenohumeral joint are joint conformity, the labrum, adhesion, the vacuum effect, and the capsule/ligament complex. Because the glenohumeral joint has a tremendous amount of movement, joint constraint is minimal. The shoulder arthroscopist sees the glenohumeral joint not as a ball-and-socket joint, but as a basketball sitting on a coffee-cup saucer.

The labrum provides soft tissue extension of the glenoid, thereby increasing the contact area by an estimated 25%.

As the two cartilaginous surfaces glide by one another, stability is provided by the physical property of adhesion.

Another contributor to passive glenohumeral stability is the joint capsule vacuum effect. Experiments have revealed that subluxation occurs when the normal, resting negative intra-articular pressure is released.

The importance of the glenohumeral ligaments as static stabilizers has been well documented.[124,128] The primary stabilizer limiting anterior translation of the 90° abducted shoulder is the inferior glenohumeral ligament complex. The MGHL, the anterior band of the IGHL, and the subscapularis tendon provide the primary restraint against anterior translation at lower angles of abduction.

ACTIVE STABILIZERS

Active glenohumeral joint stabilizers include the scapular muscles, the deltoid, the rotator cuff, and the biceps. The scapular muscles include serratus anterior, trapezius, and latissimus dorsi. These muscles primarily function to rotate the scapula, thereby keeping the glenoid underneath the humeral head (Fig. 12–3). As the arm is raised in the overhead or throwing position, the humeral head rotates and the scapula glides along the chest so that combined scapular and glenohumeral rotation produces complete and effective overhead arm elevation and activity. When the scapular rotators are not functioning optimally, the scapula lags behind glenohumeral movement and normal scapulohumeral rhythm is disrupted. Consequently, greater stress is placed on the passive and the other active stabilizers of the glenohumeral joint (Fig. 12–4).

Deltoid force results in upward shear, but by working effectively with the

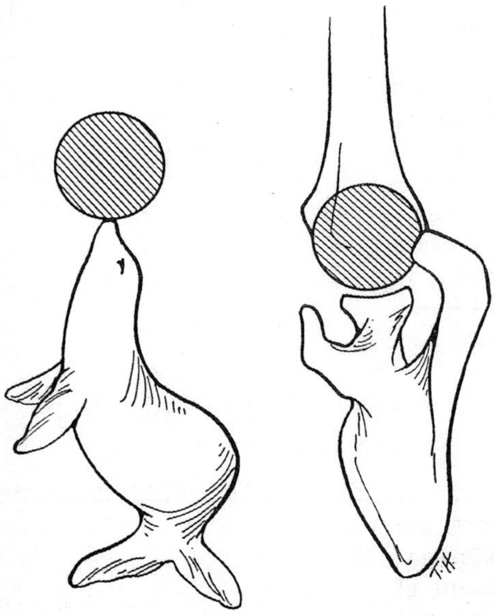

FIG. 12–3. Scapular movement attempts to keep the glenoid "under" the humeral head like the seal attempts to remain "under" the ball.

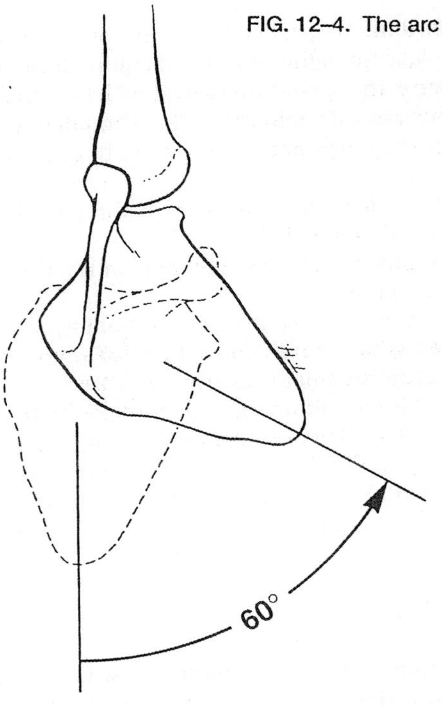

FIG. 12–4. The arc of scapular motion.

rotator cuff, the humeral head is centered in the glenoid, thereby facilitating elevation.

Rotator cuff muscles have a critical role in glenohumeral instability. Though they are smaller and less powerful than the deltoid muscle, rotator cuff tendons are located closer to the center of rotation. The force vector of all rotator cuff musculature is primarily one of compression. The rotator cuff functions to "cinch" the humeral head in the socket while the deltoid provides the power of movement. Loss of rotator cuff strength can aggravate instability by altering the force relationship between the deltoid and the rotator cuff. The posterior deltoid is a larger muscle and has a moment arm that acts at a greater distance from the center of rotation than does the infraspinatus and teres minor. The posterior del-

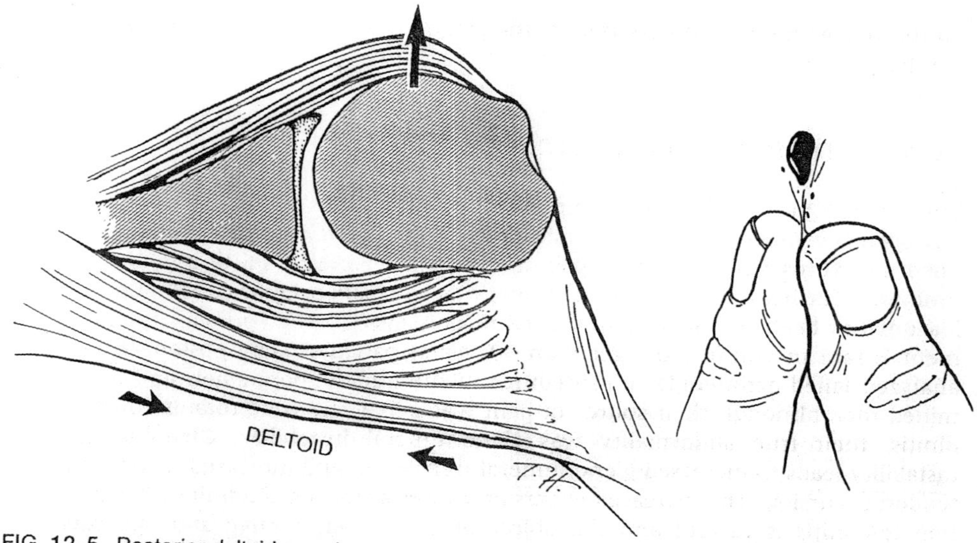

FIG. 12–5. Posterior deltoid muscle contracture results in an anteriorly directed force.

toid exerts a significant anterior shear force on the glenohumeral joint. With a strong, dynamic, and coordinated rotator cuff, the humeral head is centralized. As the rotator cuff weakens because of insufficiency or tear, the stabilizing effect of the rotator cuff is lost, and an increased anteroinferior translation can result (Fig. 12–5).

The biceps has long been regarded as a humeral head depressor. Experimental work has focused on the role of the biceps in anteroinferior instability and has documented the instability caused by an experimentally created biceps tendon lesion.[129] This role definition is supported by the clinical experience of many shoulder surgeons who have noted the relationship between a biceps tendon-labrum tear (SLAP lesion) and patients with clinical findings of anteroinferior instability.

SUBSCAPULARIS MUSCLE

The relationship between the subscapularis and glenohumeral stability has been investigated by Glousman and associates.[130] Loss of strength and coordination of the subscapularis muscle decreases dynamic stability. Increased stress on the static stabilizers results.

BODY MECHANICS

Multiple factors that do not involve the shoulder contribute to glenohumeral stability in the athlete who throws. Body position, throwing mechanics, and leg and trunk strength are all factors that allow a stable glenohumeral joint to function effectively. Abnormalities in any or all of these factors place greater demand on the active and passive stabilizers of the glenohumeral joint and lead to shoulder dysfunction.

CUFF-INSTABILITY CIRCLE (FIG. 12–6)

The relationship between glenohumeral instability and rotator cuff symptoms has been the subject of recent publications.[131,132] The failure of acromioplasty, open or arthroscopic, to relieve pain and return an individual to athletics has prompted further investigation. The work of Glousman, Jobe, and their colleagues has been of critical importance in emphasizing that primary impingement is rare in young (younger than 30 years) patients. They postoperatively analyzed failed acromioplasty procedures in the athletic population and determined that, although their source of pain was perceived to be rotator cuff tendinitis, their true abnormality was glenohumeral instability. Glenohumeral instability leads to increased glenohumeral translation and increased rotator cuff tendon excursion. The increased excursion causes a traction tendinitis. This traction tendinitis is painful and the object of much conservative and operative treatment. When treatment is directed at the rotator cuff and the true source is ignored, clinical failure results. Correction must be directed at the underlying instability, which is corrected with a rehabilitation program or with surgical intervention. Occasionally, instability may lead to the actual tearing of the rotator cuff tendon, most often in the anterior distal portion of the supraspinatus. Repair of the rotator cuff tendon, along with correction of the instability, is then required.

The reverse situation also appears true in that primary rotator cuff problems can lead to glenohumeral instability. Decreased rotator cuff strength causes a loss of dynamic stability that leads to increased load on the static stabilizers. These stabilizers may stretch and allow increased translation of the humeral

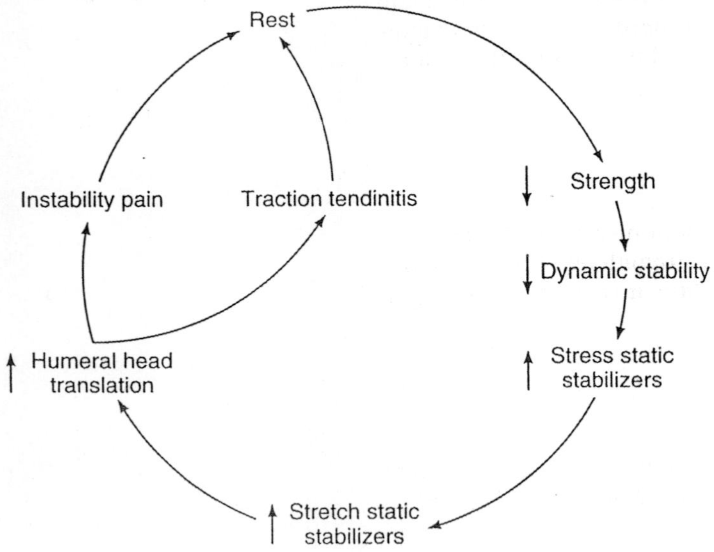

FIG. 12–6. The "vicious" cycle of rest, instability, and tendinitis.

head. Correction of the rotator cuff tendinitis eliminates the pain, allows the rotator cuff to recover its role as a dynamic stabilizer, and thereby also controls the instability process. Rotator cuff insufficiency that causes instability is probably less appreciated than the reverse condition because instability caused by rotator cuff insufficiency rarely is symptomatic, whereas rotator cuff tendinitis produced by instability is quite painful. Instability rarely develops following rotator cuff injury in an individual with normal glenohumeral translation. The individual who is more likely to develop instability has asymptomatic *bilateral* shoulder laxity. If an examination could be performed before the injury occurs, one would see increased excursion of the humeral head on the glenoid caused by the laxity in the passive restraints. The joint is *potentially unstable*. The joint is *functionally stable*, however, because the dynamic stabilizers of the glenohumeral joint, primarily rotator cuff tendons, serve to contain the humeral head within the glenoid cavity during activities of daily living, work, and sports. When this individual injures the rotator cuff, the painful shoulder is rested and a period of deconditioning occurs. The dynamic stabilizers are weakened and, with the pre-existing deficiency of passive stabilization, the situation becomes critical. Without the normally strong dynamic stabilizers, *increased* excursion occurs and the *asymptomatic laxity* becomes *symptomatic instability*.

Most often the symptoms are controlled by correction of rotator cuff insufficiency with rest and rehabilitation. Occasionally, instability increases in severity with prolonged periods of rotator cuff insufficiency. The passive restraints stretch to such an extent that, even when rotator cuff insufficiency is eliminated (the dynamic stabilizers are brought back to their normal condition), the static stabilizers have become so lax that symptomatic glenohumeral instability results.

Our concept of shoulder instability has advanced from the simple division into stable and dislocatable categories. At present, subtle instabilities can be appreci-

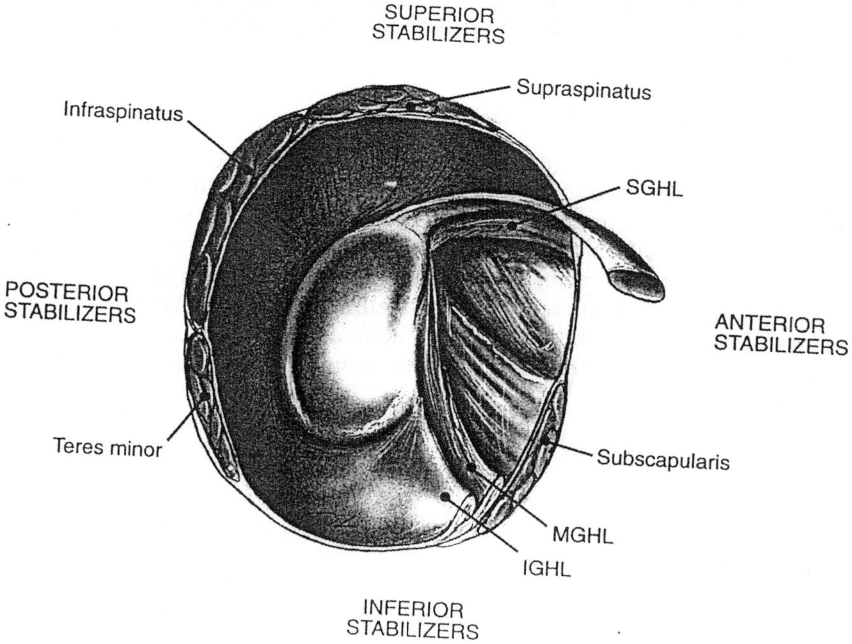

FIG. 12–7. The static and dynamic stabilizers of the shoulder.

ated. Glenohumeral stability is viewed as a "ring" concept (Fig. 12–7). Excessive anteroinferior translation results from a deficiency in the anteroinferior static stabilizers combined with a deficiency in the superior stabilizers. Posteroinferior instability is accompanied by a deficiency in the superior static stabilizers.

The relationship between rotator cuff disorders and glenohumeral instability is circular. Glenohumeral instability can allow increased glenohumeral excursion, increased traction on the rotator cuff, and a rotator cuff traction tendinitis. Similarly, a primary rotator cuff deficiency can lead to glenohumeral instability.

A thorough understanding of the anatomy and pathophysiology of this area is required before sufficient clinical data can be obtained from a patient's history, physical examination, and supplemental tests to allow the orthopedic surgeon to make an appropriate diagnosis and choose appropriate treatment for glenohumeral instability. Within the context of this book, the determination of proper treatment means the determination of whether or not the instability can be managed arthroscopically. Each question, physical examination maneuver, or imaging technique is directed toward determining whether arthroscopic treatment would be a viable approach for a particular patient.

CLINICAL INFORMATION

HISTORY

Certain information should be documented in the history. The mechanism of injury, arm position, and amount of force required to create the instability are noted. The reduction method, presence of neurologic symptoms, previous treatment, and family history also are recorded. Positions and activities that are painful and/or cause instability symptoms are documented.

The history is taken to determine the degree and direction of instability, and more importantly, it helps to identify the abnormality causing the instability. The *type of abnormality* determines whether the shoulder can be treated arthroscopically.

MECHANISM OF INJURY AND ARM POSITION

The mechanism of injury and arm position can be considered together. The individual whose arm is taken into forcible external rotation when abducted 90° develops anterior glenohumeral instability (Fig. 12–8). A similar instability pattern can result from a fall on the outstretched arm because the arm is forcibly abducted without adequate external rotation. Direct distraction mechanisms point to an anteroinferior or inferoanterior instability pattern (Fig. 12–9).

An individual who falls on the outstretched hand and thus drives the humeral head posteriorly or posteroinferiorly has examination results consistent with the posterior instability pattern.

AMOUNT OF FORCE

The amount of force required to create the instability is important. The atraumatic or minimally traumatic event that leads to instability is usually subluxation. Ligament substance attenuation instability is the arthroscopic finding. Individuals who sustain dislocation from significant force are more likely to show findings of ligament insertional instability.

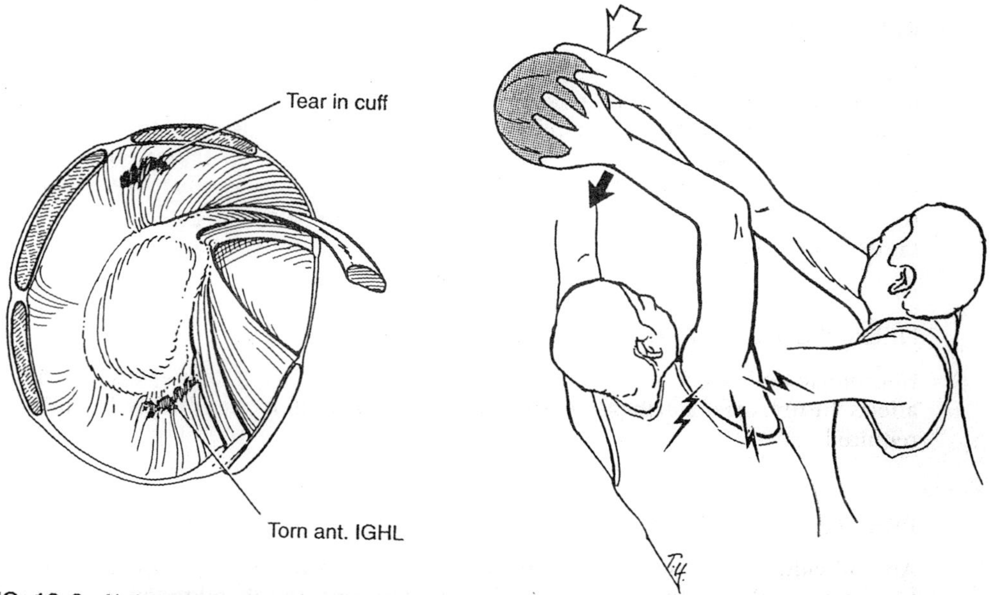

FIG. 12–8. Abduction external rotation injury resulting in damage to the anteroinferior glenohumeral ligament and the posterosuperior rotator cuff.

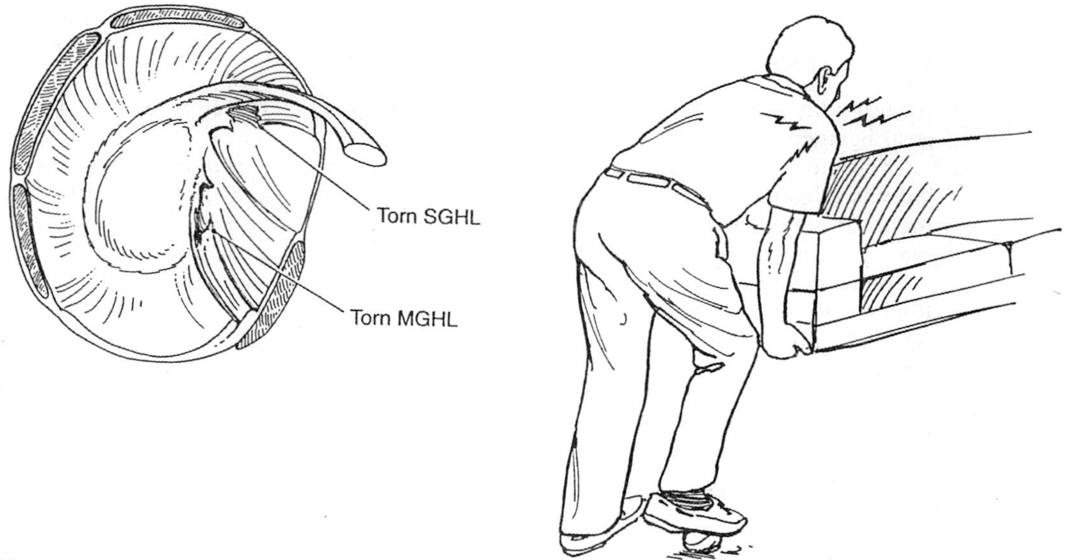

FIG. 12–9. Inferior distraction causes damage to the superior and middle glenohumeral ligaments.

REDUCTION

The mechanism by which the dislocation was reduced provides certain relevant information. Individuals who require reduction by another individual (physician in the emergency room or athletic trainer on the field) have sustained a dislocation of the glenohumeral joint and are more likely to have ligament insertion findings. Those whose "dislocations" spontaneously reduced or were self-reduced may have ligament insertion lesions, but are more likely to have sustained a subluxation rather than a true dislocation.

NEUROLOGIC DISORDERS

Neurologic deficiency that persists after the reduction of a shoulder dislocation affects future care. Further investigation of the persistent neurologic lesion is required.

PREVIOUS TREATMENT

An individual may have recurrent symptomatic instability because previous treatment, such as immobilization and activity protection rehabilitation, may not have been adequate. Appropriate rehabilitation exercises for scapular muscles, deltoid, and rotator cuff may not have been performed or, more commonly, were discontinued once the patient "felt better."

FAMILY HISTORY

A family history of glenohumeral instability or of patellofemoral problems suggests ligamentous laxity.

The history is taken by the surgeon to understand whether the patient's instability is a ligament insertion problem, which is amenable to arthroscopic treatment, or is a ligament-capsule attenuation problem, which at present is not well managed arthroscopically and is best treated by an open surgical procedure.

The work of Rockwood and Matsen has been helpful in clarifying this issue.[133] Rockwood has described two types of anterior instability referred to as TUBS and AMBRI. Patients with **T**raumatic, **U**nidirectional instability are likely to have a **B**ankart lesion and are commonly managed **S**urgically. Patients with an **A**traumatic injury may have **M**ultidirectional instability, usually have **B**ilateral instability, and should respond to a **R**ehabilitation program. However, if conservative treatment fails and surgery is required, an **I**nferior capsular shift is performed (Table 12–1).

TABLE 12–1. CHARACTERISTICS OF INSTABILITY TYPES

TUBS	AMBRI
Trauma	Minimal or no trauma
Dislocation reduced in Emergency Room	Spontaneous reduction
No family history	Family history
No other joint laxity	Generalized laxity
No sulcus	Sulcus

Although no historical information or physical findings are pathognomonic, this classification system is helpful in counseling patients on the advisability of an arthroscopic approach. An arthroscopic examination can determine the presence or absence of an arthroscopically treatable lesion, but patients should be provided preoperatively with as much information as possible regarding the arthroscopic treatment of their problem.

PHYSICAL EXAMINATION

The diagnosis of glenohumeral instability is rarely made in the absence of any historical information provided by the patient. Certainly, various degrees of laxity may be identified on physical examination without any relevant complaints, but *symptomatic* glenohumeral instability is most often diagnosed by history and *confirmed* by physical examination. The physical examination determines whether laxity is present, whether that laxity is greater than that in the opposite shoulder, and whether the laxity is indeed the source of the patient's complaints. An individual may demonstrate greater, equal, or lesser degrees of laxity in one shoulder compared to the other, but only by combining the patient's history with the results of the physical examination can the examiner determine whether laxity is symptomatic instability.

Laxity must be differentiated from *instability*. Instability is defined as the symptomatic expression of excessive translation (laxity). Thus, although an individual may be lax in various directions, he may be unstable in only one. For example, an individual may demonstrate posteroinferior, inferior, and anteroinferior laxity on examination, but is only symptomatic when the shoulder is examined for anteroinferior translation. The operative approach is aimed at the direction of instability, not necessarily at all directions of laxity.

The initial evaluation can be directed toward a determination of generalized laxity. Recurvation of the knees and elbows can be observed. Metacarpal-phalangeal hyperextension (thumb to forearm) can be measured and documented.

The presence of generalized ligamentous laxity is most likely in an individual with multidirectional instability. These individuals rarely have any intra-articular disorder that is amenable to arthroscopic treatment. They generally have capsular laxity that requires open surgical reconstruction when a rehabilitation program is unsuccessful.

The range of motion of both shoulders should be documented. Elevation (flexion in the scapular plane) is generally equal in each shoulder. External rotation with the arm at the side and external rotation with the arm at 90° of adduction can be significantly different. Our experience shows that the amount of external rotation is not predictive of intra-articular lesions. Diminished internal rotation measured with the arm in 90° of abduction, and/or decreased cross-body adduction (Fig. 12–10) and behind-the-back internal rotation, are manifestations of posterior capsular and/or posterior rotator cuff contracture. Any significant degree of posterior contracture causes an obligatory anterosuperior translation, which aggravates the instability.[134]

Posterior capsular contracture is a condition that generally can be corrected by a well-supervised stretching program. The presence of anterior subluxation with a tight posterior capsule should encourage the surgeon to pursue nonoperative care. Restoration of a normal range of motion with reversal of the posterior contracture can eliminate subluxation. The individual who has subluxation but does

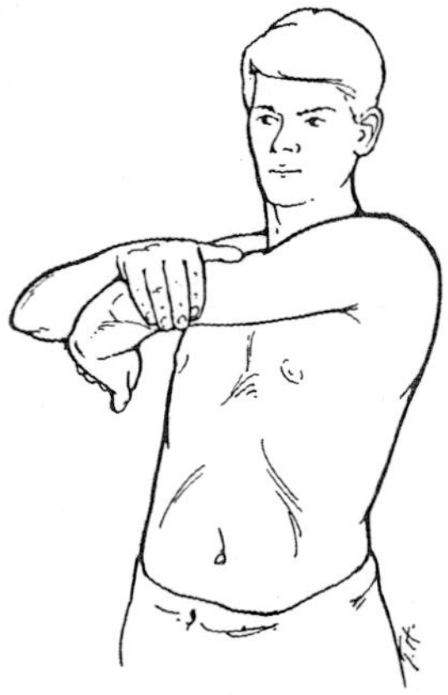

FIG. 12–10. Diminished cross-body adduction indicates posterior capsular contracture.

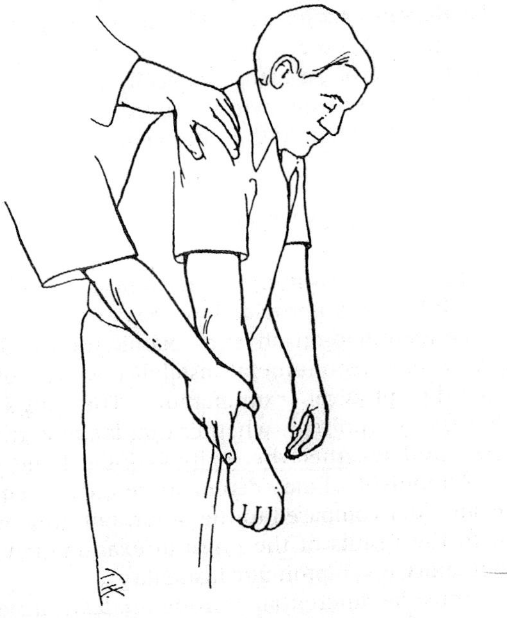

FIG. 12–11. A slight bend at the waist allows the arms to relax and aids in the examination of antero-inferior translation.

not have a posterior contracture is less likely to respond to nonoperative care.

The neurologic and circulatory status should be documented. A routine neurologic evaluation includes shoulder shrugging for proximal brachial nerve lesions (dorsal scapular), examination of the deltoid (axillary nerve) and biceps (musculocutaneous nerve), and distal sensibility and motor function for radial, median, and ulnar nerve lesions. The management of common instabilities rarely requires an extensive circulatory investigation. Vascular investigation is more often warranted with severe traumatic injuries to the shoulder girdle.

Various impingement signs are then performed to document the degree of rotator cuff involvement. A full-thickness tear can occur in patients with glenohumeral instability, particularly in those whose first dislocation occurred after the age of 45.[135]

In younger individuals, diffuse weakness, often bilateral, may be indicative of rotator cuff insufficiency resulting from poor conditioning. Rotator cuff testing may be painful and may indicate a traction tendinitis. Positive impingement signs, and even a positive impingement test, *do not* rule out glenohumeral instability as the underlying cause of the shoulder pain.

INSTABILITY TESTS

Numerous instability tests have been described, and all have a place in the patient evaluation. Examination for instability requires the patient's cooperation and relaxation. The contralateral asymptomatic shoulder is examined first to provide the examiner with an estimation of the patient's range of motion, strength, and stability. Perhaps the least painful and stressful test to the patient is arm distraction with the body bent slightly at the waist. We have chosen to call this the Rowe test, as it has been popularized by Carter Rowe. Often, the patient associates complaints of instability with the arm in the throwing position; consequently, an examination in that position is limited by the patient. With the Rowe test, the patient is rarely in discomfort; thus, relaxation is easy to achieve and the degree of inferoanterior laxity can be easily appreciated (Fig. 12–11).

The "drawer" test is performed next. The examiner stabilizes the scapula with one hand and grasps the humeral head between the thumb and long finger with the other hand. Anterior and posterior stresses are applied. The amount of translation and any symptoms, or lack of, are recorded.

The "sulcus sign" is then elicited with the arm distracted in the adducted position. External rotation is first measured with the arm at the side, and then the arm is raised so that external rotation stresses can be applied in various degrees of abduction. Apprehension, pain, and/or instability are recorded. While the arm is in 90° of abduction and external rotation, the patient is asked to perform a resisted throwing maneuver (Fig. 12–12). A sharp posterior joint pain is appreciated when the shoulder is unstable anteriorly. The shoulder is then tested for posterior instability. Occasionally, the shoulder can be dislocated posteriorly. Usually, the posterior subluxation is little appreciated by the patient, but as the arm is taken into extension, the shoulder reduces and the patient's symptoms can be reproduced. We commonly perform posterior instability tests with the patient supine because this position provides a smooth transition to the next test.

The relocation test has proved to be helpful in diagnosing subtle anterior instabilities (Fig. 12–13).[131] With the patient supine, the arm is taken into abduction/external rotation, and an anterior stress is applied until the patient's apprehension is reproduced. Posterior stress is then applied by pressing against the upper arm. This maneuver reduces the subluxation if present, and the patient's apprehension often is dramatically decreased. This decrease in apprehension is a positive test.

RADIOGRAPHIC STUDIES

Standard radiographic views in the instability series include anteroposterior glenoid, axillary, supraspinatus outlet, and apical oblique views. Findings on the anteroposterior glenoid study, made with the arm in internal rotation, include the presence of a Hill-Sachs' lesion. The axillary projection can occasionally demonstrate anterior or posteroinferior calcifications consistent with instability, but such calcifications are more commonly seen on the Westpoint and/or apical oblique views, in which the beam is tilted to project the anteroinferior glenoid edge away from superimposed bone structures. The glenoid version is an unreliable aid to diagnosing the direction of instability. Increased anteversion is of concern during arthroscopic corrections of anterior instability because the fixation devices may slide off the bone if the insertion angle is unacceptably high. The supraspinatus outlet view provides information in patients with rotator cuff findings or complaints.

If additional information is required, other imaging techniques are available. A CT-arthrogram with contrast evaluates capsular volume and ligament insertion disruptions, as well as labrum tears. MRI seems particularly sensitive for labrum

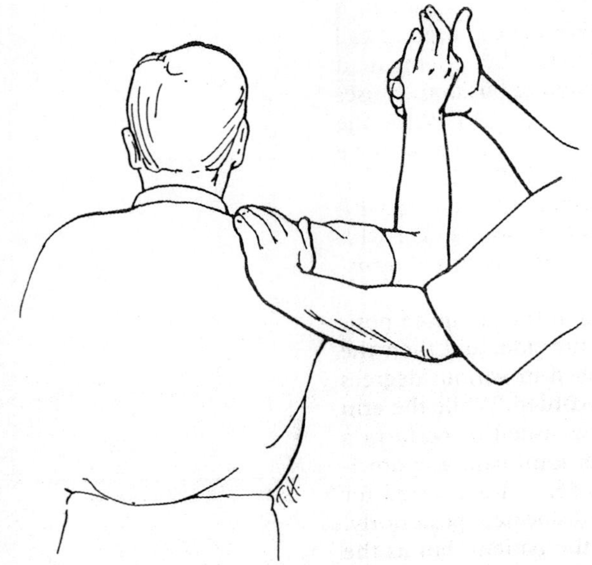

FIG. 12–12. Subtle instabilities can be diagnosed with a stress test. As the patient attempts to "throw" the examiner's hand, posterior joint line pain is produced.

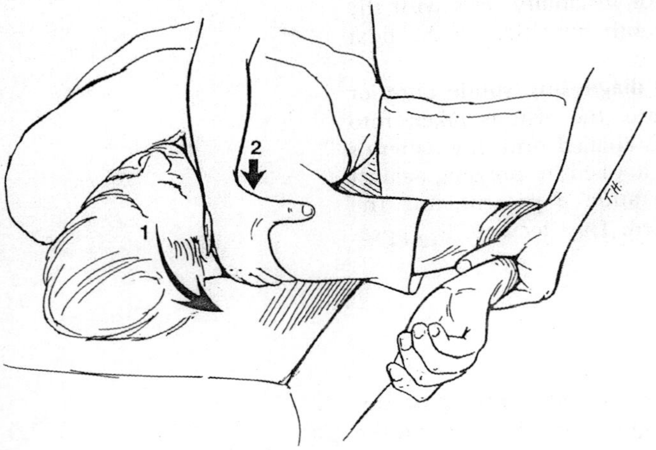

FIG. 12–13. Anterior stress (1) to the abducted externally rotated arm reproduces the patient's pain. Posterior force (2) reduces the subluxation and diminishes the pain.

tears. Stress views and examination under fluoroscopy can also be used if the degree and direction of instability are not clear.

CONSERVATIVE CARE

ACUTE DISLOCATIONS

A great deal has been written on the management of an acute anteroinferior shoulder dislocation.[136–141] The shoulder should be protected against distraction and external rotation stresses for 6 weeks. One common approach calls for constant immobilization of the shoulder in a sling for a period of 3 weeks. The sling is removed only for bathing, elbow

TABLE 12–2. CHARACTERISTICS THAT SUGGEST PROBABLE OUTCOMES OF CONSERVATIVE REHABILITATION

SUCCESS	FAILURE
1. Atraumatic onset	1. Traumatic onset
2. Initial dislocation at age 30 or older	2. Initial dislocation at age 20 or younger
3. Recurrent subluxation	3. Recurrent dislocation
4. Ligament laxity	4. No ligament laxity
5. Multidirectional instability	5. Unidirectional instability
6. Posterior capsular contracture	6. No posterior capsular contracture
7. Weak rotator cuff	7. Strong rotator cuff
8. No prior rehabilitation program	8. Good prior rehabilitation program

motion, and gentle shoulder elevation performed to prevent stiffness. The sling is then discarded, and the patient voluntarily limits distraction and external rotation stress for an additional 3 weeks. As soon as the pain has subsided, usually within the first week, the patient is started on a shoulder girdle rehabilitation program that strengthens the 3 parts of the deltoid, the scapular muscles, and the rotator cuff. Return to sports is limited until the patient regains range of motion and strength in the injured shoulder. The recurrence rate varies, but it can be as high as 90% in a high-risk population, such as young (20 years old or younger) athletes who are required to participate in vigorous physical exercise.[142]

RECURRENT INSTABILITY

Patients with recurrent instability may respond to the appropriate conservative care and rehabilitation program just outlined. Certainly, all patients, regardless of their diagnosis, can be put on a 6-month period of exercises. Individuals who respond favorably to a rehabilitation program seem to share certain characteristics (Table 12–2). For these patients, the onset of symptoms either is atraumatic or occurs with minimal trauma. These individuals subluxate rather than dislocate and are more likely to have multiaxial instability rather than unidirectional anteroinferior dislocations.

Characteristics that predict a less successful response to conservative care are essentially opposite to those just listed. Individuals who sustained a dislocation as a result of significant trauma and do not have ligamentous laxity are more likely to suffer from unidirectional anteroinferior instabilities. Individuals without any posterior capsular contracture, who have normal rotator cuff strength, and who have attempted a well-supervised rehabilitation program also are not likely to respond.

Although most patients are interested in trying a conservative care program, patients are equally interested in knowing whether their chances of success are great or small. Individuals are entitled to an opinion regarding not only the types of treatments available, operative and nonoperative, but also regarding their chance of success with each treatment.

ARTHROSCOPIC TREATMENT OF GLENOHUMERAL INSTABILITY

13

Arthroscopic evaluation begins with an examination of the patient's range of motion under anesthesia. *Both* shoulders are examined, and direction and degree of translation are recorded. Increased translation is possible in all patients under anesthesia, but a difference in degree should be noted between the symptomatic and the asymptomatic shoulder.

Anteroposterior stability is assessed with the arm abducted 90° and in neutral rotation. The degree of movement is graded 0 to 3+ (0, no appreciable translation of the humeral head relative to the glenoid; 1+, movement of the humeral head to the glenoid rim but not over it; 2+, subluxation of the humeral head over the glenoid rim with spontaneous reduction after manual pressure is released; 3+, frank dislocation of the humeral head over the glenoid rim with locking after manual pressure is released). Inferior translation is also assessed on a 0 to 3+ scale. Inferior distraction on the adducted arm is graded as follows: 0, inferior translation of the humeral head relative to the glenoid of less than 0.5 cm; 1+, inferior translation of 0.5 to 1.0 cm; 2+, inferior translation of 1 to 2 cm; and 3+, inferior translation of greater than 2 cm (Fig. 13–1).[143]

Appreciation of whether posterior subluxation occurs or whether the shoulder is resting in an anteriorly subluxated position and posterior stress merely reduces the subluxation is difficult to achieve. For this reason, direct observation of the humeral head under anesthesia has proved beneficial.

Once the arthroscope enters the shoulder, further information can be obtained. Individuals with recurrent instability have large capsules that are easy to enter and take a greater volume of fluid. Excessive posterior capsular laxity often allows the trocar to merely invaginate the capsule between the humeral head and glenoid, thereby giving the tactile impression that the instrument is located intra-articularly when actually it is in an extra-articular site (Fig. 13–2). After the arthroscope is inserted, the humeral head can be directly observed. The shoulder is subjected to anterior, inferior, and posterior stress with the arm moved in various positions of abduction and external and internal rotation. An attempt should be made to reproduce the symptomatic position to observe whether significant instability does occur. The normal humeral head translates at least 50% of the glenoid surface width. Humeral head displacement *over* the glenoid rim (dislocation) is always considered significant. Humeral head displacement *to the level* of the glenoid rim is considered significant only with confirmatory findings of labrum tearing in that area and with a clinical history and

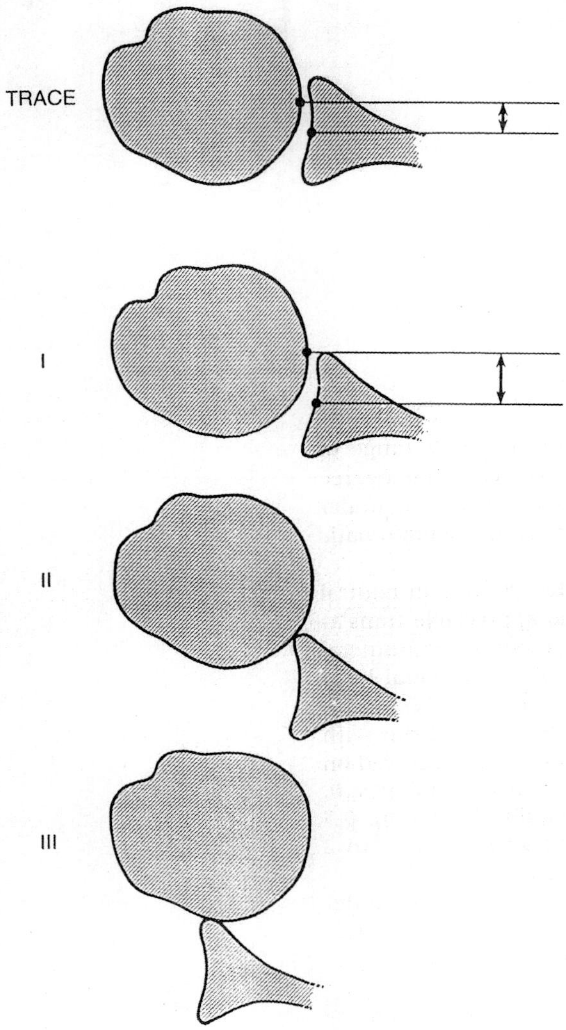

FIG. 13–1. A system to grade the amount of humeral head translation.

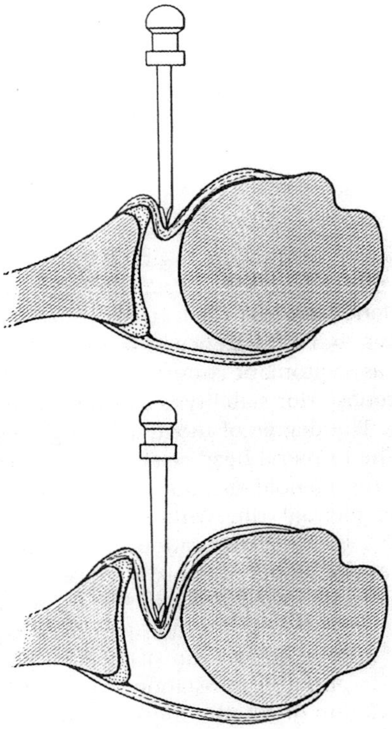

FIG. 13–2. The trocar can remain extracapsular yet give the impression that the joint has been penetrated.

physical examination consistent with that direction of instability. The arthroscope should be moved to the anterior portal, where these maneuvers are repeated.

ARTHROSCOPIC FINDINGS CONSISTENT WITH INSTABILITY (TABLE 13–1)

LABRAL LESIONS

Common labral findings consistent with glenohumeral instability include labra that are torn, shredded, separated, and/or recessed.[126,144–146]

TABLE 13–1. ARTHROSCOPIC FINDINGS

	TUBS	AMBRI
Biceps	SLAP	Normal
Cuff	Posterosuperior partial tear	Normal, atonic
Loose bodies	Yes	No
Labrum	Frayed, detached, torn	Normal, may be atrophic or absent below equator
Superior glenohumeral ligament	Normal	Normal
Middle glenohumeral ligament	Normal, torn	Attenuated
Anteroinferior glenohumeral ligament	Bankart	Normal
Hill-Sachs' lesion	Yes	No

Although glenohumeral compression injuries and repetitive throwing motions can result in torn labra, this finding is most commonly caused by glenohumeral instability. Labral shredding combined with direct observation of humeral head movement over the area of the labral disorder is confirmatory evidence of glenohumeral instability. Labral separation in the area of the Bankart lesion is diagnostic of anteroinferior instability. Individuals with recurrent subluxation often have an attenuated, small, or even absent labrum, particularly below the equator. Whether this characteristic is a normal variant, is the result of repeated instability episodes that "wear down the labrum," or is a congenital abnormality that predisposes an individual to instability is unknown. Nonetheless, the absence of labrum from the 4 o'clock to the 8 o'clock position is a quite consistent finding in individuals with anteroinferior subluxation.

ROTATOR CUFF

Rotator cuff findings consistent with instability include loss of tone, a partial tear, and an interval tear. Atonic cuffs are seen in individuals with multidirectional instability. The entire shoulder capsule is hyperelastic, and although no physical disruption can be seen within the rotator cuff, palpation with the probe allows appreciation of loss of normal muscle tone. Partial tears in the rotator cuff, particularly in the posterosuperior portion, are consistent with an anteroinferior instability pattern. Interval lesions are more consistent with an inferoanterior instability pattern. The findings of an interval lesion include tear or attenuation of the superior glenohumeral ligament, fraying of the biceps tendon, superior partial fraying of the subscapularis tendon, and/or partial tearing at the most anterior border of the supraspinatus tendon where the biceps tendon exits the glenohumeral joint (Fig. 13–3).

LOOSE BODIES

Loose bodies in the glenohumeral joint are almost pathognomonic of glenohumeral instability. In the absence of any arthritic or synovial condition, a loose body should alert the orthopedic surgeon to search for underlying instability.

HILL-SACHS' LESION

The Hill-Sachs' lesion, located at the posteroinferior margin of the humeral head, is diagnostic of an anteroinferior dislocation. One cannot be certain of the

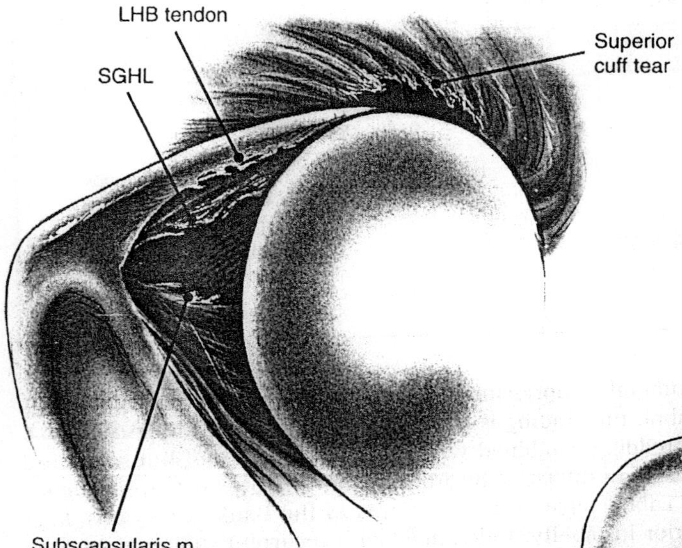

FIG. 13–3. Lesions of the rotator interval may include tearing of the superior glenohumeral ligament (SGHL), fraying of the subscapularis and/or biceps tendons, and a tear of the most anterior portion of the supraspinatus tendon. LHB = long head of the biceps.

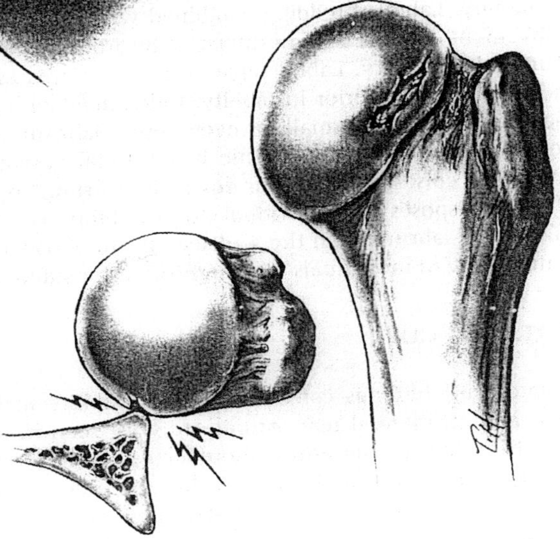

FIG. 13–4. The location of the Hill-Sachs' lesion on the humeral head is more medial than that of the normal bare area.

cause of the Hill-Sachs' lesion, but its presence documents instability. Care should be taken not to confuse the Hill-Sachs' lesion with the normal bare area of the humerus (Fig. 13–4).

AXILLARY RECESS

Although we have not been able to quantify the size of an axillary recess, the arthroscopist with experience can appreciate the normal contour of the inferior pouch. Individuals with multiaxial instability demonstrate a large inferior recess.

SUBSCAPULARIS BURSA

The subscapularis bursa should be inspected for loose bodies. A large subscapularis bursa can also provide confirmatory evidence of instability because this characteristic can indicate an enlarged glenohumeral joint capsule.

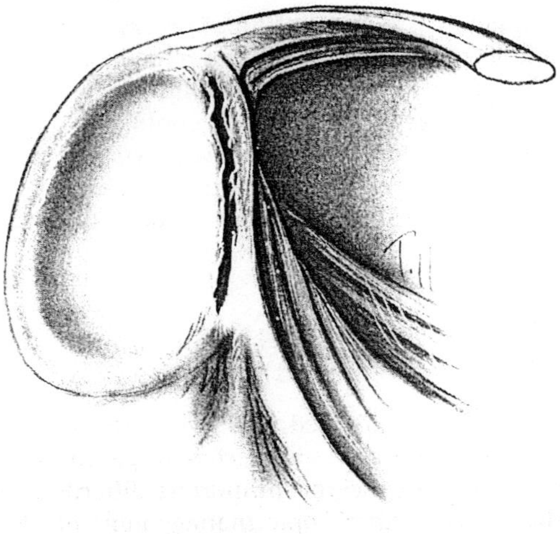

FIG. 13–8. Rarely, the anteroinferior glenohumeral ligament inserts to the superior margin of the glenoid. Detachments of this type function as Bankart lesions.

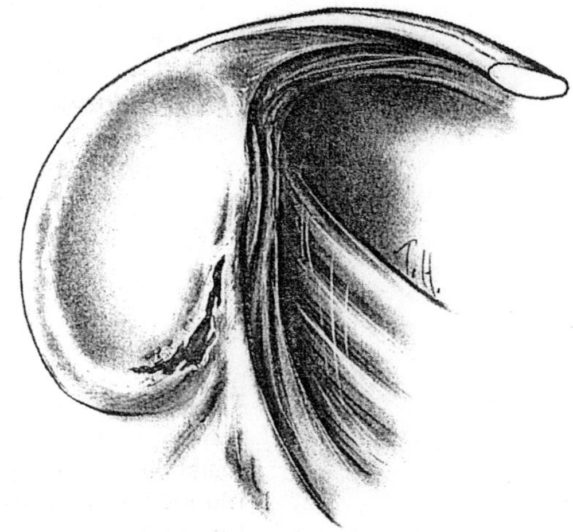

FIG. 13–9. The classic Bankart lesion involves ligament-labrum separation in the inferior quadrant.

scopic treatment, but are more likely to improve with open surgical reconstruction. The third encompasses individuals who will likely benefit from surgery, open or arthroscopic, but in whom the small differences in recurrence rates may be crucial.

The first group of patients includes voluntary dislocators who can perform the dislocation maneuver without experiencing pain. These instability maneuvers, performed in multiple directions and, often, with the arm positioned at the side, are evoked by patterns of muscle contraction and relaxation. This group may have psychologic problems, and the results of open reconstructive surgery in these individuals have been notoriously poor. Because these individuals do not improve with any type of reconstruction, arthroscopic surgery should be avoided. Individuals, however, who must maneuver the arm to produce a painful dislocation do benefit from surgical correction.

The second group of individuals have multidirectional instability and generally do not have a Bankart lesion. The abnormality is capsular laxity, which is treated with a Neer inferior capsular shift. Our experience with the arthroscopic capsular tightening procedures for capsular laxity was poor,[147] because we were not able to estimate reliably the amount of capsular tightening required. We regard as investigative the arthroscopic management of multidirectional instability and do not recommend its use until further clinical and experimental work has been presented.

The third group of individuals includes those with ligament-labrum insertion lesions (Bankart lesion). This group of individuals can be treated successfully using conventional open techniques, as well as arthroscopic techniques. Even in the most experienced hands, arthroscopic techniques seem to have a 10 to 15% lower success rate than that for open procedures, and this failure rate is higher for orthopedic surgeons learning the arthroscopic technique. The monetary cost of repeated surgery may not be acceptable to many individuals, and the possibility of an additional procedure should be discussed. For some individuals, *time* cost is more significant. In athletes, a recurrence can mean a lost season, which is a significant proportion of the athlete's professional life. For example, if the arthroscopic repair is performed and a recurrence follows the rehabilitation period, a second surgery, which must be followed by more rehabilitation, may result in 1 to 2 years of missed competitive athletics. This situation could prove devastating to the patient. Such a situation can occur with open reconstructive techniques as well, but at present, based on the average recurrence rates of open and arthroscopic techniques, the chances for recurrence are smaller with open surgery.

ARTHROSCOPIC TECHNIQUES

The arthroscopic surgical technique section is divided into two parts. The basic technique is common to all arthroscopic operations that control glenohumeral instability. A second part has been added to include numerous different techniques available to the orthopedist in the arthroscopic management of glenohumeral instability. At present, no one technique is superior to another.

PATIENT POSITION

The decubitus position has the advantage of providing better distraction and arm control with suspension so that an assistant is not required to manipulate the arm. The disadvantage is that conversion to an open reconstruction involves moving the patient to the supine position. The beach chair position is converted more easily to the open procedure should the arthroscopic approach prove unsuccessful. The disadvantage of the beach chair position is the need for an assistant to manipulate the arm and to provide distraction as needed. Each position has its supporters. We favor the decubitus position for subacromial surgery and the beach chair position for instability repairs.

BASIC TECHNIQUE

The shoulder is entered through the posterior portal, and the joint is filled with saline. A brief inspection is then carried out, and an anterior portal is created with a Wissinger rod. We favor an anterosuperior portal entering immediately anterior to the exit of the biceps from the glenohumeral joint. This position allows a good view of the anterior glenoid rim, as well as provides adequate space for an anteroinferior portal.

If gravity inflow is used, the tubing is connected to the anterior cannula and the cannula is used as a palpation probe. If necessary, a pump can be attached to the arthroscope and a probe can be inserted through the anterior portal.

DIAGNOSTIC EVALUATION

A systematic inspection of the glenohumeral joint is performed, and a comment is made about whether each structure is or is not associated with instability, as described previously.

THE DECISION TO PROCEED

After the diagnostic part of the procedure is concluded, certain decisions must be made.

1. Is the diagnosis of instability correct?
2. Does this instability require surgical correction?
3. If surgical correction is required, is this best performed arthroscopically or with open surgical techniques? Or, is either method appropriate?

If the steps just outlined have been followed, beginning with a complete history and physical examination and then an examination under anesthesia and under arthroscopy, a determination of whether the patient's complaints of pain are related to glenohumeral instability should be easily made.

The decision as to whether the instability requires surgical correction depends on the exact findings at surgery and also on when the individual had undergone arthroscopic surgery. An individual who has recently sustained a first-time acute dislocation and demonstrates a midsubstance glenohumeral tear may heal with conservative care, whereas an individual with repeated dislocations and a Bankart lesion is unlikely to improve with conservative care and, therefore, requires surgical care.

The third question is more difficult to answer. The literature comparing open and arthroscopic techniques is scant. Of course, much of the decision must be based on whether the orthopedic surgeon has advanced arthroscopic skills within the shoulder and is familiar with an appropriate arthroscopic technique.

We have been most successful in confining our surgery to anteroinferior instability of the insertional type, or Bankart lesions. The labrum, anteroinferior glenohumeral ligament, and/or middle glenohumeral ligament should be assessed, and if, in the surgeon's opinion, the structure is sufficient to hold the fixation device, arthroscopic treatment is appropriate. Anytime a criterion such as bulk, substance, or structure strength is used, an element of subjectivity is inserted. At present, however, we know of no better way to define the ability of tissue to hold the fixation device. We make similar determinations during open reconstructive surgery involving the rotator cuff or glenohumeral ligaments. The percentage of individuals with adequate structures in terms of type (insertional) and integrity (ability to hold a fixation device) is approximately 33 to 50%. An individual with an insertional type of instability with adequate soft tissue structures can be treated either arthroscopically or with conventional open surgical techniques.

Once the decision has been made to proceed with arthroscopic correction, *adequate flow* must be achieved. If an arthroscopic pump system is utilized, adequate flow for the arthroscopic procedure can be obtained without additional portals. If gravity inflow is utilized, the anterosuperior portal previously created can be used as an inflow portal. We prefer this portal to the superior portal. Once adequate inflow has been established, the arthroscope is kept in the posterior portal, advanced anteriorly, and rotated inferiorly to *view the anterior recess.* Occasionally when the anteroinferior portion of the joint cannot be visualized with this technique, the arthroscope is moved to the anterosuperior portal. The arthroscope is then repositioned posteriorly after the lesion has been inspected.

An alternative technique is the use of a 70° arthroscope. This technique requires an additional arthroscope, but more importantly, the improved viewing angle is diminished by the accompanying distortion.

An *anteroinferior portal is then created.* This portal should be made *just* superior

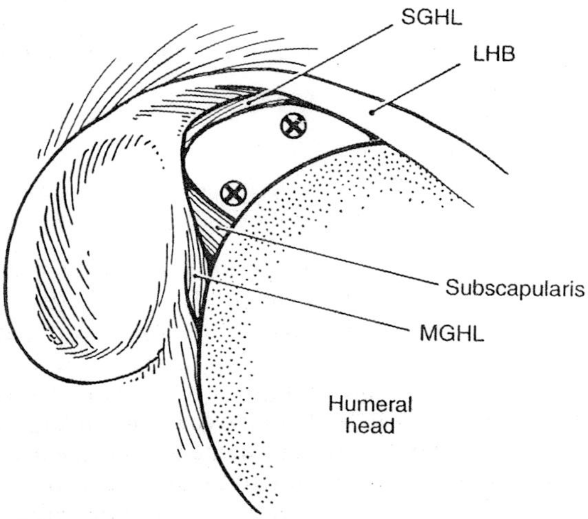

FIG. 13–10. The anterosuperior and anteroinferior portal sites. MGHL = middle glenohumeral ligament; LHB = long head of the biceps; SGHL = superior glenohumeral ligament.

to the superior edge of the subscapularis tendon (Fig. 13–10). The anteroinferior portal must be kept superior to the subscapularis tendon and as medial as possible while remaining lateral to the coracoid. Although placement of the inferior portal directly opposite the ligament detachment site is tempting, the neurovascular structures would be at risk.

A needle can be inserted until the precise spot for trocar entrance is found. The trocar is then introduced into the joint, and a soft tissue resector is inserted.

Three goals must be accomplished in all instability operations.

1. The anteroinferior ligament complex, if not freed, must be dissected from its site of false attachment and must be freely movable.
2. The anterior scapular neck must be abraded until cancellous bone is visible. Such abrasion allows for soft tissue/bone contact and permanent healing, as well as allows penetration of the implant.
3. Superior anteroinferior glenohumeral ligament movement must obliterate the Bankart lesion.

The first step is to *remove any fibrous tissue* from the anterior glenoid rim to help to *create a cancellous bone surface* for permanent ligament healing. In the normal situation, the anteroinferior glenohumeral ligament is detached from the anteroinferior rim. Thus, the soft tissue resector is easily placed, and soft tissue covering the anterior scapular neck is removed.

Debridement should be performed at least 1 to 1.5 cm medial to the articular surface and throughout the entire area of ligament detachment (Fig. 13–11).

A more difficult situation is noted when the ligament is only minimally displaced. Often the ligament has healed with a weak soft tissue attachment and must be forcibly separated from the glenoid. A small rasp or curette accomplishes this task. Ligament dissection should continue until the *ligament is freely movable.* A probe or an arthroscopic instrument can be used to grasp the ligament and draw it superiorly, thereby demonstrating *obliteration of the Bankart lesion* (Fig. 13–12).

Once the ligament is freely movable, *the bone should be prepared.* A small round bur is utilized. Keep the protected side of the bur against the ligament structures.

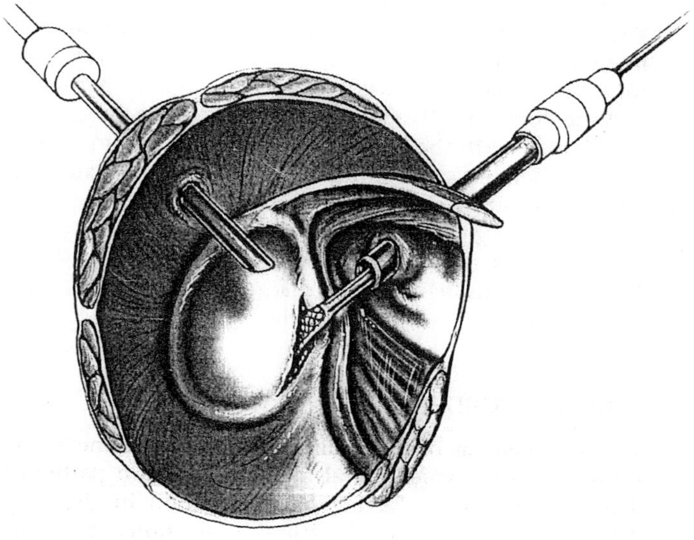

FIG. 13–11. Preparation of the anterior scapular neck may be performed with motorized or hand instruments. Always protect the soft tissues with the instrument guard.

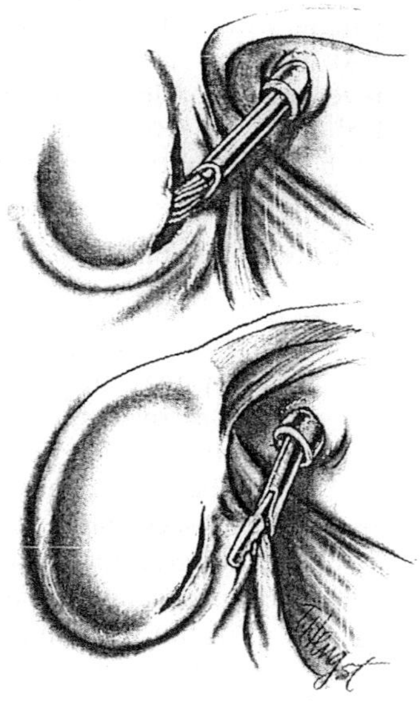

FIG. 13–12. Superior traction should demonstrate elimination of the Bankart lesion.

The entire area of soft tissue debridement should undergo decortication, which involves removing approximately 1 mm of bone. Two goals are accomplished. A cancellous bone surface is created for ultimate permanent soft tissue healing, and the bone surface allows easier penetration by the surgeon's choice of fixation device. With the scope held posteriorly, the most anteroinferior portions of this debridement can be difficult to visualize, particularly in larger individuals or when a longer operative time has allowed increased soft tissue swelling, which limits the surgeon's ability to advance the arthroscope anteriorly. If such swelling occurs, the arthroscope should be moved to the anterosuperior portal. The instruments remain in the anteroinferior portal, and an excellent view is obtained.

LABRAL DISORDERS

The management of labral disorders in glenohumeral instability involves decisions regarding which labral abnormalities are pathologic and which require debridement. Minor fraying of any portion of the labrum does not require debridement. Bucket-handle labral tears should be debrided to eliminate any mechanical source of pain and/or instability. A separated labrum should not be debrided, because doing so results in further instability. Altcheck and colleagues reported on their results with labral debridement.[144] Their study included 40 patients, 30 with anterior labral disorders (4 detached and 26 torn) and 10 with posterior labral disorders (2 detached and 8 torn). Of the patients, 85% were rated excellent to good in the early evaluation, but when they were examined later, the failure rate was 90%. Glasgow and associates also noted good results with labral debridement in stable shoulders and generally poor results in patients with labral tears and anterior instability.[145]

At this point, loose bodies have been removed, other areas of labral disorders have been debrided, a cancellous bed has been created, and the glenohumeral ligament has been dissected free so that it is movable in a superior direction and can be placed at the glenoid articular rim.

Technical Problems

1. Insufficient ligament. At this stage the surgeon may determine that the ligament is insufficient to allow arthroscopic reattachment. This insufficiency may be determined from the anatomic findings or may result from an overaggressive debridement.
   Solution:
   a. Abandon the procedure and convert to an open reconstruction.
   b. Dissect more anteroinferior glenohumeral ligament from the anteroinferior scapular neck to use in the repair.
   c. Incorporate the middle glenohumeral ligament or the superior border of the subscapularis in the repair. (This option does not reliably end in a successful result.)

2. Anterior portals too close.
   Solution:
   a. Abandon the procedure. The difficulty that can result from two anterior portals can be minimized if portals are created with the largest possible distance between them. This distance is attained by placing

the initial portal at the most anterosuperior portion as is possible (immediately anterior to the anterior supraspinatus border) and the anteroinferior portal at the superior edge of the subscapularis. Such placement almost always results in sufficient working distance so that the dissection and surgery can proceed with minimal difficulty.

b. If the procedure has been done without success, replace the portals correctly (see previous paragraph).

ALTERNATE SURGICAL TECHNIQUES

Multiple surgical techniques are currently used to re-establish the ligament attachment to the glenoid, and no particular technique is universally agreed upon. The techniques can be divided into two basic groups, those involving sutures and those involving fixation devices. The suture techniques include the single suture technique of Morgan and Bodenstab,[148] the multiple suture technique of Caspari,[149] and variations by Maki.[150] The Mitek implant can be used to attach sutures to the anterior scapular neck.[151] The implant techniques involve a staple,[152–154] a cannulated screw (Dyonics, Wolf), or a biodegradable tack.[143]

MULTIPLE SUTURE METHOD

This technique is an arthroscopic adaptation of the method described by Reider and Inglis.[155] Multiple sutures can be placed in the ligament/labrum complex. Tension is adjusted by pulling on various sutures until the ligament is in the precise position. If one of the sutures breaks, other sutures are still in place. A disadvantage of this technique is that the sutures must be tied posteriorly over the infraspinatus fascia. A separate posterior incision is required, and the possibility exists that tension on the sutures could be lost when swelling diminishes in the postoperative period.

TECHNIQUE

After the anterior scapular neck has been prepared, a 1/4-inch Steinmann's pin is passed through the anterior cannula and drilled across the glenoid neck to exit posteriorly in the infraspinatus fossa. Care is taken to angle the pin medially so that it exits close to the medial scapula border. This angle is necessary to avoid putting in jeopardy the suprascapular nerve branch to the infraspinatus, which passes approximately 1 to 2 cm medial to the glenoid rim (Fig. 13–13). The Steinmann's pin is then removed from the bone. A 1/0 monofilament suture is introduced into the suture channel, and the suture wheel is turned to feed the suture through the needle. The wheel is reversed until the suture is just within the hollow needle point. The suture punch (or curved awl) is then inserted through the anteroinferior cannula and placed into the joint. The most inferior suture is placed first. The needle pierces the ligament and is pushed through until the needle point is *clearly* visible puncturing the ligament. The suture wheel is then turned until at least 25 cm of suture are in the joint. The instrument is then removed from the joint. The intra-articular portion of the suture remains in view to avoid pulling the suture from the ligament and removing it from the joint, thereby causing repetition of the sequence just described. The two ends of

FIG. 13–13. Attempt to angle the transglenoid pin medially and inferiorly.

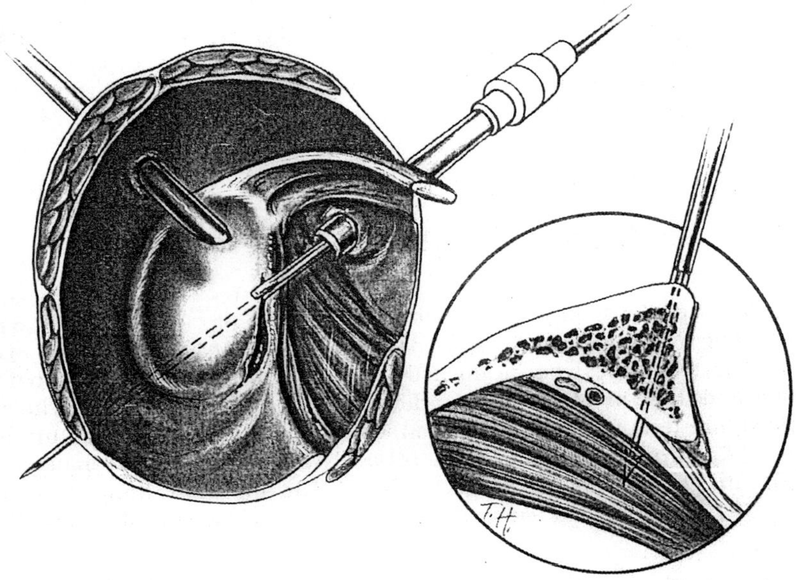

FIG. 13–14. Suture placement in the detached ligament-labrum complex.

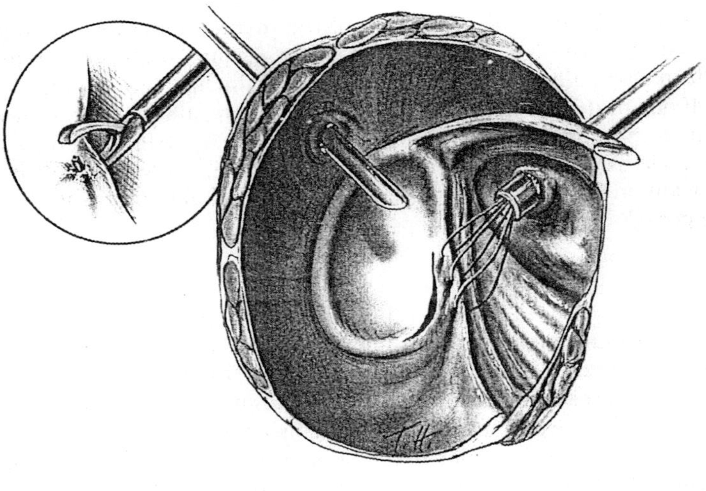

the suture are then grasped with a hemostat. This process is repeated two to six times; sutures are placed in the ligament from inferior to superior (Fig. 13–14).

After all the sutures have been placed in the labrum, a smaller Steinmann's pin with a hole at the end is passed through the anterior cannula into the previously drilled glenoid neck hole. All the suture ends are fed through the pin hole and pulled through the cannula into the bone hole. They are then delivered posteriorly through the puncture wound in the infraspinatus fossa (Fig. 13–15).

If the patient is in the decubitus position with arm suspension, the weight is released and the arm is brought into internal rotation. This maneuver releases tension on the ligaments and allows their anatomic reattachment.

Although placing the arm in the position of risk (abduction/external rotation)

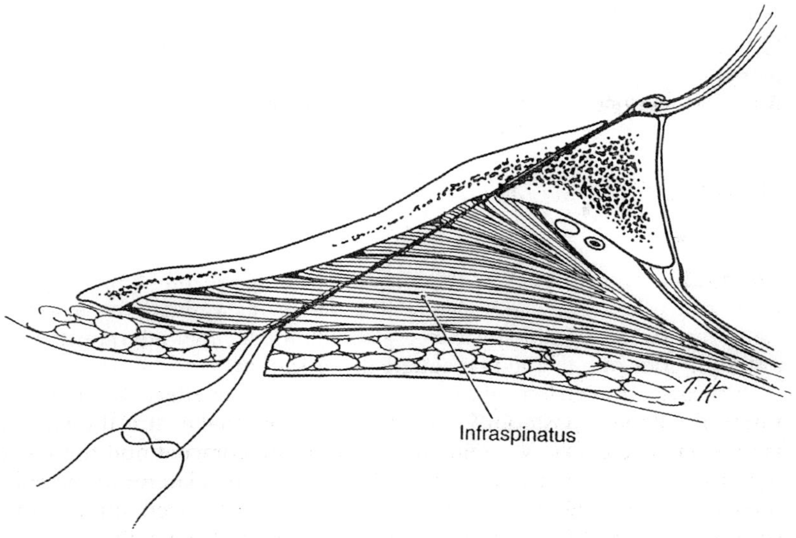

FIG. 13-15. The sutures are tied over the posteromedial infraspinatus.

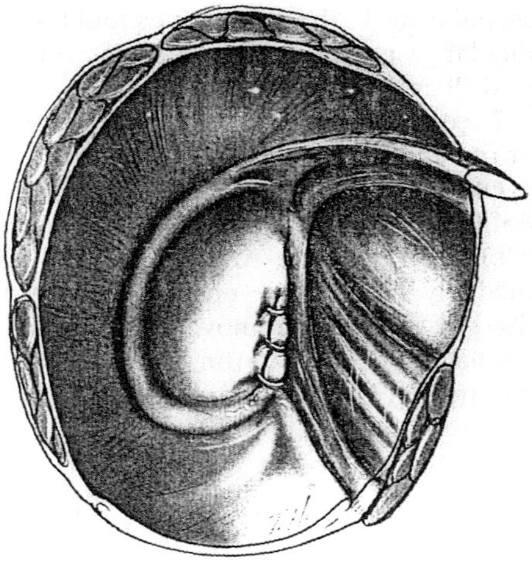

FIG. 13-16. Tension on the sutures reapproximates the Bankart lesion.

and then applying maximal tension to the ligament might seem desirable, the arthroscopic reality is that the ligament complex cannot be advanced when the arm is placed in this position.

The sutures are then separated into two equal bundles and are pulled taut to approximate the detached labrum/ligament complex to the glenoid neck. The sutures are tied into a standard square knot after passing one bundle through a piece of infraspinatus fascia with a standard round needle.

Arthroscopic inspection from either the posterior cannula or the anterosuperior portal should demonstrate firm coaptation of the glenoid labrum/ligament complex to the glenoid neck, thereby reconstituting the competency of the anteroinferior glenohumeral ligament. The labrum/ligament complex should be located at the margin of the glenoid rather than medially on the anterior scapular neck (Fig. 13-16). The ligament/labrum complex may be advanced as far superiorly as possible.

The shoulder then is thoroughly irrigated with saline and drained. All cannulas are removed, and puncture wounds are closed with simple sutures. A sterile bandage is applied and may be replaced with an adhesive bandage within 24 hours. The arm is immobilized in a sling for 3 weeks.

TECHNICAL PROBLEMS

Pin

Pin Slides Medially. A problem occurs when the pin fails to penetrate the bone and slides medially across the anterior scapular neck (Fig. 13–17). Causative factors include increased glenoid anteversion, lateral placement of the anteroinferior portal, and inadequate decortication.

Excessive anteversion cannot be corrected, but its effect can be minimized by tilting the patient posteriorly. The surgeon must make sure the pin portal is as far medial as possible, yet remains lateral to the coracoid and the musculocutaneous nerve. The appropriate entry site for the pin is lateral to the coracoid and medial to the glenoid rim. The pin should be advanced until it touches the scapular neck and then should be advanced by mallet tapping, because drilling causes the pin to spin medially. Once the tip of the pin has securely engaged the scapular neck, the whole pin should be levered medially to position it as perpendicular as possible to the scapula. The pin then may be advanced with a mallet or drill as desired.

Excessive lateral placement can be corrected with the procedure just described or the anteroinferior portal may be moved more medially.

Often the pin site is located more superior on the scapular neck than the Bankart lesion. For this reason, the superior scapular neck is not decorticated. When the scapular neck is not decorticated, however, the pin tends to slide medially because the tip of the pin cannot penetrate the bone. Consequently, the pin should be removed and a small starter hole should be prepared 5 mm medial to the glenoid rim. The pin can be placed in this hole under direct vision and further tapping or drilling can be accomplished.

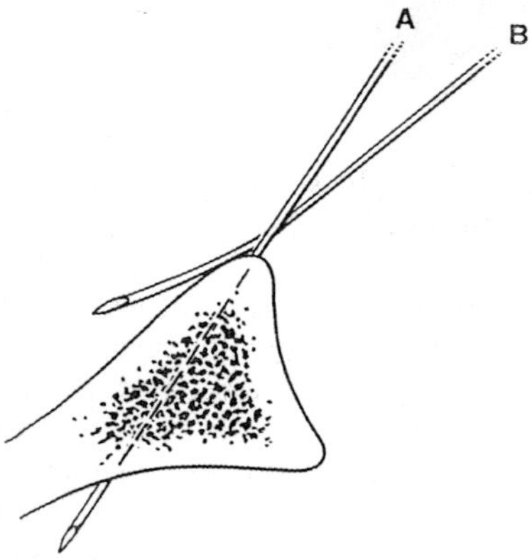

FIG. 13–17. When the approach of the pin is too tangential, it slides medially. A perpendicular angle is best.

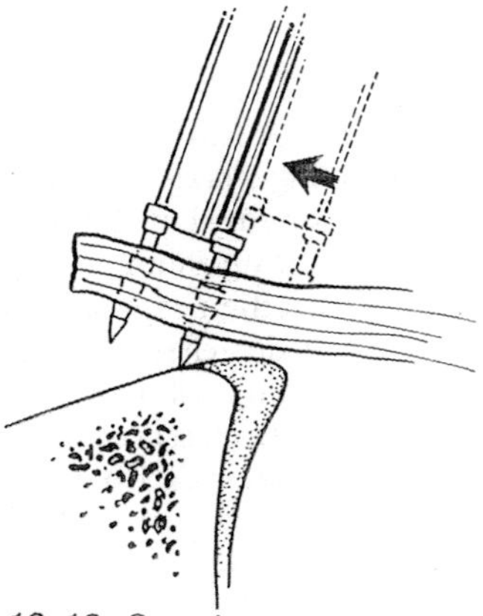

FIG. 13–18. Superior movement tightens the detached ligament.

Pin Scores Cartilage. Cartilage injury can occur with the transglenoid suture technique, as well as with the use of implants. When the anterior cannula is not placed medially enough or is not angled medially enough, the transglenoid pin can score the cartilage. Care must be taken to ensure that the cannula is *translated,* not merely *angled,* medial to the glenoid rim before any drilling takes place. The risk of this injury obviously becomes greater with the increase in pins required.

Lost Pin Hole. Because the pin hole is drilled prior to suture placement, soft tissue and bone debris can combine to obscure the site. Thus, the arthroscope should be in the anterior portal. Attach suction to the scope and look in the area of the hole. The suction removes loose bone and causes the soft tissue to shift away from the anterior scapular neck to allow the site of the pin hole to be seen. Another technique is to place a smaller-diameter suture passage pin in the hole before the sutures are placed in the ligament. Push the pin so that it barely exits posteriorly. When the time for suture passage occurs, push the pin anteriorly and into view.

Suture

1. Only monofilament suture should be used at this time. Braided suture does not advance in the suture passer.
2. Do not attempt to advance the suture into the joint until the needle tip has clearly penetrated the ligament.
3. The suture can be pulled out of the ligament if enough of the suture is not advanced into the joint (20 to 25 cm). Once enough suture is coiled in the joint, the suture hook can be safely withdrawn.
4. The suture or suture needle can pull out of the ligament if insufficient ligament is grasped. At least 3 to 5 mm of ligament should be seen on each side of the suture.

STAPLE METHOD[153]

TECHNIQUE

After the scapular neck has been prepared, the staple, either metal or biodegradable, is inserted through the anteroinferior portal. The detached tissue, generally the superior band of the anteroinferior glenohumeral ligament, is impaled with the staple. The staple and impaled tissue are then moved superiorly to re-establish tension in the ligament capsule complex (Fig. 13–18). Further tension can be created by staple rotation, which twists and tightens the ligament (Fig. 13–19). This maneuver should be performed in a clockwise direction because counterclockwise rotation could unscrew the staple from the inserter. Medial placement of the staple (medial to the articular cartilage rim) is done to minimize the chances of contact between the humeral head and the metal staple, as well as to shift the ligament insertion site to increase tension. Traction is removed from the arm, and the mallet is used to drive the staple into the scapular neck until the head protrudes slightly. The impactor device is unscrewed and removed from the joint. A probe should be inserted to make sure the ligament/labrum complex is firmly attached to the scapular neck. Placement of

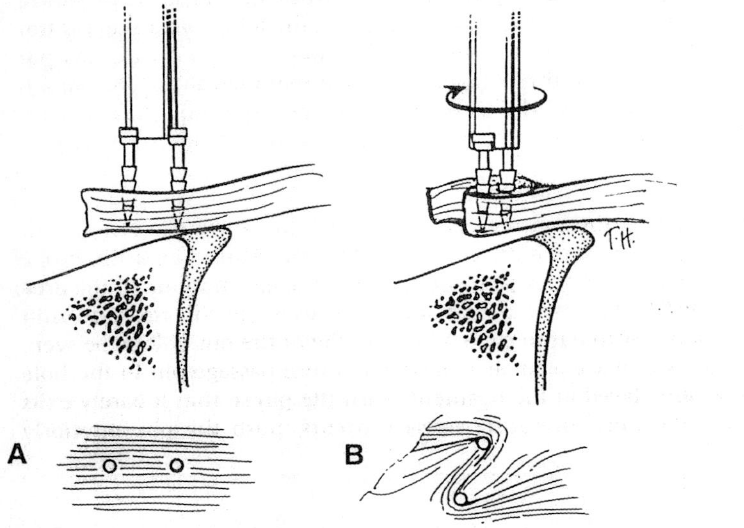

FIG. 13–19. A and B, Rotation of the staple can increase tension in the ligament.

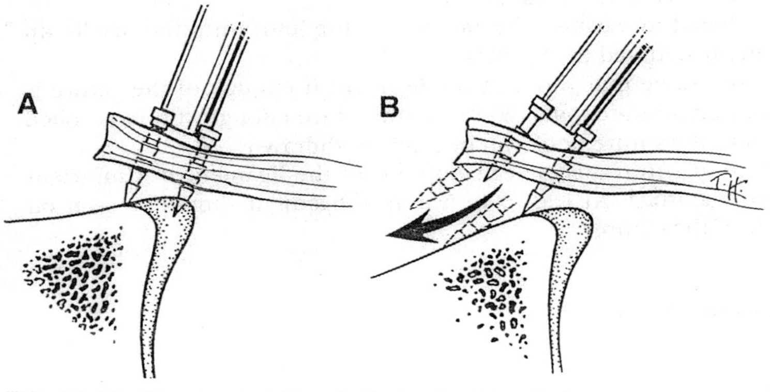

FIG. 13–20. Placement of the staple too far laterally is a common error (A). Correction involves translation of the staple medially. Attempts to increase the angle of the staple only cause the staple to slide across the scapular neck (B).

the arthroscope in the anterosuperior portal helps to obtain a final inspection after ligament reattachment has been completed.

TECHNICAL PROBLEMS

Angle of Approach

The staple shares many technical difficulties with the multiple suture technique. The staple may be angled too medially, thereby failing to penetrate the scapular neck, or may be angled too laterally, thereby scoring the articular cartilage (Fig. 13–20). The solutions are also similar.

Staple Depth

When the staple is driven too deeply, the soft tissue is amputated. The staple should be driven until the tines are imbedded and the staple head can still be seen. When soft tissue is amputated, the staple must be removed; if sufficient ligament remains, *another* staple is used for reattachment. When placed too superficially, the staple can pull out. After the staple is impacted, it should be checked by *probe palpation while the staple head is in direct view.*

Ligament Placement

If the staple is placed medially, away from the glenoid cartilage and humeral head, safety is increased; however, the staple must be placed laterally to replace the ligament in its anatomic location at the level of the glenoid rim. This lateral position is precariously close to the surface of the glenoid articular cartilage. The conflict between these two goals, medial placement for safety and lateral placement for anatomic repair, causes difficulty during the arthroscopic management of recurrent instability with a metal or biodegradable staple.

ADDITIONAL ALTERNATE METHODS

Warren is currently investigating a biodegradable tack (Fig. 13–21).[143] Preliminary results are encouraging. Because the tack is biodegradable, the implant does not permanently remain in the joint.

If the tack is placed in an inappropriate location (most commonly too lateral on the scapular neck so that the tack protrudes over the glenoid rim), a bur can be used to remove that portion of the tack. The tack is made of a material softer than the metal of the staple; thus, humeral head/tack contact should cause minimal problems. The biodegradable staple can be modified in a similar fashion.

Maki has reported the development of a clever intra-articular method that avoids the tying of a knot over the posterior soft tissues.[150] The anteroposterior drilling of the large Steinmann's pin is also avoided by arthroscopic Mitek fixation (Fig. 13–22).[151]

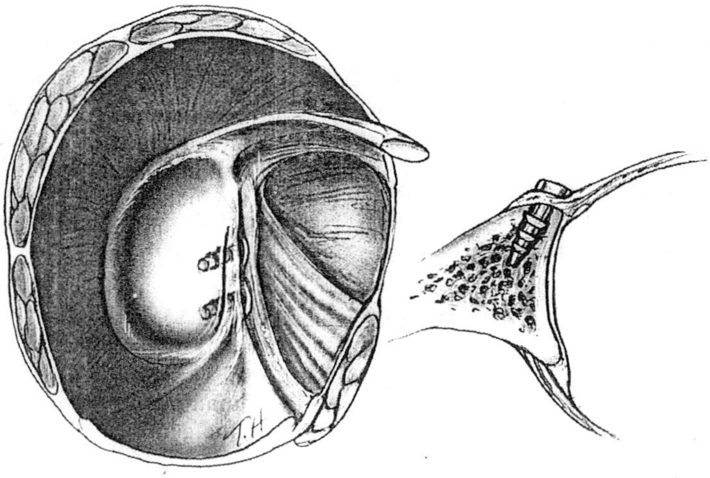

FIG. 13–21. The biodegradable tack.

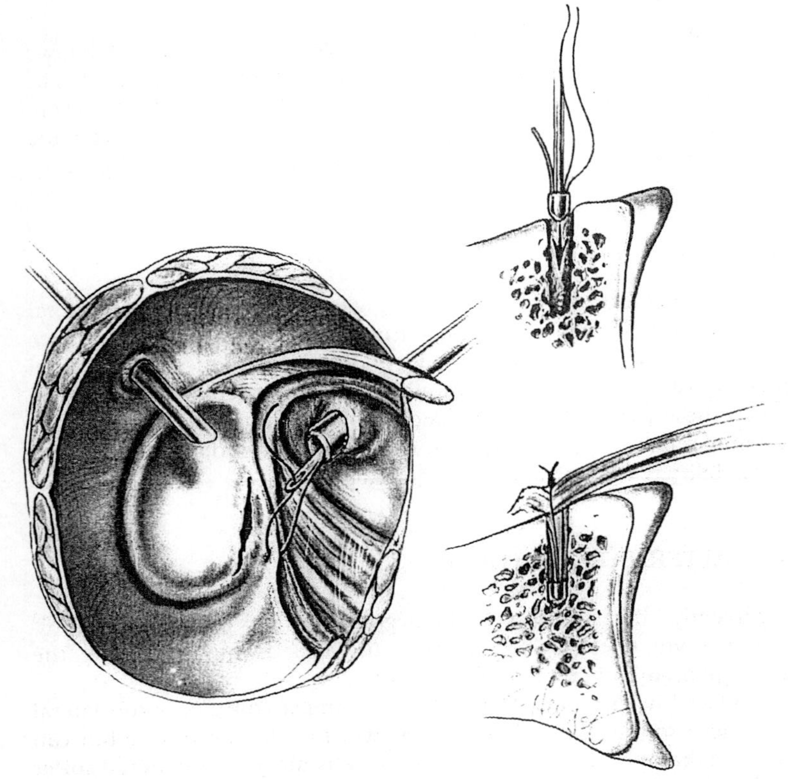

FIG. 13–22. Arthroscopic repair of the Bankart lesion achieved with the Mitek device.

INTRAOPERATIVE EXCLUSIONS

The arthroscopic management of glenohumeral instability is a difficult undertaking, and the surgeon should not hesitate to abandon the arthroscopic technique if difficulties encountered during surgery make the procedure too difficult or unsafe. The surgeon should be aware of the elapsed time and set a limit. If sufficient progress has not been made after 1 1/2 to 2 hours, alternatives to the procedure include abandoning the arthroscopic surgery and converting to an open repair or stopping the surgery entirely and trying again on another date.

Common reasons for abandoning the arthroscopic technique are an absence of appropriate soft tissue structures, excessive soft tissue swelling, poor cannula placement, and technical ability. Arthroscopic management of instability is not and will not be the procedure of choice for all instabilities or for all orthopedic surgeons. Each surgeon must make an individual decision for each patient in regard to whether the arthroscopic techniques are appropriate.

POSTOPERATIVE CARE

A sling or shoulder immobilizer is worn for 3 weeks. The sling is only removed for bathing and elbow range of motion. Codman pendulum exercises are started 3 weeks after surgery. The sling is removed and gentle active movement is started. As the patient's pain and general status allow, a strengthening program is undertaken. Grip, triceps, and biceps strengthening can be started quickly. Isometric exercises are followed by isokinetic strengthening to the deltoid, rotator cuff, and scapular musculature and are continued until normal motion and strength have returned. Passive stretching is avoided.

RETURN TO ACTIVITY AND SPORTS

The same criteria are used after arthroscopic surgery as are used after open reconstruction. Return to contact sports is allowed 6 months after surgery if strength has returned to normal. This determination is most accurately made by objective measurements. Experts disagree as to whether this procedure should be performed in athletes involved in collision sports. Warren has allowed his patients to return to collision sports, whereas Johnson has found the high failure rate unacceptable.[143,153] Caspari advises his patients to abstain from contact sports for 9 to 12 months.[149]

RESULTS OF REPAIR

The reported results after arthroscopic repair have been excellent. Caspari has reported 96% excellent results with his technique.[149] In their initial report Morgan and Bodenstab had 100% excellent results.[148] Morgan subsequently reported on 153 patients after a 1- to 6-year follow-up and had 94% excellent and 6% poor results.[125] After an initial 16% failure rate, Hawkins began to immobilize his patients for 3 weeks.[152] Since doing so, he has reported 100% success. Johnson experienced a high dislocation rate (29%) with minimal (less than 3 weeks) immobilization.[153] When the period of immobilization was increased to 3 weeks, the failure rate was reduced to less than 10%. Not all investigators report such excellent results. Matthews and associates reported a 24% failure rate with the staple.[154] Grana and colleagues reported a 44% failure with the transcapular suture technique.[156] Wolin reported a 27% recurrence rate,[157] and Maki reported a 23% reoperation rate with similar techniques.[150]

RANGE OF MOTION

Morgan and Bodenstab describe 100% of their patients with "full, active range of motion."[148] Johnson reports "no more restriction of motion than the most recent pre-operative measurement" in all patients.[153] Caspari reports 100% return of movement.[149] Matthews and associates reported a 9° loss of external rotation.[154]

RETURN TO ACTIVITIES

Morgan and Bodenstab report 100% return to "pre-injury level of activity, including contact and throwing sports, without symptoms of pain or instability."[148] Patients were allowed to return to sports 6 months after surgery.

COMMENTS

These exceptionally good results must be put into some perspective. All authors report the short-term nature of follow-up and acknowledge that relatively few patients were studied. All the reporting investigators are experienced arthroscopic surgeons who possess a high degree of skill. They are all pioneers in the development of arthroscopic techniques for glenohumeral stabilization. The less experienced arthroscopists are far less likely to achieve 100% success. Nonetheless, arthroscopic approaches are promising, although some practitioners may consider them "investigational." We emphasize caution when adding these techniques to the surgical methods available. Though arthroscopic techniques offer some advantages, surgeons performing few arthroscopic procedures on the shoulder may be unwilling to abandon successful open techniques.

Our experience with the arthroscopic management of instability has not been as rewarding as those previously reviewed. Approximately 40% (6 of 14) of patients in whom a cannulated screw and ligament washer were used to reattach the anteroinferior glenohumeral ligaments developed either recurrent subluxation or metal impingement. The single suture technique of Morgan and Bodenstab did not appear to provide adequate fixation of the ligament. The most successful technique has been the multiple suture approach advocated by Caspari. Our 76% (19 of 25) success rate, however, did not appear to justify the continued use of this technique when we were experiencing a 95% success rate with open reconstruction. Nonetheless, the arthroscopic techniques appear promising and their appropriate place will be determined in the future.

COMPLICATIONS AND PROBLEMS

Perhaps the most significant problem in the arthroscopic management of glenohumeral instability involves its technical difficulty. When viewing a videotape from an expert, few can appreciate the amount of judgment, experience, and psychomotor skill that is required. Few practicing orthopedic surgeons have had any experience with this technique during their training, and most are learning at instructional courses. For most orthopedic surgeons, the surgical management of glenohumeral instability is not a daily occurrence, and obviously, learning a new technique is difficult when it is not practiced with frequency. The orthopedic surgeon also must realize that complications and failures are highest during the steep portion of the learning curve. Each individual must decide whether to abandon successful techniques that involve open surgery to embrace newer, yet unproven, difficult techniques because they are arthroscopic.

Complications and problems related to arthroscopic techniques can be divided into several areas: failure of thought, failure of technique, failure of the implant, rehabilitative failure, postoperative trauma, and failure of concept.

FAILURE OF THOUGHT

Failure can occur when an instability operation is performed for an inappropriate diagnosis. Certain lesions, such as the anterosuperior labrum tear and the SLAP lesion, may mimic instability findings.

A more common area of failure involves the preoperative contraindications previously discussed. An arthroscopic operation on an individual with capsular laxity and multidirectional instability usually is not curative.

Another common error is operating on the inappropriate direction of instability. The direct observation of the humeral head and the glenoid should eliminate the problem of confusing posterior and anterior instability. In this situation, the humeral head is subluxated anteriorly and the "posterior dislocation" produced is, in actuality, a reduction of an anterior subluxation.

FAILURE OF SOFT TISSUE TENSIONING TECHNIQUE

A great deal of subjectivity is involved in adjusting the soft tissue tension. Clearly defined markers are not available, and few well-established guidelines allow the surgeon to position the detached ligament/labrum complex appropriately. The wonderful visualization provided arthroscopically creates a paradox. The surgeon can place the ligament with unparalleled precision, yet cannot be sure as to the location of that precise spot.

The ligament complex can be placed under inadequate tension, but also can be overtightened and consequently restrict motion. For patients in the seated position, this overtightening most commonly occurs when the arm is placed across the chest in internal rotation. When the ligament is placed under maximal tension with the arm in internal rotation, regaining external rotation can be quite difficult. Ligament tension should be adjusted with the arm in neutral rotation.

Soft tissue tensioning is most advantageous in the multiple suture technique. Many sutures can be placed in various portions of the ligament, and the tension can be precisely adjusted. If one of the sutures does not create enough tension, it can be replaced or discarded. Similarly, if one of the sutures, particularly the most inferior, appears to tighten the capsule excessively, it simply can be removed by pulling on one end or by using arthroscopic scissors to divide it intra-articularly. The multiple suture technique appears to give the surgeon the most flexibility in establishing tension in a superoinferior direction.

FAILURE OF IMPLANT

MULTIPLE SUTURES

One problem with the multiple suture technique is that the implants (sutures) are tied over the posterior soft tissue. Only one complication of pseudocyst formation has been reported,[158] but skin, wound, and pressure problems are more frequent. The theoretic disadvantage of distension of the posterior soft tissue fixation point at the end of the arthroscopic procedure is also worrisome. As soft tissue swelling diminishes, the tension on the ligaments theoretically could decrease and allow soft ligament bone separation.

SINGLE IMPLANTS

One of the limitations of the staple is that, as a single implant, it offers only one-point fixation. Size of the staple and the angle required for its correct placement make placement of a single staple difficult. A staple can also inadvertently cut the ligament when the ligament/labrum complex is grasped and pulled superiorly or can divide the ligament if it is impacted too deeply. The staple tine may

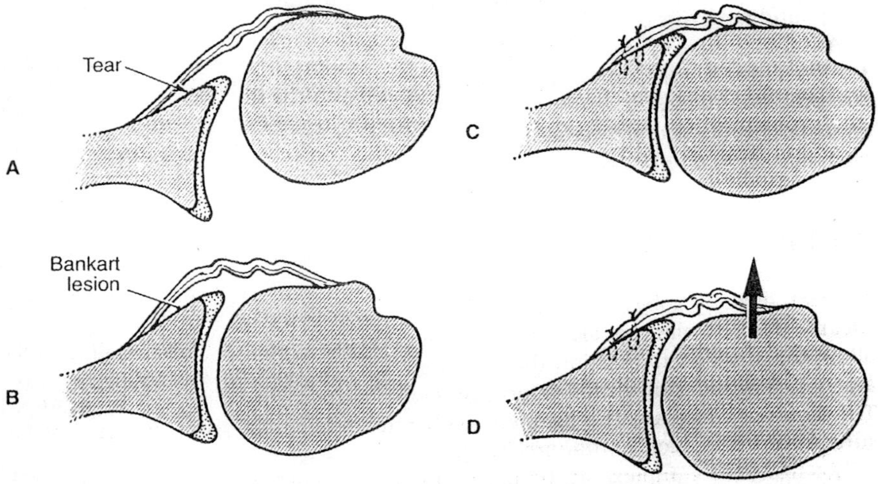

FIG. 13–23. Repair of a Bankart lesion without correction of midsubstance ligamentous laxity continues to allow subluxation.

bend or break, particularly when inadequate bone preparation has occurred. The problems of metallic implants around the shoulder are well described.[159,160]

BIODEGRADABLE IMPLANTS

Biodegradable implants have the fewest known implant problems. No long-term studies or large patient populations have been reported because the device was investigational until recently. The theoretic problems are obvious. The implant may dissolve too quickly, before ligament bone healing has occurred. Conversely, the implant may dissolve too slowly, and if it is placed in an "at-risk position" (too close to the glenoid rim), impingement against the implant could result.

REHABILITATIVE FAILURE

Rehabilitation problems that result in failed arthroscopic surgery are no different from problems encountered with open surgical reconstruction. The length of immobilization may be too long or too short. The individual may be allowed back to work or vigorous sports before the return of strength, motion, coordination, and timing has been complete.

Before returning our patients to competitive sports or heavy labor, we require a return to within 10° of normal motion in elevation and external rotation at 90° of abduction. Normal strength must be documented by dynamometer measurements. Whether an individual should return to contact or collision sports is controversial. Johnson, with his staple capsulorrhaphy, does not allow return to contact sports and does not advocate performing this operation on individuals who desire to return to contact sports.[153] Warren, on the other hand, allows patients to return to contact sports.[143]

We allow the individual to return to contact or collision sports as desired. We believe that a good operation should satisfy the patient's needs. If it cannot do so, the operation should be abandoned.

POSTOPERATIVE TRAUMA

Repetitive microtrauma that causes failure has not been reported following arthroscopic repairs. Only time will reveal whether these arthroscopic repairs are sufficiently secure and anatomic to allow an individual to return to prolonged competitive overhead athletics without recurrence of symptoms.

FAILURE OF CONCEPT

One of the most interesting arguments against arthroscopic reconstruction is that the repair may be "too anatomic." With superb visualization afforded by arthroscopic examination, and the surgeon's ability to repair the ligament complex within millimeters of its desired location, excellent results from this procedure would seem unavoidable. Unfortunately, excellent results are not the norm, and we often speculate on the causes of this disappointing outcome. Some evidence reveals that, in addition to the ligament insertion detachment, a stretching of the ligament fibers occurs at the time of the acute traumatic dislocation.[161] This stretching of the ligament, even in the face of a Bankart lesion, could also occur with repeated instability episodes. When the ligament insertion is placed in its anatomic location, soft tissue laxity diminishes but is not eliminated because of the relative incompetence of the ligament structure (Fig. 13–23).

This laxity is overcome during open procedures by the inevitable shortening that occurs when a structure is divided, moved, and reattached. Also, at the time of an open reconstruction, many surgeons tighten the capsule if excessive laxity exists after the Bankart lesion has been repaired. Such tightening is difficult to achieve arthroscopically.

ACUTE DISLOCATIONS

Open surgical reconstruction for the acutely dislocated shoulder is rarely performed. Indications for surgery are failure to achieve a reduction because of interposition of the biceps tendon or osteochondral fracture fragments.

Historically the treatment of an individual with a recently reduced acute dislocation has been nonoperative. The arm is immobilized in a support device, and once pain diminishes, strengthening exercises are started.

The success of this treatment is variable. Patients who dislocate their shoulder and are less than 20 years of age do poorly. With conservative management, 33 to 50% of such patients dislocate again.[142]

Traditionally these high-risk patients are not offered an alternative method of care. No standard orthopedic text advocates early surgery. The patient is not offered a choice between 95% success with surgery or 50% success without surgery.

The approach to the shoulder seems fundamentally at odds with the approach to the knee. Individuals frequently undergo major knee ligament reconstructions near the time of injury to minimize pain and allow an active lifestyle; yet, the surgeon is reluctant to operate on the patient's shoulder, although a successful surgical option exists.

Baker's pioneering work has helped to classify the disorder at the time of dislocation.[126] Three groups were identified. Group 1 (6 of 45) had capsular tears with no labral lesion. These shoulders were stable under anesthesia and had no or minimal hemarthrosis. Group 2 (11 of 45) had capsular tears and partial labral detachments. These shoulders were mildly unstable and had a mild hemarthrosis. Group 3 (28 of 45) had capsular tears with labral detachments. These shoulders were grossly unstable and had large hemarthrosis. This knowledge allows the examiner to predict which individuals may go on to repeated dislocation and, thus, to offer those individuals a surgical cure.

Few investigators have reported their results of treating acute shoulder dislocations with arthroscopic repair.[141] Not surprisingly, although the series is small, the success rate is excellent. Structure is less distorted after a single traumatic event. Repeated episodes of instability have not caused continued labrum wear, loose body formation, and capsular/ligament attenuation. Bankart lesions are repaired anatomically. Midsubstance ligament or capsular tears are treated conservatively. An early repair should have the highest degree of success.

Although arthroscopic surgery for acute dislocations is not a common procedure, we believe it will become routine in the future.

OPEN REPAIR OF GLENOHUMERAL INSTABILITY

14

OPEN SURGICAL REPAIR PROCEDURES

The techniques described in this chapter have proved effective for successful open surgical reconstruction of anteroinferior glenohumeral instability. Our goal is to accomplish anatomic repair of abnormalities found at surgery. Different findings require different surgical solutions.

Bankart lesions are repaired with reattachment of the ligament/labrum complex. Individuals with a lesser degree of ligamentous insufficiency but without a Bankart lesion are treated with an anterior capsular reconstruction (Fig. 14–1). Multiaxial instability is corrected with a Neer inferior capsular shift.

GENERAL SURGICAL TECHNIQUE

General endotracheal anesthesia is utilized and the patient is placed in a semisitting position. The shoulder area is prepared and draped routinely. An anteroinferior skin incision is utilized (Fig. 14–2), and dissection is carried down through skin and subcutaneous tissue. The deltopectoral interval is identified, and the cephalic vein is dissected along its medial aspect. The deltopectoral interval is then entered carrying the cephalic vein laterally with the deltoid. The clavipectoral fascia is then identified and incised. This incision should be made along the lateral muscular border of the conjoined tendon rather than along its more medial tendinous portion. Dissection continues superiorly until the coracoacromial ligament is identified. When any symptoms of rotator cuff tendinitis exist preoperatively, a Darrach elevator is placed under the coracoacromial ligament and the ligament is divided. The musculocutaneous and axillary nerves are then palpated (Fig. 14–3). A self-retaining retractor is placed to retract the deltoid laterally and the conjoined tendon medially. The subscapularis tendon is then exposed.

One or more of the surgical techniques described in the following sections is performed next.

After the surgical technique(s) has been performed, the wound is closed by repairing the deltopectoral fascia with absorbable sutures. Subcutaneous tissues are then reapproximated, and a running subcuticular 4-0 absorbable suture

FIG. 14–1. Insertion tear and treatment (A through C); midsubstance tear and treatment (A′ through C′).

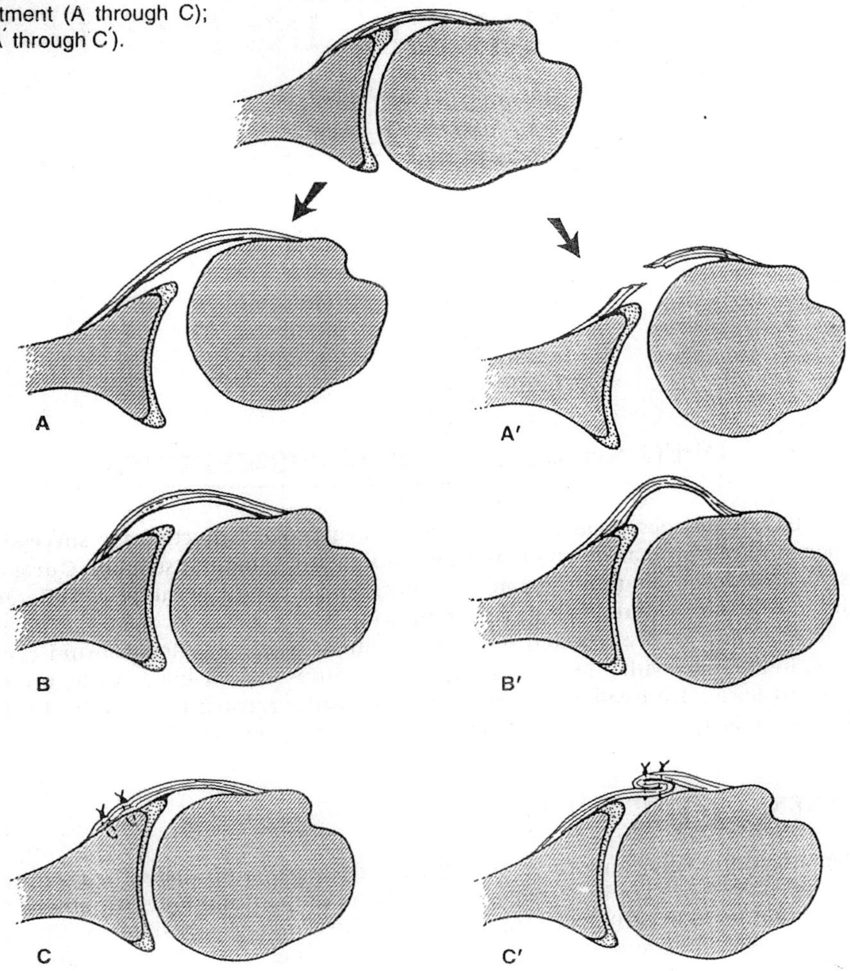

FIG. 14–2. Anteroinferior skin incision.

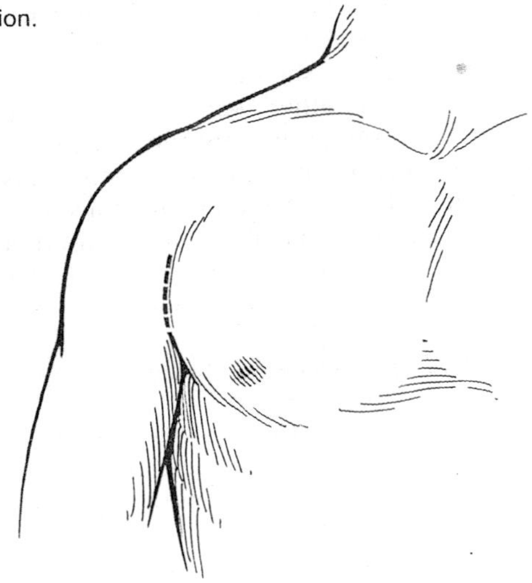

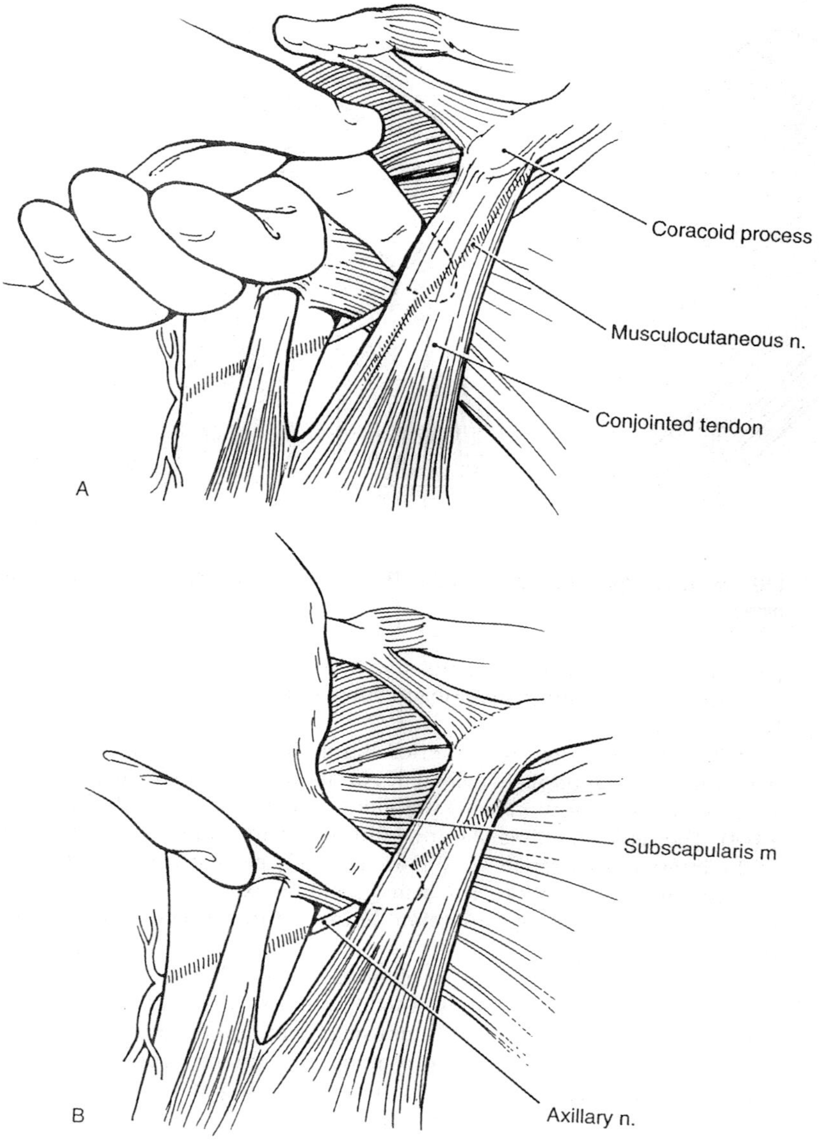

FIG. 14–3. Palpation of musculocutaneous (A) and axillary (B) nerves.

approximates the skin. Skin repair is supported with sterile adhesive strips. A hemovac drain is placed anterior to the subscapularis muscle and is removed the next morning. The arm is placed in a sling, and the patient is transported to the recovery room.

NEER CAPSULAR SHIFT

Individuals who require this procedure demonstrate a significant inferior component to their instability. If inferior translation is greater than 1 cm when the

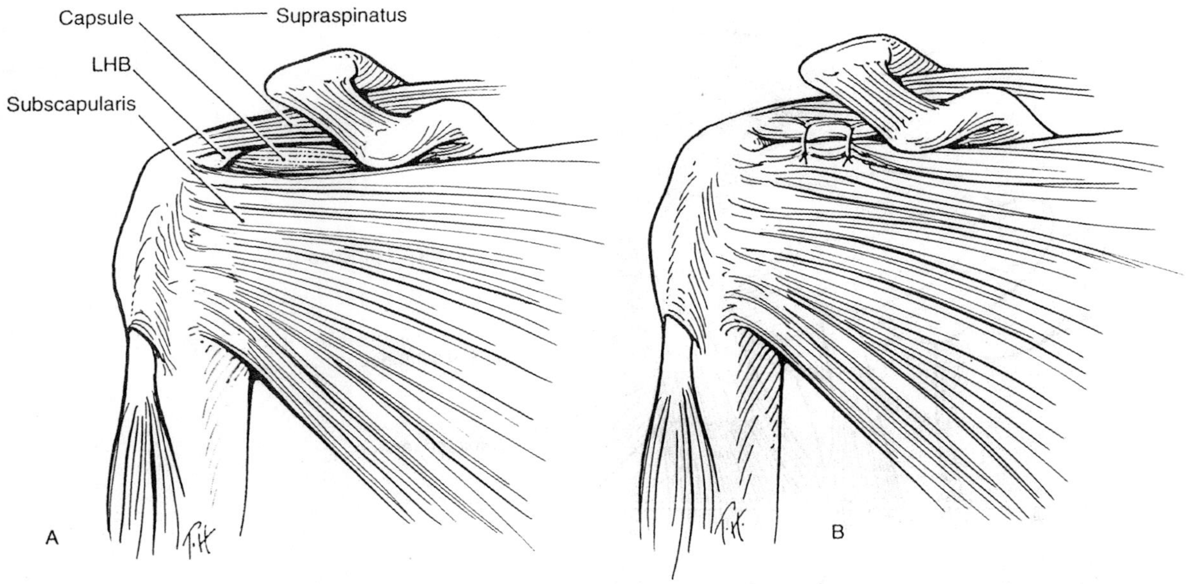

FIG. 14–4. A, Open interval lesion. B, Repair of interval lesion. LHB = long head of the biceps.

patient is awake, or if any significant inferoposterior or posteroinferior component to the instability exists prior to subscapularis division, a Neer capsular shift is performed.[162]

The interval between the anterior supraspinatus border and the superior border of the subscapularis is palpated. An abnormally enlarged (> 1 cm) interval or direct communication with the glenohumeral joint should be repaired (Fig. 14–4). The repair requires placement of only 1 to 2 sutures in the lateral portion of the interval. Any repair done more medially permanently restricts both elevation and external rotation. The arm should be externally rotated 45° during the repair. Failure to appreciate interval lesions results in persistent inferior translation.

The subscapularis tendon is divided perpendicular to its fibers midway between the musculotendinous junction and the lesser tuberosity. The tendon is dissected free from the capsule; approximately one third of the tendon remains attached to the capsule as reinforcement. The tendon is placed deep to the self-retaining retractor. The capsule is then incised longitudinally, and a lateral "T" incision is created (Fig. 14–5). A Fukuda retractor is placed within the wound, and the glenoid, labrum, and ligament insertion sites are inspected. In the rare instance when a Bankart lesion is present, a Bankart repair is performed (see description that follows). More commonly, no ligament insertion lesion is noted at the glenoid. The Fukuda retractor is removed, and attention is turned to the capsular reconstruction. The superior flap is incised laterally to the level of the superior border of the capsule. The inferior flap is also incised laterally along the humeral neck. The degree of inferior capsular release is determined by the degree of inferior instability. Generally, the capsule is released to the 6 o'clock position. Inferoposterior and posteroinferior instability patterns are corrected by continuing the dissection around the humeral neck posteriorly. The axillary nerve should be protected with a retractor.

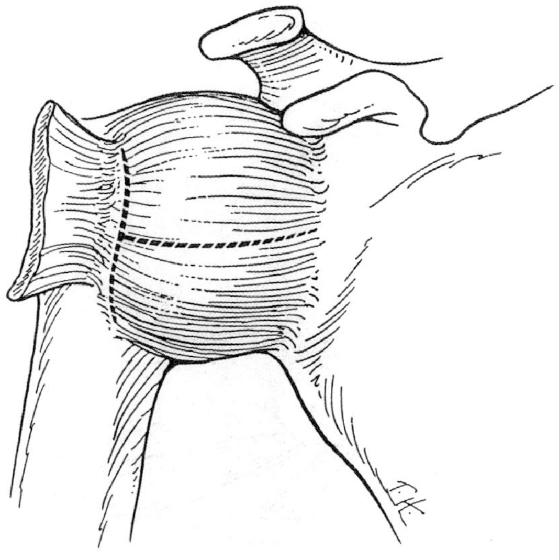

FIG. 14–5. Lateral "T" incision created in capsule.

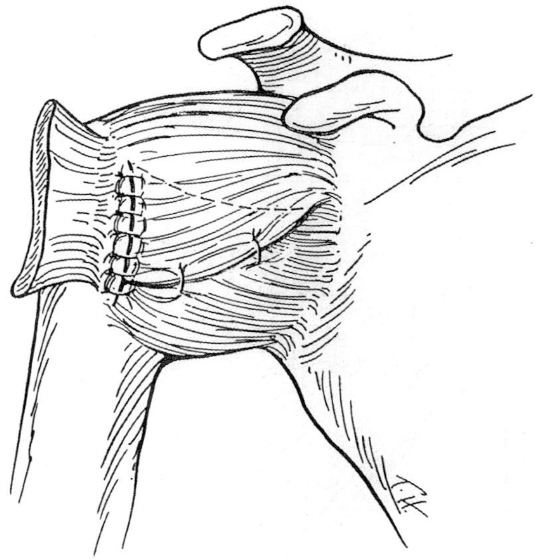

FIG. 14–6. Flaps sutured in place.

Inferior capsular release must continue until the inferior and anterior recesses are obliterated. Total obliteration is tested by placing a blunt probe in the inferior recess and applying superior traction on the flap.

At this point, a power bur or curette is used to create a cancellous bed as a site for permanent capsular attachment. The extent of the cancellous bed is identical to the extent of the capsular dissection (Fig. 14–6).

Maximum tension is placed on the inferior flap, which is sutured with the arm in abduction (35°) and external rotation (35°). The arm is then brought into adduction and neutral rotation, and the superior flap is sutured.

The subscapularis is then reattached anatomically and securely. No attempt at shortening or advancement is made.

BANKART REPAIR

Individuals with unidirectional, anteroinferior instability findings on history, physical examination, and examination under anesthesia are likely to require a Bankart repair[163] or an anterior capsular reconstruction.

When the subscapularis is exposed, the surgeon can grasp the humeral head directly and confirm that the predominant direction of instability is antero-inferior.

The subscapularis is divided in line with its fibers. The incision begins at the junction of the upper two thirds and the lower one third (Fig. 14–7).

Dissection is started as far medially as possible, and blunt elevators are used to spread subscapularis fibers and to identify the capsule. Careful blunt dissection continues superiorly and inferiorly, thereby exposing the capsule 1 cm medial to the glenoid rim and extending as far inferiorly and superiorly as possible (Fig. 14–8). The dissection is then continued laterally until the subscapularis tendon fibers and capsule blend. A deep right-angled Gelpi retractor is then placed to

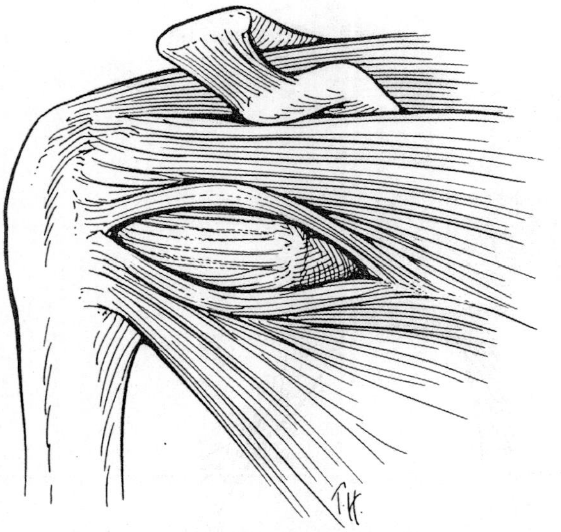

FIG. 14–7. Longitudinal division of subscapularis in preparation for Bankart repair.

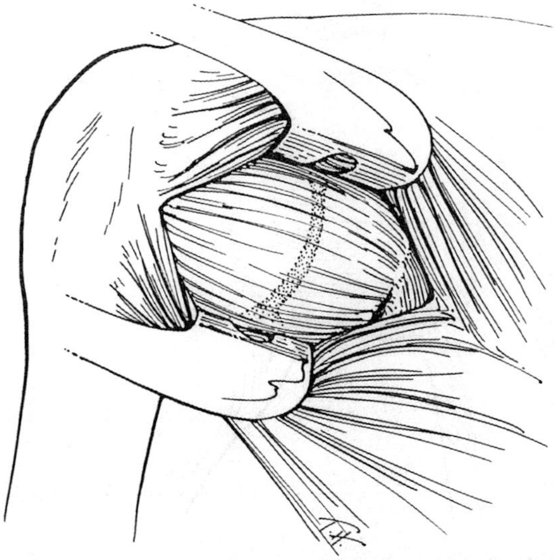

FIG. 14–8. Capsule exposed with gelpi retractor in place.

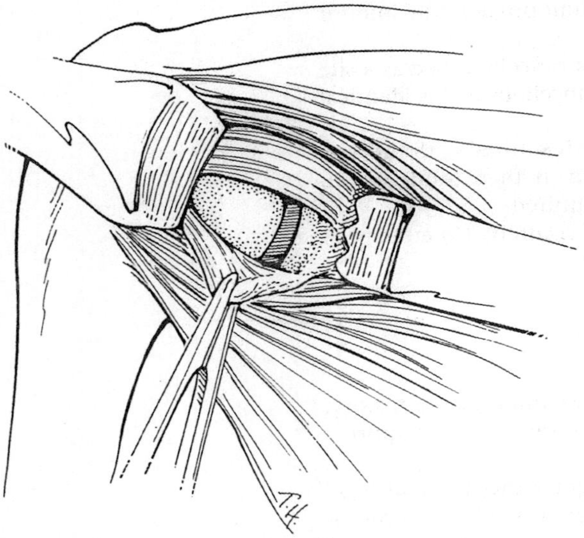

FIG. 14–9. Bankart lesion seen through open capsule.

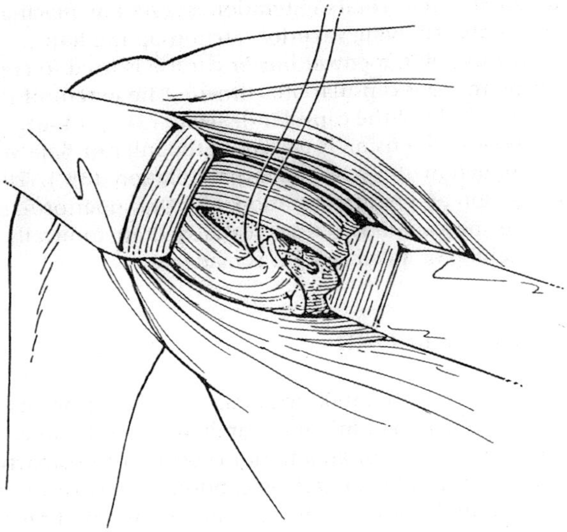

FIG. 14–10. Mitek anchors fix capsule to its anatomic site.

provide retraction, and the capsule is sharply separated from the subscapularis as required.

The arm is placed in maximum external rotation. The degree of capsular laxity is assessed by grasping and lifting the capsule. A normal capsule is tight against the glenohumeral joint and cannot be lifted. Capsular laxity is graded as mild (less than 1 cm), moderate (1 to 2 cm), and severe (greater than 2 cm).

If the surgeon grades the capsular laxity as mild to moderate in an anteroinfe-

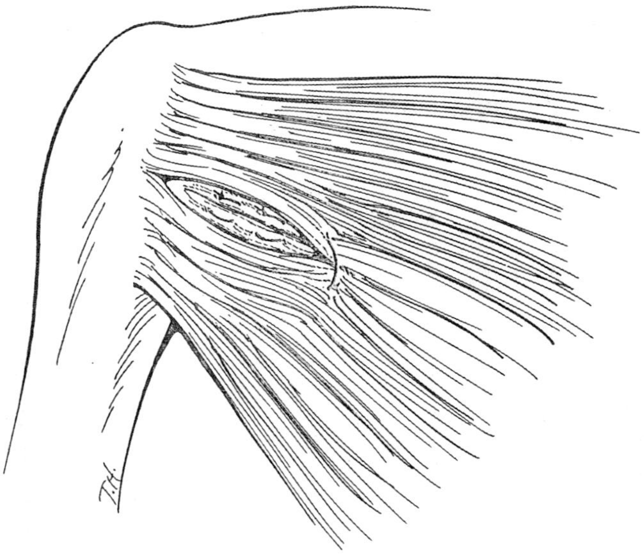

FIG. 14–11. Anatomic closure of capsule and repair of slit in subscapularis.

rior direction without any posterior or significant inferior component, the capsule can be opened parallel to the subscapularis fibers and perpendicular to the glenoid (Fig. 14–9).

If, at this point, the surgeon re-evaluates the situation and now believes that the direction of instability is predominantly inferior, this approach may be converted to the Neer capsular shift procedure (previously described) by dividing the subscapularis laterally.

Once the joint has been entered, the Fukuda retractor is inserted, the self-retaining retractor is removed, and a fork retractor is placed medially. The anterior glenoid labrum and capsular attachment are inspected for any labrum tears or a Bankart lesion.

Detachment of the Bankart lesion is usually obvious, and the bare scapular neck is easily visualized. Occasionally, limited healing has occurred, and although no Bankart lesion is apparent, minimal pressure demonstrates actual separation. "Creation" of a Bankart lesion by inserting an elevator and detaching the anterior capsule is difficult, if not impossible, in a normal situation. More commonly, a Bankart lesion is not visualized and the surgeon fails to probe. Consequently, the true site of the disorder is overlooked.

A retractor is placed deep to the detached capsule, and a cancellous bed is created. Mitek anchors are placed as needed to assure firm fixation of the capsule to its anatomic site (Fig. 14–10).

The retractor is then placed superficial to the detached capsule, and vertical mattress sutures are placed. Generally, two to three sutures are required. The capsule is then closed anatomically. The longitudinal split in the subscapularis is repaired (Fig. 14–11).

ANTERIOR CAPSULAR RECONSTRUCTION

The third common situation arises when inspection of the ligament insertion demonstrates no abnormality. These shoulders are generally subluxated rather than dislocated. No excessive inferior or inferoposterior translation is noted.

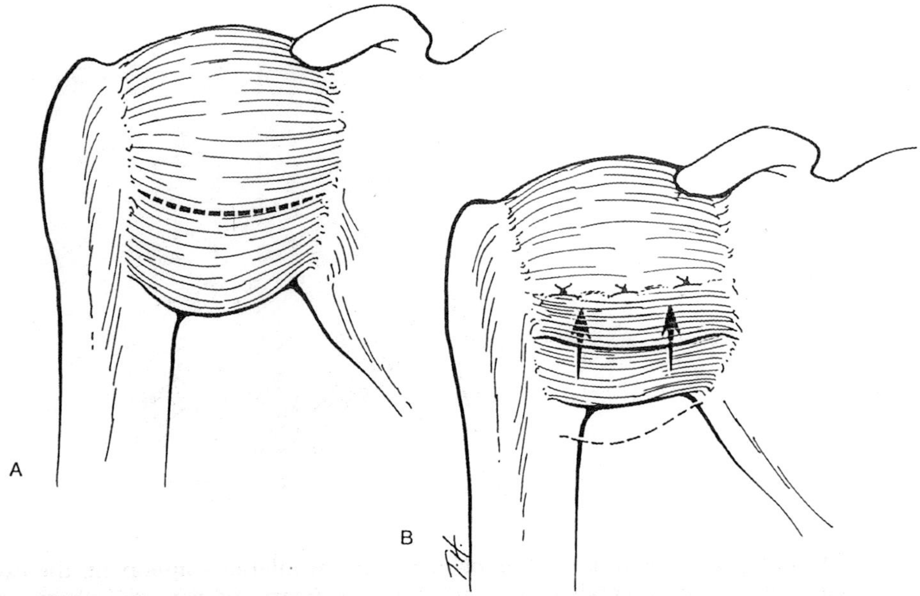

FIG. 14–12. A, Capsule divided parallel to subscapularis fibers. B, Mattress sutures used to imbricate inferior under superior flap.

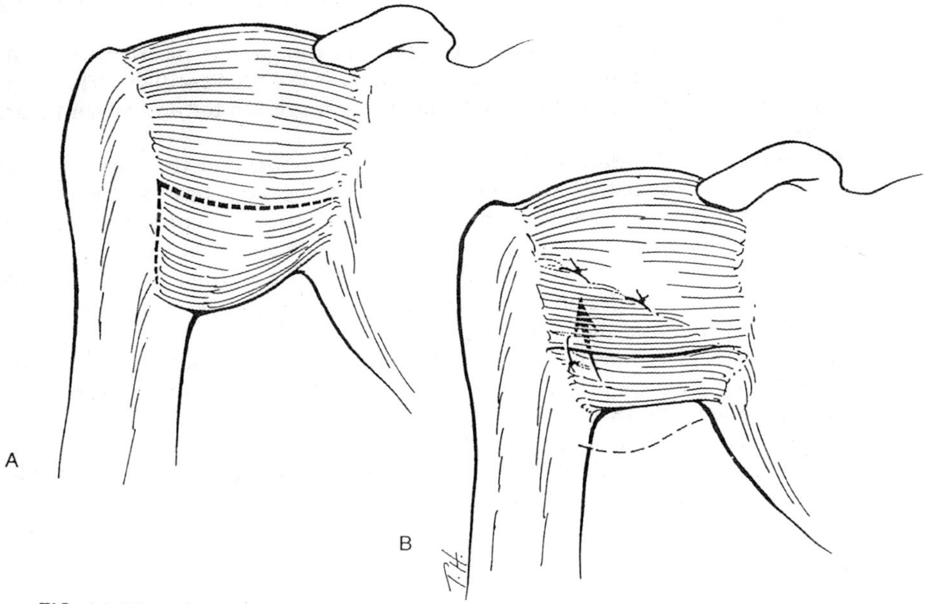

FIG. 14–13. Lateral release (A) and superior shift (B) of inferior flap for increased laxity.

These individuals have midcapsular or midligamentous stretching. We perform capsular reconstruction.

The ligament complex is firmly attached at both humeral and glenoid sites. Therefore, these sites are left untouched, and the capsule is tightened in the middle. In an effort to minimize loss of external rotation, the capsule is divided parallel to the subscapularis fibers. Imbrication of the inferior flap under the superior flap with mattress sutures eliminates anteroinferior redundancy. We tighten the capsule according to our intraoperative examination of capsular laxity. If the capsular laxity with the arm in external rotation is judged to be 1 cm, the capsule is tightened 1 cm. If laxity is judged to be 1.5 cm, the capsule is tightened by 1.5 cm, and so on (Fig. 14–12).

When the inferoanterior component of instability is greater than can be corrected by a simple imbrication, the inferior flap is detached laterally and shifted in a superior direction (Fig. 14–13). This shift allows capsular tightening in all but the most excessive cases.

In summary, we favor an anatomic repair. Excessive capsular laxity is controlled with a Neer capsular shift. A Bankart lesion is repaired with a modified Bankart procedure, and individuals with no Bankart lesion and only mild to moderate laxity undergo an anterior capsular reconstruction.

POSTOPERATIVE CARE

Patients who must undergo anterior glenohumeral reconstructions and Bankart repairs are admitted to the hospital after surgery and kept overnight. Approximately 50% stay a second night. A sling is worn for 1 to 3 weeks; the length of immobilization is inversely proportional to the patient's reliability. Patients may shower and bathe without the sling 24 hours after surgery. Gentle active motion is allowed anterior to the midaxial line in the coronal plane. Carrying objects in the hand or performing abduction/external rotation maneuvers is prohibited. When comfort allows, deltoid isometrics and grip-strengthening exercises are started. By 2 to 3 weeks after the operation, gentle active movement is allowed, and isometric and isokinetic rehabilitation exercises are started as tolerated. Strengthening is progressed through surgical tubing and light weights. Aerobic exercises are started as soon as possible, and the patient is encouraged to walk (with the sling) either outdoors or on a treadmill. Stationary bicycle riding is ideal. Nonstressful upper extremity sports (chipping, putting golf strokes) are allowed at 2 to 3 months. Athletics that involve overhead movements are allowed at 4 to 6 months, or when range of motion. has returned, the shoulder is free of pain, and normal muscle strength is documented objectively. We have allowed participation in all sports except bench-press weight-lifting. Patients who insist on performing such an activity must wait 1 year. Postoperative rehabilitation following surgery for instability is described in more detail in Chapter 25.

THE SCALPEL OR THE SCOPE? DECISION-MAKING IN GLENOHUMERAL INSTABILITY

15

Arthroscopy has two uses in the management of glenohumeral instability. Arthroscopy may serve as a diagnostic tool that helps to plan future operative or nonoperative treatment. Arthroscopy also is an option for operative correction of the instability. The two roles are interrelated, but each approach may be used selectively.

DIAGNOSTIC ARTHROSCOPY

The history and physical examination are certainly cornerstones in the diagnostic evaluation of glenohumeral instability. Although some investigators might argue that *all* glenohumeral instability can be diagnosed by a combination of history, physical examination, and appropriate radiologic studies, our experience has been different. After an appropriate evaluation, the diagnosis still is not clear in some individuals. These patients are candidates for arthroscopic evaluation. Certain individuals may not relax adequately because of pain, fear, or misunderstanding, and consequently, an adequate examination cannot be performed in the office. In other individuals, the direction of instability may not be clear. This confusion often occurs when the history and physical examination seem to point in different directions. For example, a fall on an outstretched, forward-flexed arm would indicate posterior instability, but the examination may demonstrate normal posterior stability. Another situation occurs when more than one direction of instability is suspected. Physical examination may demonstrate posteroinferior and anteroinferior instability. The degree to which each is symptomatic may be hard to determine, and therefore, the direction from which the shoulder should be surgically approached is unclear.

An arthroscopic examination may be required to look for confirmatory findings or to directly observe the direction in which the humeral head moves. Another indication for diagnostic arthroscopy is the surgeon's suspicion of other disorders. Patient complaints of pain or weakness may be suggestive of a partial or complete posterosuperior rotator cuff tear that is difficult to visualize at open surgery. Soft tissue imaging techniques (CAT scan, MRI) may demonstrate a posterior labral tear. Again, such an area is hard to reach at the time of open reconstruction, but is easily treated arthroscopically. Individuals who previously have undergone surgery can be particularly confusing, and direct observation of glenohumeral ligaments and movement of the humeral head can be invaluable in patient management.

Another situation in which arthroscopy is indicated is in the high-performance athlete. Often these individuals are suspected subluxators suffering from a rotator cuff traction tendinitis. Imaging studies are often normal. Prior to committing the athlete to a prolonged rehabilitation program that might involve missing a competitive season, an arthroscopic evaluation can help to determine the presence or absence of any significant rotator cuff lesion. Arthroscopy can also confirm the diagnosis of instability, as well as document the status of glenohumeral ligaments to determine whether a nonoperative program might be successful.

POSTERIOR INSTABILITY

The focus of this chapter is the management of anteroinferior instability. Posterior instability has received less attention because it is more uncommon, and the surgical management relies almost exclusively on open reconstructions rather than arthroscopic techniques. Arthroscopic evaluation, however, can substantially aid in the diagnosis of posterior instability.

When diagnosis is not clear and an arthroscopic evaluation must be performed, the true abnormality occasionally is discovered to be posterior instability. The humeral head can be dislocated or subluxated in a posterior or posteroinferior direction. Posterior labrum fraying can be noted, and occasionally a reverse Hill-Sachs' lesion is found. More unusual is the detection of a posterior Bankart lesion.

The situation may be surgically managed using arthroscopic techniques in two unusual instances. When a posterior Bankart lesion exists without any excessive capsular laxity (almost exclusively after a significant trauma), the arthroscopic posterior Bankart repair has been successful. We also have had experience with 2 patients in whom a large posteroinferior glenohumeral ligament was combined with moderate posterior capsular laxity. The ligament was shifted superiorly using a cannulated screw and ligament washer to control the instability.

OPERATIVE ARTHROSCOPY

Diagnostic glenohumeral arthroscopy can be performed with basic arthroscopy skills and experience. The same cannot be said for arthroscopic surgical management of glenohumeral instability. The orthopedist must decide whether arthroscopy is an effective method to use to treat glenohumeral instability and, if so, whether the surgeon has the arthroscopic skills and experience to perform this operation. Even if these questions can be answered in the affirmative, the appropriateness of arthroscopic treatment in each particular patient must be considered. Arthroscopic management of glenohumeral instability is a relatively recent phenomenon. Although numerous reports have appeared in the literature,[143,146,148-150,152-154,156,157,164-170] many more are devoted to conventional open management. Of course, this disparity does not necessarily support one technique over the other, because any new technique has less literature devoted to it than to the established technique.

Some comments appear to be common to all papers reporting on arthroscopic management of instability. The authors describe the technique as technically difficult with a complication rate higher than that for open surgical techniques. The results, in the short term, seem to be less favorable after arthroscopy than after open treatment.

Why then should the orthopedist pursue such an approach? A great deal still must be learned about the arthroscopic diagnosis and surgical management of glenohumeral instability. Invariably, as more surgeons perform these procedures, patient selection will improve, and arthroscopic techniques will be simplified. As arthroscopic techniques evolve, less tissue damage will occur, and hence, an earlier and more complete return to normal function will result. Arthroscopy also has possible advantages over the conventional technique in that certain areas of the glenohumeral joint are more easily visualized and treated arthroscopically (posterior recess, posterior labrum, posterosuperior rotator cuff).

Arthroscopy also affords the surgeon precision in injury identification. Whereas isolated lesions of the superior glenohumeral ligament or middle glenohumeral ligament are identifiable arthroscopically, these same lesions are not well appreciated with open techniques.

ARTHROSCOPY VS. OPEN TREATMENT

A comparison of the many facets of arthroscopy and open treatment is offered in Table 15–1 and reviewed in the following sections.

SUCCESS RATE

A summary of recent publications leads to the conclusion that the present success rate of the arthroscopic treatment of instability is less than that of open reconstruction. Three factors appear to be involved. One, with arthroscopy the surgeon is learning a new technique, and errors are more likely to occur during the steep phase of the learning curve. Two, an understanding of which instabili-

TABLE 15–1. COMPARISION OF OPEN VS. ARTHROSCOPIC TECHNIQUE

	OPEN SURGERY	ARTHROSCOPIC SURGERY
LOS	–	+
Cosmesis	–	+
Cost	–	+
Pain	–	+
Patient demand	–	+
Muscle		
Subscapularis	–	+
Deltoid	=	=
Cuff	+	–
Immobilization	+	–
Rehabilitation	+	–
Technical ease	+	–
Complications	+	–
Associated lesions	+	–
Success	+	–

LOS means length of stay; + means preferred procedure; – means less preferred procedure; = means equally preferred procedures.

ties are best managed with arthroscopic techniques is just beginning to take shape. Prior investigations report on all anteroinferior glenohumeral instability without any significant selection according to the particular anatomic structure of the patient. Third, the security of implant fixation does not appear to be as great with arthroscopic methods as with the open technique. Most authors advise an increase in immobilization time compared to that required for open surgical procedures.

TECHNICAL EASE

The open Bankart repair is not a technically simple process. Few surgeons who perform arthroscopic reconstruction, however, do so on the basis of its simplicity. To those on the steep part of the learning curve, the arthroscopic technique is significantly more difficult.

COMPLICATIONS

The increased complication rate in arthroscopic surgery relates to the problems with implant devices discussed in Chapter 13, as well as to the increased time required for the surgery and thus for the anesthesia.

IMPLANT PROBLEMS

Implant problems are common to both arthroscopic and open techniques for shoulder reconstruction.[160] The metallic fixation device, in and of itself, is probably not the cause of the high complication rate. Instead, the surgeon is likely to experience difficulty in achieving accurate placement and in securing fixation with metallic implants.

REHABILITATION

The rehabilitation exercises for the postoperative management of both arthroscopic and open surgical reconstruction are identical. The only difference appears to be that most surgeons start rehabilitation earlier after open techniques than after arthroscopic repairs.

ASSOCIATED DISORDERS

The arthroscope is more effective in the treatment of labrum tears and loose bodies. The open surgical technique is better able to manage such associated problems as rotator cuff tendon tears, rotator interval tears, or excessive capsular laxity.

COSMESIS

The arthroscopic approach is almost always perceived by the patient to be cosmetically superior. Certainly most arthroscopic cannula wounds heal well, particularly when compared to the healed anterosuperior saber incision. When an anteroinferior axillary incision is used, a cosmetically appealing scar results. Also, the patient may not understand that arthroscopic approaches involve multiple puncture wounds and that these are clearly visible in the superior aspect of the shoulder. The 7-cm anteroinferior scar from an open procedure should be compared to one posterosuperior wound for the arthroscope, one anterosuperior wound for the inflow cannula, one anteroinferior wound for the fixation device, and one 2-cm posteroinferior wound for pull-through sutures required by the arthroscopic approach.

COST

One might assume that the arthroscopic outpatient approach is more cost effective. At present, however, the cost benefits are not great. The majority of the cost for a hospital stay occurs during the first day. A great percentage of this cost is related to surgery and recovery room costs. Most orthopedic patients stay in the hospital 1 to 2 nights and receive little intensive medical care. The daily room charge is a small proportion of the patient's total bill. Time required to complete arthroscopic techniques is longer than that needed for open techniques. The increase in time means an increase in anesthesia time, longer operating room and recovery rooms stays, and, thus, correspondingly greater charges.

Arthroscopy is a high-technology field with significant expenses related to cameras, video equipment, and disposable instruments.

TISSUE DAMAGE

Arthroscopy requires no extensive soft tissue dissection, division, or splitting of the subscapularis muscle. Although the amount of swelling in the immediate perioperative period is impressive, this swelling disappears rapidly. The appearance of the shoulder is more acceptable and the amount of pain experienced by the patient is lesser with arthroscopic techniques than with open surgical techniques.

PATIENT DEMAND

Most patients prefer an arthroscopic outpatient procedure to an open reconstructive inpatient procedure. If this were the only criterion upon which a decision was to be based, the arthroscopic approach would clearly be superior. All the previously mentioned factors must be taken into consideration, however, when discussing the choice of surgical approach with the patient. Perhaps the greatest factors are the skill, experience, judgment, and training of the surgeon.

FUTURE DEVELOPMENTS (TABLE 15–2)

The surgical management of glenohumeral instability will certainly change. Our current experience with both open and arthroscopic surgical techniques continues to be analyzed in detail, and indications for each treatment method will

TABLE 15–2. COMPARISON OF OPEN VS. ARTHROSCOPIC TECHNIQUES IN THE FUTURE

	OPEN SURGERY	ARTHROSCOPIC SURGERY
LOS	–	+
Cost	–	+
Patient demand	–	+
Muscle		
Subscapularis	–	+
Deltoid	–	+
Cuff	–	+
Immobilization	=	=
Rehabilitation	=	=
Technical ease	=	=
Complications	=	=
Associated lesions	=	=
Success	=	=

LOS means length of stay; + means preferred procedure; – means less preferred procedure; = means equally preferred procedures.

become more clearly defined. Current levels of knowledge and experience suggest that future arthroscopic techniques will be most useful in the two following situations:

1. In acute traumatic dislocation in high-risk populations.
2. In individuals with unidirectional, anteroinferior glenohumeral recurrent dislocations in whom the anteroinferior glenohumeral ligament is of sufficient quality to support a fixation technique.

Recurrent subluxations and multidirectional instabilities will probably continue to be treated with open surgical techniques.

The success rate of arthroscopic repairs should eventually increase to equal or better the level of open surgical management as the technique becomes less traumatic and more precise.

An increased use of arthroscopic techniques in the shoulder, as well as a refinement in current surgical techniques for arthroscopic instability management, will result in increased technical ease. As technical skills advance, anesthesia and surgery time will correspondingly decrease. A combination of improved indications and improved implant technology will allow more secure fixation, thereby accelerating arthroscopic rehabilitation to the level of open surgical reconstruction. Hopefully, improved techniques will allow for fewer portal sites and improved cosmesis.

Should an individual surgeon perform an arthroscopic evaluation or arthroscopic surgical reconstruction on a particular patient? This question is obviously complicated, and the answers that hold true in our experience may not be valid for other practitioners. The moderate approach to the arthroscopic treatment of glenohumeral instability that is taken in our practice is reflected in this chapter.

SECTION

THE ARTHRITIDES AND MISCELLANEOUS AFFECTIONS

GLENOHUMERAL ARTHRITIS

Degenerative joint disease (osteoarthritis) and rheumatoid arthritis are the most commonly encountered types of glenohumeral arthritis. The role of arthroscopy in the treatment of these two conditions and a variety of other arthritides is the subject of this chapter.

Shoulder arthroscopy has led to often unexpected encounters with the earliest manifestations of joint disease. The arthroscope offers direct inspection of the articular surfaces under gross magnification. Thus, pathologic variations may be delineated long before they otherwise would have been discovered. The review that follows is based on our observations and preliminary evaluation of the results of treatment of disorders that inexorably lead to joint destruction. Modification of the pathologic changes by synovectomy or debridement of cartilaginous detritus or loose bodies may have little long-term effect on the outcome of the disease. In the short term, benefits may be judged based on relief of pain and improvement in function. Longer-term results await further study.

DEGENERATIVE JOINT DISEASE (OSTEOARTHRITIS)

The pathogenesis of degenerative joint disease is generally regarded as part of the general aging process. The condition is hastened by excessive functional demand and a decreased efficiency of blood supply. The earliest pathologic changes are collagenization of the synovial membrane and stenosis of its fine vascular network (Fig. 16–1A). Changes that develop in the intracellular chondroid produce crevices and fissures (Fig. 16–1B). The chondroid atrophies and disappears, particularly in stress-bearing areas. Thus, the joint surface becomes increasingly irregular and the thickness of the cartilaginous plate diminishes. As stress trajectories shift, the cartilage at the joint margin grows outward, thereby producing marginal lipping. The resultant spurs, along with narrowing of the joint, are the basis for the roentgenographic diagnosis of degenerative joint disease.[171]

The changes just described may be precipitated in varying degrees by repetitive stressful activities, musculoligamentous instability, or trauma.

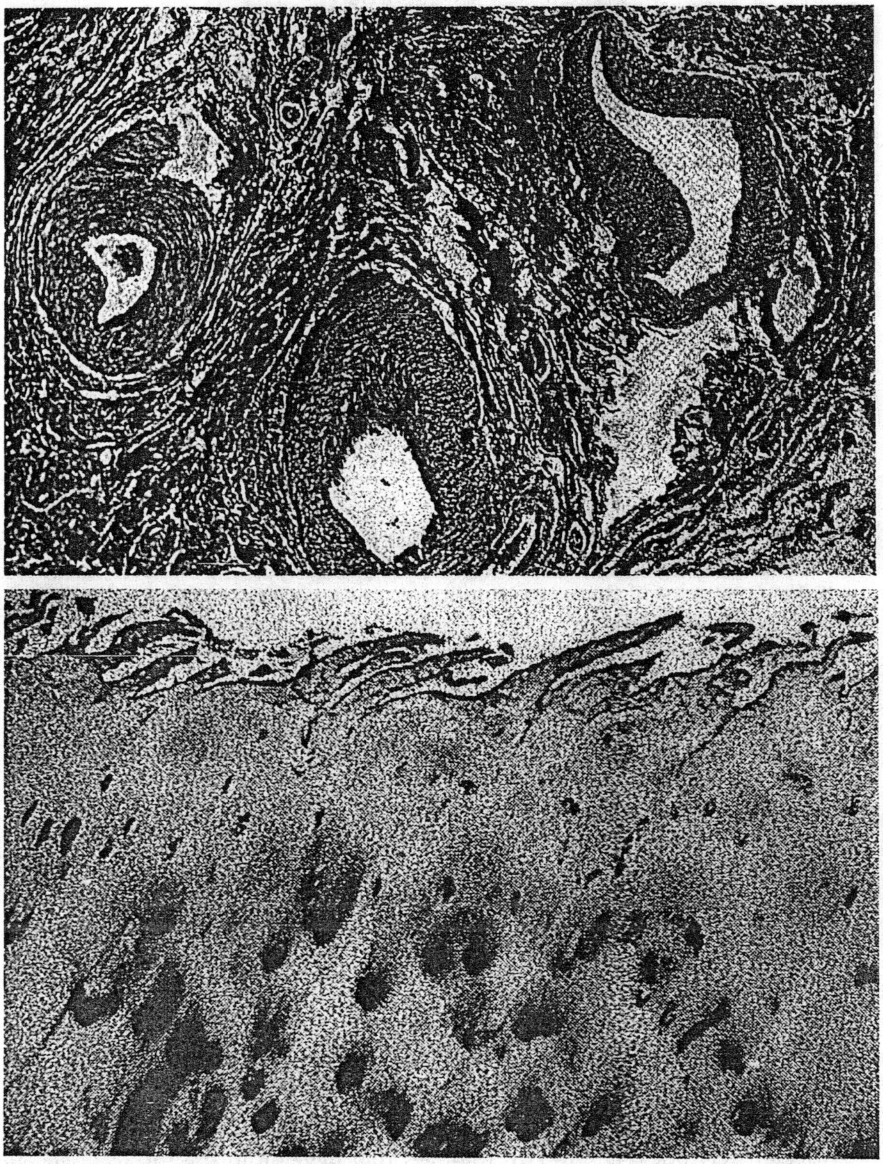

A

B

FIG. 16–1. A, Osteoarthritis: Collagenization of the synovial membrane and stenosis of its fine vascular network are the earliest signs of degenerative joint disease. (From Aegerter, E., and Kirkpatrick, J.A., Jr.: Orthopaedic Diseases. 4th Edition. Philadelphia, W.B. Saunders, 1975.)
B, Chondroid atrophies in stress-bearing areas, and joint surface becomes irregular (fibrillation). (From Harris, N.H. (Ed.): Postgraduate Textbook of Clinical Orthopaedics. Oxford, Butterworth-Heinemann Limited, 1983).

EARLY DEGENERATIVE JOINT DISEASE (CHONDROMALACIA)

The crevices and fissures that accompany early chondral destruction can be seen with an arthroscope. As cartilage is eroded, subchondral bone is exposed (Fig. 16–2A). These changes develop in stress-bearing areas. The location of the defect on the humeral head varies. The defect is more central and superior in primary osteoarthritis, and more inferior and posterior when joint laxity is present (Fig. 16–2B). When subluxation is significant, a cartilaginous lesion on the anteroinferior glenoid accompanies the humeral defect (Fig. 16–2C). We refer to these changes as "subluxation arthropathy" to differentiate their cause from primary osteoarthritis. The cartilage peripheral to the expanding defect is usually undermined and loosened for 3 to 5 mm; it resembles an unstable flap of tissue ready to crack off and fall into the joint. Indeed, small fragments of cartilage found within the joint attest to this occurrence (Fig. 16–3). Much of this material must disintegrate and dissolve because enough loose cartilage to fit into the defect is seldom found. Some of these articular fragments may remain and grow into cartilaginous loose bodies of considerable size. Eventually, central ossification occurs, and the osteochondral loose body becomes apparent on plain radiographs.

TREATMENT

Both anterior and posterior portals are required. The anterior portal is established just above the level of the coracoid process by using a transfer rod (Fig. 16–4). The rod penetrates the capsule just above the upper border of the subscapularis. The point of exit is made without endangering the axillary vessels. Switching sticks should be available or a cannulated arthroscopy system should be used to allow easy interchange of instruments from front to back.

Inspection

A 4.5-mm serrated suction shaver (Dyonics Turbotrimmer 3529) or a 4.5-mm full-radius resector (Dyonics 3443) initially vacuums the joint to eliminate small fragments of cartilaginous detritus. Large chunks of cartilage are morselled with a basket forceps before removal. The joint is then systematically inspected to identify the location and extent of cartilage loss. When both glenoid and humeral head lesions are present, the shoulder is rotated and abducted to determine the position in which the two areas of erosion approximate each other. In primary osteoarthritis, the contact area is more central on both the humeral head and the glenoid, and contact occurs at 60 to 70° of abduction. Subluxation arthropathy produces defects along the anteroinferior portion of the glenoid and the posteroinferior aspect of the humeral head. The lesions of instability require greater abduction and external rotation for contact than do the lesions in primary osteoarthritis. When pressure is exerted from behind, the head is seen sliding anteriorly in the unstable joint. The labrum usually appears worn, frayed, and attenuated in the lax joint. Minor fissures develop in the labral insertion into the glenoid. The labrum in the patient with atraumatic subluxation is not torn from the anterior glenoid to the extent that it is torn in the patient who experiences acute traumatic dislocation.

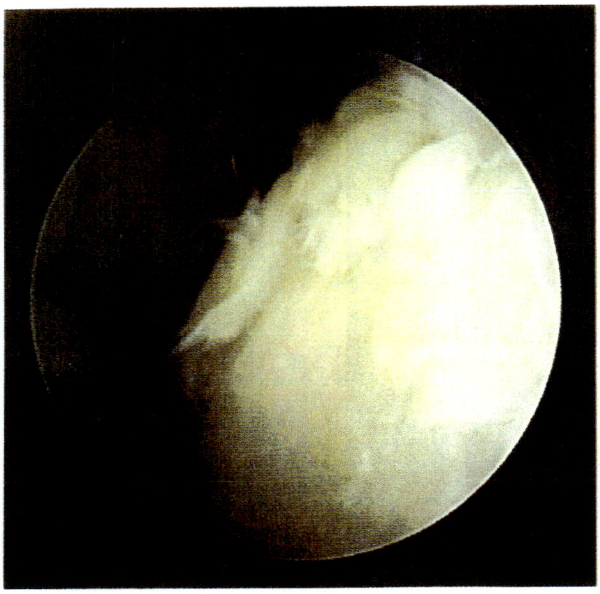
A

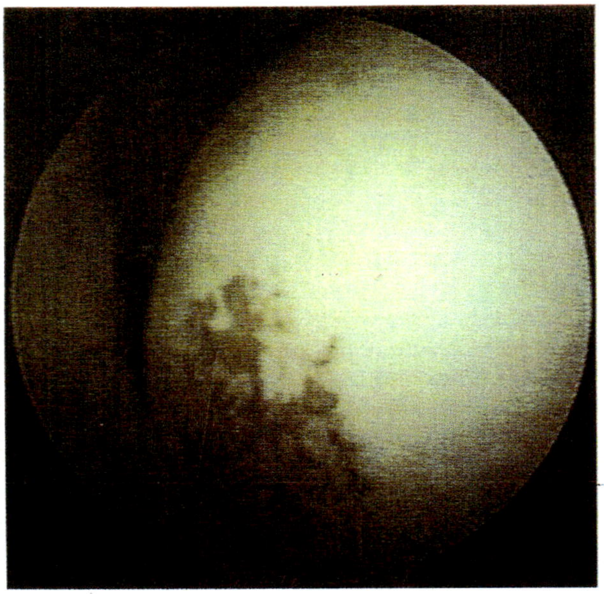
B

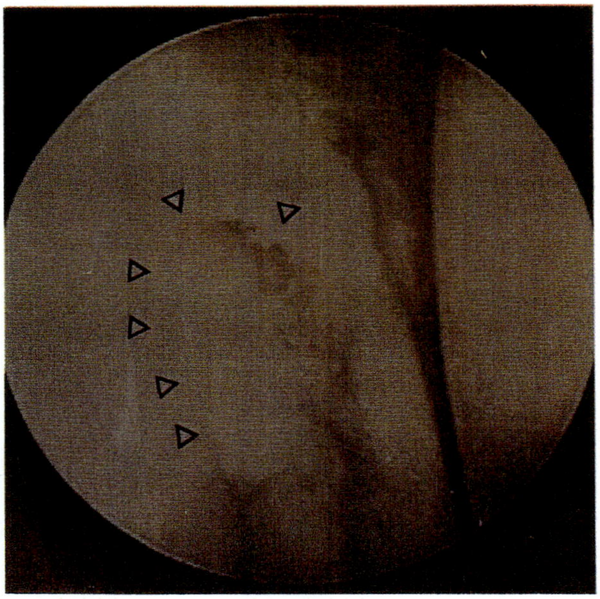
C

FIG. 16–2. A, Chondromalacia: Humeral head seen from posterior portal shows erosion of cartilage and central exposure of subchondral bone.
B, Area of chondromalacia on inferoposterior aspect of humeral head is associated with joint laxity.
C, Chondromalacia (open arrows) at anteroinferior aspect of glenoid is associated with "subluxation arthropathy."

Modified Chondroplasty

The area of chondromalacia is often difficult to access. The humeral head must be rotated and manipulated in various directions to make the lesion accessible to the rigid instruments that pass through a confined portal. A superior portal may be necessary. Instruments are often exchanged between portals to gain access. Then, the loosened cartilage at the periphery of these lesions must be trimmed away to leave a stable margin. Trimming is done with a motorized shaver or an

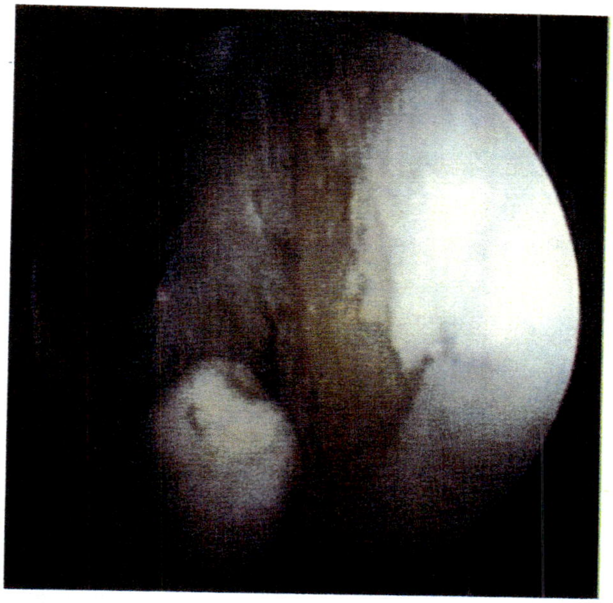

FIG. 16–3. Unstable cartilage at periphery of lesion has broken off to produce a loose body.

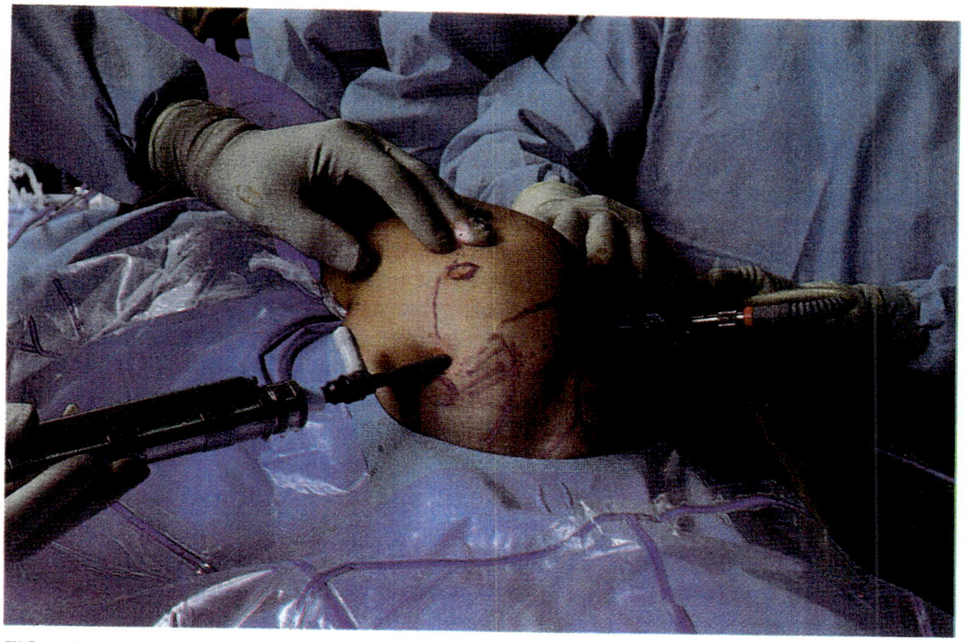

FIG. 16–4. Anterior portal has been established just above and slightly lateral to the coracoid process.

open curette (Fig. 16–5). The exposed subchondral bone is lightly curetted and smoothed with the shaver. An irregular area may be burred lightly to make it level. The modified chondroplasty does not include burring through the chondral surface to expose bleeding cancellous bone or drilling the area of defect.

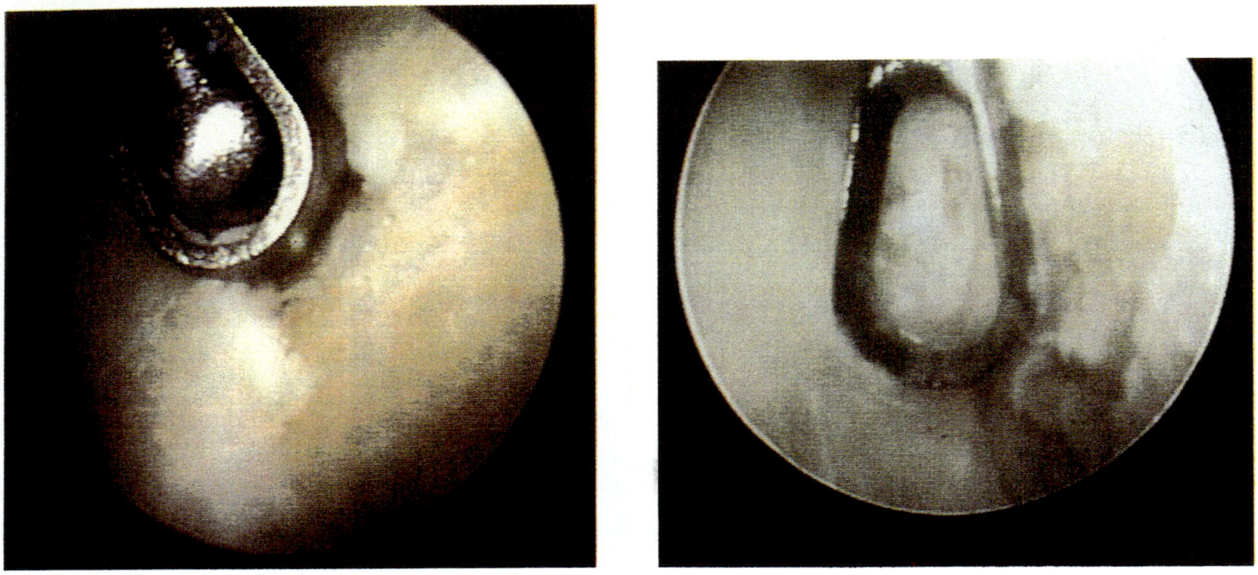

A B

FIG. 16–5. A, Motorized shaver trims the loose cartilage from margins. B, Open curette lightly curettes the subchondral space.

Synovectomy

Reactive synovitis may be present to varying degrees in focal areas. Resection of pathologic synovium is reserved until the end of the chondroplasty to avoid the troublesome bleeding that accompanies synovectomy.

On the first postoperative visit, the patient with chondromalacia is invited to view the video or photographs that display the cartilaginous defects. Patients are routinely advised that high-impact stress loading adversely affects their prognosis. Viewing the defect often promotes the activity modification necessary to retard progression. When the early changes of subluxation arthropathy are discovered, capsular stabilization should be considered.

RESULTS

Our preliminary results indicate that when chondromalacia is encountered in the absence of radiographic evidence of degenerative joint disease, arthroscopic debridement is beneficial at least in the short term (3 to 5 years). When objective evidence of impingement syndrome accompanies the finding of chondromalacia, a subacromial decompression is also performed. The criteria for performing the decompression include arthroscopic visualization of cuff disease (articular or bursal surface partial tears), hypertrophic bursal stroma consistent with chronic impingement in the subacromial space, and often fraying on the anterior undersurface of the type II or type III acromion.

We have some concern that the relief of accompanying impingement symptoms may allow some patients with chondromalacia to resume high-impact activities that will encourage further development of degenerative joint disease. When cartilage has been denuded over an extensive area, the relief of pain from debridement and lavage diminishes as joint degeneration continues.

ADVANCED DEGENERATIVE JOINT DISEASE

Once the joint has deteriorated to the point that deformity is recognizable, as evidenced by joint narrowing, subchondral irregularity, and marginal osteophytosis, any relief obtained by joint lavage and debridement is probably transitory. Our experience, and that of other authors,[107] with arthroscopic intervention in more *advanced* degenerative joint disease suggests that the procedure has little to offer.

LOOSE BODIES

Osteochondral loose bodies commonly accompany degenerative joint disease. They result from metaplastic ossification of cartilaginous fragments that have fallen into the joint. Nourished by synovial fluid, they may grow to significant proportions. The loose bodies that accompany *primary osteoarthritis* are rarely capable of producing episodes of locking in the later stages of the disease. The loose bodies are too large and the joint space too narrow to enable them to intervene between the opposing articular surfaces. Instead, they congregate in the inferior subscapular or subacromial recess, where they are confined as their size increases and glenohumeral motion decreases. Attempts to remove loose bodies in this circumstance are not likely to benefit the patient.

On the other hand, the loose bodies that accompany instability of the shoulder have an extensive area in which to forage. An *acute dislocation* may create cartilaginous or osseous fragments quite abruptly. The chondromalacia associated with *subluxation arthropathy* creates many more fragments. These fragments may become sizable and produce locking episodes. Because of the capacious capsule, the loose bodies accompanying subluxation arthropathy can interpose themselves between the joint surfaces more freely than can the loose bodies accompanying primary osteoarthritis. In these circumstances, removal of the loose body is often indicated (Fig. 16–6). The technique of loose body removal is described in Chapter 17.

CALCAR SPURS

The development of marginal spurs occurs in osteoarthritis as stress trajectories shift. In the shoulder the head appears to flatten slowly and a spur develops at the junction of the articular cartilage of the humeral head with the neck (Fig. 16–7). These spurs may grow to amazing proportions. In the earliest form, the spur is a minor bulge or blunting that when recognized is a reliable indicator of early degenerative joint disease. The spur often can be seen before any joint narrowing is evident. This spur is the result of, and not the cause of, joint degeneration. Removal of the spur by arthroscopic means has no logical benefit for the patient.

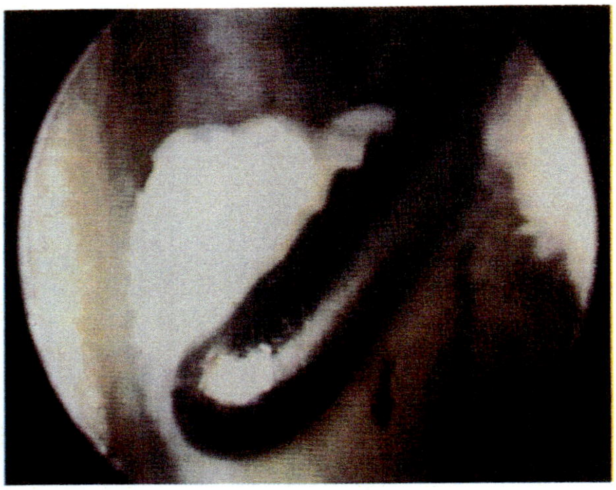

FIG. 16–6. Removal of large osteochondral loose body from shoulder with subluxation arthropathy.

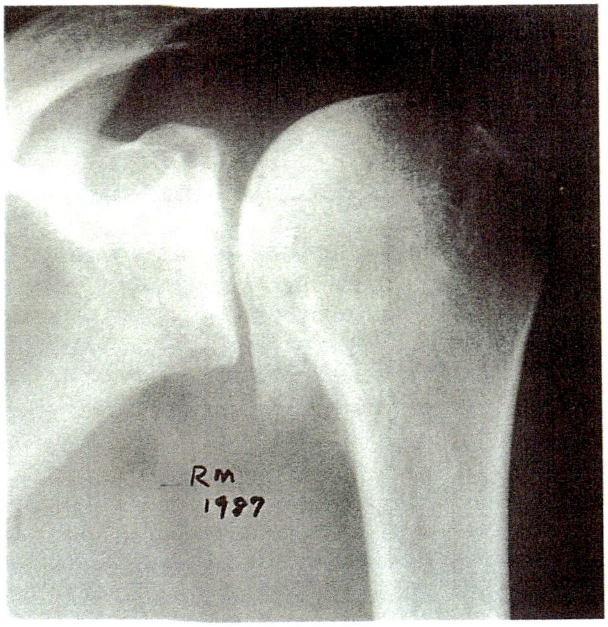

FIG. 16–7. A large spur has developed in a shoulder with degenerative joint disease. Removal has no logical benefit.

RHEUMATOID ARTHRITIS

Among the many ways to treat the diseased shoulder, arthroscopic treatment has perhaps the greatest potential to diminish the effects of rheumatoid arthritis. The shoulder joints are commonly involved in the polyarthritis that accompanies systemic rheumatoid disease. As the disease progresses, treatment is usually directed toward the weight-bearing joints. Meanwhile the patient manages to adapt to the progressive shoulder dysfunction until the joint is nearly destroyed. By that time, shoulder replacement arthroplasty may be the only viable surgical consideration.

The literature abounds with reports on synovectomy of the knee (open and closed), elbow (open and closed), and other joints, yet little has been written about this procedure in the shoulder.[172] The extensive exposure required to permit an open synovectomy in the shoulder has undoubtedly discouraged investigation. The minimally invasive potential of arthroscopic synovectomy is worthy of exploration.

SYNOVECTOMY IN JOINTS OTHER THAN THE SHOULDER

Synovectomy in other joints has been most beneficial when carried out early in the disease, before extensive local destruction has occurred. The procedure also benefits those in whom activity of the disease in subsequent years can be controlled. The destructive rheumatoid synovium must be removed before cartilage and bone have been destroyed, or before the rotator cuff has been ravaged by pannus.

Patient selection is based on the Steinbrocker Radiographic and Functional Classification.[173] The patient is classified according to the stage of involvement prior to the start of treatment and is later reassessed at intervals to determine the progression of disease. The classification is summarized as follows:

RADIOGRAPHIC CLASSIFICATION

Stage I: No destructive change. Osteoporosis and soft tissue change only.
Stage II: Mild/moderate erosive change or joint space reduction.
Stage III: Joint markedly narrowed (less than 1 mm); extensive erosion and subluxation.
Stage IV: Fibrous or bony ankylosis.

FUNCTIONAL CLASSIFICATION

Class I: Full function.
Class II: Adequate function despite pain and limited motion.
Class III: Very limited function.
Class IV: Wholly incapacitated.

The response to treatment is assayed in four categories:

Grade I: Complete remission.
Grade II: Major improvement.
Grade III: Minor improvement.
Grade IV: No improvement or progression.

Patients belonging in the first two radiographic stages and the first two functional classes have the best chance of benefitting from synovectomy, based on studies of other joints.

The results of synovectomy and debridement in rheumatoid arthritis involving the knee were reviewed. From 1923 to 1967, 17 authors with 3 months to 5 years of follow-up reported an average of 80% improvement. The frequency of recurrence following knee synovectomy (as reported by 14 authors published between 1926 and 1966) was 20% after 2 to 6½ years of follow-up. The continued use of systemic disease-modifying agents is required to maximize the benefits following synovectomy.

Inglis and colleagues studied the results of elbow synovectomy and found that 25 of 28 (89%) patients improved after 3½ years. They considered that the "basis of the destructive process . . . caused by rheumatoid arthritis is a proliferative and exudative synovitis."[174]

Rheumatoid arthritis may involve all three joints in the shoulder girdle. The acromioclavicular joint may be involved in as many as one third of the patients with glenohumeral disease; subacromial bursal involvement is estimated to occur in one of every five patients. The sternoclavicular joint is rarely involved.

TECHNIQUE OF ARTHROSCOPIC SYNOVECTOMY

PORTALS AND BASIC INSTRUMENTS

The lateral recumbent position is preferred. Standard anterior and posterior portals are established (see Chap. 3). Because bleeding often accompanies this procedure, additional fluid inflow is required and is introduced through the superior portal. Although a synovectomy can be performed with gravity inflow, we regard the arthroscopy pump as invaluable during this procedure. The intra-articular pressure and rate of fluid influx are controlled precisely with the pump. The pump can be set up with a sensor directly on the end of the scope, or a small Varies needle with an intra-articular pressure-sensing device can be introduced through the superior portal under arthroscopic control. Fluid from the pump is attached to the right-angle arm of the plastic operating cannula. A large-bore cannula facilitates fluid ingress when the shaver is in the cannula and also facilitates the removal of larger pieces of tissue when a grasping forceps is used. Because the position of the arthroscope and other instruments is frequently changed from one portal to another, an interchangeable cannula system greatly simplifies this process. Alternatively, switching sticks are used. All cannulas should have dams to maintain joint distention as instruments are inserted and withdrawn. A synovectomy requires a great deal of soft tissue removal, and motorized resectors are essential. Grasping forceps to remove loose bodies are useful.

CONTROL OF BLEEDING

Electrocautery is essential during the performance of synovectomy. Areas of obvious vascularity are cauterized prior to the use of the motorized resector. As bleeding occurs, the electrocautery instrument can be rapidly brought to this area to control bleeding before the field becomes obscured. Intra-articular pressure may be increased to control bleeding by elevating the fluid bags or adjusting the pump. The pressure is lowered again after hemostasis has been obtained. The areas that require synovectomy should be inspected, and the order of resection should be from least vascular to most vascular (white areas to red areas). When the areas of highest vascularity are approached first and bleeding becomes a problem, the remainder of the operation becomes exceedingly difficult. If, however, the areas of avascularity or minimal vascularity undergo synovectomy early in the surgery, a great deal can be accomplished before the problem of bleeding is encountered. Nursing personnel must remain alert to keep bags of fluid from emptying totally before new bags have been opened. A constant flow of fluid at an adequate pressure is essential during synovectomy. Epinephrine in the solution has a small effect on bleeding and is rapidly absorbed. A more helpful technique is the maintenance of systolic blood pressure below 90 mm Hg when doing so can be safely tolerated.

The loss of an established portal creates a serious problem if it cannot be relocated. The joint cannot be adequately distended if fluid is allowed to escape through an unoccupied portal. Extensive periarticular distention also develops.

AREAS OF SYNOVECTOMY

All areas of the glenohumeral joint and subacromial space should be inspected and should undergo systematic synovectomy (Fig. 16–8A). We prefer to start with the arthroscope in a posterior position and the instruments in an anterior position. The synovectomy begins with the biceps tendon and the superior rotator cuff and moves to the interval between the subscapularis and the biceps tendon (Fig. 16–8B). Particular attention should be paid to the anterior capsule and the subscapularis recess (Fig. 16–8C and D). Because loose bodies may be lodged within this recess, the arthroscope should be passed directly into this recess and a thorough inspection should be made. Labrum abnormalities are dealt with as required. The arthroscope is then inserted anteriorly and the motorized resector is inserted posteriorly. This configuration allows an inspection and debridement of the posterior labrum, the posterior glenoid recess or gutter, and the posteroinferior capsule. The arthroscope can then be directed to evaluate the anteroinferior aspect of the glenohumeral joint. By varying the position in which the arm is extended and rotating the arm, the surgeon can gain access to all areas of the shoulder. Although the procedure is often tedious when a great deal of proliferative tissue is present, or when bleeding is excessive (Fig. 16–8E), an extensive synovectomy can be performed through several tiny portals.

The subacromial space should not be neglected in patients with rheumatoid arthritis. Bursal proliferation, particularly within the subacromial space, may produce chronic impingement (Fig. 16–9). Debridement and occasionally acromioplasty or acromioclavicular joint resection may be required.

POSTOPERATIVE MANAGEMENT

A suction drain is often employed postoperatively for 24 hours. The patient is hospitalized following this procedure to allow for better pain control, as well as to coordinate medical management. Range-of-motion exercises are started on the day following surgery. The patient is encouraged to resume activities of daily living as soon as tolerated.

Although our experience with arthroscopic synovectomy is limited, we believe that the role of early synovectomy in the treatment of rheumatoid disease in the shoulder will increase. When synovectomy is performed prior to the development of cartilage or bone destruction, pain is relieved and the potential to extend the functional integrity of the joint is quite real. A long-term clinical study adhering to the established criteria for evaluating therapeutic results is in progress.[173] In the past, the greatest advance in the treatment of the rheumatoid shoulder was the development of a successful prosthesis to replace a destroyed joint. The future offers the technology to resect the proliferative, exuberant synovitis that destroys the joint with minimal disturbance to the surrounding tissue structures. Physicians and surgeons involved in the treatment of rheumatoid arthritis must be aware of the frequency of shoulder involvement and provide the patient with an opportunity for treatment in the early, rather than the later, stages of this insidious disease.

SYNOVIAL CHONDROMATOSIS

Synovial chondromatosis involves the shoulder in approximately 4% of patients. Men are involved more frequently than women (3:1). The radiographs may show only mild degenerative changes or may be normal if the lesions are purely cartilaginous. Occasionally, the multiple ossified lesions may be seen on an x-ray study. If the radiograph is not diagnostic, the arthroscope may allow the diagnosis to be made on inspection as well as with synovial biopsy.

The portals for loose body removal and synovectomy are established as previously described. A large-bore cannula is desirable. Cartilaginous loose bodies tend to agglutinate into large clumps. With ossification, a remarkable size may

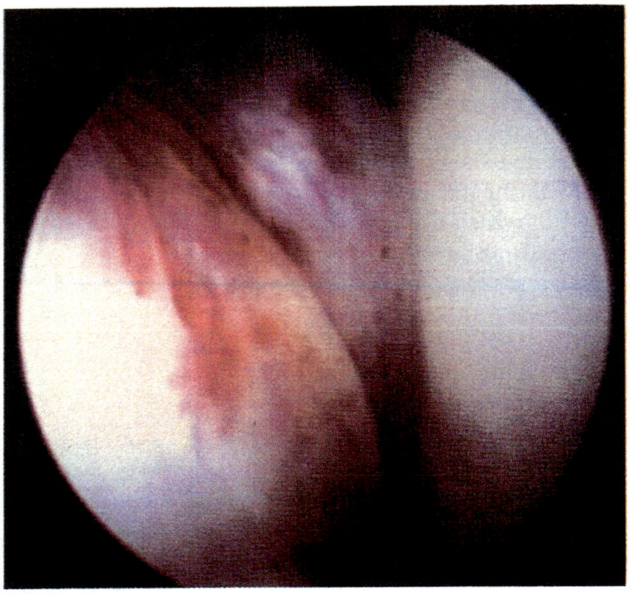

A

FIG. 16–8. A, Area of proliferative synovitis in a patient with an established diagnosis of rheumatoid arthritis.
B, Synovectomy begins above the long head of the biceps to remove pannus from the undersurface of the rotator cuff.
C, The subscapularis recess is inspected prior to synovectomy. The long head of the biceps is above; the humeral head is on the right.
D, Synovectomy of subscapular recess nearly completed.
(continued)

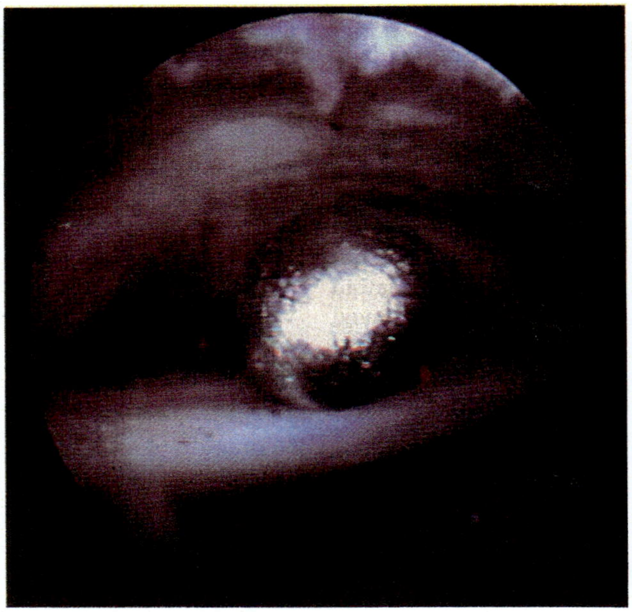

B

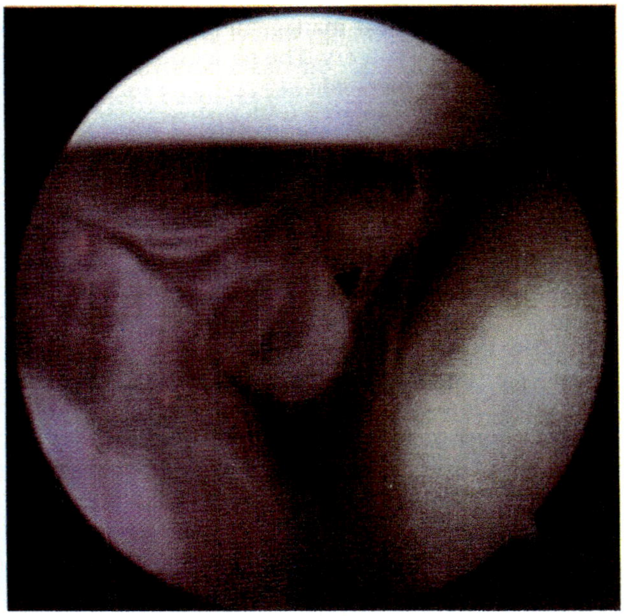

C

be achieved. Hundreds of loose bodies may require evacuation, and the largest feasible cannula is helpful. Larger fragments may have to be morselled before removal.

After loose bodies are removed, the synovium is inspected. Areas of metaplastic synovitis are resected. An extensive synovectomy retards recurrence.

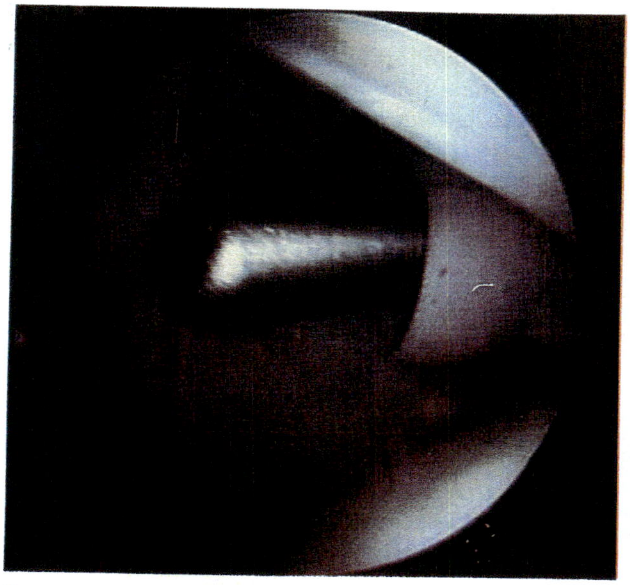

D

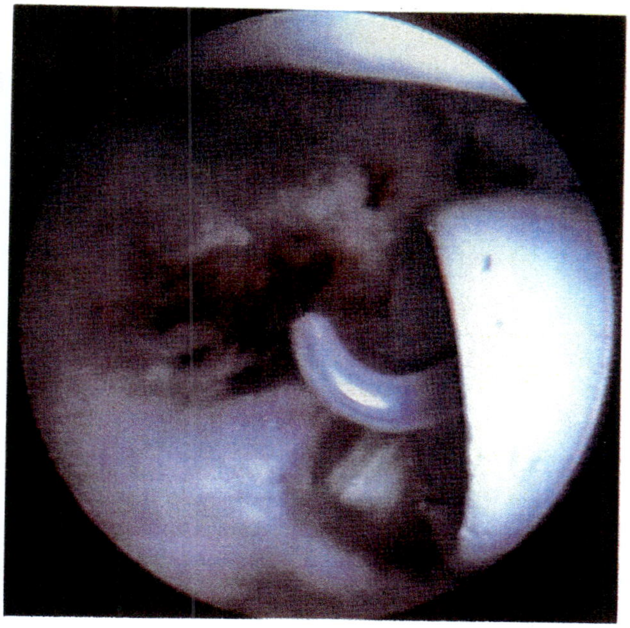

E

FIG. 16–8 (continued)

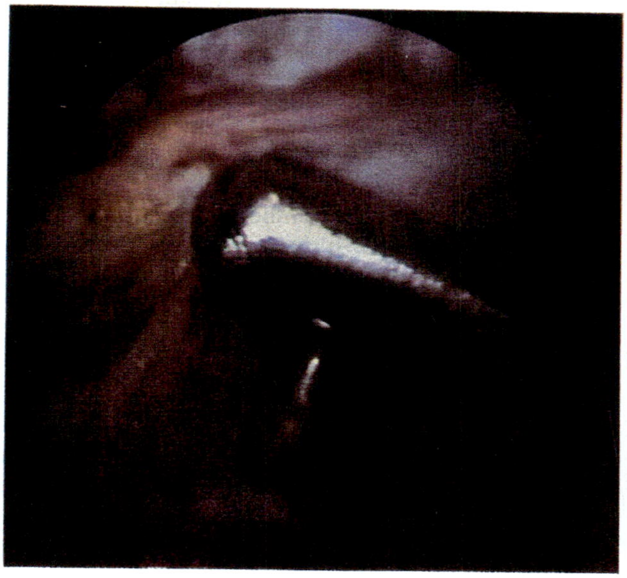

A

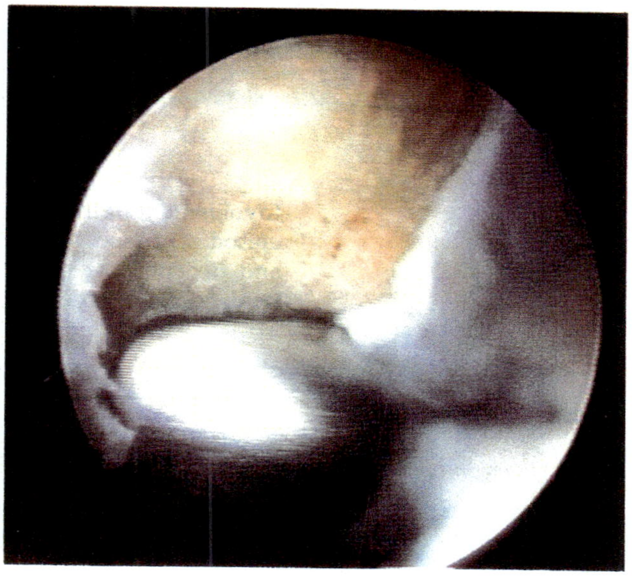

B

FIG. 16–9. A, Subacromial space shows significant rheumatoid bursitis. B, Note the clean sub-bursal tissue after shaving.

PIGMENTED VILLONODULAR SYNOVITIS

Involvement of the shoulder in this condition is rare—less than 1%. Swelling and decreased range of motion with mild pain are noted. Men and women are equally affected. The arthroscope can provide visual confirmation and a pathologic specimen to establish the diagnosis. The treatment of pigmented villonodular synovitis is synovectomy. Though tedious because of the amount of diseased tissue, the procedure can be performed arthroscopically.

CRYSTALLINE ARTHRITIS

Crystalline arthritic conditions rarely require arthroscopic evaluation or treatment. *Gout* (sodium monourate disease) is more common in men than in women. The shoulder is an unusual site for the primary presentation of gout; however, it is slightly more commonly affected in the flare-up of postoperative gout. Tophi may be noted, and the gout may affect the subacromial space, but because the disease can be medically controlled so effectively, arthroscopic evaluation is rarely needed to make the diagnosis or to treat the disease. *Pseudogout* (calcium pyrophosphate disease) involves men and women equally and is more common than gout in the shoulder. Chondrocalcinosis may involve the shoulder in approximately 50% of patients with this disease. Again, because the condition can be diagnosed and managed medically, the arthroscope is rarely required. *Calcium hydroxyapatite deposition* occurs in the "Milwaukee shoulder syndrome." The findings in this condition are similar to those described by Neer and Foster [162] as "cuff arthropathy."

HEMOPHILIA

Involvement of the shoulder is common in the hemophilic adolescent. Recurrent episodes of bleeding lead to a synovial reaction, ultimate cartilage destruction, and degenerative joint disease. Medical control is obviously the mainstay of treatment, but occasionally synovectomy is required.

OCHRONOSIS (ALKAPTONURIA)

This rare inherited condition may produce characteristic deposits of brown-black pigment in cartilage. The gross appearance of these deposits when viewed arthroscopically is quite distinctive. Little can be done to reverse the slowly progressive arthropathy associated with this disease.

AMYLOIDOSIS

Rarely, amyloid deposits in the glenohumeral joint may cause a destructive arthropathy. Amyloidosis develops in patients with chronic disabling illnesses. Patients who have undergone dialysis treatments for many years are prone to this disorder. Arthroscopy is of little value other than diagnostic.

AVASCULAR NECROSIS

In the early stage of avascular necrosis, the articular surface may appear intact, but the plain radiograph or magnetic resonance imaging study can provide a definitive diagnosis. When collapse of the humeral head develops, the changes may be visualized by the arthroscope, but arthroscopy has little to offer therapeutically.

CONCLUSION

The cause, presentation, medical management, and precise indications for arthroscopic treatment of all the conditions described in this chapter are quite varied. The arthroscope can be of value in both diagnosis and treatment. When the diagnosis is unclear, arthroscopy can provide an excellent view of the glenohumeral joint and subacromial space and allows the surgeon to obtain tissue for microscopic analysis. Evaluation of the status of the rotator cuff and any damage to the articular cartilage helps to plan appropriate treatment.

Therapeutic applications described in this chapter include debridement of cartilaginous debris and loose bodies in early degenerative joint disease and stabilization of loosening marginal cartilage. Synovectomy is the treatment of choice for synovial chondromatosis and pigmented villonodular synovitis and appears to be of value in the early stages of rheumatoid arthritis, either juvenile or adult, prior to significant destruction of the cartilage or bone.

MISCELLANEOUS INTRA-ARTICULAR CONDITIONS

17

LOOSE BODIES

CAUSES

The primary cause of loose body formation in the shoulder is glenohumeral instability. Other significant causes are osteoarthritis, osteochondritis dissecans, and foreign bodies.

INSTABILITY

Pieces of bone, cartilage, or labrum can be sheared off to form loose bodies either during initial dislocation or during further episodes of subluxation or dislocation that result in instability.

Excision of loose bodies in instability falls into three groups: (1) loose bodies that may be removed during arthroscopic evaluation and arthroscopic repair of instability; (2) loose bodies that may be found at diagnostic arthroscopy when the diagnosis of instability is not certain; and (3) the loose body that results in a functional instability because the position of the loose body does not allow the humeral head to fit securely in the glenoid.

Loose bodies must be removed prior to any attempt at repair of instability. The chasing of loose bodies after the completion of a difficult instability repair is frustrating.

The most common sites of origin are the anteroinferior glenoid cartilage and the anteroinferior glenoid labrum. Occasionally, the posterior lateral humeral head cartilage is the source of loose body formation when the Hill-Sachs' lesion engages the anterior glenoid during a dislocation. The site of origin usually is not clearly defined because with time the divot or crater created by the loose body has been smoothed.

Loose bodies may be hidden in the subscapularis bursa, inferior recess, or posterior gutter. All areas should be carefully viewed. In addition, suction should be placed on the arthroscope in an attempt to draw any loose pieces into view.

When diagnostic arthroscopy is performed and the cause of shoulder pain is in doubt, the presence of a loose body should alert the arthroscopist to the possibility that glenohumeral instability is the cause. The arthroscopist, therefore, should examine the superior, middle, and anteroinferior glenohumeral ligaments for integrity, size, and attachment. The area of the Hill-Sachs' lesion should be inspected also. Although exposed bone may not be identified, more subtle signs, such as cartilage fragmentation or flattening, may suggest instability. Careful attention should be paid to the anteroinferior glenohumeral ligament. Inspection alone is not sufficient. A probe must be inserted anteriorly and the attachment site must be palpated. An apparently well-attached anteroinferior glenohumeral ligament may, with gentle probing, demonstrate the classic Bankart lesion.

Perhaps the rarest type of instability is the functional instability first described by Pappas and associates.[175] In this instance, a structural abnormality, such as a loose body or bucket-handle labrum tear, is interposed between the humeral head and glenoid, thereby creating in the patient the sensation that the shoulder "is not in place." Examination under anesthesia demonstrates a stable shoulder, whereas the arthroscopic evaluation demonstrates a large loose body or labrum tear that creates a mechanical abnormality. The ligaments are normal in attachment and integrity, and removal of the fragment completely resolves the patient's symptoms.

OSTEOARTHRITIS

Loose bodies frequently occur in patients with osteoarthritis. The arthroscopic management of both early and late degenerative joint disease is reviewed in the preceding chapter. Although arthroscopic intervention appears to be of little value in the late stages of the disease, the removal of a loose body is indicated on occasion. Removal is necessary when episodes of locking, accompanied by sharp, stabbing pain, are superimposed on the generalized ache and discomfort of the osteoarthritic condition. Removal of the loose body has been helpful in these circumstances and is usually accompanied by a limited synovectomy and debridement.

OSTEOCHONDRITIS DISSECANS

A third cause of loose bodies is osteochondritis dissecans. These rare lesions in the shoulder can arise from either the glenoid or the humeral head. Our treatment has been limited to removal of loose pieces and smoothing of the cartilage edge. When larger lesions are encountered, drilling and temporary fixation with metal implants are feasible arthroscopically. The use of biodegradable implants eliminates the necessity for a second operation to remove the implant.

FOREIGN BODIES

We have removed bullets, needles, staples (placed arthroscopically or with open surgical technique), arthroscopic knives, broken curettes, pieces of powered arthroscopy burs, fragments of plastic, and even the diaphragm from an operating cannula.

TECHNIQUE FOR REMOVAL

The technique for removal of a loose body can be divided into three phases: visualization, stabilization, and extraction.

Finding the loose body involves knowing where the loose pieces are most likely to reside. The most common area is in the axillary pouch of the glenohumeral joint. Other possible sites include the subscapularis bursa, posterior recess, and deep to the middle glenohumeral ligament.

The subscapularis bursa is present in most individuals and is located immediately superior to the subscapularis tendon. A good view can be obtained with the arthroscope in the posterior portal by advancing the scope anteriorly past the anterior glenoid rim and then rotating the arthroscope inferiorly. Suction applied through the arthroscope may bring loose pieces into view.

Continue to sweep the arthroscope along the anterior glenoid rim and inspect the middle glenohumeral ligament. If a foramen is located between the ligament and the subscapularis tendon, insert the arthroscope in that foramen and search for the loose body. If none is found, withdraw the arthroscope until it is at the level of the anterior glenoid rim. Distract the arm to allow the arthroscope to pass under the humeral head without injury to either the cartilage or the lens of the arthroscope. The arthroscope is now in the axillary recess.

The recess can also be approached from the posterior glenoid rim by maneuvering the arthroscope until the biceps tendon insertion is in the center of the viewing field. Gently withdraw the arthroscope as far as possible without pulling out of the joint. Rotate *and* angle the scope inferiorly until the posterior and inferior aspects of the joint are seen.

Once identified, the loose piece must then be stabilized. A grasper can be used. This instrument should be passed through a cannula if at all possible. Because the loose bodies are almost always an irregular size, grasping them is difficult. Usually, they can be maneuvered against the humeral head or glenoid, stabilized, and then grasped.

Occasionally, other techniques may be needed. An accessory portal can be created to insert a second grasping forceps. This addition allows bimanual technique to stabilize the loose body. On rare occasions, a spinal needle may be inserted to pierce the loose body and hold it against the glenoid or humeral head so that it can be grasped. A magnetized rod can be used to remove metallic objects. This rod is particularly useful with arthroscopy knife blades or pieces of power or hand equipment.

Once the loose body has been identified and stabilized, it should be removed through the cannula. A great deal of soft tissue exists between the anterior joint capsule and the skin. A loose piece can be lost anywhere in this area if it is not brought through the cannula system. If the loose body cannot be removed through the anterior cannula, the cannula should be exchanged for the largest-diameter cannula possible to avoid pulling the loose fragment through the soft tissue unprotected.

On occasion, large pieces that cannot pass through the cannula system are encountered. The choice then must be made either to bring the piece out whole or to divide the loose body into smaller pieces to facilitate removal. When a large loose body is grasped (no matter how firmly), it most likely will not pass through the joint lining. The joint capsule must be incised with a knife or basket forceps to allow the loose piece to pass unimpeded through that opening. If the loose body is bone and the surgeon decides that the piece should be made smaller, a small round power bur can be used. The loose body can be held in place against the glenoid rim or even the anterior soft tissue while it is divided. A hand-held punch can also perform this task quite effectively.

Once completed, loose body removal is almost always rewarding. The actual removal can be tedious and can challenge the psychomotor skills of the surgeon. Rapid identification, stabilization, and extractions of loose bodies are facilitated by these principles.

SEPTIC ARTHRITIS

Pyarthrosis of the glenohumeral joint is an uncommon indication for arthroscopy. In our experience, however, the arthroscope has greatly facilitated the management of this difficult condition. Treatment goals include joint decompression, functional recovery, and minimal morbidity. Repeated needle aspirations may not remove all joint debris, loculations, or infected clots. Arthrotomy accomplishes complete removal, but with increased morbidity.

In a recent review, Calhoun and associates reviewed 35 septic shoulders.[176] Of these, 23 were from adults, and the causes were traumatic (37%), hematogenous (27%), idiopathic (22%), and previous surgery (17%). The most frequently cultured organisms were *Staphylococcus aureus* (61%) and *S. epidermidis* (17%), followed by *Pseudomonas aeruginosa* and *Proteus mirabilis*. Four anaerobic bacteria were cultured, and polymicrobial infections were frequent (67%). Osteomyelitis occurred in approximately 33% of the patients and was treated with arthrotomy, debridement, and long-term antibiotics. Patients without osteomyelitis received shorter-term parental antibiotics and underwent joint aspiration. At follow-up, however, only 33% demonstrated a good functional range of motion and were pain free.

Gelberman and associates evaluated 15 patients with 16 septic glenohumeral joint infections and noted significant underlying medical conditions, such as alcoholism, liver disease, malignant disease, heroin addiction, or renal failure, in each patient.[177] They also reported a significant decrease in the functional outcome when treatment was delayed longer than 4 weeks. Leslie and colleagues have also reported on septic arthritis of the shoulder.[178] They reviewed 18 patients and found generally poor functional results. They noted 4 patients with major tears of the rotator cuff found at arthrotomy and 2 additional patients with clinical manifestations of rotator cuff tears. Numerous review articles on septic arthritis have cited an incidence of 3 to 12% in the shoulder. Leslie and colleagues also noted that only 1 patient did not have a major associated medical condition. Although no firm conclusions could be given, the authors believed that the patients who had been treated operatively had a better range of motion of the shoulder than did those who had been treated with aspiration alone. Also, they proposed that the patients who were initially treated with aspiration but later had operative drainage did better than those who had aspiration only.

If glenohumeral infection is suspected, the patient should be surgically prepared and positioned routinely, but preoperative antibiotics should not be administered. The trocar enters the joint easily when it is distended by the infectious process. The trocar is withdrawn leaving the cannula in place. Prior to the installation of any irrigating fluid, appropriate cultures should be taken for various agents, such as aerobic, anaerobic, tuberculous, and fungal organisms. At this point, the arthroscope should be reinserted and the anterior portal created. Biopsy specimens of soft tissue or bone should be sent for analysis. Fluid inflow can then be introduced anteriorly to irrigate the joint thoroughly. The amount of joint destruction that accompanies these infections is impressive. Massive rotator cuff tears, significant synovitis, and cartilage fragments have been found.

Any necrotic areas of tendon, synovium, or labrum should be debrided. Any loose flaps are smoothed at this time. A synovectomy is performed routinely. With the arthroscope inserted posteriorly, a drain is placed through the anterior cannula and the cannula is removed. A second drain is placed through the posterior cannula and then that cannula is also removed.

The goals in the management of glenohumeral pyarthrosis are identification of infection, identification of the infecting organism, irrigation and lavage of the joint, mechanical debridement of necrotic tissue, and placement of drainage catheters. These goals can be accomplished rapidly and effectively by using arthroscopic techniques and thus minimizing trauma.

On the rare occasion that sepsis is confined to the subacromial space, the rotator cuff is intact. The principles of arthroscopic treatment in this instance are the same as those for arthroscopic treatment of pyarthrosis involving the glenohumeral joint.

TOTAL SHOULDER REPLACEMENT

Shoulder arthroscopy is valuable in identifying the source of pain after an individual has undergone total shoulder replacement or hemiarthroplasty.

Arthroscopically identifiable sources of pain in these individuals are component loosening, rotator cuff tears, instability, sepsis, synovitis, and the presence of cement debris.

The preparation and set-up for arthroscopy in these individuals is standard. When a prosthesis is examined arthroscopically, prophylactic antibiotics are always administered after tissue or bone samples have been taken for culture and sensitivity.

Special attention should be given to ensure atraumatic entry to avoid scratching the component. We routinely use only plastic cannulas and trocars in this situation.

Rotator cuff tears and loose pieces are identified using the techniques described elsewhere. An instability examination can be performed to detect the degree and direction of instability. The location of wear on the glenoid component is often helpful in determining patterns of instability. Loosening of the glenoid component is easily diagnosed by inserting a probe and palpating the glenoid/bone interface. Loosening of the humeral head is difficult to confirm. The best area for visualization is the posterosuperior aspect of the humeral head. The arthroscope is inserted anteriorly and a probe is inserted posteriorly to identify the metal/bone interface and observe any movement. Synovitis can be identified, and biopsy specimens can be taken as needed.

FRACTURES

The role of the arthroscope in the management of intra-articular fractures is limited at this time. At times, the amount of intra-articular involvement and displacement with glenoid fractures and fracture dislocations may be critical. This situation has always occurred in combination with a question of stability. The arthroscopic examination allows documentation of the degree of cartilage damage and bone displacement, as well as allows the stability to be tested under direct visualization.

LABRUM LESIONS

The increased use of shoulder arthroscopy has focused attention on the glenoid labrum. Prior to the advent of arthroscopy, glenoid labrum lesions were mentioned rarely and, in general, only as they related to glenohumeral instability. Pappas and associates focused attention on significant glenoid labrum lesions that led to interposition between the humeral head and glenoid, thereby giving the patient the feeling of "instability," when in actuality, no true ligamentous damage existed.[175] Pappas termed this concept "functional instability" and noted significant improvement with removal of these labrum lesions during open arthrotomy.

The glenoid labrum is so well visualized arthroscopically that minor abnormalities are assigned more importance than is warranted on the basis of scientific evidence. We are beginning to understand which labral abnormalities are simply the consequence of the aging process and are of no clinical significance and which signify an underlying pathologic condition of the shoulder.

Minor abnormalities of the labrum are common and appear to be either age related or of no clinical significance. These include minor fissures that occur longitudinally along the glenoid labrum, fraying of the leading edge, or areas of local separation. In an autopsy study by Kohn,[179] minor abnormalities occurred in 76% of the specimens. Such minor abnormalities could not have caused any clinical condition resulting in shoulder pain.

Labral abnormalities that are truly pathologic but are actually manifestations of underlying disease are more common. Such abnormalities are associated most frequently with glenohumeral instability. Several investigators have noted labrum lesions in from 70 to 90% of their patients with glenohumeral instability. Of individuals undergoing arthroscopy for full-thickness rupture of the rotator cuff or partial-thickness rupture of the rotator cuff, 30% have labral abnormalities, whereas in individuals with impingement, the incidence of significant labral abnormalities is less than 5%. These labral abnormalities are characteristic. Their structure should be noted and should alert the surgeon to search for the underlying cause of shoulder pain. Labral abnormalities occurring with instability generally involve the inferior half of the glenoid and consist of fraying of the leading edge, fissuring, or a separation between the labrum and glenoid (the soft tissue Bankart lesion).

Posterior Bankart lesions are rare. More commonly, labral signs of posterior instability consist of fraying at the posteroinferior quadrant of the glenoid. Patients with multiaxial instability may have labrum fraying at both the anteroinferior and the posteroinferior locations.

Altcheck and colleagues reported their results on arthroscopic labral debridement in 40 patients.[180] All their patients were involved in competitive sports and complained of persistent shoulder pain without complaints of instability. Anteroinferior labral detachments were noted in 4 patients; tears were noted in 26 patients (16 inferior quadrant, 10 superior quadrant). Posterior labral detachments in the inferior quadrant were noted in 2 patients, and 8 patients had tears in the posteroinferior quadrant. Of all the patients, 85% reported good initial pain relief and return to sports following arthroscopic debridement of labral tears. At a 2-year follow-up, however, the pain had recurred and function had diminished in 90% of all patients. Poor results were seen in all patients with labrum detachments (signs of the Bankart lesion). The authors concluded that labral lesions result from translational increases of the humeral head across the glenoid. Debridement with extensive rehabilitation may allow temporary relief of pain, but continued participation in sports causes eventual recurrence of symptoms in most patients. The authors also believed that debridement of labral detachment is unlikely to provide even temporary relief. Similar results were noted by Glasgow and associates.[181]

Labral abnormalities in an individual with a full-thickness rotator cuff tear are related not only to the increased age of these individuals, but also to the abnormal translation and shear forces that exist in the glenohumeral joint with an abnormal rotator cuff. Although minor fraying and fissuring are of little clinical significance and do not require arthroscopic debridement, interposable labral tears or bucket-handle lesions may cause symptoms after rotator cuff repair, and therefore, excision is worthwhile.

One labrum abnormality is most often noticed in the anterosuperior quadrant of the glenoid. This abnormality should not be confused with the Bankart lesion because it exists in a different portion of the glenoid and most likely represents an anatomic variant. Kohn also described this area as a common site of labrum separation that is unlikely to be of clinical significance and that possibly is related to the different embryologic development of this portion of the labrum.[179]

This anterosuperior labral separation should not be confused with the labral detachment or bucket-handle tear that occurs in swimmers. McMaster correctly pointed out that this anterior labral lesion may mechanically catch during the swimming movement, thereby producing pain and often a click.[182] Although most competitive swimmers have ligamentous laxity, the orthopedist must not necessarily conclude that the instability must be corrected to eliminate the patient's pain. Often the instability in swimmers is clinically silent, and the removal of just the mechanical abnormality allows the patient to return to preinjury status.

SUPERIOR LABRUM TEARS, ANTERIOR AND POSTERIOR (SLAP)

A particular labral abnormality is the SLAP lesion, which involves the labrum from its anterosuperior margin to the posterosuperior margin. Snyder and coworkers have stated that, although the SLAP lesion is not common, it is a source of significant disability when it occurs.[183] The lesion is difficult to diagnose without arthroscopy, and arthroscopic treatment of these patients has been successful. Their review of 700 shoulder arthroscopies performed by a group of orthopedic surgeons revealed 27 patients with a significant disorder of the superior labrum.

Two distinct mechanisms of injury were apparent. The most common mechanism was a compression force applied to the shoulder, usually the result of a fall on the outstretched arm with the shoulder positioned in abduction and slight forward flexion. A second mechanism of injury was traction on the arm, either as a result of a sudden pull or as a result of a throwing motion. All patients complained of pain, and a "catching" sensation was noted preoperatively in approximately half of their patients. Various preoperative evaluation techniques were utilized, including magnetic resonance imaging and computed tomographic arthrography, but none accurately defined the superior labral disorder.

Four types of SLAP lesions have been described. In type I, the superior labrum has marked fraying with a degenerative appearance, but the peripheral labrum edge remains firmly attached to the glenoid and the attachment of the biceps tendon to the labrum is intact. Type II injuries involve fraying and degenerative changes similar to those of type I, but in addition, the superior labrum and attached biceps tendon are stripped off the underlying glenoid, thereby rendering the labrum/biceps anchor unstable. The type III injury involves a bucket-handle tear in the superior labrum. The central portion of the tear can be displaced into the joint. A type IV injury has a bucket-handle tear, but in addition, the tear extends into the substance of the biceps tendon.

The occurrence of each type of lesion in the review by Snyder and colleagues was type I–3 patients (11%), type II–11 patients (41%), type III–9 patients (33%), and type IV–4 patients (15%).

Treatment depended on the type of lesion. Type I lesions were treated by debridement of the torn and frayed labral tissue while carefully preserving the labrum attachment and biceps tendon. Type II lesions were treated by abrading the superior glenoid neck below the biceps anchor to promote healing of the avulsed labrum to the underlying bone. Current treatment, according to Snyder, involves the use of an absorbable fixation tack to reattach the superior labrum.

Field and Savoie also reported good results with arthroscopic repair using multiple sutures.[184] Type III lesions were treated with excision of the bucket-handle tear, and type IV lesions were treated in a similar fashion but also underwent resection of the split portion of the biceps tendon. If the biceps tear involved more than 50% of the tendon and the patient had symptoms referable to the biceps tendon, a biceps tenodesis was performed.

Also of interest was the high incidence of associated injuries. Of the injured patients, 26% had partial rotator cuff tears, 15% had full-thickness rotator cuff tears, 15% had anterior instability, and 11% had acromioclavicular joint arthritis.

The follow-up period in this group has been relatively short, but the authors state that most patients were satisfied with their surgery.

Minor labral fraying exists in approximately 20% of shoulders and is rarely the cause of any shoulder joint pain. The type I lesion most likely is the result of age rather than of a specific injury. We debride and smooth any excessive fraying in the labrum, but we also search for an underlying cause of the shoulder pain and do not ascribe pain to what seems to be a relatively minor condition.

The type II lesion, separation of the labrum from the glenoid, raises similar issues. Is this a pathologic entity or simply a variation of normal anatomic structure? Detrisac and Johnson have studied normal labral anatomy extensively.[185] They have found that the labrum is always attached to the underlying glenoid peripherally, with varying attachment of the central edge. Cooper and associates studied 23 fresh frozen cadaver specimens and found that the structure of the superior labrum was distinctly different from that of the inferior labrum.[186] The superior and anterosuperior labra appeared meniscal with a *loose* attachment to the glenoid, which allowed the labrum to be quite mobile.

These findings concur with our clinical experience with separation of the superior labrum from the glenoid. When history of trauma or signs of injury within the joint are lacking, the separation probably represents a normal anatomic variant.

The biceps labrum separation occasionally appears to be the result of trauma, possibly from the mechanism described by Snyder (a fall on the outstretched arm with the humeral head moving superiorly and displacing the biceps labrum complex). In our experience, types II, III, and IV SLAP lesions have often been associated with anteroinferior glenohumeral subluxation or dislocation.

Rodosky and colleagues have demonstrated the stabilizing effect of the biceps labrum junction.[187] In a cadaver study, the biceps labrum junction was divided and an increase in anteroinferior instability was noted. Thus, two or more mechanisms may be involved in a biceps labrum separation—distraction instability or compression avulsion, each of which requires a different treatment.

When the instability is corrected surgically (without treatment of the SLAP lesion) the results have been good. SLAP lesions that exist without glenohumeral instability are repaired arthroscopically. Our results and technique are similar to those of Field and Savoie,[184] who described 20 consecutive patients who obtained a good or excellent result. Other techniques employ a metallic staple, biodegradable SurTac, or Mitek implant suture method. The lesion is exceedingly difficult to repair by open surgical techniques.

In summary, when the SLAP lesion is the result of glenohumeral instability, repair of the instability relieves the patient's symptoms and no specific treatment directed toward the SLAP lesion has been performed. Whether repair of the SLAP lesion in addition to repair of the instability would improve the end result is unknown. When instability is not found, the SLAP lesion should be repaired.

Type III and type IV SLAP lesions cause mechanical symptoms, and thus excision of that portion of the labrum is required. The bucket-handle tear in the superior labrum probably is a result of a compression injury of the humeral head against the glenoid rather than an anteroinferior instability mechanism.

ADHESIVE CAPSULITIS

The orthopedist rarely misses a full-blown case of adhesive capsulitis characterized by severely restricted active and passive motion, insidious onset, and an arthrogram that demonstrates a small capacity joint with obliteration of the axillary recess. The orthopedic surgeon is more likely to be confused by an individual who is either in the beginning or in the end of the adhesive capsulitis process. These individuals have small losses of external rotation at both 0° abduction and 90° abduction. The loss of external rotation does not allow greater tuberosity clearance during arm elevation, and "impingement" results. Treatment is not by acromioplasty but rather by intervention designed to regain normal shoulder movement, biomechanics, and function. If the patient is developing adhesive capsulitis and an acromioplasty (arthroscopic or open), is performed, the surgery is followed by a prolonged postoperative course. The stiffness that was about to occur as part of the natural progression of this disorder is now blamed on the orthopedic surgeon.

Signs of adhesive capsulitis that should alert the surgeon to the true nature of the problem include a decreased range of motion under anesthesia and a difficult entrance into the joint with the cannula. The contracted joint makes movement of the instruments difficult and increases the risk of cartilage damage. Intra-articular signs of adhesive capsulitis include a small axillary recess with or without inflammation.

No distinct scar tissue bands within the joint can be divided because the entire capsule is contracted. Division of the anterior or inferior capsule with a knife is possible but seems dangerous because of the proximity of the neurovascular structures. If manipulation is the surgeon's treatment of choice, the arthroscopy can be performed and a switching stick can be left in the joint. The manipulation then is performed without possible damage to the arthroscope or the joint surfaces. The cannula is introduced over the switching stick and the arthroscope is inserted. This method can confirm that the joint has been located and allows inspection of the rotator cuff for tears.

Adhesive capsulitis remains a challenging clinical problem, and arthroscopy has not contributed significantly to the determination of its etiology, to its diagnosis, or to its management.

ACROMIOCLAVICULAR JOINT ARTHROSCOPY

18

Acromioclavicular joint pain is a common cause for a visit to the orthopedist. When acromioclavicular joint disease is related to a specific injury, the patient can localize the pain to the superior and/or anterior aspects of the joint. The patient may also localize the pain to the joint with demonstrations of painful arm positions used in routine activities of daily living.

Direct palpation of the joint on its anterior and superior surface reproduces the patient's pain. Placing the arm in cross-body adduction or horizontally extending the abducted arm also causes pain in the joint.

Common patient complaints are joint pain experienced while washing the opposite axilla or while attaching the chest portion of a seatbelt. Pain is also reported during pushing activities, such as weight-lifting. Such actions as reaching behind the back to fasten a brassiere or reaching for a wallet in the back pocket place the arm in extension and adduction and can be painful.

None of these symptoms is pathognomonic for acromioclavicular joint disease, but they are useful when combined with appropriate findings from the physical examination.

Common mechanisms of injury are a fall or a direct blow to the lateral or superior aspect of the joint. Probably the most common area of symptomatic overlap exists with rotator cuff disease. Rotator cuff disease may mask a true acromioclavicular joint disorder, an acromioclavicular joint disorder may mask rotator cuff disease, or the two conditions may co-exist.

Rockwood and Matsen have described six types of acromioclavicular joint injury (Fig. 18–1).[188] Acromioclavicular joint dislocations rated type III or higher are not appropriately treated arthroscopically and therefore are not reviewed here.

Type II injuries represent a spectrum of disease and therefore are a gray zone in terms of treatment. If the subluxation is less than 25%, arthroscopic techniques may be considered. If the subluxation is greater than 25%, the arthroscopic approach becomes too technically difficult to be considered reliable because the superior clavicle border is more difficult to resect. More importantly, the pain in primary acromioclavicular joint arthritis is exclusively caused by joint incongruity, but when the injury results in dislocation, instability also comes into consideration.

This added degree of difficulty that accompanies instability is most obvious in the type V injury. The symptoms are not from joint incongruity (the medial

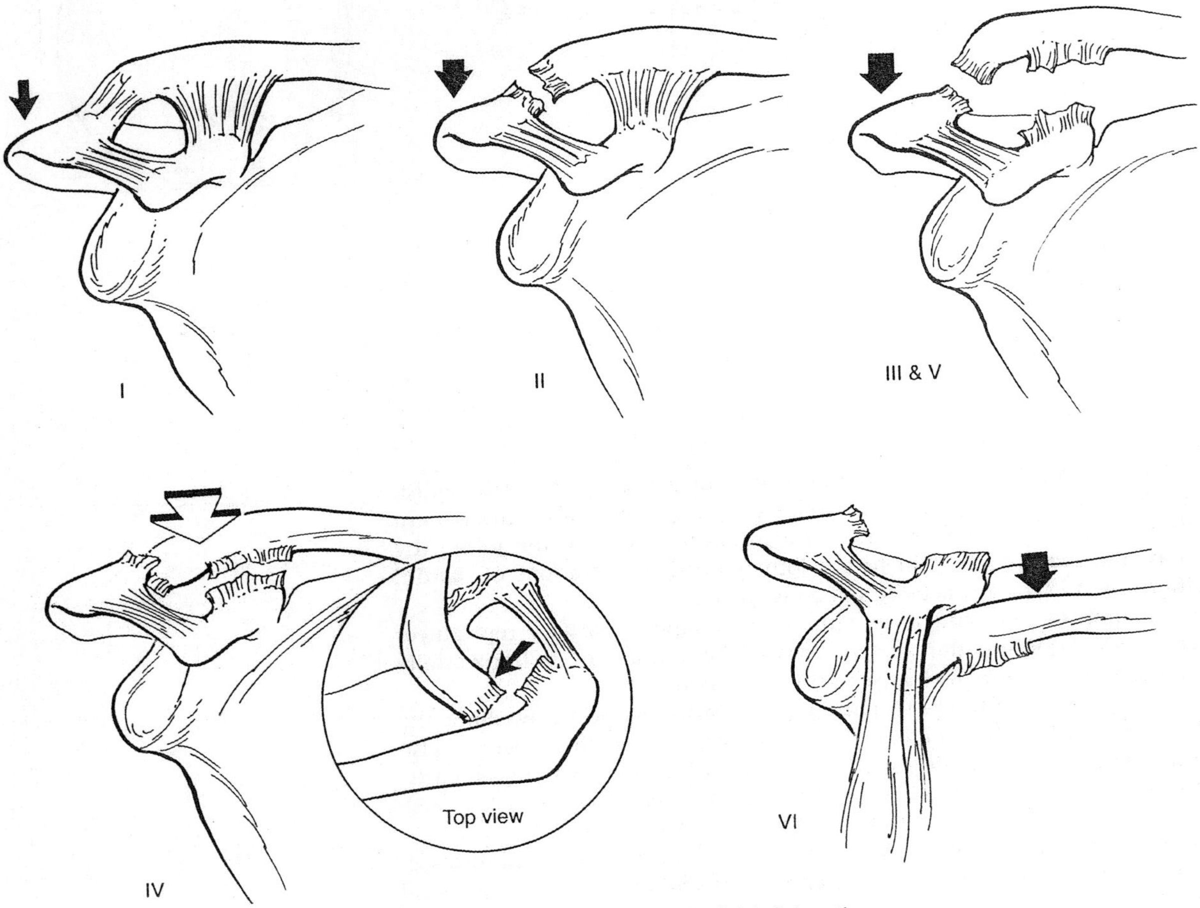

FIG. 18–1. Type I-6 achromoclavicular joint dislocation.

acromion and distal clavicle are not in contact at all), but rather are from the "disconnection" of the arm from the body. The only true joint connection of the arm to the axial skeleton (through the acromioclavicular joint) is lost. In this situation, both the joint integrity and the coracoclavicular ligaments have been destroyed. Thus, the remaining soft tissues in the upper extremity must now support the entire arm. This burden on the remaining soft tissues causes the patient to complain of arm heaviness, pain, or weakness.

Cure requires the re-establishment of distal clavicular stability. Because the arthroscopic approach addresses only joint incongruity, it cannot be recommended for this type of acromioclavicular injury. The successful treatment of type III and type V injuries relies on the repair of the ruptured deltoid-trapezius aponeurosis and the re-establishment of the coracoclavicular connection. Such repair also is not an arthroscopic procedure. Finally, neither type IV injuries (posterior dislocation) nor type VI injuries are treated arthroscopically.

Only the painful type I injury (post-traumatic arthritis), the type II injuries previously described, primary osteoarthritis, rheumatoid arthritis, septic arthritis, and osteolysis of the distal clavicle seem amenable to arthroscopic treatment.

Appropriate arthroscopic treatment requires that the the joint is not dislocated, the coracoclavicular ligaments are intact, and the source of pain is the incongruous joint.

DIAGNOSIS

IMAGING

Acromioclavicular joint disorders are commonly diagnosed with plain radiographs. A 10° acromioclavicular cephalic tilt view demonstrates the increased distance between the clavicle and the coracoid that can accompany injuries. A direct anteroposterior view of the clavicle more accurately projects inferior acromioclavicular joint osteophytes. The axillary radiograph is necessary to determine any significant anterior or posterior displacement, such as the dislocation that might accompany a type IV injury.

As the use of magnetic resonance imaging (MRI) increases, the understanding of its role in the diagnosis of acromioclavicular joint arthritis also increases. At present, the MRI accurately images the acromioclavicular joint but seems oversensitive. Many asymptomatic individuals receive MRI reports of acromioclavicular arthritis.

The clinical diagnosis of acromioclavicular arthritis requires that the history and the physical examination correlate with the radiographic findings. Many patients with joints that appear arthritic on radiographic and MRI studies are asymptomatic and do not require treatment.

INJECTION

The diagnoses of acromioclavicular joint arthritis and rotator cuff disease sometimes are difficult to separate. One method of differentiation requires the selective injection of lidocaine into each area. If all the patient's pain is relieved with a subacromial injection, rotator cuff disease is the likely problem. If the pain is not completely relieved, the acromioclavicular joint then should be injected.

The technique for acromioclavicular joint injection varies from that used to inject the subacromial space. A 25-g short-barrel needle is used, because a longer needle could penetrate the inferior joint capsule and result in an inadvertent subacromial space injection. The skin overlying the superior aspect of the joint is cleaned with a topical disinfectant soap, and the joint then is injected with a local anesthetic. Joint orientation should be gained from radiographs because the acromioclavicular joint may slope or tilt in different directions. The needle is advanced, and if bone is felt, the needle is withdrawn slightly and redirected until the joint is entered. The application of gentle pressure on the plunger allows one to feel the change in resistance after the joint has been entered. Approximately 1 to 2 ml of 2% plain lidocaine is instilled. The joint is so small that only 1 to 2 ml can be injected, and therefore, a stronger anesthetic is used.

The maneuvers in the physical examination that produced the pain in the joint (cross-body adduction, adduction in extension, or horizontal extension of the 90° abducted arm) are then repeated, and the elimination or diminution of the pain is noted. The impingement signs should also be repeated and the effect of this injection recorded. The injection test is positive if the pain is eliminated or markedly reduced. A positive test is strongly suggestive of symptomatic acromioclavicular joint disease.

CONSERVATIVE TREATMENT

Once the diagnosis has been established by appropriate historical, clinical, and radiologic means, treatment is initiated. Most acromioclavicular arthritic conditions can be treated nonoperatively. No long-term prospective or retrospective studies analyzing the natural history of this condition exist, however.

The mainstay of conservative treatment is selective rest. The positions and activities that are painful should be avoided. Certain vocational or avocational activities may require modification or avoidance. The patient is told that the body should remain active, but the injured part, the shoulder, should rest.

Patient education is most beneficial. Patients should be warned against "working through the pain" because the inflamed joint must be allowed to recover. Patients often incorrectly assume that the painful acromioclavicular joint is a muscle strain that should be worked out.

Perhaps the most difficult part for both the patient and the physician is the length of time required for the resolution of symptoms. The patient often assumes that symptoms lasting for 2 to 3 months imply that the condition is permanent and therefore requires a solution. We try to convince the patient that additional time may allow resolution of the symptoms.

The pain of isolated acromioclavicular joint arthritis in our experience is rarely disabling when the conservative care program is followed. The pain may disrupt activities and sleep, but generally the level of pain is moderate enough that the patient can allow conservative treatment to proceed. For this reason, a nonoperative approach is generally tried for a minimum of 6 months.

SURGICAL INDICATIONS

The surgical indications for arthroscopic acromioclavicular joint resection follow.

1. Pain interfering with activities of daily living, work, or sports has been unresponsive to appropriate conservative care for a minimum of 6 months.
2. The acromioclavicular joint has been identified as the source of the disorder by patient history, physical examination, plain radiographs, and, when appropriate, more advanced imaging studies.
3. Preferably a positive injection test.

SURGICAL CONTRAINDICATIONS

Acromioclavicular joint dislocations of types III through VI are not appropriate for arthroscopic acromioclavicular joint resection. An absolute contraindication is the presence of cellulitis or any other skin infection that might allow contamination of the deeper soft tissues.

A relative contraindication is the type II acromioclavicular dislocation in which a determination as to whether the patient is symptomatic from joint incongruity, joint instability, or a combination of these two factors is difficult to make.

OPERATIVE TECHNIQUE

The surgical treatment of acromioclavicular joint arthritis has traditionally been open resection of the distal clavicle. This treatment accomplishes two goals. The abnormal clavicular articular surface is removed, and enough space is created between the medial acromion and the remaining distal clavicle to eliminate painful contact between these two bones during shoulder movements. The arthroscopic approach similarly involves removal of the clavicular articular surface but also creates space by removing a small amount of medial acromion and correspondingly less bone from the distal clavicle (Fig. 18–2). We have termed this procedure arthroscopic resection of the acromioclavicular joint.

Patient preparation, set-up, and instrumentation for glenohumeral arthroscopy are described in Chapter 3. All patients undergo diagnostic evaluation of the glenohumeral joint and operative arthroscopy of intra-articular lesions as appropriate. The acromioclavicular joint is approached through the subacromial space rather than by a direct transcutaneous entry as advocated by Flatow and associates.[189] A large cannula and trocar are inserted into the subacromial space through the posterior skin incision. The positions of the cannula and trocar are confirmed by palpation of the acromial undersurface. A long blunt rod is inserted through the posterior cannula to exit the anterior skin incision. The anterior cannula is inserted over the rod and the fluid inflow is connected. An inspection of the subacromial space is performed. If the subacromial space is clearly visualized, a spinal needle is placed to confirm the precise spot for entry of the lateral cannula, and an incision is made. The cannula and trocar are inserted, and the instruments are brought in through the lateral cannula.

If the subacromial space is not clearly visualized because of subacromial fibrosis and/or bursitis, the space is cleared as described in Chapter 4. The motorized soft tissue meniscal cutter is inserted through the lateral portal and the anteromedial aspect of the acromion is identified (Fig. 18–3). The introduction of spinal needles to identify the margins of the acromion may be helpful. Soft tissue is removed from the acromial undersurface until the bone is clearly visible

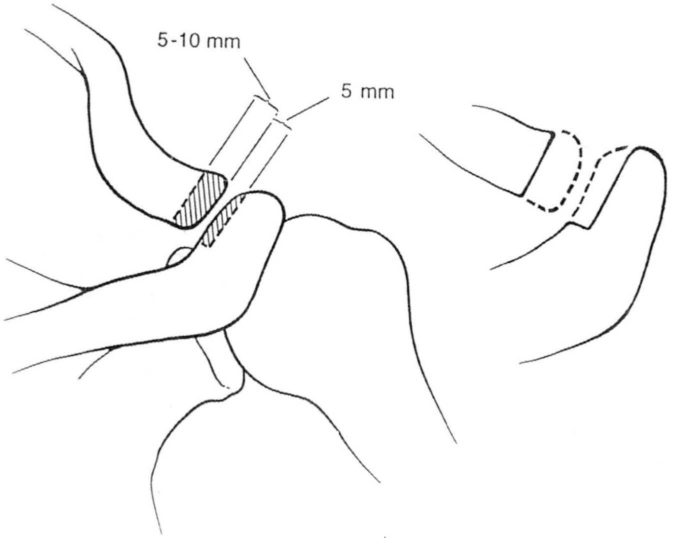

FIG. 18–2. Hatched area represents desired bone removal.

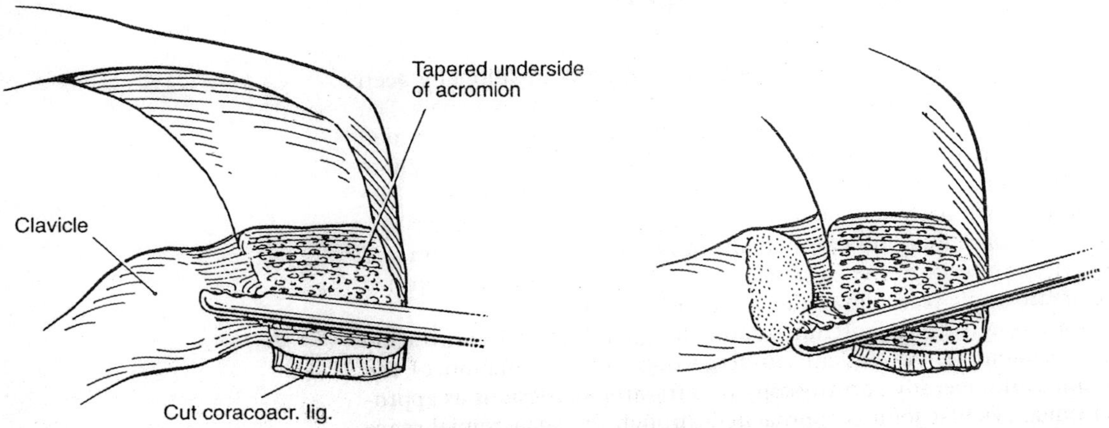

FIGS. 18–3 and 18–4. Acromioplasty and acromioclavicular joint resection combined. Inferior acromioclavicular joint ligaments removed to expose acromioclavicular joint.

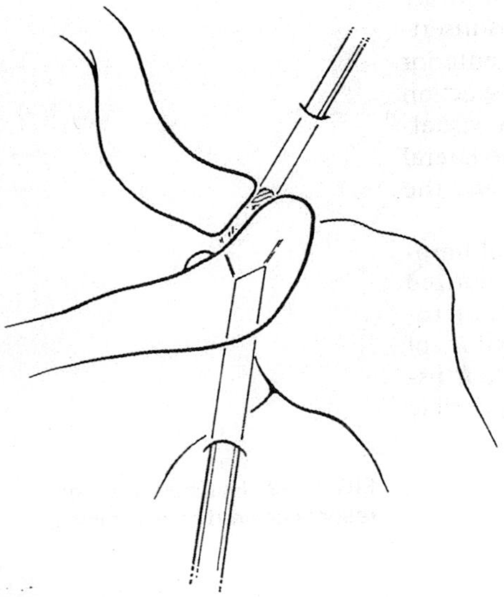

FIG. 18–5. Bur placement anterior to acromioclavicular joint and parallel to joint surfaces.

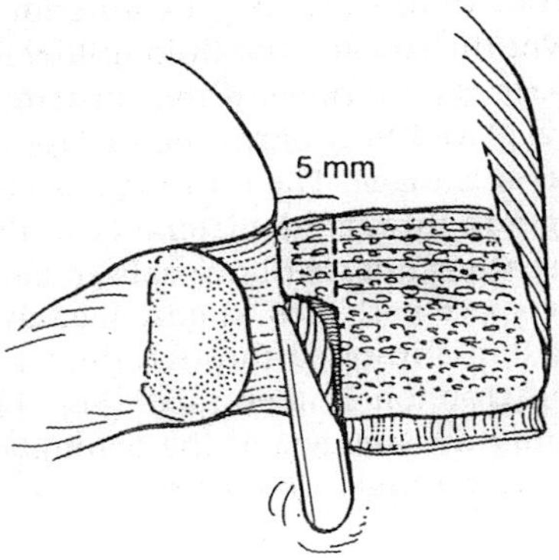

FIG. 18–6. Bur removes 5.5-mm strip of medial acromion.

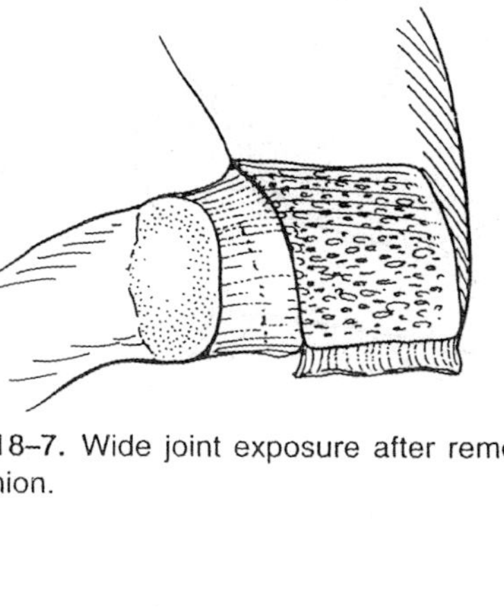

FIG. 18–7. Wide joint exposure after removal of medial acromion.

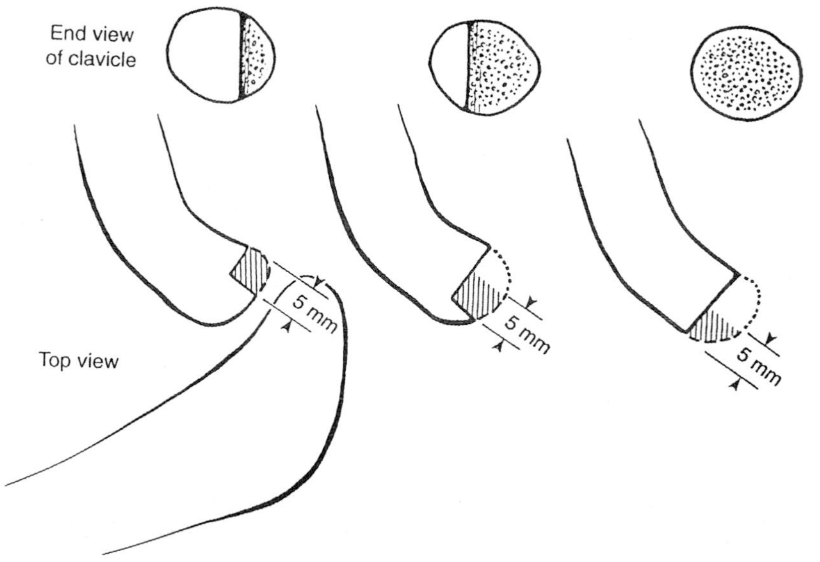

FIG. 18–8. End view of the distal clavicle demonstrating the sequential removal of bone from anterior to posterior.

(Fig. 18–4). Bleeding is controlled by using electrocautery, adjusting fluid pressure, and maintaining the patient's blood pressure at a systolic level of less than 90 mm Hg. Once the medial acromial border is identified and the soft tissue under the acromioclavicular joint is noted, electrocautery is used to coagulate any identifiable vessels near the undersurface of the joint. We have found that coagulation of this quite vascular area prior to entering the joint is helpful.

Once the medial border is identified and the area has been coagulated, the meniscal cutter is removed. The inflow cannula is moved to the lateral portal and the acromionizer bur is inserted anteriorly (Fig. 18–5). Acromial bone is resected from the anteromedial border of the acromion to the posteromedial border. When the acromial (medial) border of the acromioclavicular joint is removed, two goals are achieved. The first goal is the creation of a 5.5-mm (1 bur width) space between the distal clavicle and the remaining acromion (Fig. 18–6). The second and most important goal is the complete visualization of the distal clavicle from the subacromial space. Once the medial acromion is removed, the distal clavicle can be clearly visualized (Fig. 18–7).

Soft tissue elements that obscure the distal clavicle are removed with an appropriate motorized cutter. Once the bone surface of the distal clavicle is visualized, its anteroposterior, superior, and inferior margins can be located. A bur's width of bone (5.5 mm) from the anterior border of the distal clavicle is removed from its inferior cortex to the superior cortex. Resection of the distal clavicle is continued in an anterior to posterior direction while always attempting to keep the amount of bone removal constant (Fig. 18–8). Once bone removal has been completed, any inferior clavicular osteophytes are removed. The superior acromioclavicular joint capsule and ligaments remain intact. This procedure creates an 11-mm space between the distal clavicle and the medial acromion (Fig. 18–9).

The arthroscope is then placed in the anterior cannula, which now occupies the space of the resected acromioclavicular joint. The space is viewed directly, the arm is taken through a range of motion, and any contact area is noted. If more bone removal is needed, a spinal needle is inserted percutaneously though

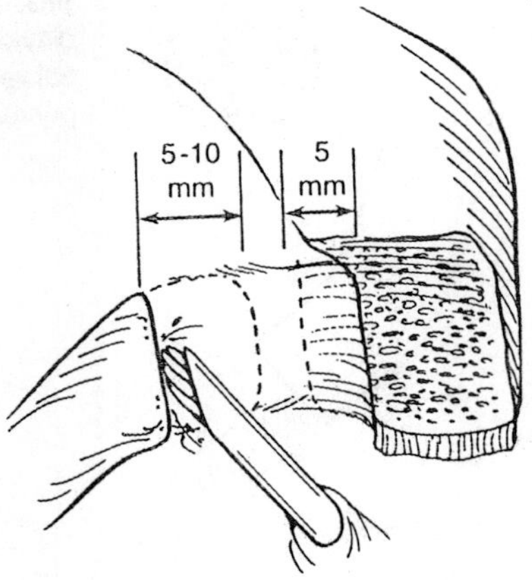

FIG. 18-9. Further bone may be removed to achieve the desired space between the distal clavicle and the medial acromion.

the posterior aspect of the joint, a small incision is made, and a cannula and trocar are introduced. A 4-mm oval bur is inserted and bone is removed as necessary.

The distal clavicle occasionally is difficult to see if soft tissue swelling becomes excessive. As the swelling increases, both the distance and the angle from the arthroscope to the clavicle are altered. This problem occurs more often in large (>100 kg) individuals, in older patients >65 years), and with prolonged operating time (>45 min). When this situation occurs, the arthroscope is moved to the lateral cannula and the inflow cannula is placed through the posterior portal. The end of the clavicle is then seen directly, and bone resection is performed more easily.

Arthroscopic acromioclavicular joint resection is complete when the following six criteria have been met.

1. A strip of medial acromion measuring 5.5 mm in width and extending in length from the anterior border to the posterior border of the distal clavicle has been removed.
2. 5.5 mm of the distal clavicle have been removed.
3. Any inferior projections of the distal clavicle have been removed.
4. No sharp edges have been left on the anterior, posterior, superior, or inferior surfaces of the distal clavicle.
5. The superior surface of the clavicle has been clearly visualized and the superior acromioclavicular joint fibers have been identified but not excised.
6. A 5- to 15-mm space has been created. No impingement from the distal clavicle to the acromion is noted when the arm is adducted across the chest to check anterior clearance and is horizontally extended to check posterior clearance. This observation is made with the arthroscope directly in the joint.

The arthroscope and cannulas are removed, and the incisions are closed with simple sutures. A sterile dressing is applied. The surgery is performed on an outpatient basis unless medical conditions warrant inpatient admission.

OPERATIVE FINDINGS

Common operative findings include a thickened subacromial bursa that requires resection, complete or partial loss of cartilage covering the distal end of the clavicle, cystic changes in the distal clavicle, and meniscal fragmentation. Meniscal abnormalities are most common in younger patients. Whether these younger patients with meniscal disorders can be treated by meniscus excision alone or whether distal clavicle excision is always needed is not known. At present, the data to support soft tissue resection alone are not adequate. We have chosen to always combine meniscus excision with distal clavicle resection.

INTRAOPERATIVE COMPLICATIONS

Intraoperative complications are infrequent. We have never seen any nerve or vascular injuries or ectopic bone formation. One of our patients developed a superficial wound infection that cleared with oral antibiotic management.

TECHNICAL TIPS FOR OPERATIVE PROBLEMS

Most operative problems are technical difficulties related to the position of the cannula, inadequate inflow, bleeding, bur/lens contact, and inappropriate area or amount of bone resection.

POSITION OF CANNULA

Three portals are used for this procedure. The posterior portal is the viewing portal through which the arthroscope is placed. The lateral portal and the anterior portal each have dual roles. The lateral portal is initially a working portal through which the soft tissue cutter, electrocautery instrument, and then the power bur are placed and may be used as a viewing portal. The anterior portal starts out as an inflow portal, then becomes a working portal, and ends as a viewing portal. As in any arthroscopic operation, the position of the cannulas is important, and small errors in their placement can lead to technical difficulties during surgery.

The operative procedure just described used a gravity inflow system. The use of an arthroscopic pump simplifies this procedure greatly by eliminating the inflow portal and allowing pump-controlled changes in pressure and flow rate to improve visualization.

POSTERIOR PORTAL

Problem: Too medial. Small changes in the placement of a portal cause altered views of the desired area. When the cannula is placed too far medially, the joint is viewed tangentially. Consequently, resection of the posterior aspect of the medial acromion and exposure of the posterior aspect of the acromioclavicular joint become difficult. The surgeon discovers that increased torque is required to keep the joint in view.

Solution. If a 30° scope is being used, a switch to a 70° scope gives the desired view. A better solution, however, is the creation of a new posterolateral portal as described in Chapter 2.

Problem. Too inferior. This problem starts when the initial portal into the glenohumeral joint is placed in the posterior soft spot. Although this portal affords an excellent view of the joint, use of this skin incision to enter the subacromial space and work on the acromioclavicular joint forces the surgeon to angle the arthroscope sharply in a superior direction. The acromion is well visualized, but the scope cannot be directed medially enough to get a clear view of the acromioclavicular joint.

Solution. Place the initial posterior portal more superiorly. Placement of the skin incision 1 cm medial and 1 cm inferior to the posterolateral corner of the acromion allows an excellent view of the glenohumeral joint and also allows a more parallel entry into the subacromial space. If the initial portal is made too inferiorly or the cannula position is unsatisfactory because of the soft tissue swelling that can accompany this procedure, this portal should be abandoned and a separate posterolateral portal should be created.

General Comments. These problems can be minimized by performing the initial soft tissue resection and then rapidly moving the arthroscope to the lateral portal and using the posterior portal for inflow. The posterior viewing portal has not been abandoned in favor of the lateral portal for several reasons. The surgeon uses the posterior portal during all other arthroscopic procedures. Thus, orientation is maintained. This portal arrangement allows excellent visualization for an initial inspection of the subacromial space, clearing of the pathologic subacromial bursa, identification of the acromioclavicular joint, and initial bone resection. With the arthroscope in the posterior rather than the lateral portal, the scope can be directed more superiorly, and the superior margins of the resected anterior acromion and clavicle can be well visualized. These critical areas can be difficult to view when the arthroscope is in the lateral portal.

LATERAL PORTAL

As noted previously, the lateral portal is placed 1 cm posterior to and 2 to 3 cm distal to the anterior acromial edge. If the cannula is placed too distally, the axillary nerve is in jeopardy. Placement of the lateral portal too far posteriorly is rarely a significant problem.

Problem. Placement of the lateral portal too far anteriorly interferes with visualization of the anterior distal clavicle and particularly of the anterosuperior edge of the medial acromion. As the operation progresses, soft tissue swelling accentuates this problem and results in inadequate bone resection.

Solution. Switch the arthroscope back to the posterior portal to obtain a good view of the anterosuperior aspect of the joint. Create a new lateral or posterolateral portal.

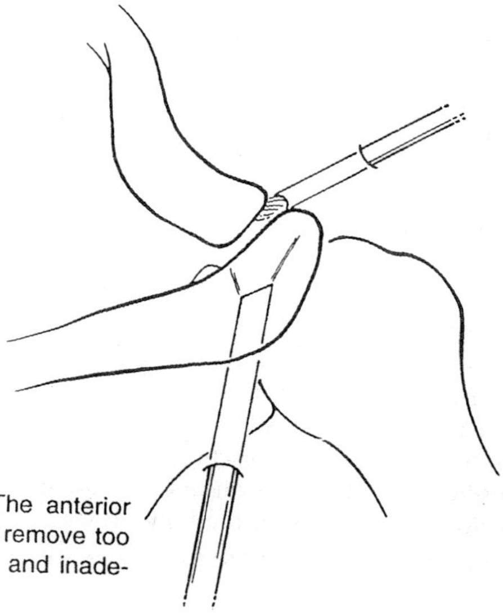

FIG. 18–10. Inappropriate bur placement. The anterior portal is too lateral. The surgeon will tend to remove too much bone from the posterior distal clavicle and inadequate bone from its anterior aspect.

ANTERIOR PORTAL

Problem. The most frequent difficulty with anterior portal placement is that the portal is made too far laterally. This location causes the instruments to approach the acromioclavicular joint obliquely. Thus, excessive bone resection anteriorly and inadequate bone resection posteriorly occur (Fig. 18–10).

Solution. Avoid the problem. Mark the acromioclavicular joint with a surgical pen prior to making the skin incision or identify the joint with a spinal needle. Replace the cannula directly anterior to the acromioclavicular joint.

INFLOW

Good fluid inflow is mandatory. A large inflow cannula provides excellent visualization but care must be taken to continually check the position of the cannula. Movement of the instruments and distention of soft tissues may allow the cannula to withdraw from the subacromial space, thereby resulting in extravasated fluid that may contribute to the surgeon's difficulty.

An arthroscopic pump simplifies this problem. The surgeon, however, should not try to compensate for poor placement of the cannula or for poor hemostasis by making nonphysiologic alterations in the pump pressure.

BLEEDING

The major areas of bleeding particular to this procedure are the inferior and posterior aspects of the acromioclavicular joint. Before any soft tissue is resected near the medial acromial border, the entire area should be cauterized by using the coagulating current of the electrocautery device. After the soft tissue has been resected and the medial acromion has been removed, the distal clavicle is visualized well. Again, observe the inferior aspect of the distal clavicle, but at this point, pay greater attention to the inferoposterior aspect and cauterize this area prior to any bone resection.

The other area of bleeding involves coracoacromial ligament resection, which is covered in Chapter 4.

BUR/LENS CONTACT

One of the difficulties that accompanies arthroscopic work in the subacromial space is the proximity of motorized instruments to the lens of the arthroscope. As a general rule, the distance from the scope to the instruments should be maximized by taking advantage of the scope angle. This increase in distance results in increased safety, as well as in a less magnified, wider field of vision. Always try to begin the bone resection close to the lens and then cut away from the arthroscope. Because the distance is small, spinning of the bur always should start prior to contact with the bone. If started while in contact with the bone, the bur may "jump" and consequently nick the scope lens.

BONE RESECTION

The relationship between the acromioclavicular joint and the distal clavicle is difficult to grasp when viewed from the subacromial space. The best way to appreciate the true location of the joint is to start with a routine subacromial decompression. At the end of the procedure, identify the anteromedial border of the acromion and the medial acromial wall. With the acromionizer bur in the lateral portal, start to resect bone in a medial direction beginning just posterior to the anteromedial acromial border. After 1 to 5 mm of bone have been resected, the sensation of "breaking through" occurs and meniscal soft tissue or the distal clavicle cartilaginous surface is seen. At this point, the remaining medial acromion is easily removed in a posterior to anterior direction. The location of the joint and the angle at which the clavicle approaches the subacromial space can then be appreciated. When repeated four to five times, this procedure facilitates a formal arthroscopic acromioclavicular joint resection.

Each of the following steps in the acromioclavicular joint resection can be simplified with a few comments. These steps are (1) identification of the anteromedial acromial border, (2) identification of the portion of the medial acromion that marks the posterior limit of bone resection (posteromedial margin), (3) resection of the superior margin of the anteromedial acromion and anterior distal clavicle, and (4) estimation of the amount of bone resected.

1. Identification of the anteromedial border. One way to identify this area is to insert a spinal needle percutaneously prior to the start of the procedure. The acromioclavicular joint is palpated, and a needle is inserted directly through the anterior aspect of the joint or just anterior to the joint. When the subacromial space is well visualized, the needle can be seen clearly and serves as a guide to bone resection. Visualization of the medial aspect of the subacromial space to find the anterior border of the acromion may be done as easily. An inferior osteophyte often projects toward the rotator cuff. If the joint area cannot be seen immediately, start with the motorized cutter and begin to remove soft tissue at the area you believe to be the anterior margin. Once the soft tissue has been

removed, the acromion can be identified easily and followed to its anteromedial margin.

2. Identification of the posteromedial margin. The posterior limit of medial acromial resection is approximately 2 mm posterior to the posterior aspect of the distal clavicle. Usually this site can be seen with the arthroscope in the posterior portal and always can be visualized with the arthroscope in either the posterolateral or the lateral portal. The amount of bone resected must be sufficient to ensure that the posterior aspect of the distal clavicle will not impinge upon the posterior portion of the medial acromion.
3. Resection of the superior margin. The superior border of the distal clavicle and the medial acromion may be incompletely resected because of a lack of visualization. If this area is palpated with the bur and bone is felt, more resection is needed. If only soft tissue is felt, bone resection may be complete, but palpation alone is not a reliable guide. The area should be viewed directly to confirm adequate bone removal (see Fig. 18–7).
   If the area cannot be seen when the scope is inserted maximally and rotated to look directly at this area, the surgeon has two options: (1) To switch to a 70 or 90° arthroscope, or (2) to create a portal at the posterosuperior aspect of the acromioclavicular joint and insert the scope at that location. These options give a direct view of the desired area, as does a view from the anterior cannula.
4. Estimation of the amount of bone resected. This area is often of most concern to surgeons beginning their experience with either arthroscopic subacromial decompression or distal clavicle resection. Two approaches are helpful. The surgeon must decide preoperatively how much bone to remove. This decision is based on the plain radiographs. Initially, we resected 15 to 20 mm of bone in an attempt to duplicate arthroscopically the traditional open distal clavicle resection. As our experience has increased, the amount of bone we resect has decreased because we have been able to produce successful clinical results with only 5 to 10 mm of bone removal.

The surgeon should keep in mind the amount of desired bone removal, and should remove the bone according to the techniques previously described. The amount of bone removed is measured by placing an object of known size, commonly the 5.5-mm acromionizer bur, into the area and judging the quantity of bone removed on the basis of bur diameter, e.g., 1 diameter = 5.5 mm, 2 diameters = 11 mm, 1.5 diameters = 8.25 mm.

POSTOPERATIVE MANAGEMENT

A sling is worn for 1 day, and the patient is started on exercises beginning on the first postoperative day. Pendulum exercises are advised as a gentle warm-up. Active and passive elevation and external rotation movements are aided with a dowel rod. The patient is encouraged to use the arm as normally as possible, but is discouraged from overhead work or sports until discomfort is minimal and movement and strength have returned. The patient is started on a program of isometric and isokinetic strengthening 1 week postoperatively and is permitted to resume work or sports under the previously mentioned conditions. The stretching program advances to internal rotation (behind the back) and cross-body adduction as tolerated to regain posterior capsule and rotator cuff flexibility.

CLINICAL RESULTS

Because this technique is new, the literature is relatively scarce. Evidence reveals that an adequate resection of the distal clavicle can be performed in a laboratory setting utilizing arthroscopic techniques.[190] Flatow and colleagues,[189] Whipple,[191] Snyder and co-workers,[192] and Detrisac and Johnson[185] have been early contributors to the literature. One study reported good results in 17 of 20 patients. The 3 failures were all caused by lack of adequate bone resection, which was a finding documented at the time of open conventional surgery. Resection of the remaining bone converted these failures to good results.[193]

Arthroscopic acromioclavicular joint resection seems to be well founded in theory, and the early clinical results seem supportive.

SECTION

RELATED CONSIDERATIONS

SPORTS INJURIES

Shoulder injuries that occur during sports should not be isolated from the entire spectrum of shoulder problems.[132,194–199] The pathologic processes that involve the shoulder structures are similar whether the condition started in a baseball game or by raising a garage door. Nonetheless, specific abnormalities regularly occur in certain sporting activities.

GOLF

Shoulder problems related to golf can be divided into those that involve the dominant shoulder and those that involve the nondominant shoulder.[200]

NONDOMINANT SHOULDER

Golfers commonly complain of posterior shoulder pain that occurs during the backswing. Posterior capsule and rotator cuff tightness causes two problems. First, the contracted structures sustain traction lesions because they are not pliable enough to allow the desired movement. Second, posterior capsule contracture results in increased anterosuperior translation of the humeral head and rotator cuff tendons. This translation causes the tendons to contact the rigid coracoacromial arch and thereby produces impingement.

This condition is treated with a stretching program to regain flexibility in the posterior rotator cuff and capsule. The traction stress on the posterior structures is diminished, and the elimination of the posterior contracture decreases the obligate humeral head translation and minimizes or eliminates impingement symptoms. Occasionally, this approach is unsuccessful; arthroscopic treatment consisting of acromioplasty then is performed.

IMPINGEMENT

The obligatory impingement that results from a posterior contracture, if untreated, may lead to fibrotic changes within the rotator cuff and subacromial bursa that result in stage II impingement. This result most often occurs with structural abnormalities already present in the shoulder, such as a prominent anterolateral acromial osteophyte, inferior acromioclavicular joint osteophytes, or a type III acromion. At this point, even though flexibility in the posterior cuff and capsule has been regained, an arthroscopic decompression is required.

ADHESIONS

Occasionally, either with a single traumatic event or with repeated inflammation, the posterior cuff and deltoid become adherent and lead to persistent complaints of posterosuperior shoulder pain during the backswing. The joint is normal when viewed arthroscopically. The adhesions are plica-like and are seen in the subacromial bursa. Usually the arthroscope is inserted anteriorly to allow the surgeon to visualize the posterior structures more easily. One or more fibrous bands are noted and can be easily resected. Whether these adhesions represent inflammatory response to a traction tendinitis or are the result of a bursal surface partial rotator cuff tear is unclear.

ACROMIOCLAVICULAR JOINT

Another nondominant shoulder problem involves the acromioclavicular joint. This problem occurs during the backswing as the arm is adducted across the chest. The golfer attempts to limit pain by raising the arms in front of the body rather than by raising them in the adducted position. This adjustment causes an outside-to-inside swing path, and the resulting slice is infinitely more painful than the localized tenderness noted on examination of the acromioclavicular joint.

SUBLUXATION

A complete follow-through places the nondominant shoulder in a position of abduction and external rotation. A subtle instability may become symptomatic at this time. The patient may experience the sensation of the shoulder "slipping out of place," but more commonly, pain is noted in the area of the posterior glenohumeral joint line. Attempts to limit the amount of external rotation require increased abduction and inhibit squaring of the clubface at impact. Shots pushed to the right result.

DOMINANT SHOULDER

IMPINGEMENT

Impingement is most commonly noted during the full follow-through. As the arm is brought into flexion, the rotator cuff can contact the subacromial arch. Lack of posterior flexibility aggravates this problem, but unless significant structural bone abnormalities as previously described are present, a conservative program generally is effective.

SUBLUXATION

In an individual with ligamentous laxity, the power of the golf swing creates a distraction force of sufficient magnitude to cause anteroinferior subluxation and a labral tear. This injury results in pain from a mechanical source within the joint. Arthroscopy allows correction of the labral abnormality. In the rare instance when the subluxation occurs at the completion of the swing, posterior subluxation can result as the arm is rapidly brought into a position of adduction and internal rotation. Treatment involves a good rehabilitation program that pays particular attention to external rotation strengthening. The arthroscopic findings are minimal, and if the problem is refractory to conservative care, an open reconstruction is generally required.

ROTATOR CUFF INTERVAL

An interesting area of pain in the golfer's dominant shoulder is localized anterosuperiorly. The pain is more anterior than the classic pain from impingement and is more superior than the pain caused by subluxation or anterior labrum tears. The golfer may have a history of striking the ground hard with the golf club either during an attempt to produce extra power or as an angry reaction to a poor shot. The physical examination demonstrates normal stability and rotator cuff strength, but pain is produced during resisted internal rotation, thumb-up abduction, and palm-up flexion (Speed's test). Findings of the arthroscopic examination are localized to the rotator cuff interval, which is the area between the superior border of the subscapularis and the anterior border of the supraspinatus. Tears are seen in the superior glenohumeral ligament, the superior edge of the subscapularis, the biceps tendon, or the anterior border of the supraspinatus. Most individuals do not improve with arthroscopic debridement or acromioplasty and thus require an open repair of the rotator cuff interval.

PITCHING

SUBLUXATION

Most shoulder pains in the athlete who performs throwing motions are caused by rotator cuff problems secondary to instability and may range from traction tendinitis to partial or full-thickness rotator cuff tears.[130,201–205] The throwing action is so rapid that the patient's perception of exactly when in the throwing cycle the pain occurs may not be valid. More accurate data have been provided by videotape and electromyographic analysis.

Posterosuperior pain during the end of the cocking and the beginning of the acceleration is the result of anteroinferior subluxation. The mechanism for this problem, although not clear, probably relates to traction of the posterior capsule or labrum compression. This abnormality should not be confused with a posterior subluxation or a rotator cuff tendinitis. Pain localized posteriorly during the examination with the arm placed in abduction and external rotation helps to confirm this diagnosis. More subtle instabilities can be brought out by the resisted throwing test and the relocation test described in Chapter 12. Arthroscopy may be indicated in these individuals for arthroscopic correction of a Bankart lesion, diagnosis of a capsular problem that requires open surgical treatment, or diagnosis of co-existing labral and partial rotator cuff tears on the articular and/or bursal surfaces.

Posterior shoulder pain may not always be the result of anterior subluxation and the resulting traction tendinitis to the rotator cuff. Posterior subluxation can occur during the follow-through as the arm is decelerated and brought into a position of cross-body adduction and internal rotation. Arthroscopy can help to confirm the diagnosis of posteroinferior instability and may be corrective if labral tears and/or loose bodies have created a mechanical source of pain.

LOOSE BODIES

Occasionally a loose body is noted. Unless proved otherwise, these bodies are secondary to instability, and although their arthroscopic removal may occasionally give temporary symptomatic relief, surgical reconstruction to correct the instability is generally required. Labrum tears found in stable shoulders can be successfully treated by arthroscopic debridement, but when these tears are secondary to instability, debridement alone is not sufficient.

SLAP LESION

The SLAP lesion has 3 causes in the athlete who throws: (1) the lesion results from a traumatic subluxation, (2) the lesion is a response to anterior instability, and (3) the lesion is a result of avulsion from a fall on the elbow or outstretched arm.

1. The lesion may be a result of a traumatic subluxation or dislocation in which the anterior ligaments are torn from their glenoid attachments and the tear continues superiorly to involve the superior labrum. Correction requires stabilization of the anterior ligaments. Whether the SLAP lesion must also be repaired is not known, but we advise doing so.

2. The microtrauma of repetitive throwing can lead to increased anterior laxity and translation. Because biceps labrum detachment allows increased translation, increased humeral head translation probably causes increased stress on the labrum attachment site.

3. A SLAP lesion that is the result of macrotrauma by direct compression of the humeral head into the glenoid or superior displacement from a fall on the elbow is treated differently. These individuals have stable shoulders. The symptoms are caused by the labrum lesion, which is best treated with arthroscopic repair of the SLAP lesion as described previously.

WEIGHT-LIFTING

LABRUM TEARS

The highly compressive stress placed on the shoulder during weight-lifting can result in labrum tears to the anterior and posteroinferior glenoid labrum.[206] Pain from mechanical irritation of the labral fragment can be corrected by arthroscopic debridement. An evaluation can be made during arthroscopy as to the presence of posterior subluxation.

ROTATOR CUFF

The weight-lifter often has difficulty determining whether the pain experienced during the sport is resulting in increased muscle strength or is causing damage. Adequate warm-up, appropriate training, and proper lifting techniques are essential. If a stage II impingement does not respond to nonoperative care, arthroscopic decompression can be useful. Full-thickness rotator cuff tears pose additional problems. In general, these athletes require all available strength, and thus, rotator cuff repair, open or arthroscopic, seems advisable. Arthroscopic debridement without repair may benefit individuals who complain only of pain but do not experience any loss of strength and/or individuals for whom the time required to recover from rotator cuff repair is prohibitive.

BICEPS TENDON

Biceps tendinitis can occur without subacromial impingement in the weight-lifter. During arthroscopy, inflammation can be seen in the intra-articular portion of the tendon. More commonly, however, the abnormality is in the extra-articular area, which can be brought into the joint by pulling on the tendon with the anterior cannula. Biceps tenodesis may not be desired because small amounts of strength loss can be critical. Tenosynovectomy or transverse humeral ligament division are alternatives to biceps tenodesis.[207]

ACROMIOCLAVICULAR JOINT

Osteolysis and localized acromioclavicular joint arthritis occur in weight-lifters. If not improved with appropriate conservative care, surgical treatment for these problems is appropriate. Resection of the distal clavicle is curative, but the resultant decrease in strength may not be acceptable. Resection of the medial aspect of the joint, the medial acromial border, may diminish pain while allowing maintenance of clavicle length and, hopefully, strength.[208]

INSTABILITY

Instability is commonly seen in the weight-lifter's shoulder, particularly during the bench press. The arm is placed in the position of abduction, and if balance is lost and the weight moves superiorly, the arm is brought into external rotation and horizontal extension. A traumatic subluxation or dislocation can occur. Recurrent instability hampers performance and could prove damaging if another dislocation occurs with a heavy load. Surgical correction is advised if the individual wishes to continue participating in this sport.

Posterior instability can occur as the shoulders are adducted and internally rotated during certain exercises.

More subtle instabilities are brought out by a combination of posterior capsular tightness and relative weakness of the rotator cuff. The posterior capsular contracture increases anterior translation. The weight-lifter increases the strength of the deltoid without a parallel increase in cuff strength. The shoulder is therefore "out of balance," and instability can result. Arthroscopy may confirm the absence of any significant intra-articular findings that could hinder a cure effected through a well-supervised rehabilitation program of stretching and strengthening.

ARTHRITIS

Perhaps the most unusual finding in the weight-lifter's shoulder is the presence of arthritic changes. These changes may range from localized areas of damage to severe advanced arthritis of the glenohumeral joint. Advanced arthritis is seen on a plain radiograph, but early degenerative changes that are not detectable can occur in the glenohumeral joint. Out experience has ranged from patients with small chondral defects in otherwise normal cartilage to those with significant degrees of cartilage thinning and larger areas of cartilage loss. Arthroscopy helps to make this diagnosis and thus allows effective counseling to be performed. Loose cartilage, labrum fragments, or loose bodies can be removed to provide some temporary relief.

VOLLEYBALL

SUBLUXATION

Rotator cuff pain during serving and/or spiking motions may be secondary to underlying instability. The extremes of external rotation in the 90° abducted position seen in the volleyball serve and spike place great stresses on the glenohumeral joint. If the static restraints are not intact, a traction tendinitis develops. Arthroscopic findings are minimal in terms of the rotator cuff. The glenohumeral ligament attachments usually are normal, but a common finding is laxity of the middle glenohumeral ligament. Open capsular reconstruction is required in refractory cases.

A particular problem for the volleyball player involves posterior pain during the "bump." The downward traction during the "bump" can tear the inferior glenohumeral ligaments anteriorly or posteriorly. More likely, prolonged traction over a period of time can gradually attenuate the glenohumeral ligaments and capsule, thereby causing instability. Arthroscopic findings demonstrate a large inferior recess. Correction is accomplished by open surgical capsular repair.

SUPRASCAPULAR NERVE

Suprascapular nerve problems have been described in the volleyball player and may result in decreased cuff function.[209]

The resulting decreased humeral head depression may result in the symptoms of "impingement." Arthroscopy may help to document the absence of any "impingement signs" in the subacromial space or glenohumeral joint. Suprascapular nerve palsy and/or entrapment are best documented with electromyography.

SWIMMING

Shoulder problems in competitive swimmers are common,[210–214] but problems requiring arthroscopic evaluation are rare.

LABRUM LESIONS

McMaster has described the anterior labral lesion in competitive swimmers.[182] The swimmer notes pain when the hand enters into the water, and the patient can often recall an episode of the shoulder "going out." Physical examination demonstrates pain when the arm is adducted and internally rotated. The patient is not apprehensive when the arm is stressed during the instability examination. The arthroscopic finding is a torn anterior labrum without glenohumeral ligament detachment. Debridement has been uniformly successful.

INSTABILITY

Most competitive swimmers have substantial shoulder joint laxity, and without proper rotator cuff, deltoid, and scapular muscle conditioning, problems of instability can result. Excessive translation occasionally leads to subluxation, consequently causing a labrum tear. Symptoms of anterior joint pain, grinding, and pain with translation can be confirmed arthroscopically as arising from a torn labrum. Good relief of pain can be accomplished through arthroscopic debridement, as previously mentioned, but the relief in this instance is only temporary because the labrum tear is not the sole cause of pain, but is a result of instability. The challenge to the orthopedist is to determine which shoulders are painful solely as a result of the labrum tear and which shoulders are painful from labrum damage that is itself merely the result of an underlying pathologic process.

IMPINGEMENT

Most shoulder complaints in the swimmer are caused by rotator cuff tendinitis. A primary injury to the rotator cuff rarely is the cause. More commonly this "pseudo-impingement" is the result of trapezius muscle fatigue, which produces a lack of scapular synchrony and contact of the rotator cuff against the acromial edge. Arthroscopic examination may help to define the status of the rotator cuff and the glenohumeral joint in the high-level competitive swimmer, but it is unlikely to prove curative. The condition is not treated by subacromial decompression but rather by a well-organized rehabilitation program aimed at restoring strength to the scapular muscles.

GYMNASTICS

The gymnast shares a similar situation with the swimmer. The high demand of the sport is combined with a patient population that has greater-than-normal ligament laxity.

The high impact and muscular forces generated during competitive gymnastics can result in labrum injuries and partial rotator cuff tears diagnosed and managed arthroscopically as previously described. Temporary benefit is the rule, but caution must be applied because these problems may be the result of instability that will require surgical correction.

SKIING

Injuries to the shoulder that occur while skiing are numerous and include dislocation, rotator cuff tears, acromioclavicular joint separations, and isolated fractures.[215] These injuries can be managed as previously described.

GREATER TUBEROSITY FRACTURE

Most minimally or nondisplaced greater tuberosity fractures heal uneventfully. Persistent pain may require further investigation. In an individual with a type III acromion, minimal displacement may be sufficient to cause impingement that is refractory to nonoperative care. Arthroscopic subacromial decompression then is necessary.

Individuals with a greater tuberosity fracture may also have significant partial articular-surface rotator cuff tears that were not identified on arthrogram or MRI investigation. Persistent pain in spite of the healing of the tuberosity and the completion of a rehabilitation program should alert the orthopedist to the possibility of such tears.

TENNIS

Shoulder problems related to tennis are divided into those affecting the backhand stroke and those affecting the forehand stroke and serve.[216,217]

BACKHAND

Problems involving the dominant shoulder during the backhand stroke are similar to those involving the nondominant shoulder during the golf swing. In both instances, the arm is fully adducted across the chest.

ACROMIOCLAVICULAR JOINT

Cross-body adduction may aggravate acromioclavicular joint arthritis. Diagnosis and treatment are the same as those previously reviewed.

IMPINGEMENT

Posterior capsular and rotator cuff contracture may lead to traction lesions and posterior pain. As previously noted, the contracture increases the obligate anterosuperior translation of the humeral head, thereby causing symptoms of impingement.

FOREHAND STROKE AND SERVE

Problems with the forehand and serve are similar to those of the throwing action of the pitcher.

SUBLUXATION

Pain in the posterior joint line during the serving motion is characteristic of anterior subluxation. Players may attempt to compensate by altering the position of the ball toss and changing hip rotation to diminish the amount of abduction and external rotation required for a power serve. Evaluation of serving mechanics, with particular attention paid to body mechanics, combined with a rehabilitation program to strengthen the scapular muscles and the rotator cuff may be curative. When persistent instability remains, a capsular reconstruction allows return to tennis activity.[218] Arthroscopic treatment is reserved for those few patients whose symptoms suggest a mechanical abnormality within the joint.

IMPINGEMENT

Pain localized to the subacromial area or to the deltoid insertion during the serve or overhead stroke is typical of impingement. Often the posterior capsule is tight, and its correction can be accomplished with a stretching program. Arthroscopic subacromial decompression allows a return to the sport.

ROTATOR CUFF TEAR

Many individuals with degenerative full-thickness tears of the rotator cuff are unwilling to forego the sport and instead pursue activities that take place below shoulder level. Patients who complain of pain *and* loss of strength, particularly when no evidence of structural impingement is present (type II acromion, no inferior acromioclavicular joint osteophytes), should be treated with repair of the tendon.[219] Individuals who complain of pain but have no weakness and in whom structural acromial arch abnormalities exist (type III acromion, inferior acromioclavicular joint osteophytes) may be treated with arthroscopic subacromial decompression. When a partial-thickness tear involves more than one-half the thickness of the cuff (Grade 3), it is often advisable to excise the defect and perform a mini-open repair after arthroscopic decompression to avoid return of symptoms when strenuous serving is resumed.

BOXING

ANTERIOR SUBLUXATION

Anterior subluxation occurs with the jab. The nondominant shoulder is affected. The punch is thrown straight ahead and often occurs simultaneously as the boxer pulls away from his opponent.[220] This movement produces distraction and may cause anterior subluxation in an individual with mild laxity. The condition almost always responds to rehabilitation. Arthroscopic findings are usually minimal.

POSTERIOR SUBLUXATION

Posterior subluxation occurs in the dominant arm as the power punch or "cross" is thrown. The movement is similar to the follow-through of the pitcher. Rapid deceleration of the adducted and internally rotated arm may cause a posterior inferior subluxation. Localized pain of a mechanical nature can suggest a posteroinferior labrum tear, which is responsive to arthroscopic debridement. Symptomatic instability refractory to nonoperative management is best treated with an open posterior capsular reconstruction.

ARCHERY

Shoulder complaints are common among competitive archers.

SUBLUXATION

The nondominant shoulder is held in a position of abduction and slight horizontal flexion. This position can cause posterior instability in an individual with preexisting laxity.[221] Arthroscopic findings are minimal, and persistent pain requires an open posterior reconstruction.

IMPINGEMENT

As Mann and Littke have noted, the male archer pulls a 45-pound bow 75 times a day for 4 days during an international event.[222] The equivalent is approximately 1500 kg pulled in a single day. This motion requires placing the dominant arm in abduction and internal rotation and maintaining that position while aiming at the target. Persistent symptoms may require arthroscopic subacromial decompression.

SUMMARY

This chapter has focused on the shoulder without regard to the significant role of training, technique, warm-up, and lower extremity function. Management of shoulder injuries in the competitive athlete is challenging. Precise diagnosis aids in the treatment. Arthroscopic surgery is highly successful when the lesion is *mechanical* (labral lesions leading to pain or functional instability),[145,223,224] *structural* (acromial impingement, coracoacromial ligament hypertrophy), or causes *incongruity* (acromioclavicular joint arthritis). Arthroscopic surgery is less predictable when *reconstruction* is needed for the correction of instability or rotator cuff tears. Reproducing the exact amount of movement required for the competitive athlete without allowing any excessive translation remains a challenge. Accomplishing this goal within the time constraints placed upon the athlete's career is difficult.

20 WORKERS' COMPENSATION EVALUATION

Workers' compensation, and its attendant medical and legal characteristics, has an effect on clinical practice. This area of practice deserves separate attention. Although injuries may differ in terms of how and where they occur, either internal or external to the workplace, the basic types of injuries incurred by both groups appear similar. Both groups may suffer from single injury macrotrauma or from repetitive overuse microtrauma. The banker with stage II impingement syndrome of the shoulder brought on and aggravated by overhead tennis strokes suffers the same pain as the boilermaker who works continually at or above shoulder level. A biopsy specimen of the rotator cuff and bursa in each patient probably would show identical histology. Each individual's quality of life, however, may be affected differently by the same injury.

Most companies employ physicians to screen and evaluate industrial injuries. These physicians can deal with most shoulder girdle problems, but they cannot reasonably be expected to have the time, training, or temperament required to treat complex shoulder conditions. Most shoulder-related problems are classified at the initial evaluation as "muscle strain" or "bursitis." The patient is referred to a shoulder specialist when the condition does not resolve in what the industrial physician considers to be an appropriate length of time. Therefore, the first obstacle encountered by the patient is a delay in reaching the appropriate physician.

Upon initial patient evaluation, prior shoulder injuries or problems frequently are not reported because the patient wants to be sure that the industrial injury is blamed for the shoulder pain. In addition, the patient may not have told the employer about a prior shoulder problem for fear of being refused employment.

Language and cultural barriers that exist between physician and patient can be minimized if an interpreter is available.

Patients also often exaggerate the amount of shoulder pain they are experiencing. Because visible evidence of injury, such as a laceration or fracture, is not present, the patient's complaints may have been ignored on previous occasions. Consequently, the patient may feel the need to exaggerate the amount of pain and incapacity. The physician can minimize this problem most effectively by creating an atmosphere of genuine concern and also by communicating the fact that the physician believes a shoulder problem exists. Once the patient realizes that the physician is sympathetic, complaints become more reasonable and specific.

Careful documentation is especially important in a workers' compensation case. The events that lead to shoulder pain in the general patient population may be described briefly as "shoulder pain noted after opening heavy garage door." The physician's purpose for making such a description in this instance is merely to note that the shoulder pain occurred after a traumatic event of sufficient magnitude to damage shoulder structures. The individual with a workers' compensation complaint presents additional problems, however. Characteristically, this patient goes into great detail describing the circumstances of the injury. These patients do not merely slip on the floor and strike their shoulder; instead, they focus on the fact that the floor was slippery because the new employee was careless and did not dry up the soapy water. Individuals under these circumstances do not hurt their shoulders twisting a heavy valve. Instead, they hurt their shoulders twisting a valve so heavy that two people are normally required to turn the valve, but on that particular night, because of company policy, procedure, lay-offs, financial difficulties, etc., only one person was available to turn the valve, and consequently, the shoulder problem occurred for that reason.

Of course, whether the patient injured his arm turning a heavy valve that was stuck or that required two people to turn is medically unimportant. No medical difference exists among falls caused by soapy water, by oil, or by poor lighting. Nonetheless, the circumstances of the injury have significant legal impact on the patient and must be recorded. The physician does not have to determine the accuracy of these events. The events were not witnessed directly. Our practice has been to document the patient's description of the accident in detail and to preface the text by noting *the patient stated* the floor was slippery or *the patient stated* two people are required to turn the valve. Such complete documentation greatly simplifies the management of the case and is valuable when any legal or disability determinations must be made.

Physical examination at the initial visit also has some unusual characteristics. Again, probably in an attempt to increase credibility, the patient may exaggerate the amount of pain experienced by various shoulder maneuvers. Initially, the shoulder "may be too painful to move." Any attempt to touch or move the arm may bring on severe pain inconsistent with the examiner's prior experience. Each orthopedist treating shoulder injuries is familiar with the amount of pain associated with each of the common shoulder conditions, and when patient complaints exceed those boundaries, the physician is alerted. Most often these exaggerations can be minimized and a good physical examination performed.

When an occasional examination proves to be essentially inconsistent, we document that the examination, or a portion thereof, cannot be considered reliable. For example, an examination of instability may not be performed because of the patient's complaints of pain, but rotator cuff strength can be evaluated well. A more accurate impression sometimes can be made during repeated visits. The physician may see the individual for an independent medical examination, and comments regarding such become part of the medical record. Inflammatory statements, such as "obvious patient malingering," should be avoided. Such statements may sound biased or lacking in compassion when questioned by an attorney at a deposition.

A determination is made as to whether the patient has a problem, whether that problem involves the shoulder area, and whether that problem falls within the physician's training. For example, an individual may have shoulder pain from a brachial plexus stretch injury that requires neurologic evaluation. The patient may have shoulder pain from a rhomboid-trapezius spasm that can be treated by a physical medicine and rehabilitation specialist.

The patient's job performance must often be decided before all diagnostic testing can be completed. Unless the shoulder injury is extensive or other body parts are involved, the patient is not totally incapable of performing *any* type of work. Vague statements, such as "return to light or limited duty work," should be avoided unless a work capacities form that relates directly to that patient's specific job is available. Rather, the better approach describes the limitations the patient currently has and allows return to work only if these limitations can be met. These limitations may include unlimited shoulder use, restricted work below shoulder level, limited lifting, or even one-handed duty.

The patient often states that light duty is not available at work. In this instance, we inform the patient that our function is merely to state the circumstances under which the patient may return to some work. Whether or not this work exists depends on the particular job situation. Most patients can accept this explanation. We also share with the patient (in writing) the circumstances under which we believe a return to work is acceptable and when we believe these circumstances will occur. When further requests from the company are received, we forward a copy of both the request and our reply to the patient. Such sharing of information avoids misunderstandings and strengthens the patient-physician relationship.

Standard diagnostic techniques are used for the patient covered by workers' compensation. The pressure to diagnose and treat the problem, however, is greater for these patients than for the general patient population. Although the banker described in our original example may simply modify his tennis game, the individual unable to work and receive a paycheck is distinctly more interested in resolving the problem with greater speed. In this sense, the injured worker is treated more like the professional athlete than is the business executive. Because time is a much more important factor, the physician may reach a precise diagnosis more rapidly. When the injured worker is not interested in returning to work, recovery from injury is slow.

The longer the worker is kept from his original job, the less likely that individual is to return in a full capacity. Job retraining or vocational counseling should be instituted. Every attempt should be made to return the injured worker to his prior occupation as rapidly as possible.

ROLE OF ARTHROSCOPY

The role of arthroscopy in the patient covered by workers' compensation is similar in many respects to its function in all other patients. The greatest difference is, however, that arthroscopy in this patient group more often is an attempt to furnish objective information about subjective complaints. Arthroscopy is equally valuable in determining and documenting whether some objective shoulder findings are present.

ABSENCE OF OBJECTIVE FINDINGS

The examiner can also evaluate both shoulders under anesthesia for range of motion and stability. If no findings consistent with disease or injury can be identified, this absence should be stated. If the physician believes that the patient has real pain, but no objective findings can be seen, referral for further evaluation may be appropriate. Options include an orthopedic surgeon specialist (e.g., shoulder, cervical spine), neurosurgeon, neurologist, physical medicine and rehabilitation specialist, or pain clinic.

PRESENCE OF OBJECTIVE FINDINGS

Objective findings are corrected if necessary. If objective signs are found, but the surgeon believes the lesion may heal with further conservative care, this conclusion should be documented. The patient should be informed of the required healing time so that unrealistic expectations do not occur. The workers' compensation carrier should also be informed of the estimated time for full recovery and of when the individual can return to limited duty. A complete job description, if not available, should be requested at this point. The carrier also should be informed of when maximum medical improvement is anticipated and of whether permanent impairment can be expected. A rehabilitation agency should be involved, if appropriate, because the patient may recover, but not to a level that allows return to heavy labor. If that is the case, vocational counseling should be initiated as soon as possible.

If the abnormalities found at arthroscopy are correctable only by open surgery, two options are available. If the need for open surgery has been discussed with the patient and carrier, and all have agreed to the procedure, the surgeon may move directly from the arthroscopic procedure to the open surgical correction. By doing so, the time between the two surgeries is minimized. The disadvantage is that the initial preoperative explanation must necessarily involve possibilities, probable procedures, and possible outcomes. Although the separation of the arthroscopic examination and the open surgery increases the cost, the length of treatment, and the number of anesthesias, it allows the physician to state more precisely the nature of the surgical procedure, the length of recovery, and the possible impairment. This complete discussion may also provide the patient with other options. For example, the patient may wish to take early retirement or may not wish to undergo open rotator cuff reconstruction if the likelihood of returning to a heavy-labor job is not likely.

INCIDENCE OF SURGERY

Patients with shoulder injuries who were seen by referral for the last 4-year period were reviewed. Approximately 4900 patients were seen. Of these, 1600 were covered by workers' compensation. At some point in their care, approximately 500 (31%) of the patients with workers' compensation had surgery (350 arthroscopic and 150 open reconstructive). In the noncompensation group, approximately 800 (24%) had surgery (400 arthroscopic and 400 open).

The higher percentage for surgery (31% vs. 24%) in the patients covered by workers' compensation is multifactorial. The patients covered by workers' compensation generally have the more physically challenging jobs, and the light-duty work available is limited. Access to different types of work is restricted, as is the ability to modify the work environment.

Secondary gain, which may also be involved, appears to be more emotional than financial. The amount of money available to settle workers' compensation claims is usually limited by statute. Secondary gain may be a factor for the individual who engages in passive aggressive behavior against the company. This behavior seems more common in the older employee who has worked in a sedentary, supervisory position. When moved to a more labor-intensive job, this individual resents the addition of tasks or the increased physical duties.

ARTHROSCOPIC FINDINGS

The two most common shoulder injuries requiring arthroscopic evaluation are rotator cuff injuries and glenohumeral instability. The other common shoulder conditions, such as acromioclavicular joint or glenohumeral arthritis, do not require diagnostic arthroscopic evaluation.

ROTATOR CUFF

Arthroscopy is not required to diagnose full-thickness tears of the rotator cuff tendon. Less invasive radiographic techniques are currently available and widely accepted. Both the arthrogram and magnetic resonance imaging (MRI) techniques provide high accuracy and sensitivity. Occasionally, when pain persists but the radiographic study is negative, arthroscopic examination demonstrates a full-thickness rotator cuff tear. In our experience, however, this outcome is unusual. The most common findings at arthroscopy that are not identified radiologically are (1) partial-thickness tears of the rotator cuff on both the articular and bursal surfaces and (2) longitudinal interval tears in the rotator cuff tendons between the supraspinatus and subscapularis tendons.

PARTIAL-THICKNESS TEARS

The arthrogram underestimates the number of partial-thickness tears. The MRI has a greater ability to identify partial-thickness tears, but the false-negative and false-positive results remain high enough to require occasional arthroscopic evaluation.

ARTICULAR SURFACE TEARS

Articular surface tears are most often located in the anterior supraspinatus tendon near the tendon insertion into the humeral head. Tears decrease in frequency from anterior to posterior locations. Consequently, isolated articular surface tears of the infraspinatus and teres minor are approximately 10% of the total that occur in the supraspinatus tendon. The partial articular surface tear should be identified, and its location, size, and depth should be estimated as well as possible. Probes may be inserted into the joint to measure the tear, and minimal debridement may be required to determine the extent of damage.

BURSAL SURFACE TEARS

Bursal surface tears comprise only 15% of all partial tears. They appear almost exclusively in the supraspinatus tendon near the rotator cuff insertion. They range from small tears (less than 1 cm) of minimal depth to larger bursal surface flap tears in which bone is exposed but a probe cannot be passed into the glenohumeral joint.

INTERVAL LESIONS

Longitudinal tears between the anterior border of the supraspinatus and the superior border of the subscapularis constitute a large portion of radiographically negative, arthroscopically positive rotator cuff lesions. Most commonly, these tears are the result of a violent distraction mechanism, but they can also occur from a fall on the elbow that drives the humeral head in a superior direction. The supporting structures binding the rotator interval split and cause a mixture of instability complaints (feelings of looseness, arm slipping, deep-seated joint pain) and impingement findings (positive impingement tests, positive biceps signs). The injury to the coracohumeral ligament is difficult to evaluate arthroscopically. Findings within the glenohumeral joint interval lesion include abnormalities in structures bordering the interval. These abnormalities include fraying of the superior border of the subscapularis tendon, superior glenohumeral ligament tears, and fraying of the biceps at the exit from the joint. Fraying at the most anterior border of the supraspinatus tendon is also consistent with this lesion.

INSTABILITY

The findings of instability are no different from those noted in Chapter 6 and range from capsular-ligament laxity, Bankart lesions, loose bodies, labrum tears, and lesions of the rotator interval.

MANAGEMENT

ROTATOR CUFF LESIONS

Management of these lesions is multifactorial. Significant factors include the patient's occupation, the acromial type, the mechanism of injury, pre-existing shoulder disease, and the level of the pain. Individuals with partial rotator cuff tears, heavy laboring jobs, type III acromions, and increasing pain 4 to 6 months after injury should undergo surgical correction. Individuals with partial tears and structural abnormalities (type III acromions, inferior acromioclavicular joint osteophytes, acromial spurs) suffer from an *extrinsic rotator cuff tendinopathy* and benefit from arthroscopic surgery because the tendon injury is aggravated by the structural abnormality. Removal of the structural abnormality should allow a previously normal but acutely damaged tendon to heal. Alternatively a traumatic partial-thickness rotator cuff tear superimposed on a previously damaged or degenerating tendon without any extrinsic structural abnormality (a type I or type II acromion) should be thought of as an *intrinsic rotator cuff tendinopathy*. Arthroscopic decompression generally is unsuccessful because an extrinsic structural abnormality is not present. In these individuals, open surgical resection of the partial tear and tendon repair are required.

The individual's job can influence the treatment to some extent. An individual who can be placed in a less physically stressful position has a chance to continue gainful employment while the shoulder condition is observed. An individual with the identical problem but who does not have the option to change jobs may require surgical correction at an earlier date.

INTERVAL TEARS

These lesions are managed by open surgical repair of the rotator interval.

INSTABILITY

At present, we do not perform arthroscopic procedures in individuals at the time of the acute trauma; a period of months normally elapses before arthroscopic evaluation is indicated. By that time, signs of acute trauma have disappeared. The presence of any hemorrhage or tissue staining that might have accompanied the original injury is unlikely now, and the orthopedist must identify the secondary signs of shoulder instability as previously described. The separation of the anteroinferior glenohumeral ligament-labrum complex from the anteroinferior glenoid rim is a sign of instability. This condition is unlikely to improve with conservative care, and surgical correction is required. Whether this correction is open or arthroscopic depends on the surgeon's preference. Individuals in whom more subtle signs of instability have been found (mild laxity on physical examination, thinning of the middle glenohumeral ligament, minimal displacement or a healing Bankart lesion) may be treated conservatively with physical therapy to determine whether the shoulder will heal.

MEDICAL REPORTS

Medical reports for the injured worker covered by workers' compensation require more documentation than do those for other patients. This increased documentation necessitates additional physician and secretarial time. Certain information that is always required may not always be specified by the insuring agency. This lack in communication results in frequent phone calls and letters between the physician's office and the insurance carrier. The simplest method is to answer all questions at one time rather than to respond in piecemeal. The following outline can serve as a guideline to minimize paperwork and to help to clarify some simple medical-legal issues.

INITIAL VISIT

1. History of the occupational injury. The *circumstances* of the injury are described. The *source* of this information should be noted. The source is commonly the patient's version of the events but may also include reports from a supervisor or prior treating physician. Any *treatment* received by the patient since the injury should be listed. The patient's *chief complaint* and *activity limitations* are recorded.

2. Significant past medical history. The absence of any *prior significant* shoulder problems should be stated. If the patient has experienced any prior shoulder problem of significance, clearly state when that problem started and ended. Was it the same type of problem for which the patient is now being evaluated? A prior rotator cuff strain that had resolved completely has no bearing on an acromioclavicular joint injury. Note the *pain-free interval*, if one existed, and state whether the patient was able to perform his *usual and customary* job between the two incidents.

3. Clinical assessment. Record areas of tenderness, range of motion, strength, and stability as *objectively* as possible.

4. Radiographic and imaging tests. Record dates, location, and test *results.*

5. Clinical impression.

6. Accident-complaint relationship. State whether in your opinion the accident described to you by the patient was the *direct cause* for the problem currently under treatment. Did the accident *aggravate* a pre-existing condition? These statements are derived from the *subjective history* provided to the physician by the patient and are *based on reasonable medical probability.* Medical probability is usually defined as likely to occur more than 50% of the time.

7. Treatment plan. List any additional diagnostic tests required, the *reason* the tests are required, and *how the results of the test will affect* the treatment or eventual outcome. If physical therapy is advisable, state whether the therapy is a home exercise program or requires visits to a therapist. State the *frequency, length of time,* and *expected goals* of the therapy.

8. Referrals. State whether consultation with any other physician or health care professional is needed.

9. Medication.

10. Return to work. The estimated date for the patient's return to *limited* work should be provided. Limitations for lifting, pushing, pulling, and carrying should be given. Restrictions for work *at or above shoulder level* are important. An estimate for a return to *full* duty should be made if possible. If an estimate cannot be made, the inability to do so should be stated. Such reporting also applies to the time for *maximal medical improvement.*

11. Current Procedural Terminology (CPT) codes. These codes should be included with the initial report.

FOLLOW-UP VISITS

1. CPT code. Change the diagnostic CPT code if necessary. For example, the initial code may have been for rotator cuff strain. If an arthrogram performed since the initial visit has demonstrated a complete tear, a *re-coding* of the diagnosis alerts the carrier to the more extensive nature of the problem.

2. Clinical assessment. Include the worker's subjective impression of his condition, and record any objective tests performed, e.g., range of motion, impingement, strength, or stability.

3. Treatment plan. Describe any *changes* required or the reason for continuing current treatment.

4. Referrals. Describe any necessary referrals to physical therapy, physical medicine, neurology, orthopedic specialist, etc.

5. Medications.

6. Patient *compliance.*

7. Return to work. Estimate the date for return to *limited duty.* Describe the *restrictions* under which the individual can work in terms of *type of activity* (how much lifting, etc.) as well as *number of hours* per day.

Estimate the date for return to *regular duty.* The physician may have to obtain a job analysis. Determine whether the individual can return to his regular job for a limited number of hours. The physician does not have to determine the availability of such work, but only *what type* of work can be done, for *how long,* and as of *what date.*

8. Maximum medical improvement. Record the estimated date when the patient should reach maximum medical improvement with nonoperative or operative care.

FINAL EVALUATION

1. Onset and clinical course. Describe *briefly*.

2. Description of the most recent clinical examination. Record patient's *subjective complaints*, if any. Record results of last physical examination.

3. Maximum medical improvement. *Date* at which individual reached maximum medical improvement.

4. Impairment rating. An impairment rating is not a disability rating. An understanding of the difference is critical. Impairment is a medical estimation based on the American Medical Association Guides to the Evaluation of Permanent Impairment.[225] Most of the impairment rating is based on *lost motion and strength*. Some subjectivity is involved because the patient may be unwilling to allow shoulder movement, thereby falsely increasing the amount of impairment. On the other hand, a shoulder with good movement may lack adequate strength to function normally. Also, strength and movement may be normal but pain may prohibit activity. Nonetheless, the impairment rating is made and may be confined to the shoulder, to the arm, or may be related to the whole person. Only *objective* findings of impairment are included.

The report should also state whether the impairment is *permanent* or *temporary*.

Information that contains the level of impairment, the limitations of the individual, the length of time these limitations of the individual, the length of time these limitations have existed, and *estimates* of disability is helpful. An example of an entry might be, "The individual has a 10% permanent partial impairment in the shoulder. This is based on range of motion lost (50° elevation, 3%, and 40° external rotation, 2%) added to a 5% impairment based on strength loss (range of motion against gravity and some resistance). This *translates* to a 3% impairment to the whole person. At this time, the patient may return to all activities except those activities involving lifting, pushing, pulling, or carrying more than 30 pounds or those requiring prolonged work at or above shoulder level. The patient may have 0 to 100% disability with these findings based on the exact nature of their prior occupation."

DISABILITY EVALUATION

Note the ambiguity of this disability statement. Disability is more closely related to the individual's *specific* job. Two individuals with the same amount of impairment may have widely differing disabilities. The typist with chronic impingement syndrome and a 20% shoulder impairment based on loss of overhead motion may have 0% disability, but that same individual, if required to stock boxes overhead, may have 100% disability.

Disabilities are either *permanent or temporary* and should be stated as such with the realization that, with certain limited exceptions (massive irreparable rotator cuff tear), any objective statement of permanence is not possible and that the answers are subjective in nature.

The opinion of the orthopedic surgeon is usually confined to impairment. We make comments on disability *only in response to direct questions* from the carrier or attorney and then do so only when a *complete job analysis* has been provided. We can then offer our opinion whether the patient *can or cannot* perform the specific tasks listed.

COMPLICATING FACTORS

PRE-EXISTING CONDITIONS

If the patient has had *no prior* significant shoulder problems, the situation is simplified. Occasionally patients have had *prior shoulder problems* or surgery. If medical records are available, they can be reviewed to ascertain whether the condition truly involved the shoulder or represented a cervical or rhomboid-trapezius strain. If the prior condition was *intrinsic* to the shoulder, a determination must be made whether the prior condition was essentially the same as the current condition or the prior condition *predisposed* the patient to this present condition. If the past and present shoulder conditions are similar, the amount of pain and the work status of the individual in the time period *between the two events* are critically important. If this time period is short and/or the patient was never free from pain and thus restricted work, the two injury episodes are related. The most accurate statement that can be made is that the second injury aggravated the first. No objective way is available to determine which injury is the most significant or to apportion a percentage of the problem to each injury.

If the time period between the two injuries is greater than 1 year and/or if the individual states that he had recovered completely from the first injury and worked at his regular job without pain, as a general rule one can state that, on the basis of medical probability and based on the subjective statements of the patient, no cause-and-effect relationship exists between the two injuries.

QUESTIONS REGARDING WORK-RELATEDNESS

The orthopedist is commonly questioned about the exact cause of the patient's problem. Does proof exist that the work injury caused the damage? Could this injury have been the result of a sporting injury that took place outside the work environment? The surgeon should not be placed in the position of judging which of these two situations is primarily responsible. An appropriate response for the orthopedist is that the damage found at surgery (or arthrogram, etc.) is consistent with the type of work injury described by the patient. Based on the patient's history of no similar problems prior to the work incident and of pain after the work incident, medical probability supports that the work accident was the direct cause of the patient's problem.

NATURAL DEGENERATIVE CHANGES

Another line of inquiry commonly pursued during a deposition revolves around whether an accident caused an injury or was coincidental with a naturally occurring degenerative process. Such questioning frequently happens with rotator cuff tears, glenohumeral arthritis, and acromioclavicular joint arthritis. The carrier or an attorney may ask for proof that a previously asymptomatic individual with one of these problems became symptomatic as a result of the alleged work accident. *Let the attorneys argue* this point. The physician can reasonably state that, although certain shoulder conditions do occur with the aging process, the patient has stated that pain was not experienced prior to the accident and that pain developed after the accident. Consequently, reasonable medical probability points to the conclusion that the work accident described by the patient was the direct cause of the problem under discussion.

CONCLUSION

The shoulder surgeon assumes additional roles when workers' compensation is involved. The general patient population requires physicians to diagnose, treat, and rehabilitate. In the workers' compensation situation, surgeons take on different roles. They may be patient advocates. They interrelate with attorneys for both the defendant and the plaintiff. They function as impairment raters and occasionally as disability raters. They play a large role in the distribution of pension and retirement funds. They are the guardian of the insurance funds. Their decisions may have profound effects on insurance rates and the business environment. Physicians have not been formally trained for any of these tasks.

Scant literature is available documenting specifically how individuals with shoulder problems fare when they return to work. Reports on treatment for injuries of the rotator cuff have documented poor results in the workers' compensation population both in the United States and Canada. The reasons for these poor results have never been fully analyzed and are multifactorial. In this regard, the laborer has much in common with the professional athlete—how many *uninjured* laborers (or baseball pitchers!), if taken off work for 1 to 2 years, could then return to their jobs at their prior level of performance?

Although the shoulder surgeon rarely treats a professional baseball player, the injured worker is frequently a patient. Patients injured in the workplace, and the pressures and problems that result from this situation, have created a dimension to clinical practice that is of great importance. This topic undoubtedly will benefit from further study, clarification, and research.

ARTHROSCOPY TO EVALUATE FAILED SURGERY

The shoulder surgeon is faced with a unique challenge when the patient has had previous open reconstructive shoulder surgery yet continues to complain of pain. The history may be difficult to clarify, the examination complicated by prior surgery, imaging techniques unreliable because of scarring, and both the physician and the patient frustrated by the experience of a previous failed operation. Certainly the mainstays of routine orthopedic care, an accurate history, physical examination, and appropriate imaging techniques, allow accurate diagnosis and appropriate treatment to be carried out in most of these patients. The arthroscope, however, can prove to be a valuable diagnostic and therapeutic tool in these difficult situations. Many of these patients have had their surgery performed by another surgeon, and some unsuccessful procedures are personal failures. In either instance, one should begin with a new diagnostic evaluation.

In all these situations, the orthopedic surgeon must determine whether or not the patient is believable. Most of our patients complain of pain or dysfunction—subjective statements on the part of the patient. An ongoing assessment is made throughout the process to determine whether the problem is in the shoulder girdle, whether an organic problem elsewhere is causing shoulder pain, or whether no such problem can be identified. When no abnormal findings can be identified, a judgment must be made regarding whether further investigation is warranted and what type of investigation is appropriate. Options may include referral to another orthopedist for examination of the shoulder girdle, to an orthopedist specializing in spinal disorders, to pain clinics, to rehabilitation agencies, to psychologists, or to neurologists.

HISTORY

The essential elements of the history in these patients are unchanged from those of a patient with no previous surgery. When did the problem begin and under what circumstances? Where is the pain? What factors, positions, and/or activities make the pain better or worse? These types of questions are common to all. The difference in previously treated patients is that now *two* histories exist. The first history is the patient's story of the problem up to the time of the initial surgery. The second history covers events from the index operation to the present.

Often, the surgeon must exercise great patience to elicit this information because the patient is often frustrated, resentful, and suspicious. Records of previous treatment should be reviewed again if the surgeon performed the original surgery. If another surgeon performed the first operation, then *all* records, including records from the emergency room and the operating room (surgery *and* anesthesia), should be requested. Office notes, as well as imaging, laboratory, or consultant's reports, should be reviewed. When possible, the original radiologic studies should be requested and reviewed. Occasionally, the surgeon's review of the actual arthrogram or MRI study differs from the interpretation of the radiologist or previous surgeon.

The description of the problem prior to and after the surgery generally falls into one of three groups. The two stories may be identical, similar, or seemingly unrelated. Whatever the relationship, valuable information is gained by a careful delineation of the two descriptions of pain.

IDENTICAL HISTORIES

Patients in this group state quite clearly that a problem in their shoulder led them to have the first surgery, the problem was unaffected by the first operation, and they are essentially unchanged. Four questions must now be answered.

1. Was the original diagnosis correct?
2. Was the appropriate surgical procedure chosen?
3. Was that operation performed well?
4. Were the postoperative course and rehabilitation appropriate?

The accuracy of the original physician's diagnosis is not of great importance in this group because the patient's original problem was unaffected by prior surgery. The present surgeon must make a diagnosis and proceed with treatment. If the conventional method of history, physical examination, and diagnostic imaging fails to achieve a diagnosis, arthroscopy is considered. Arthroscopy is often used in this group because these patients may not be willing to undergo repeated arthrograms or MRIs because of discomfort or cost. Insurance carriers are often reluctant to approve expensive tests that did not lead to problem resolution the first time. Although arthroscopy certainly is a costly way to diagnose the problem, radiologic imaging in the patient who has undergone previous surgery may prove unrewarding. A "direct" look at the problem area becomes more appealing, particularly if the injury can be corrected at the same time.

Once the diagnosis has been determined, the appropriateness of the previous surgery is more easily clarified. For example, if the current diagnosis is acromioclavicular joint arthritis and the previous operation was an acromioplasty, the next step is straightforward. This situation develops most commonly with the erroneous diagnosis of "subacromial impingement" in the athlete who throws, when the correct diagnosis is glenohumeral instability with secondary traction rotator cuff tendinitis. In this instance, when an open acromioplasty is performed, the patient's pain continues. Often the correct diagnosis can be made with a good history and physical examination combined with appropriate hindsight. If the diagnosis is not clear, arthroscopy allows an examination under anesthesia and an observation of glenohumeral ligament detachment or insufficiency.

If the previous surgeon made the correct diagnosis and selected an appropriate procedure, the next part of the decision process requires a determination of whether that procedure was well performed. This determination is made most easily when the current surgeon also performed the original procedure. Often, however, dissatisfied patients seek help from a second surgeon who must use secondary means to determine whether the procedure was well performed. Common mechanisms used to evaluate the procedure include radiographs (demonstrating inadequate, excessive, or inappropriate bone resection), operative records, or videotapes. Anesthesia records are surprisingly useful. The surgeon rarely documents particularly difficult procedures, but when the actual time of surgery, as noted in the anesthesia record, is excessive, one can bet that the procedure did not go as smoothly as the surgeon had wished.

If the operation was regarded as well performed, some additional cause for failure must be uncovered, and often the answer lies in the postoperative management.

A detailed description should be obtained as to the exact type and length of immobilization, when passive and active movement were started, and what types of strengthening exercises were performed. Patients who underwent procedures to correct instability and/or rotator cuff injuries may have been immobilized too long, thereby allowing adhesions to develop. This situation commonly resolves with time and further rehabilitation, but may require arthroscopic adhesion resection. These patients generally note resolution or diminution of their original problem (instability or rotator cuff pain), but describe a new problem (stiffness and a different type of pain) that developed after the first surgery. Alternatively, patient movement may have started too soon, thereby causing a tear of the cuff or an injury to the ligament attachment site. Patients in this group are more likely to note no change in their pain pattern. Arthroscopy may serve to document the area of detachment and possibly to allow its correction.

SIMILAR HISTORIES

This group of patients describe "partial improvement" in their situation. The initial diagnosis and treatment selection probably were correct, and the failure occurred in surgical performance and postoperative management.

Common areas of failed surgical technique involve failure to do an adequate acromioplasty in rotator cuff surgery and failure to correct inferior capsular laxity during an anterior instability operation. These errors result in incomplete resolution of the patient's pain. Arthroscopy can demonstrate signs of impingement in the subacromial space and allow for a further decompression. The procedure also can demonstrate excessive inferior laxity in the face of a well-performed Bankart procedure.

Postoperative pain is similar in nature to the preoperative situation in an individual with a rotator cuff repair whose rehabilitation was inadequate. The shoulder muscles are not allowed to regain their normal strength and a type of "impingement" results from muscular insufficiency. The inadequately strengthened rotator cuff muscles do not effectively "depress" or "contain" the humeral head during arm elevation. Consequently, the rotator cuff tendons contact the acromion. The patient often perceives the pain as more mild than that of the original preoperative situation, but describes a similarity in its quality. Further efforts at rehabilitation generally cure this condition, but arthroscopy may be required to determine the adequacy of the repair.

Two situations found during arthroscopy can explain partial but incomplete improvement of the patient's symptoms. A small full-thickness tear that did not appear on radiologic studies or a partial articular surface tear that was not appreciated at the time of open surgery may be present. This area of partial tearing may be just medial to the site of repair or may exist in another area of the cuff altogether. We have seen areas of posterior partial tearing when the full-thickness tear was at the supraspinatus-subscapularis junction. Management of these two situations is covered in Chapters 6 and 7.

DIFFERENT HISTORIES

The patient who describes a pain complex that was eliminated by prior surgery but then was replaced by a new type of pain or disability is particularly difficult to treat. Obviously, the problem is simplified if a significant injury has intervened. An individual with a prior Bankart repair may fall and injure the acromioclavicular joint, or an individual with a successful Mumford procedure may fall off a horse and dislocate the glenohumeral joint. These instances provide relatively straightforward situations, and arthroscopy rarely is needed for diagnosis, although arthroscopic correction may be appropriate. Frequently, however, no obvious trauma was involved. Patients with pain in the shoulder that differs in quality from the pain they suffered prior to their open shoulder surgery can be placed into one of two large groups—patients with pain after an instability operation and patients with pain after subacromial space surgery (e.g., rotator cuff repair, decompression for impingement, acromioclavicular joint resection).

PAIN AFTER SUBACROMIAL SPACE SURGERY

Intact Rotator Cuff

Adhesions. Two types of adhesions, massive and isolated, can be found at arthroscopic exploration. The patient with massive adhesions rarely undergoes arthroscopy because the profound loss of movement that occurs makes the diagnosis obvious. The individual with the massive adhesions and the extreme loss of movement often undergoes an open surgical procedure also because of contractures in the glenohumeral joint capsule and coracohumeral ligament. These structures are more safely released under direct visualization rather than arthroscopically.

A patient may appear after rotator cuff surgery with persistent pain that occurs at the extremes of movement in cross-body adduction or abduction/external rotation. This complaint is in contrast to the more common preoperative complaint of pain with abduction/internal rotation. These individuals have fibrous bands between the rotator cuff and the undersurface of the acromion or deltoid fascia. The fibrous band produces traction on the rotator cuff as the arm is moved. These bands form as a result of immobilization after surgery and must be differentiated from the normal bursal structures, particularly from the posterior bursal curtain. Band resection has proved successful in relieving pain.

Instability. As previously noted, instability is more likely to masquerade as impingement. As a result, an individual continues to have the same complaints that led to the first (incorrect) surgery. Occasionally instability may develop after rotator cuff surgery, thereby causing a different type of pain from that caused by the original problem. This replacement of old pain with new pain occurs in individuals with asymptomatic laxity in their shoulders. Often the condition is bilateral. This laxity is compensated for by a strong, functional rotator cuff, which provides dynamic stability to the glenohumeral joint. When a lesion is sustained that requires rest or surgery, both cuff strength and coordination are abnormal. The dynamic stabilizers of the shoulder can no longer center the humeral head in the glenoid during activity. Arthroscopy documents a large inferior capsular recess and/or a small or absent middle glenohumeral ligament. A Bankart lesion is found rarely.

Torn Rotator Cuff

When postoperative pain differs in quality from the preoperative pain caused by a completely torn rotator cuff, the situation can be similar to that for stage II impingement previously described. In addition, degenerative arthritis, acromioclavicular joint disorders, and lesions of the biceps tendon can occur.

A deep-seated, aching pain present at rest can signal degenerative changes in the glenohumeral joint. When the radiographic signs are present, the diagnosis is clear. On occasion, the radiographs are normal, however. In these individuals, the arthroscope provides clear information about the extent and site of the disorder. The arthritis may be widespread but superficial in depth or may be deep but well localized to either a portion of the glenoid or the humeral head. Acromioclavicular joint arthritis may cause problems in two ways. The acromioclavicular joint may have been symptomatic at the time of rotator cuff repair but went unrecognized and therefore untreated. Alternatively, the acromioclavicular joint may have become symptomatic in a manner unrelated to the prior surgery, may have sustained injury at the time of surgery, or may have been subjected to increased forces during the rehabilitation period.

The diagnosis of acromioclavicular joint disorder is rarely made arthroscopically. The diagnosis of acromioclavicular joint instability (coracoclavicular ligaments cut during the cuff repair) or acromioclavicular joint arthritis is made on the basis of the physical examination and routine radiographs. Complete ruptures of the biceps tendon are usually noted at the time of open surgery, but in our experience, deep-seated pain in the shoulder after a repair of the cuff can occur from complete or partial tears of the intra-articular portion of the biceps tendon. These lesions may not be noted on the arthrogram or MRI study and can often only be visualized arthroscopically. Management is discussed in Chapter 10.

PAIN AFTER INSTABILITY SURGERY

Most commonly, individuals who appear with problems after an instability operation have *identical* preoperative and postoperative complaints. Evaluation demonstrates a failure of the first surgery to correct the condition (Bankart lesion not healed). Patients with *similar* preoperative and postoperative complaints often demonstrate a partially healed Bankart lesion or a healed Bankart lesion but uncorrected inferior capsular laxity that allows inferior translation. Patients who complain of pains or dysfunction that are *different* after an instability operation from those that occurred before the surgery may have problems with instability, metallic hardware devices, bone impingement, or arthritis.

Bristow

Pain of a different quality after a Bristow operation can be the result of screw penetration into the joint. This penetration either can cause mechanical symptoms or may lead to a generalized arthritic condition within the joint. If a coracoid process placed too laterally acts as a bony block to motion, impingement of the humeral head against this bone can result in pain. Defects in the anterior aspect of the humeral head may be noted at the time of arthroscopy.

Magnusson/Putti-Platt

These procedures can result in significant loss of motion and degenerative arthritis. They can also result in excessive excursion in a posterior and/or inferior direction. The resulting iatrogenic posterior and/or inferior instability can be observed and documented at the time of arthroscopy, thereby providing an explanation for a pain pattern that differs substantially from the preoperative situation.

Bankart

Postoperative problems that occur after the Bankart procedure can also develop when the surgery is performed properly, but unrecognized recurrent posterior subluxation becomes symptomatic as the anterior structures are tightened. Difficulties with metallic fixation devices likely increase with the number of modifications in the original procedure and the increase in the types of fixation devices available to the orthopedist.

TECHNIQUE

The technique of arthroscopic evaluation in the individual who previously has undergone shoulder surgery has some slight modifications from the technique used in other individuals. Entry into the joint must be precise and atraumatic. Sharp trocars should not be used. The surgeon must note whether the damage is a result of a prior surgery or of an unrecognized injury or pathologic process. Articular gouging during the arthroscopic surgery confuses the issues. Documentation is essential and may be done in the form of systematic complete operative reports, VCR recordings, or still photographs from the compact disc. A systematic visualization of all structures within the glenohumeral joint *and* the subacromial space is mandatory with appropriate manipulation of the shoulder structures as required. If instability is suspected, the glenohumeral ligaments must be palpated for tension and substance and must be examined while the shoulder is stressed in the appropriate direction. The rotator cuff should be inspected in full abduction and various positions of rotation to ensure that portions are not missed.

RESULTS

Arthroscopy in 71 patients was performed for evaluation and/or treatment after one or more open surgical procedures on the shoulder had failed. These patients reflected an incidence of approximately 7% of all shoulder arthroscopic surgeries performed. Most of the patients had undergone prior surgery for impingement or rotator cuff tear. Only 13 were evaluated after a failed instability procedure.

The findings in the group of patients with rotator cuff problems ranged from massive irreparable tear to continued impingement without full-thickness tear. The success of the arthroscopic procedure was good when an identifiable, correctable lesion could be found, but was poor in individuals in whom no obvious source of pain could be seen. The individuals with a preoperative diagnosis of failed instability correction underwent arthroscopy for diagnostic purposes. These patients were all large men averaging 6 feet and 180 pounds. This shared characteristic might account for the difficulty in making the diagnosis in the office. The most common finding was inferior subluxation after an open anterior reconstruction for dislocation.

Arthroscopic evaluation in a patient who has undergone one or more prior open reconstructive surgeries is challenging. A logical evaluation sequence has proved useful.

COMPLICATIONS

22

The growing popularity of shoulder arthroscopy has been accompanied by an increase in the number of presentations and publications devoted to arthroscopic complications.[226-231] A 1988 survey from the Arthroscopy Association of North America reported an overall complication rate of 1%.[232] Complications were lowest in diagnostic shoulder arthroscopy and highest (5.3%) with anterior staple capsulorrhaphy. Arthroscopic subacromial decompression has a 2 to 3% complication rate when both major and minor complications are included.[233-235]

In a large series of shoulder arthroscopies from a single institution, Curtis and associates reported an overall 6% complication rate.[229] Arthroscopic procedures alone had a 4.45% rate, and combined arthroscopic and open procedures had an 8.1% rate. Several points deserve emphasis. The combination of diagnostic arthroscopy and open stabilization did not increase the morbidity of either procedure. The highest complication rate was with combined open and arthroscopic procedures in and around the subacromial space (11.6%). They also reported no infections, acromion fractures, or axillary nerve injuries.

Complications of shoulder arthroscopy are broadly grouped into common and uncommon complications. More common complications include injury to nerves, articular surfaces, tendons, vascular structures, and ligaments. More uncommon complications are infection, compartment syndrome, venous thrombosis,[236] cyst formation,[158] and reflex sympathetic dystrophy.

Each complication is reviewed with respect to its nature, pathogenesis, prevention, and management.

NERVE INJURY

ANESTHETIC RELATED

Two types of anesthesia techniques are used during shoulder arthroscopy—general and regional. Complications caused by general endotracheal anesthesia are not specific to shoulder arthroscopy. Anesthetic-related nerve injuries occur during regional anesthetic techniques that require the introduction of needles and solutions. When regional anesthesia is employed, the patient should receive an explanation of the possible risks of complete or partial, permanent and/or temporary injury to the brachial plexus. The explanation should be documented.

POSITION RELATED

Two positions are commonly used in shoulder arthroscopy. The lateral recumbent is the more traditional approach; the semi-sitting or "beach chair" position is gaining popularity.

LATERAL RECUMBENT

Patients in the lateral recumbent position are susceptible to stretch injuries of the brachial plexus from a combination of arm distraction, arm position, joint distention, fluid extravasation, and neck position. Greater than 15 pounds of traction in certain individuals may produce enough humeral head displacement to result in stretch injuries to the brachial plexus. This result is best prevented by using a minimal amount of weight (<10 pounds). The surgeon should think of the arm as being suspended rather than distracted. If a small amount of flexion is maintained in the elbow, the surgeon can minimize the amount of pull that occurs across the neurovascular structures.

Arm position affects brachial plexus stretch also. Extreme positions of adduction and extension should be avoided because these two positions are known to produce excessive strain on the plexus.

Most series report a low incidence of clinically diagnosed neurologic injuries. Pitman and associates, however, recorded somatosensory-evoked potentials and documented abnormal findings of the musculocutaneous nerve in all 20 patients.[237] These findings were produced upon initial joint distention in 16 patients and by traction in 11 patients. In 10 patients, varying combinations of median, ulnar, and radial nerve involvement resulted. Two cases of clinical neurapraxia were recorded, both of which resolved in less than 48 hours.

In a laboratory study, Klein and co-workers concluded that 45° of forward flexion combined with either 90° or 0° of abduction produced 2 positions that afforded excellent visualization of the glenohumeral joint and minimal brachial plexus strain.[238] The combination of 0° flexion and 10° abduction produced high strain readings. The neck should be supported on a headrest so that excessive lateral bend and increased plexus strain do not occur.

We use the lateral recumbent position, 5 to 15 pounds of weight, and an arm position of 15° of forward flexion, with abduction varying from 20 to 55°. No significant nerve palsies have been noted in approximately 2000 patients.

Brachial plexus lesions may be diagnosed with a thorough neurocirculatory examination performed in the recovery room. Electrodiagnostic studies document the location and severity of the palsy.

Patients in the lateral recumbent position are also susceptible to cutaneous nerve injuries of the upper and lower extremities. The radial sensory nerve to the dorsum of the hand can be affected through the use of the suspension gauntlet or wrapping. The nerve is subcutaneous and particularly vulnerable to pressure. Injury is best prevented by padding the area well and minimizing the amount of traction weight as previously described. Management is generally conservative; surgical intervention is reserved only for refractory cases.

The contralateral lateral femoral cutaneous nerve of the thigh or the peroneal nerve as it courses around the fibular neck may also be involved. These lesions are caused by pressure in some susceptible individuals. They are best prevented by using thick foam padding under the iliac crest, knees, and ankles. Management is similar to that for the sensory nerve injury in the wrist.

SEMI-SITTING POSITION

The semi-sitting position may result in injury to the brachial plexus or to the cranial nerves. The plexus is susceptible to complete or partial injury in the semi-sitting position. The head is fixed with tape or a secure headrest. Arm distraction can produce stretch injury that is prevented best by minimizing manipulation, traction, and distraction to the shoulder. The position of the head should be checked frequently by the anesthesia staff.

One rare complication that occurs is transient palsy of the posterior auricular nerve. The patient awakens and notes numbness in the area around the ear. In our experience, this numbness resolves completely in a period of 1 week to 3 months.

Hypoglossal nerve palsy also has been reported and resolves spontaneously.[239]

PROCEDURE RELATED

SUPRASCAPULAR NERVE

The suprascapular nerve is injured in four ways. During many stabilization procedures, a hole must be made in the glenoid. The nerve can be injured as the drill or Steinmann's pin is passed from an anterior to a posterior site. This complication occurs as the suprascapular nerve passes within 1 to 2 cm of the glenoid rim.[240] If the drill is not directed medially, the pin may exit laterally, close to the articular margin, and thereby pierce the suprascapular nerve. This misplacement most often affects the branch to the infraspinatus muscle and is best prevented by angling the drill in a medial direction so that the pin exits in the middle or medial portion of the scapula. When this complication occurs, weakness and atrophy in the infraspinatus may be recognized. If improvement is not noted by 6 weeks, electrodiagnostic studies should confirm the site of injury. The neurologic damage to the infraspinatus muscle may be significant, and operative exploration, neurolysis, repair, and/or grafting should be performed.

The suprascapular nerve may also be injured during stabilization procedures as the two bundles of sutures are tied posteriorly. The suprascapular nerve branch to the infraspinatus may be compressed if the nerve is caught between the two suture groups.

The third type of suprascapular nerve injury occurs during joint entry. As the cannula and trocar are used to palpate the posterior joint line, care must be exercised not to stray too far medially and possibly contuse or lacerate the nerve branch. The trocar should be used to gently palpate the interval between the medial glenoid margin and the humeral head.

The fourth type of suprascapular nerve injury occurs with the introduction of a superior portal. This complication results when the cannula and trocar are angled too medially. The suprascapular nerve is vulnerable in this location as it exits from under the suprascapular notch. Prevention of this complication relates to surgical technique. The precise point and angle for entry to the joint should be determined with a spinal needle before the trocar is used to palpate the interval between the humeral head and glenoid. This step helps to assure that the cannula does not enter medial to the glenoid. Management of this injury is similar to that previously described.

AXILLARY NERVE

The axillary nerve can be injured with portal placement in the anterior, posterior, or lateral locations commonly used during operative shoulder arthroscopy.[241]

The axillary nerve may be injured posteriorly either by placing this portal too far inferiorly and damaging the axillary nerve as it exits from the quadrilateral space or by placing the arm in excessive abduction, thereby relatively translating the nerve from an inferior to a superior position and placing it in harm's way. Both complications can be prevented by selecting an appropriate site for portal entry and avoiding extreme arm positions.

The nerve can be injured anteriorly by an excessively inferior portal placement. This error in placement most commonly occurs as the surgeon attempts to gain access to the anteroinferior glenoid during an instability repair. Prevention is possible by placing the anterior portal superior to the superior edge of the subscapularis tendon.

The axillary nerve can be injured in lateral portal placement and most commonly occurs in subacromial decompression or acromioclavicular joint procedures. This complication results from the excessively distal placement of the lateral portal. Burkhead and colleagues have shown that the axillary nerve can be located significantly less than the accepted 5 cm from the acromial border.[242] As the surgeon places the portal more laterally to gain parallel entry into the subacromial space, nerve injury can occur. This problem is best prevented by placing the entry site of the cannula within 3 cm of the acromion.

MUSCULOCUTANEOUS NERVE

The musculocutaneous nerve is injured through the excessively medial placement of the anterior portal. Its injury is best prevented by keeping the anterior portal lateral to the coracoid process.[243]

The location of the coracoid process should be noted. The skin can be marked with a pen if necessary. When a Wissenger rod is used to create the anterior portal, a fingertip can be placed on the coracoid to help to guide the rod laterally. If a direct anterior entry is desired, the precise location of the coracoid should be determined, and the spinal needle should be placed lateral to this site. Direct observation of the entry of the needle into the joint should precede placement of the trocar.

Partial palsies of the musculocutaneous nerve have been managed conservatively, and all have resolved within 3 months. Failure to improve at 6 weeks should prompt electrodiagnostic evaluation and surgical management as indicated.

BONE INJURY

Complications related to bone removal are inadequate bone removal and excessive bone removal.

INADEQUATE BONE REMOVAL

ACROMIOCLAVICULAR JOINT

Inadequate bone removal is covered more completely in Chapter 18. Primarily, this complication involves failure to remove enough distal or anterior clavicle during arthroscopic acromioclavicular joint resection. Failure to remove the superior edge of the clavicle and the superior medial acromion border is also covered in Chapter 18.

ACROMIOPLASTY

In an arthroscopic subacromial decompression, the surgeon may fail to remove the anterior acromial protuberance. This portion of the acromion projects anterior to the anterior border of the acromioclavicular joint, and failure to perform the "anterior acromial recession" as described in Chapter 5 may lead to persistent impingement symptoms.

Another common complication that occurs during arthroscopic subacromial decompression is the performance of a medial rather than a lateral acromioplasty. This complication occurs when the posterior portal is placed too far laterally. Such placement directs the scope in an anteromedial direction, and the surgeon consequently may confuse the midportion of the anterior acromion with its lateral border. This error is best prevented by correctly placing the posterior portal. A secondary check is also advisable. The surgeon should be convinced that proper subacromial space orientation has been achieved. The instrument in the lateral portal should be moved medially, and medial movement should be confirmed on the monitor. Anterior and posterior movement should be similarly observed. The anterolateral corner of the acromion then should be identified, and the *lateral* border should be palpated for a distance of at least 5 mm. These steps assure the surgeon that the anterolateral corner is actually being visualized.

If this complication is recognized during surgery, replacement of the cannula or redirection of the arthroscopic view anterolaterally corrects the problem. More commonly, the problem is discovered in the postoperative period when the patient does not recover satisfactorily. Axillary radiographs reveal *medial* acromial thinning, and a repeated scapular outlet view demonstrates the continued presence of a downward-sloping acromion, which should be managed by revision surgery, open or arthroscopic.

EXCESSIVE BONE REMOVAL

Another potential complication is acromial fracture. The acromion that recently has been treated by acromioplasty is thinned and therefore more susceptible to fracture. The acromion usually heals with conservative care, but a malunion in a downward-tilted position may cause repeat symptoms of impingement that require either osteotomy and internal fixation or repeat acromioplasty. Another complication of excessive bone removal involves significant acromial thinning that causes the acromion to deform plastically and tilt downward. This result may cause impingement symptoms. We have been able to manage this problem only with repeat surgery and further removal of anterolateral acromion.

True intraoperative fracture of the acromion is rare and actually represents a misplacement of the acromioplasty. The surgeon mistakenly begins the inferior acromioplasty at some point posterior to the anterior acromial margin and burs through the superior cortex. A "fracture" results. A prominent anterior protuberance, or ossification of the coracoacromial ligament, can make identification of the anterior acromion difficult.

This type of "fracture" can be prevented in one of two ways. Before the acromioplasty is started, the surgeon should be absolutely satisfied that the anterior acromion is well seen. Adequate visualization of this structure often requires resection of the coracoacromial ligament and visualization of deltoid muscle fibers. If any doubt exists, the arthroscope should be inserted laterally and the bur positioned posteriorly. The bur is placed flat against the acromial surface, and the acromioplasty is performed. This technique is preferred by some surgeons.[244,245] The complication can be managed conservatively, but as previously noted, a malunion with downward tilt may result in persistent symptoms that eventually require repeat surgery.

LIGAMENT INJURY

INCOMPLETE RESECTION

Incomplete coracoacromial ligament resection may result in continued impingement symptoms. This complication can occur when the surgeon fails to visualize deltoid fibers from the lateral acromial margin to the acromioclavicular joint. Prevention requires adequate resection as described in Chapter 5. Management may require repeat surgery to completely excise the ligament if impingement symptoms continue.

EXCESSIVE LIGAMENT RESECTION

Resection of the superior, middle, or inferior glenohumeral ligament leads to complications. A surgeon rarely resects the ligaments deliberately because instability results. This complication is most often the result of inadvertent ligament resection during labrum debridement. A flap or fraying in the glenoid labrum may be noted, and overvigorous debridement of this labrum can result in separation of the labrum-ligament complex from the glenoid, thereby rendering the glenohumeral ligament ineffective. An actual ligament transection can also occur.

This complication is best prevented by clear and direct visualization of the debridement area. We maintain the synovial resector above the labrum and allow suction to bring the frayed or separated part of the labrum into the resector. This approach is in contrast to the placement of the resector directly in contact with the damaged labrum. If contact is made, even the slightest amount of force could cause excessive soft tissue resection.

If this complication is recognized arthroscopically, management may require immediate arthroscopic or open repair if the ligament debridement results in significant instability. Mild to moderate degrees of instability may be managed conservatively with immobilization, but care should be taken to observe the patient for any instability problems in the postoperative period.

CORACOCLAVICULAR LIGAMENT

Coracoclavicular ligament resection can occur during coracoacromial ligament resection or during acromioclavicular joint resection. If coracoacromial ligament resection continues medially until the coracoid is visualized, the resector can be moved posteriorly along the superior coracoid surface to transect the coracoclavicular ligaments and cause acromioclavicular joint separation. This result can be avoided by stopping the coracoacromial ligament resection at the medial acromial border. Symptomatic acromioclavicular separation may require either immediate repair or late reconstruction.

ACROMIOCLAVICULAR LIGAMENT

Acromioclavicular ligament resection occurs while removing an inferior osteophyte that projects from the acromioclavicular joint. The medial acromial and inferior distal clavicle surfaces are resected, and therefore, the inferior aspect of the acromioclavicular joint and its ligament are also removed. In most individuals, this procedure does not result in acromioclavicular joint instability or symptoms, but problems develop on occasion. The reason for this sporadic occurrence is unclear. Prior injury may have rendered the joint potentially unstable, or the patient's pain may be the result of arthritis aggravated by intra-articular surgery and injury.

After acromioplasty, patients should be evaluated for acromioclavicular joint symptoms and treated appropriately.

VASCULAR INJURY

Two types of vascular injury are common complications of shoulder arthroscopy. The first is injury to the cephalic vein; the second is injury to the acromial branch of the thoracoacromial artery.

Occasionally, a branch of the cephalic vein, or even the cephalic vein itself, may be injured when the anterior portal is created. The Wissenger rod or cannula may nick the vein and result in hemorrhage. The presence of the cannula generally tamponades the vein, and bleeding is most often noted with skin closure as blood flows from the skin portal. No "fool-proof" method can prevent this complication. The best way to minimize the problem is the use of a Wissenger rod. Once the rod has exited the joint, it should be advanced slowly with gentle rotation to try to protect the vein from puncture if encountered.

If brisk bleeding is encountered and cannot be controlled with simple pressure, the skin portal must be enlarged to allow identification and coagulation of the vein.

THORACOACROMIAL ARTERY

The acromial branch of the thoracoacromial artery is most often injured during subacromial decompression procedures. The artery lies adjacent to the coracoacromial ligament and is most often lacerated during division or resection of that ligament. A dilute (1:300,000) epinephrine solution helps to control oozing but does not adequately control arterial bleeding.

Two methods can be used to prevent the complication. The first method involves electrocautery. When electrocautery is used with coagulation current and the ligament is detached from its lateral aspect, thereby leaving the more vulnerable medial coracoacromial ligament for last, bleeding can be minimized. If bleeding is encountered, the electrocoagulation instrument is available.

The second method requires dissection of the coracoacromial ligament from the acromion with the acromionizer bur.[245a] When acromioplasty is performed prior to coracoacromial ligament resection, the bone insertion of the coracoacromial ligament is removed and the ligament is displaced toward the rotator cuff. The entire ligament then is easily visualized and can be resected with less risk of vascular injury.

If significant arterial injury does occur, bleeding can delay or even prevent arthroscopic subacromial decompression. Brisk bleeding can generally be controlled with electrocautery. Good inflow must be maintained to tamponade the vessel. The inflow pressure is decreased to allow identification of the bleeding point and then is quickly increased to stop the bleeding. The electrocautery unit then can be applied appropriately. A combination of increased inflow resulting in tamponade and use of electrocautery allows control of most bleeding. The cannula may also be used as the surgeon's "finger" to directly apply pressure to a bleeding area and maintain hemostasis. Attention should also be directed at the patient's blood pressure. Maintenance of the systolic blood pressure below 90 mm Hg helps to keep the operative field clear.[246]

Occasionally, another technique is utilized because bleeding may continue as high flow washes off newly formed blood clots. Suction is used to withdraw all fluid from the subacromial space. A period of rest without any flow allows the clots to mature. Two to 3 minutes are allowed to pass, and then the subacromial space is filled with fluid. If these techniques fail, the arthroscopic procedure should be stopped. An incision is made to identify the site of arterial injury directly. The artery should be controlled with conventional open techniques. The operation may then continue with open or arthroscopic techniques at the surgeon's discretion.

VENOUS THROMBOSIS

One case of venous thrombosis has been reported as a complication of shoulder arthroscopy. Burkhart suggests that the presence of venous thrombosis should alert the orthopedic surgeon to the presence of a hypercoaguable state or an extrinsic mass causing venous compression.[236] In the one case reported, further investigation identified a Hodgkin's lymphoma. This mass was the source of the venous occlusion.

ARTICULAR INJURY

Articular injury during shoulder arthroscopy may occur with portal placement, drilling, electrocautery, and metal implants. The type of irrigating solution also may have some effect.

PORTAL PLACEMENT AND DRILLING

The posterior aspect of the humeral head is the area of cartilage most commonly injured. The humeral head is damaged during the initial insertion. We routinely use only blunt trocars, but in spite of this precaution, articular injury may occur if the trocar is forced between the humeral head and the glenoid. This complication is prevented by entering the glenohumeral joint in a more superior location so that the cannula can pass just superior to the superior glenoid margin, between the humeral head and rotator cuff tendons. This space is larger and minimizes the risk of inadvertent penetration. The surgeon should gently use the blunt trocar to palpate the posterior glenoid and then the humeral head. The humeral head is movable with arm rotation, but the glenoid is not. Joint entry is facilitated by placing the trocar on the glenoid and moving it laterally rather than by placing the trocar on the humeral head and moving it medially.

Articular damage may also occur through placement of the anterior cannula if the cannula is inserted by palpation techniques alone. With the arthroscope in the posterior portal, the entry site is first identified with a spinal needle. The cannula then can be precisely inserted under direct vision to minimize the chance of articular damage. Another method uses a Wissenger rod to guide placement of the anterior cannula and to minimize the chance for damage to the articular surfaces.

Articular damage may be decreased by the use of plastic rather than metal cannulas. Plastic cannulas are softer and, therefore, less likely to score the articular surface. The cannula must be rigid enough, however, to allow its use as a palpating tool.

Articular damage also may occur during operations for glenohumeral instability. As noted in Chapter 13, these operations commonly require preparation of the anterior glenoid neck site to allow healing of the detached labrum-ligament complex. Articular damage occurs through the use of a bur and excessive inferior debridement, which can be prevented best by using the bur under direct vision. The posterior portal allows a good view of the bur as it comes over the articular surface, but placement of the arthroscope in the anterosuperior portal and the bur in the anteroinferior portal allows excellent visualization of the anterior glenoid neck and allows the surgeon to stop before glenoid articular damage occurs.

Any of the surgical techniques that require a drill hole across the glenoid neck for suture passage may cause cartilage damage. Most commonly, the damage is a result of a superficial drill hole that damages subchondral bone. This damage can lead to articular collapse. The drilling pin may also dissect the cartilage from the subchondral bone or place a gouge or trough in the cartilage surface. This complication occurs as a result of excessive lateral placement of the anterior portal. The farther lateral or superior the anterior drilling portal is made, the easier the portal can be made. This location, however, creates an acute angle between the capsular entry site and the anterior glenoid neck. Fluid extravasation into the soft tissues further displaces the anterior cannula, thus making the drilling angle more acute and the entry into bone even harder. The pin may slide down the anterior scapular neck without entering the bone.

Prevention is best accomplished by strict adherence to technical details in the placement of the anterior cannula. The cannula must be positioned just superior to the superior edge of the subscapularis tendon. The placement should be made under direct vision. The superior leading edge of the subscapularis tendon should be pierced if an appropriate cannula position must be assured. Piercing of the tendon by the cannula has the disadvantage of limiting movement of the cannula during the procedure because the cannula is tethered by the strong tendon rather than loosely contained by the anterior capsule. The cannula cannot be placed inferior to this position because damage to the axillary nerve or brachial plexus may occur. Medial placement of the cannula allows a more perpendicular approach to the glenoid, but is limited by the safe boundary lateral to the coracoid and musculocutaneous nerve.

ELECTROCAUTERY

Articular surface damage may also result from the use of the electrocautery unit. Superficial cartilage damage is caused by thermal necrosis and is best prevented by coagulating only under direct vision with both the tissue and the electrocautery unit placed in the center of the arthroscopic field.

Cautery is most effectively performed in nonconductive solutions, such as water. Thus, the surgeon must switch irrigating fluids each time cautery is required. Another option is the use of plastic-coated electrode tips that are effective in isotonic solutions. Use of these tips eliminates the need to switch from conductive to nonconductive solution (physiologic saline or Ringer's solution to water) during the procedure but requires a higher power setting on the electrocautery unit, thus increasing the possibility of soft tissue thermal damage.

Management of articular surface damage is limited at present to removal of loose articular fragments that may cause mechanical damage. If the cartilage is damaged and a piece is floating free, it should be removed. Cartilage flaps that result from gouges or scoring of the articular surface also should be removed. Minor scuffing of the articular surface does not seem to require any treatment.

METAL IMPLANTS

Perhaps the most traumatic type of injury to articular cartilage occurs with metal implants placed either in the glenoid cartilage or the humeral head during instability operations.

GLENOID CARTILAGE

Glenoid damage is often related to the difficulty in placing metallic implants at the time of surgery.[160,247,248] In an attempt to bring the labrum-ligament complex up to the level of the glenoid articular surface, one of the tines of the staple can be placed directly into or gouge the articular surface. If the tine is placed in the interval between the subchondral bone and articular cartilage, the cartilage can be separated from the underlying bone. This problem can be prevented by good visualization of the staple through an anterosuperior viewing portal.

HUMERAL HEAD

Damage to the humeral head may occur during movement of the staple about the shoulder joint during the operative procedure but more commonly occurs as a result of failure to control the instability. The humeral head may subluxate or even dislocate if the operation fails to control instability completely. The humeral head can then come in contact with the metal staple wherever that staple is located on the anterior scapular neck. The result is gouging and scraping of the humeral head and damage to the cartilage.

Prevention of this situation is slightly more complex because the potential causes involve errors in technique and/or judgment. If a surgeon recognizes that an operation, such as an arthroscopic Bankart repair, is not being performed well, the procedure can be revised arthroscopically, converted to a traditional open repair, or even abandoned if the soft tissue swelling is extreme.

A more common reason for articular damage caused by metal contact, however, may be failure to recognize capsular laxity. The presence of a Bankart lesion does not eliminate the possibility of capsular or ligamentous laxity. This laxity may occur at the time of the initial dislocation or, more likely, may result from repeated episodes of dislocation and/or subluxation. The Bankart lesion may be repaired arthroscopically, but the capsular laxity is not addressed. Thus, the dislocator is converted to a subluxator. Excessive translation continues to occur, thereby causing humeral head impingement on the staple. Prevention of this complication is difficult because at present the indications for capsular tightening at the time of a Bankart repair are not precisely defined in either arthroscopic or traditional open surgical techniques. Treatment is by staple removal and open capsular reconstruction.

TENDON INJURY

Injury to the rotator cuff tendon occurs through portal insertion or excessive debridement. Damage of the deltoid muscle origin from the acromion occurs through excessive debridement during acromioplasty.

PORTAL INSERTION

POSTERIOR PORTAL

The normal entry of the posterior portal penetrates the posterior deltoid muscle and the inferior margin of the infraspinatus muscle prior to entering the joint. If the tendon itself is pierced, tendon damage and possible immediate or late tendon rupture may occur.[249] The three factors that relate to this complication are (1) arm position, (2) musculotendinous junction location, and (3) cannula direction.

As the arm is internally rotated, the more proximal muscular portion of the infraspinatus covers the posterior aspect of the joint, thereby minimizing tendon penetration. As the arm is externally rotated, the *tendinous* portion covers the posterior aspect of the joint and is more susceptible to cannula penetration. Some anatomic variation occurs among individuals, and those with a long muscle and a short tendinous unit are less likely to sustain tendon injury than are those with a shorter muscle and a longer tendinous portion of the musculotendinous unit.

As the entry point for the cannula is placed more laterally, the possibility of infraspinatus tendon injury increases. When the entry point is immediately inferior and medial to the posterolateral corner of the acromion, the risk of tendon injury is decreased. As the cannula is directed laterally toward the humeral head, the risk of tendon injury increases, and if the cannula is directed medially toward the coracoid, the risk of tendon injury is decreased.

Once the complication is recognized, the postoperative rehabilitation program should be modified to allow for tendon healing. Passive and gentle active motion can be started immediately, but strengthening exercises and full participation at work or sports should be delayed until the patient does not experience any pain when the rotator cuff muscles are tested for strength.

The late complication of a complete tear of the rotator cuff tendon generally requires surgical repair.

SUPERIOR PORTAL

The supraspinatus tendon is most often punctured during the creation of a superior portal. Because this portal is used less frequently than the standard anterior and posterior portals, the surgeon may not be quite as adept at superior portal insertion, and as the cannula is directed laterally to palpate the humeral head, the tendon can be penetrated. As noted earlier in this chapter, an excessive medial direction of the cannula may result in nerve injury. Probably the safest way to place the superior portal is under direct visualization with the aid of a spinal needle. The arthroscope is placed posteriorly and is directed at the superior portion of the cuff. A spinal needle is carefully passed into the joint to serve as a guide to appropriate medial/lateral and anterior/posterior cannula placement. Because the small spinal needle rather than the large cannuia is used until the exact placement site is determined, the risk of tendon, cartilage, and nerve injury is minimized.

ANTERIOR PORTAL

The anterior portal passes through the deltoid muscle and generally through the rotator interval, which is the space between the superior border of the subscapularis and the anterior border of the supraspinatus tendon. This area is the traditional "safe spot," where the risk of tendon injury is generally slight. If the anterior portal is placed too medially (medial to the lateral coracoid border), musculocutaneous nerve injury is possible.

EXCESSIVE DEBRIDEMENT

Excessive debridement causes tendon injury and occurs most commonly in two situations—partial tears of the rotator cuff and full-thickness tears of the rotator cuff.

PARTIAL TEARS

Debridement of a partial tear of the rotator cuff serves two functions. Flaps or frayed edges, which may cause mechanical symptoms in the joint, should be removed. Debridement of the tendon also helps to estimate the size and depth of the partial tear. No scientific evidence shows that debridement of a partial rotator cuff tear accelerates or stimulates a "healing response. Debridement of the rotator cuff until "vascularity" is seen is also unreliable. The rotator cuff is not a highly vascular structure and becomes less so with age. Also, the position of the arm and the pressure of the irrigating fluid may tamponade any bleeding. Debridement continued until vascularity is noted, although theoretically desirable, may result in excessive tendon removal. Debridement until "healthy tendon" is seen is also difficult. In general, less debridement is preferable to excessive debridement.

FULL-THICKNESS TEAR

Debridement of the complete rotator cuff tear is a controversial area in orthopedic surgery. Good results have been reported with arthroscopic debridement of irreparable tears.[250] No reports advocate debridement of a *repairable* tear as the preferred treatment method. When arthroscopic debridement is compared to repair, the results from repair are superior.[251] Undoubtedly, however, *some* patients with complete tears of the rotator cuff do well with arthroscopic debridement and subacromial decompression. At present, the indications for debridement/decompression are not well defined, and the procedure cannot be advocated as a preferred treatment option. During debridement care must be exercised to avoid converting a partial tear to a full-thickness tear or a repairable full-thickness tear to an irreparable tear.

DELTOID MUSCLE

Damage to the anterior deltoid muscle or its fascial origin occurs when the surgeon fails to recognize the difference between coracoacromial ligament and deltoid fascia. The ligament runs at nearly a right angle to the deltoid origin and inserts on the *inferior* surface of the acromion.

The middle deltoid muscle and fascial origin also can be damaged when the anterior lateral border of the acromion is not clearly defined and the acromioplasty is started laterally rather than anteriorly. The lateral deltoid fascial origin seems less firm than the anterior origin and can be excessively debrided during bone removal. Excessive removal of the deltoid origin is prevented through precise orientation in the subacromial space. The surgeon must be familiar with normal anatomic structure and have good fluid flow through well-placed cannulas. Small deltoid separations are managed by delaying rehabilitation until the deltoid has had a chance to heal. Larger areas of deltoid dehiscence present a significant challenge. Early deltoid repair or deltoidplasty may allow some recovery.

INFECTION

Infection after any arthroscopic procedure is rare, and reports range from .04 to 3.4%.[252] Data include a preponderance of knee surgery.[253,254] Infection after shoulder arthroscopy is unusual. Curtis and associates reported no infections in 711 shoulder arthroscopies, and our experience includes only 3 infections in more than 2000 patients.[229] The excellent blood supply and abundant soft tissue coverage in the shoulder may explain the generally low infection rate. Our experience in infection management has been limited to 5-day periods of oral antibiotic treatment.

FLUID EXTRAVASATION

The amount of soft tissue swelling that accompanies operative shoulder arthroscopy is impressive. Despite the rise of pressure within the deltoid muscle during surgery, the pressure drops to baseline levels shortly after the procedure is concluded. No electromyographic or clinical evidence yet shows that deltoid muscle damage occurs.[255] Extravasation should be minimized to avoid pressure damage to nerves and to prevent compartment syndromes. Also, as the soft tissues distend, bone landmarks are hard to identify and maneuvering of instruments becomes difficult.

FLUID TYPE

Physiologic saline and Ringer's lactate have been commonly used as an irrigating solution during arthroscopy. Somewhat less inhibition of proteoglycan synthesis has been found with Ringer's lactate than with saline;[256] however, both solutions have been used for many years without untoward clinical consequences. Less inhibition results with a more physiologic buffered solution, such as lactated Ringer's, thereby making its use preferable for longer arthroscopic procedures.[245a] Nonconductive solutions, such as water, were formerly placed in the joint to facilitate the use of electrocautery. These hypotonic solutions could cause chondrocyte injury, and they are used sparingly if at all in our present techniques.

A link between glycine and transient blindness has been reported in both the orthopedic and the urologic literature.[257] More physiologic solutions are being investigated for arthroscopic use.[258]

DIAGNOSTIC FAILURES

Perhaps the largest source of diagnostic failures is the patient in whom the interrelationship between instability and rotator cuff disease is not appreciated. Operations to correct instability on individuals whose primary lesion is rotator cuff disease are failures, as are operations for rotator cuff disease on patients whose underlying problem is glenohumeral instability.[259] In addition, these causes can coexist, thereby complicating diagnosis and appropriate treatment. Signs of instability include Bankart and Hill-Sachs' lesions. More subtle signs that should alert the operating surgeon are anteroinferior or posteroinferior labrum fraying, a soft tissue flap tear at the anterior glenoid margin, partial rotator cuff tears located posteriorly (usually only seen with the arthroscope inserted anteriorly), loose bodies, an absent or torn superior or middle glenohumeral ligament, and SLAP lesions.

A diagnosis of glenohumeral instability should be called into question when the following findings are noted—partial tears in the anterior portion of the rotator cuff, an absence of labrum disorders in the inferior half of the glenoid anteriorly or posteriorly, a stable examination under anesthesia, and the inability to displace the humeral head over the glenoid rim under direct vision during arthroscopy. Fraying of the biceps tendon within the joint or in the interval between supraspinatus and subscapularis is also a finding that should alert the surgeon to direct open or arthroscopic surgical correction toward the rotator cuff rather than toward instability.

ANTERIOR LABRUM DETACHMENT

As was discussed in Chapter 12, not all anterior labral detachments are consistent with instability. A labrum detachment from the anterior superior glenoid can be normal and should not be confused with a Bankart lesion. This normal detachment is always above the equator, located on the superior one half of the glenoid. The labrum may be detached with a normally positioned middle glenohumeral ligament, or the middle glenohumeral ligament may have a superior insertion on the glenoid through the anterosuperior labrum. Diagnosing this labrum detachment as an instability lesion and performing an instability operation will not be effective.

MISSING ROTATOR CUFF TEARS

The identification of full-thickness or partial-thickness tears of the rotator cuff is generally not difficult if a good view can be obtained from the anterior portion of the rotator cuff (near the biceps exit) around posteriorly to the axillary recess. Most often this view can be achieved with the arthroscope in the posterior portal, but occasionally visualization of the posterior insertion is difficult, and reversal of the instruments (placing the arthroscope anteriorly) allows a good view of the structures. Partial-thickness tears may be missed if they have healed with scar or with synovium. The use of a probe, shaver, or blunt trocar to palpate the tendon for thickness and resiliency demonstrates any partial articular surface tears.

Arm position may also cause inaccurate diagnosis. With the arm in 45° or less of abduction, the tear may appear partial because of the position of the humeral head. When the arm is moved into full abduction, the area of tendon insertion into bone is flattened and the extent of the partial tear can be documented. Any significant partial articular surface tear should prompt an examination of the bursal surface. A bursal inspection should be performed to determine whether the tear is actually a full-thickness tear. Occasionally the surgeon finds significant partial-thickness articular tears with matching significant partial-thickness bursal tears. These tears should be treated as a full-thickness tear of the rotator cuff.

DOCUMENTATION AND PATIENT EDUCATION

23

Documentation of the patient begins at the time of the first office visit and continues as the patient is re-examined in the office, is contacted by phone, or responds to a mailed questionnaire on a yearly basis. All surgeons working on the shoulder should strive to meet this goal.

INITIAL OFFICE VISIT

Certain information is common to all shoulder problems and therefore is required. Date and time of injury or onset of problem should be recorded. Was an accident involved? How was the shoulder injured? When did the pain or shoulder problem begin? This type of demographic information should be recorded because these details may have to be recalled with great specificity at a later date. Orthopedic surgeons tend not to focus on the details of an injury once the mechanics of the injury have been determined. For example, once we discover that the mechanism of injury was abduction and external rotation consistent with a traumatic dislocation, we move on as if the details of this accident, e.g., whether it occurred while throwing a football or working a winch, are of no *medical* concern. These details *are* going to make a great deal of difference to the third party payor, however. Subtle differences in injury location (e.g., in the supermarket or in the parking lot) may have profound legal ramifications. If such details are not recorded at the time of examination, the surgeon may be forced to recall (or to admit to not having recorded) these events. Typically these questions arise 1 to 2 years after the initial examination, when recollection of the patient's history has dimmed. We believe that complete documentation of an accident or injury is of great benefit to all parties concerned (Fig. 23–1).

Orthopedic surgeons take the history as outlined in Chapter 3 to arrive at an appropriate diagnosis and treatment. The data must be documented in some way. We record our data most commonly as a narrative description of the history and a brief summation of the pertinent features of the physical examination.

"John Jones is a 38-year-old competitive tennis player who first noted pain in his right, dominant arm while serving. He has had increasing pain localized subacromially for the last 2 months that interferes with overhead activities, sports, and sleep.

Accident/Injury Supplement
page 1

Patient #: __________
Problem #: ___
Date: __-__-____

Patient Name: ______________________________________

1. HOW AND WHERE WERE YOU MOST RECENTLY INJURED?
   1. at home
   2. at work
   3. at a store
   4. at friends'
   5. on a bicycle
   6. on a motorbike
   7. on an all terrain vehicle
   8. in a car
   9. as a pedestrian
   10. in an airplane
   11. in a sports accident
   12. other accident
   13. ______________________________________

2. LOCATION OF ACCIDENT:
>M 1. place: ______________________________
   2. address: ______________________________
   3. intersection: ______________________________
   4. city/county: ______________________________
   5. state: ______________________________
   6. country: ______________________________

3. WAS THERE AN ARREST OR TRAFFIC TICKET GIVEN TO YOU?
   1. yes
   2. no

4. NATURE OF MOST RECENT ACCIDENT/INJURY:
   Please describe in as much detail as possible, the events surrounding and including your accident as well as the location and/or employer.

   1. when: __-__-____
   2. where: ______________________________
   3. what happened: ______________________________
   4. how did it happen: ______________________________
   5. why did it happen: ______________________________
   6. treatment: ______________________________
   7. other facts: ______________________________

5. IF WORK RELATED, DID YOU REPORT YOUR INJURY TO YOUR EMPLOYER?
   1. yes
   2. no

6. WAS THIS YOUR FIRST INJURY TO THIS BODY PART EVER?
   1. yes - skip to question 9
   2. no - continue with next question

FIG. 23–1. Complete documentation of accident or injury is necessary and helpful when the physician is required to recall details at a later date. (Reproduced courtesy of Lanny L. Johnson.)

He has tenderness over the greater tuberosity, good cuff strength with some slight pain, and a positive impingement sign. The shoulder seems stable. The range of motion is nearly normal except for some slight loss of behind-the-back internal rotation. The radiographs demonstrate a type II acromion without any other abnormalities.

Allergies: None.

Medical conditions: None.

Diagnosis: Impingement syndrome right shoulder.

Plan: Rest the shoulder from painful activities, administer nonsteroidal anti-inflammatory medication, maintain shoulder flexibility and strength with a home rehabilitation program, re-evaluate in 6 weeks."

This narrative is probably similar to most office records kept by orthopedists and documents the essentials of the history and physical examination. By convention, the physician may choose not to record negatives, e.g., no neck pain, no generalized ligamentous laxity. Similarly, ranges of motion may be described as normal or limited rather than as measurements and degrees of motion.

When the fictional patient just described recovers, the deficits in record keeping are not noticed. Because not all conditions improve, however, a powerful argument can be made for improved methods of documentation.

Consider for a moment some alternative outcomes.

1. Mr. Jones returns in 4 months stating that the pain went away after 1 month but now has returned. The examination demonstrates change in the range of motion consistent with post-traumatic stiffness or a variation of adhesive capsulitis. Now the range of motion must be determined with greater precision so that the examiner can determine whether the patient's range of motion is getting better, getting worse, or staying the same. Degrees of elevation and external rotation should be recorded, as well as the vertebral level the patient can reach behind his back. The "slight loss of behind-the-back internal rotation" noted at the initial examination is of little benefit.

2. Mr. Jones returns in 4 months stating that the pain went away in about 1 month but now has returned. On examination today, the orthopedist notes anterior instability and apprehension consistent with a traumatic subluxation. Shoulder stability was recorded at the initial examination, but the office record merely states "seems stable." How accurate was the examination? Perhaps the shoulder was too painful to examine for instability. Perhaps the diagnosis of rotator cuff strain was so obvious that the instability examination was superficial and/or did not include the other shoulder. Is any abnormal laxity seen in the elbow or knees?

3. Mr. Jones returns in 4 months stating that the pain went away in about 1 month but has now returned. The examination is unchanged from the first visit. Mr. Jones has read, however, that a certain brand of tennis racquet has caused numerous shoulder injuries among tennis players around the country. The racquets were defective and prone to breakage during a hard serve. These circumstances reflect precisely what Mr. Jones recalls happening to him. He asks for a photocopy of the records of the original office visit, as well as a copy of the bill. Regrettably the original history does not describe whether the shoulder was injured *during the serve* or whether pain developed after the game. No mention is made of the details of the accident or even whether one occurred.

These three examples emphasize the difficulty with medical record keeping. Office dictation or handwritten notes are brief (and therefore convenient) and traditional. They are limited, however, to what is considered germane at the *moment* and are largely qualitative. Consequently, temporal comparisons are difficult if not impossible.

Many physicians use forms and protocols to document the essentials of the history and physical examination. The computerization of these records has also been tremendously helpful.

Forms range from simple (Fig. 23–2) to complex (Fig. 23–3) and may or may not be part of a computerized record keeping system. Each individual may pick and choose among the forms or may, with a small investment of time and money, custom design the form as required. All documents have the advantage of systematizing the history and physical examination; thus, this procedure becomes repetitive and therefore reproducible. Further, the documentation of ranges of motion and of negative, as well as of positive, findings simplifies the future care of individuals who do not respond to standard measures.

PREOPERATIVE COUNSELING

Patients are interested in the condition of their shoulder and are entitled to know the nature of their condition, treatment options, and the likely outcome of these options. If surgery is performed, an explanation of the benefits and risks is required. The physician should document that the patient has had these items explained and understands the options. A checklist can be created for the surgeon, and after a thorough discussion with the patient, the surgeon can document on the checklist the results of that discussion. Complements to an in-depth patient-physician discussion include handouts (Figs. 23–4 and 23–5), pamphlets (Fig. 23–6), detailed letters sent to the patient at home (Fig. 23–7), and educational videotapes.

SURGICAL DOCUMENTATION

The most common documentation mechanism of the surgical procedure is the dictated operative report. The advantages of such a system are few and the disadvantages numerous. The report may be dictated late, and consequently, details may be omitted. The report may be garbled or lost in the transcription process. The essential positive findings are probably, but not always, noted, and almost certainly, negative findings are omitted. The report has little use for research purposes unless someone is willing to read each report and transcribe the material to a database. Various options are now available to the orthopedic surgeon, and all represent an improvement over traditional methods (Figs. 23–8 and 23–9).

VIDEO RECORDING

Another type of documentation that is used in addition to the operative note (in any form) is the various methods of video representation. Arthroscopy is an ideal surgical technique for video recording. Unlike conventional surgery, the

(Text continues on p. 415)

FIG. 23–2. Shoulder evaluation form. (Reproduced with permission from The Society of American Shoulder and Elbow Surgeons.) ▶

PATIENT SELF-EVALUATION

Are you having pain in your shoulder? (circle correct answer)	Yes	No

Mark where your pain is on this diagram:

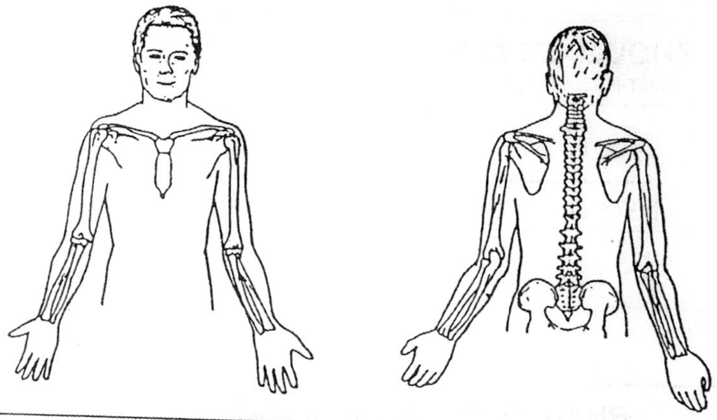

Do you have pain in your shoulder at night?	Yes	No
Do you take pain medication?	Yes	No
Do you take narcotic pain medication (codeine or stronger)?	Yes	No
How many pills do you take each day (average)?	pills	

How bad is your pain today (mark line)?

No pain at all |—|—|—|—|—|—|—|—|—|—| Pain as bad as it can be

Does your shoulder feel unstable (as if it is going to dislocate?)	Yes	No

How unstable is your shoulder (mark line)?

Very <u>un</u>stable |—|—|—|—|—|—|—|—|—|—| Very stable

Circle the number in the box that indicates your ability to do the following activities:
0 = Unable to do; 1 = Very difficult to do; 2 = Somewhat difficult; 3 = Not difficult

ACTIVITY		RIGHT ARM	LEFT ARM
1. Put on a coat		0 1 2 3	0 1 2 3
2. Sleep on your side		0 1 2 3	0 1 2 3
3. Wash back/do up bra		0 1 2 3	0 1 2 3
4. Manage toiletting		0 1 2 3	0 1 2 3
5. Comb hair		0 1 2 3	0 1 2 3
6. Reach a high shelf		0 1 2 3	0 1 2 3
7. Lift 10 lbs. above shoulder		0 1 2 3	0 1 2 3
8. Throw a ball over hand		0 1 2 3	0 1 2 3
9. Do usual work - List:		0 1 2 3	0 1 2 3
10. Do usual sport - List:		0 1 2 3	0 1 2 3

FIG. 23-2

SHOULDER ASSESSMENT FORM

AMERICAN SHOULDER AND ELBOW SURGEONS

Name:		Date
Age:	Hand dominance: R L	Sex: M F
Diagnosis:		Initial Assess? Y N
Procedure/Date:		Follow up: M; Y

PHYSICIAN ASSESSMENT

RANGE OF MOTION Total shoulder motion Goniometer preferred	RIGHT		LEFT	
	Active	Passive	Active	Passive
Forward elevation (Maximum arm-trunk angle viewed from side)				
External rotation (Arm comfortably at side)				
External rotation (Arm at 90° abduction)				
Internal rotation (Highest posterior anatomy reached with thumb)				

SIGNS

0 = none; 1 = mild; 2 = moderate; 3 = severe

SIGN		Right	Left
Supraspinatus/greater tuberosity tenderness		0 1 2 3	0 1 2 3
AC joint tenderness		0 1 2 3	0 1 2 3
Biceps tendon tenderness		0 1 2 3	0 1 2 3
Other tenderness - List:		0 1 2 3	0 1 2 3
Impingement I (Passive forward elevation in slight internal rotation)		Y N	Y N
Impingement II (Passive internal rotation with 90° flexion)		Y N	Y N
Impingement III (90° active abduction - classic painful arc)		Y N	Y N
Subacromial crepitus		Y N	Y N
Atrophy - location:		Y N	Y N
Deformity : describe		Y N	Y N

FIG. 23-2 (continued)

STRENGTH

(record MRC grade)

0 = no contraction; 1 = flicker; 2 = movement with gravity eliminated
3 = movement against gravity; 4 = movement against some resistance; 5 = normal power.

	Right	Left
Shoulder movement painful?	Y N	Y N
Forward elevation	1 2 3 4 5	1 2 3 4 5
Abduction	1 2 3 4 5	1 2 3 4 5
External rotation (Arm comfortably at side)	1 2 3 4 5	1 2 3 4 5
Internal rotation (Arm comfortably at side)	1 2 3 4 5	1 2 3 4 5

INSTABILITY

0 = none; 1 = mild (0-1 cm translation)
2 = moderate (1-2 cm translation or translates to glenoid rim)
3 = severe (> 2 cm translation or over rim of glenoid)

Anterior translation	0 1 2 3	0 1 2 3
Posterior translation	0 1 2 3	0 1 2 3
Inferior translation (sulcus sign)	0 1 2 3	0 1 2 3
Anterior apprehension	0 1 2 3	0 1 2 3
Reproduces symptoms?	Y N	Y N
Voluntary instability?	Y N	Y N
Relocation test positive?	Y N	Y N
Generalized ligamentous laxity?	Y N	

Other physical findings:

Examiner's name:

_______________________________ _______________Date

FIG. 23-2 (continued)

33. AUSCULTATION: 1. SILENT 2. N/T 3. right/left

>M 1. crepitus 1. with ______________ motion
2. popping 2. suggesting ______________
3. other ______________

34. IMPINGEMENT TESTS: 1. NORMAL 2. Abnormal 3. N/T 4. right/left
>M

	N/T	neg.	pos.	painful	neg. with local anes.	produced crepitus	produced popping	not valid due to limited motion	comment
forward flexion:	O	O	O	O	O	O	O	O	______
resisted supination (Yergason's):	O	O	O	O	O	O	O	O	______
abduction/external rotation:	O	O	O	O	O	O	O	O	______
abduction/internal rotation:	O	O	O	O	O	O	O	O	______
adduction/external rotation:	O	O	O	O	O	O	O	O	______
adduction/internal rotation:	O	O	O	O	O	O	O	O	______
palm up:	O	O	O	O	O	O	O	O	______
palm down:	O	O	O	O	O	O	O	O	______

35. MANIPULATION: 1. NORMAL 2. N/T 3. right/left
>M

	STABLE	SUBLUX	DISLOC	APPREHN	PAIN
abd, ext rotation	1. Y/N	2. Y/N	3. Y/N	4. Y/N	5. Y/N
abd, downward force	1. Y/N	2. Y/N	3. Y/N	4. Y/N	5. Y/N
add flexion	1. Y/N	2. Y/N	3. Y/N	4. Y/N	5. Y/N
add flexion, post force	1. Y/N	2. Y/N	3. Y/N	4. Y/N	5. Y/N
fixed scapula, ant force	1. Y/N	2. Y/N	3. Y/N	4. Y/N	5. Y/N
fixed scapula, post force	1. Y/N	2. Y/N	3. Y/N	4. Y/N	5. Y/N

1. abd, ext rotation ______________
2. abd, downward force ______________
3. add flexion ______________
4. add flexion, post force ______________
5. fixed scapula, ant force ______________
6. fixed scapula, post force ______________

36. STABILITY WITH ARM AT SIDE: 1. NORMAL 2. N/T 3. right/left

>M **MANIPULATION DOWNWARD TRACTION**
1. stable ______________
2. subluxation ______________
3. dislocation ______________
4. apprehension ______________

VOLUNTARY DOWNWARD FORCE
1. stable ______________
2. subluxation ______________
3. dislocation ______________
4. apprehension ______________

FIG. 23–3. Example of a complex shoulder evaluation form. (Reproduced with permission. Copyright 1985–1990, Information Health Network, Inc., Lansing, MI.)

FIG. 23–4. Information handout helps to answer patients' questions. ▶

Telephone
(713) 790-2967

Gary M. Gartsman, M.D.
Fondren Orthopedic Group
6560 Fannin St., Suite 2100
Houston, Texas 77030

ARTHROSCOPIC SURGERY
PATIENT INFORMATION

BACKGROUND Recent advances allow surgeons to do surgery inside joints without opening them in the usual way. An arthroscope is a small telescope that shows the inside of the joint (enlarged 20 times) on a television screen. Torn or abnormal tissue can be removed with special very small tools, some of which are battery powered. Every effort will be made to do your surgery through the arthroscope but, in rare cases, a small cut may still have to be made. Most of these operations are videotaped, so that the doctors can study them afterwards.

PREPARATION: Your operation will be scheduled at the Methodist Hospital. Our office will plan a date for the surgery with you. Most often the surgery will be done as same-day surgery, meaning you are not admitted to the hospital and will not stay overnight. Patients with medical problems or extensive surgery may have to stay in the hospital, but only for a few days.

COMPLICATIONS: It is important that patients having elective surgery be informed of possible complications. These rare events include bleeding, infection and nerve injury. Very rarely an instrument may break-off inside the joint and an incision must be made to remove it. The complication rate in arthroscopic surgery is less than 1%. If you have any questions, please ask me for assistance.

PREOPERATIVE TESTING: Pre-operative testing must be done within 10 days of your surgery at the Methodist Hospital Outpatient Department, located on the 5th floor of Smith Tower.

ANESTHESIA: When you arrive for surgery, you will meet one of the anesthesia doctors. They will answer your questions about anesthesia. General anesthesia is used.

INSTRUCTIONS: After surgery, a Recovery Room nurse will care for you until you wake up. When you are ready to go home, an instruction sheet like this one will be given to you along with a prescription for pain medicine and if needed, an antibiotic.

RECOVERY: Follow your post-op instruction sheet and call the office with any problems.

Thank you,
Gary M. Gartsman, M.D.

FIG. 23-4

Reconstructive Shoulder Surgery
Arthroscopy

Telephone
(713) 790-2967

Gary M. Gartsman, M.D.
Fondren Orthopedic Group
6560 Fannin St., Suite 2100
Houston, Texas 77030

POST-OPERATIVE PATIENT INFORMATION
SHOULDER ARTHROSCOPY

THE OPERATION: Your operation was done through the arthroscope. The doctor looked inside your shoulder with a small telescope. Torn or abnormal tissue was removed with special small instruments.

PAIN: You will be given a prescription for a pain pill. It may be taken every three hours as needed for the first day or so. You may place an ice bag on your shoulder if there is swelling.

DRESSING: A soft bandage has been placed on your shoulder. It will soak up any blood or fluid. You may take the bandage off the day after surgery. Bandaids should be used for a few days. If there is a lot of water in the bandage you may change your bandage tonight. The nurse will give you material for this.

WOUNDS: The two or three small holes may be sore and develop bruising over the next several days. This will go away and no special care is needed.

BATHING: The feeling of water in the shoulder is normal. It is left-over water from surgery which will go away. It is safe to take a shower or bathe one day after surgery.

ACTIVITY: You may use your sling for comfort for the first day after surgery. If you are more comfortable without the sling you do not have to wear it. Unless you are given different instructions you may use your arm as tolerated. We will show you specific exercises to do when you are seen in the office.

RESULTS: Surgery done through the arthroscope is very similar to the surgery done inside your shoulder through a larger incision. Even though the holes are small, there has been an operation inside and around the shoulder joint. Complete healing may take several weeks or months.

PRECAUTIONS: If you have a temperature, have unexpected pain, redness, or swelling in your shoulder, please contact my office immediately.

FOLLOW-UP: Please make an appointment to return to my office in about one week.

Thank you,
Gary M. Gartsman, M.D.

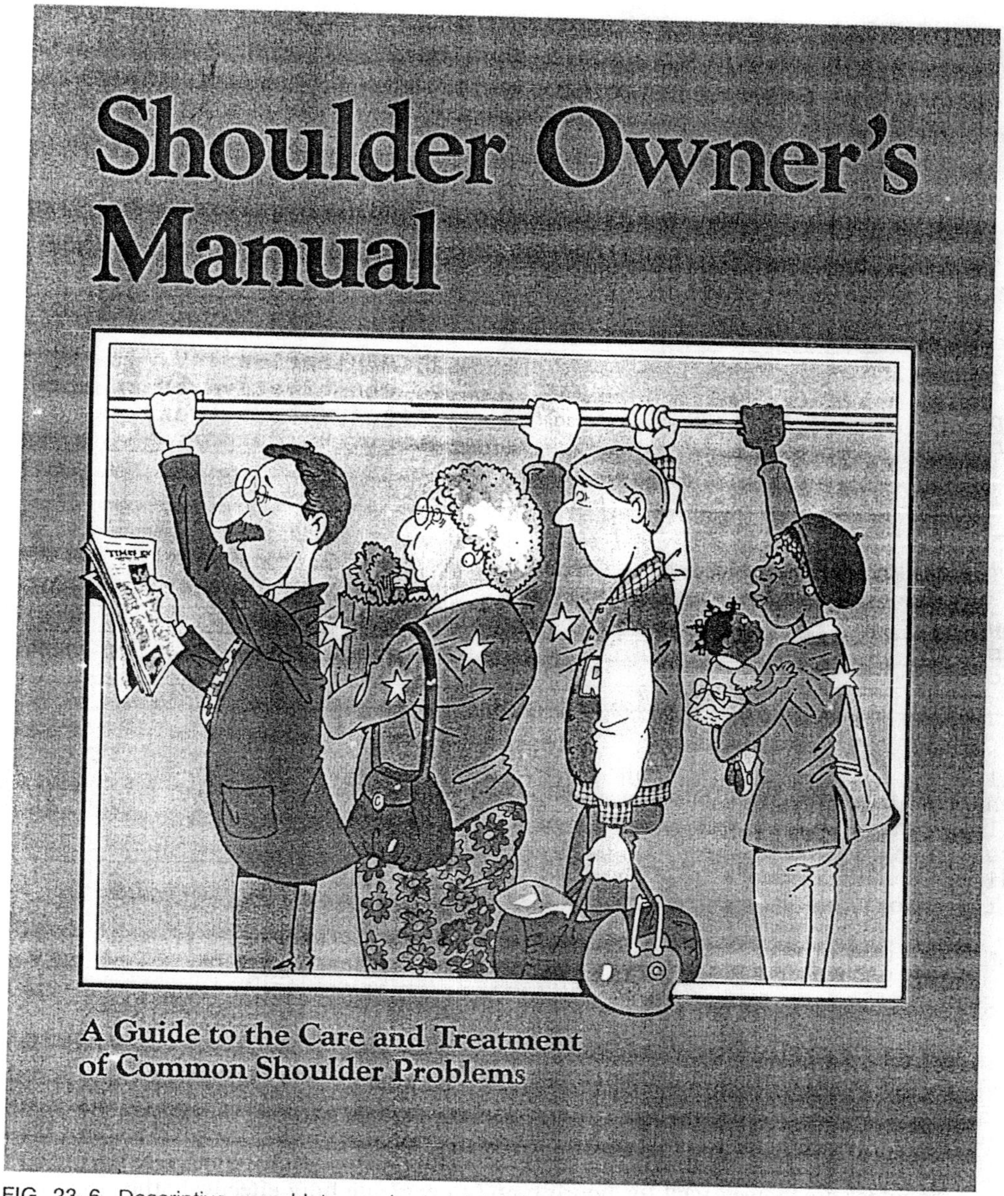

FIG. 23–6. Descriptive pamphlets can be helpful adjuncts to patient-physician communication. (Reproduced with permission. Copyright 1984, Krames Communications, San Bruno, CA.)

operation is seen on a television screen and can be recorded electronically. A videotaped record of the surgery is invaluable for documentation of the abnormalities found, of the treatment that was performed, and of the appearance of the area after treatment. We believe tape review is an excellent means of psychomotor skills education. During the procedure, the surgeon is focused on the many details involved in any surgery and consequently has difficulty in viewing his performance in an objective manner. A review of one's own videotaped per-

27. SURGICAL INDICATIONS:

>M 1. include 2. are not present 3. could develop

1. presence/persistence of:

1. pain
2. swelling
3. locking
4. giving out
5. instability
6. stiffness
7. scar tissue
8. contracture
9. fracture
10. dislocation
11. malalignment
12. numbness
13. weakness
14. ______________________

1. deformity
2. tumor
3. infection
4. implant
5. loosening
6. migration
7. ______________________

Loss of:
1. motion
2. strength
3. sleep
4. daily activities
5. work
6. sports activities
7. ______________________

Lack of improvement after:
1. medication
2. conservative treatment
3. previous surgery
4. ______________________

28. SURGICAL INDICATIONS FROM:
1. Laboratory tests indicating ______________________
2. X-Rays showing ______________________
3. Special test of ______________________
4. showing ______________________
5. (other) ______________________

29. SURGERY:

>M
1. was scheduled
2. will be scheduled
3. is medically indicated
4. is a future consideration
5. is not medically indicated
6. please call our office if you wish to schedule surgery

On your:
1. right
2. left

1. knee
2. shoulder
3. (other) ____________
4. (other) ____________

30. SURGERY SCHEDULED:
1. on __-__-____
2. at ______ o'clock
3. AM/PM

1. Please see enclosed instructions
2. Call our office for confirmation
3. Follow instructions given by our office

FIG. 23–7. Information letter sent to patient at home as part of preoperative counseling. (Reproduced courtesy of Lanny L. Johnson.)

formance helps to observe where time is wasted, to recognize what parts of the shoulder are viewed well (or poorly), and to evaluate how effectively the surgical goals have been accomplished. A video record is also helpful when a patient responds poorly to surgical treatment. The tape can be reviewed to determine whether any disorder was overlooked and/or treated suboptimally.

MACHINE AND TAPE

The most commonly utilized technique involves the VCR with standard 1/2-inch VHS tape. The improved quality of 3/4-inch tape does not compensate for its increased cost (tape and machine), decreased playing time (30 to 60 minutes compared to 2 hours), and lack of compatibility with the more numerous VHS machines.

LABRUM

42. GLENOID LABRUM ANATOMICALLY WELL DEFINED:
1. anterior
2. posterior
3. superior
4. inferior

43. GLENOID LABRUM:

>M 1. torn
2. separated
3. shredded
4. anatomically absent
5. pathologically absent
6. surgically absent
7. healed
8. absent
9. small

1. NORMAL 2. Abnormal 3. N/V

1. anterior
2. posterior
3. superior
4. inferior

44. LABRUM TEAR CHARACTERISTICS:

>M 1. recent
2. old

1. hemorrhage
2. tissue disruption
3. fracture
4. fibrosis
5. circumferential irregularity
6. healed

1. anterior
2. posterior
3. superior
4. inferior

1. correlated
2. did not correlate

1. Hill-Sach lesion
2. anterior motion
3. posterior motion
4. inferior motion

1. was extension of GH ligament bony attachments
2. was not extension of GH ligament bony attachments

45. LABRUM MOTION:
1. anterior
2. posterior
3. superior
4. inferior

1. NORMAL 2. Abnormal 3. N/T

ANTERIOR WALL

46. GLENOHUMERAL LIGAMENT:

>M 1. anterior
2. posterior
3. superior
4. middle
5. inferior

1. NORMAL 2. Abnormal 3. N/V

1. torn
2. recessed
3. contracted
4. pathologically absent
5. surgically absent
6. healed - postoperative
7. healed - posttraumatic
8. small

1. humerus
2. mid-portion
3. glenoid attachment

1. hemorrhage
2. fracture

1. recent onset
2. previous

1. continuity
2. separation
3. tear

1. atypical
2. typical

47. SUBSCAPULARIS BURSAE:
1. position
2. consistency
3. size

1. NORMAL 2. Abnormal 3. N/V

1. small
2. medium
3. large
4. obliterated

1. synovitis
2. loose body(ies)
3. foreign body

Foramen:
1. normal
2. pathologic

FIG. 23–8. Use of preprinted form reduces the likelihood of omitting important intraoperative findings from the surgical report. (Reproduced with permission. Copyright 1985–1990, Information Health Network, Inc., Lansing, MI.)

SURGIgraph OPERATIVE REPORT–ARTHROSCOPIC SURGERY *RIGHT² SHOULDER

CASE ID: ____

*DIAGNOSIS (Use Terms From Structure Column When Possible)

1. ____
2. ____
3. ____
4. ____

*Pre-Op Dx: Confirmed ☐ 64 Expanded ☐ 65 Revised ☐ 55

HISTORY

*Duration of Symptoms:
1☐ 2☐ 3☐ 4☐ 5☐ 6☐ 7☐ 8☐ 9☐ 10☐
Days☐ Weeks☐ Months☐ Years: ____
*Traumatic ☐ 3 Non-Traumatic ☐ 4
Work ☐ 5 Sport ☐ 6 Vehicle ☐ 7 Other: ____ 1
Previous Surgery: <6 months ☐ 8 6 months–1 year ☐ 9
1–2 years ☐ 10 2–5 years ☐ 11 5–10 years ☐ 12 >10 years ☐ 13

INSTRUMENTS USED

Shoulder Traction Device ☐ 14 Max. Wt. ____ 2 lbs.
Manual Traction ☐ 16
Scope: ≤2mm ☐ 17 ~3.5mm ☐ 18 ~5mm ☐ 19
~0° ☐ 20 ~30° ☐ 21 ~70° ☐ 22 ~120° ☐ 23

Powered Cutters:	Side Opening	Corner Opening	End Opening	Burr
Low Speed	☐ 24	☐ 25	☐ 26	☐ 27
High Speed (≥ 2000 RPM)	☐ 28	☐ 29	☐ 30	☐ 31

Electrosurgery ☐ 32
Knives: Banana ☐ 33 Smillie ☐ 34 Retrograde ☐ 35
Other Knives: ____ 3
Suction Punch ☐ 36 Baskets ☐ 37 Laser ☐ 204
Suture Punch ☐ 39 Staples ☐ 40
Other Instruments: ____ 4-6

*Skin Closures: None ☐ 41 Tapes ☐ 42 Staples ☐ 43
Sutures: Absorb ☐ 44 Non-Absorb ☐ 45

PROTOCOL

Position: Lateral ☐ 46 Supine ☐ 47 Beach Chair ☐ 48
*Anesthesia: General ☐ 49 Brachial/Scalene Block ☐ 50 Local ☐ 51
Agent: ____ 7
Antibiotic: ____ 8 Dose: ____ 9
Prep Type: Scrub ☐ 52 Paint ☐ 53 Spray ☐ 54
Iodophor ☐ 55 Hexachlorophene ☐ 56 Hibiclens ☐ 57
Other: ____ 10
Irrigation Solution: Ringers ☐ 58 Saline ☐ 59 Other: ____ 11
Post-Op Injection: Agent: ____ 12
Portals ☐ 60 Intra-articular ☐ 61
*Operative Time: ____ 13 min. Room Time: ____ 14 min.
Sling ☐ 62 Immobilizer ☐ 63 Abduct Splint ☐ 205
Tissue Submitted to Path. ☐ 67

COMMENTS/COMPLICATIONS

1. ____
2. ____
3. ____
4. ____

User Defined Codes: ☐ ☐ ☐ ☐ 206 207 208 209 ☐ ☐ ☐ ☐ 210 211 212 213 ☐ ☐ ☐ ☐ 214 215 216 217

POST-OP STATUS

Any Change in Range of Motion:

	Pre-op	Post-op	No Change
Flex.	____° 15	____° 16	☐ 73
Abd.	____° 17	____° 18	☐ 74
Ext. Rot.	____° 19	____° 20	☐ 75
Int. Rot.	____° 21	____° 22	☐ 76

*PORTALS USED

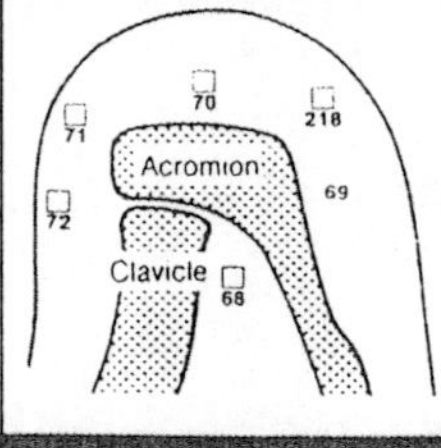

STRUCTURE / PROCEDURE

LABRUM

	Ant.	Inf.	Post.	SLAP
Irregular	☐ 77	☐ 76	☐ 79	☐ 219
Bucket Handle	☐ 80	☐ 81	☐ 82	☐ 220
Detachment	☐ 83	☐ 84	☐ 85	☐ 221

If shoulder is unstable, complete section CAPSULE/LIGAMENTS.

	Ant.	Inf.	Post.	SLAP
Partial Excision	☐ 86	☐ 87	☐ 88	☐ 222
Staple Repair	☐ 89	☐ 90	☐ 91	☐ 223
Suture Repair	☐ 92	☐ 93	☐ 94	☐ 224

No. of Sutures ____ 23
Material ____ 24
Other Procedure ____ 25
Arthroscopy ☐ 97 Arthrotomy ☐ 98 Combined ☐ 99

CAPSULE/LIGAMENTS

	Ant.	Post.	Inf.
Capsule Tear	☐ 190	☐ 191	☐ 233
Capsule Laxity	☐ 146	☐ 147	☐ 148

Exam under anesthesia displaces humeral head.
Grade I (25-50% off glenoid) ☐ 142
Grade II (50-75% off glenoid) ☐ 143
Grade III (75-95% off glenoid) ☐ 144
Grade IV (Completely Dislocated) ☐ 145
Hill Sachs Lesion:
Superficial ☐ 104 Deep (>3mm) ☐ 105

Arthroscopic Repair: Capsulorrhaphy ☐ 150
(If only Labrum reattached, complete LABRUM section.)
Open Repair: Bankart ☐ 152 Putti-Platt ☐ 153
Neer Inf. Capsulorrhaphy ☐ 154
Other: ____ 26
Augmentation: Bristow ☐ 155 Graft ☐ 156
Graft Material ____ 27
Fixation: Screws: Cancellous ☐ 157
Bicortical ☐ 158 Unicortical ☐ 159
Ligament Washer/Plate ☐ 160
Staple ☐ 161 Suture ☐ 162
Suture Material ____ 28
No. of Staples/Sutures ____ 29

ARTICULAR CARTILAGE

Note Outerbridge Grade in Appropriate Location.
1. Intact Surface–Soft or Blistered
2. Superficial Fissures
3. Deep Fissures/Fragmentation
4. Full Thickness Loss/Exposed Bone
(Indicate Grade 1, 2, 3 or 4)

Humerus ____ 30 Glenoid ____ 31

	Humerus	Glenoid
Lavage	☐ 106	☐ 107
Shave	☐ 108	☐ 109
Debride	☐ 110	☐ 111
Abrade	☐ 114	☐ 115
Drill	☐ 116	☐ 117

TENDONS

	Inflam.	Tear Part. Thick. Bursal Side	Tear Part. Thick. Artic. Side	Tear Compl. Thick.
Supraspinatus	☐ 118	☐ 225	☐ 226	☐ 120
Infraspinatus	☐ 121	☐ 227	☐ 228	☐ 123
Subscapularis	☐ 124	☐ 125		☐ 126
Biceps	☐ 127	☐ 128		☐ 129

Size of Rotator Cuff Tear:
Small (0-1cm) ☐ 229 Medium (1-3cm) ☐ 230 Large (>3cm) ☐ 231

Shave ☐ 130 Debride ☐ 131 Repair ☐ 132
Reattach: ☐ 133 Biceps Tenodesis ☐ 134
Transfer To: ____ 32
Suture Mat'l: ____ 33
Other Fixation: ____ 34
Arthroscopy ☐ 135 Arthrotomy ☐ 136 Combined ☐ 137

SYNOVIUM

Specify Lesion and Location:
____ 35
____ 36
____ 37
PVS ☐ 232

SYNOVECTOMY

Total ☐ 138
Partial ☐ 139
Local (<10%) ☐ 140
Biopsy ☐ 141

LOOSE BODY

Multiple ☐ 163
Cartilage ☐ 164
Bone ☐ 165
Completely Loose ☐ 167 ☐ 168 Adherent
Foreign Body ☐ 166
Specify: ____ 38

	Removal	Replant
	☐ 169	☐ 170
	☐ 171	☐ 172
	☐ 173	

Fixation: ____ 39

SUB-ACROMIAL SPACE

Bursa Hypertrophy ☐ 174
C-A Ligament ☐ 175
Acromial Impingement ☐ 176
A-C Osteophytes ☐ 177

Bursectomy ☐ 178 Division ☐ 179 Excision ☐ 180
Acromioplasty ☐ 181 Cheilectomy ☐ 182 Mumford ☐ 234
Arthroscopy ☐ 183 Arthrotomy ☐ 184 Combined ☐ 185

OTHER PATHOLOGY

Adhesive Capsulitis ☐ 203

	Glen. Ant.	Glen. Post.	Hum. Ant.	Hum. Inf.
Osteophytes	☐ 186	☐ 187	☐ 188	☐ 189

Effusion ☐ 194
Hemarthrosis ☐ 195 Pyarthrosis ☐ 196

Shave ☐ 197 Manipulate ☐ 198
Removal
☐ 199
☐ 201
☐ 202

*Asterisk indicates required information and must always be completed.

(HOSPITAL STAMP LOCAL USE ONLY)

Surgery Date: ____ Surgeon I.D.: ____
Name: LAST ____ FIRST ____ MIDDLE ____ Soc. Sec. No: ____ Age: ____ M ☐ F ☐
Hospital: NAME ____ CITY ____ STATE ____
Surgeon Signature: ____
Surgeon: ____ Asst: ____

Operative Report Correspondence (send to):
1. ☐ Insurer: COMPANY NAME ____ ADDRESS ____ CITY ____ STATE ____ ZIP ____
2. ☐ Referring M.D.: LAST ____ FIRST ____ MI ____ Dear- ____ ADDRESS ____ CITY ____ STATE ____ ZIP ____
3. ☐ Other: LAST ____ FIRST ____ MI ____ Dear- ____ ADDRESS ____ CITY ____ STATE ____ ZIP ____
4. ☐ Other: LAST ____ FIRST ____ MI ____ Dear- ____ ADDRESS ____ CITY ____ STATE ____ ZIP ____

FIG. 23-9

◀ FIG. 23–9. Another example of a comprehensive preprinted operative report. (Reproduced with permission. Copyright 1988, Surgical Data Management Corp., Richmond, VA.)

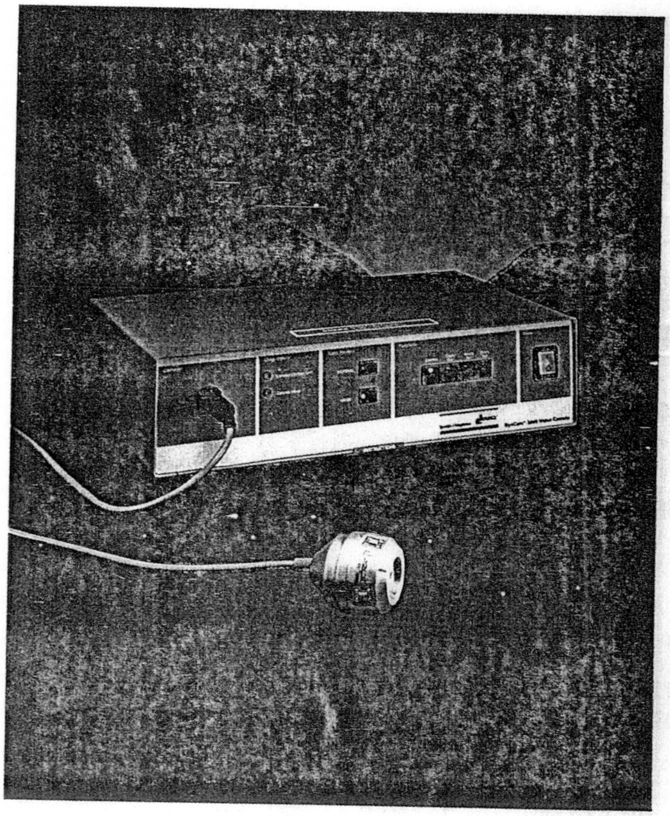

FIG. 23–10. DyoCam 3000, a new 3-chip camera. (Manufactured by Smith & Nephew Dyonics Inc., Andover, MA.)

VIDEO CONTROL

Unless the machine is started at the beginning of the procedure and remains on, video control is required. Operation of the VCR is inconvenient and at times impossible for the circulating nurse. A foot switch that can be connected to most VCRs allows the surgeon to control the unit. Alternatively, the remote control can be placed in a sterile bag and kept on the operative field. The newer arthroscopic cameras have switches directly on the camera to facilitate video control (Fig. 23–10).

FLOPPY DISC

A still picture recorder can be used in conjunction with, or in place of, the VCR. The disc can be removed and viewed after surgery on a television screen. Some or all of the pictures can be printed for documentation.

Patient #: ______
Problem #: ___
Date: __-__-____

Patient Name: ______________________________

1. THIS FORM APPLIES TO WHICH SHOULDER?
   1. right
   2. left

FOLLOWING SHOULDER SURGERY:

2. HOW LONG WAS YOUR SHOULDER IMMOBILIZED? 1. NONE
   1. in sling for ____ weeks 2. ____ days
   1. in brace for ____ weeks 2. ____ days

3. HOW LONG BEFORE YOU:
   1. returned to work ____ weeks
   2. returned to sports ____ weeks
   3. returned to unrestricted activities ____ weeks

4. DID YOU USE FORMAL POST-OPERATIVE PHYSICAL THERAPY?
   1. YES
   2. no

5. ANY COMPLICATIONS: (ask the office staff for any explanations)
   1. NONE
   2. yes (see below)

1. infection	8. atelectasis
2. thrombophlebitis	9. pneumonia
3. pulmonary embolism	10. urinary retention
4. hemorrhage-bleeding	11. ileus
5. bleeding in joint	12. extremity neurovascular problem
6. effusion	13. ligament injury
7. fistula	14. redislocation

6. PATIENT HAS PRESENT COMPLAINT: 1. YES 2. no

7. GENERAL DESCRIPTION OF SURGICAL RESULT:
   1. improved 2. same 3. worse 4. N/A

IF YOU HAVE A PRESENT COMPLAINT, CONTINUE WITH QUESTION 8.
IF YOU HAVE NO PRESENT COMPLAINT, SKIP TO QUESTION 48.

FIG. 23–11. Data-gathering forms can be mailed to patient. (Courtesy of Lanny L. Johnson.)

SLIDES

The cumbersome method of direct still photography to produce slides is being replaced by the floppy disc method. For most individuals, loss of picture clarity with the floppy disc method is more than compensated for by its ease of production.

PATIENT FOLLOW-UP

With few exceptions, the results of orthopedic treatment are either unknown, anecdotal, or based on a retrospective review. Orthopedics does not easily lend itself to prospective double-blind studies because patient variability may require many participating patients and documentation is notoriously incomplete and difficult to retrieve.

The increasing role of computers and the use of standardized protocols is helping to meet this challenge. Simple forms may be mailed to patients, and the patients' replies can be entered in the computer (Fig. 23–11). Results also may be entered at the time of yearly visits. More importantly, data should be collected regularly and completely so that information remains available for electronic review and analysis.

Only by accumulation and then analysis of these data can the effectiveness of nonoperative and operative treatments be evaluated. Such evaluation allows appropriate care for patients, and, in the future, will provide the documentation increasingly required by the federal government and third-party payors to support "outcome studies."

SECTION

REHABILITATION

REHABILITATION OF ROTATOR CUFF DISORDERS: NONOPERATIVE AND POSTOPERATIVE

24

This chapter reviews both nonoperative (conservative) and postoperative rehabilitation of rotator cuff disorders. The therapeutic exercises designed to avoid surgery are presented first. Then, the postoperative protocols for rehabilitation following various surgical interventions are presented in detail.

NONOPERATIVE REHABILITATION

Therapeutic exercises play an integral role in the conservative management of shoulder disorders. Collaboration among physician, therapist, and patient is fundamental to success. The patient must be both *instructed* and *supervised* in the prescribed exercises. The program varies with the disorder being treated.

IMPINGEMENT SYNDROME PROTOCOL

The impingement protocol is designed primarily for patients with stage I or stage II impingement without full-thickness rotator cuff tears. All exercises should be performed initially in the subimpingement range. Any exercise that brings the inflamed rotator cuff into repetitive contact with the coracoacromial arch during forward flexion or abduction is doomed to failure. The program is designed to restore balance to the rotator cuff and strengthen the musculature that controls the scapula. Postural deficiencies may need correction. Fundamental movements of the body in relation to the forequarter often require re-education. Before returning to various sports activities, the quality of stroke production must often be improved.

When impingement is secondary to instability, the instability must be successfully treated to eliminate the symptoms of impingement. Strengthening the external rotators and scapular stabilizers is emphasized when joint laxity is a factor in causing impingement.

STRENGTHENING EXERCISES

Elastic material of varying resistance is currently available (Theraband, The Hygenic Corporation). Color coding allows the patient to progress gradually as strength develops. Dental dam is a cost-effective substitute. A 20-inch length of genitourinary tubing is another inexpensive exercise device. The following exercises are "as simple as ABC."

A. External rotators (Fig. 24–1A). The patient sits with the elbows flexed 90° and held against the body. The elastic band is grasped, pulled out for a comfortable distance, and held for a 5-second count. If a coarse quiver develops, the patient is told not to pull so hard. The tension is then slowly released for a moment, and the maneuver is repeated. A set is 5 repetitions. After a brief rest, a second and third set are performed to achieve a total of 15 repetitions. This exercise strengthens the infraspinatus and teres minor. These external rotators may be surprisingly weak, even in muscular body-builders. When instability is present, external rotation strengthening is critical.

B. Abduction (Fig. 24–1B). The patient stands, and elbows are extended until the elastic device is held at midthigh level. The band is stretched by pulling the arms away from the body (abduction). The supraspinatus and lateral deltoid are the primary abductors. If shoulder pain is experienced, force should be reduced. Even the strongest pull does not permit more than 10 to 15° of abduction.

C. Forward flexion (Fig. 24–1C). The arms are elevated in forward flexion until the band reaches the level of the breast. Further elevation is likely to provoke impingement pain. The band is again stretched a total of 15 times in 3 sets of 5 repetitions in this position. The lateral and posterior deltoid, along with the cuff musculature, are the prime movers at this level.

These ABC exercises are performed in the subimpingement range. None should provoke pain of consequence. If reduction of the force applied to the stretch or of the frequency of repetitions does not eliminate pain, the exercise should be discontinued until the difficulty can be analyzed.

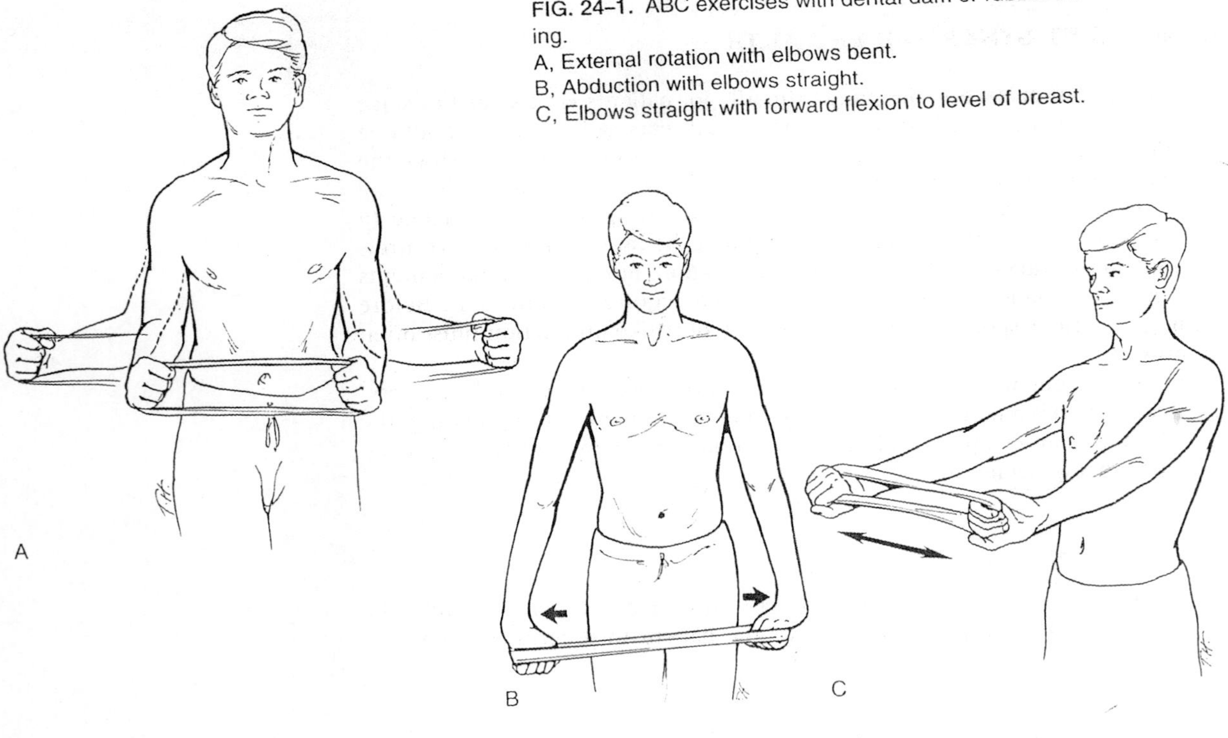

FIG. 24–1. ABC exercises with dental dam or rubber tubing.
A, External rotation with elbows bent.
B, Abduction with elbows straight.
C, Elbows straight with forward flexion to level of breast.

D. Scapular stabilizers. The scapula forms the base for synchronous shoulder motion and must be selectively mobilized and strengthened. Each of the previously described ABC exercises also challenges the scapular stabilizers. Additional scapular exercises are included in the impingement protocol.

Warm-up: Shoulder shrug (Fig. 24–2A) and scapular pinch (Fig. 24–2B) are performed 15 times each as a warm-up exercise.

Corner pushup (Fig. 24–2C: The patient faces a corner and rests the hands against the wall at shoulder level. Elbows should be extended about halfway to place the feet about 20 to 24 inches from the corner. The body should be kept straight as the elbows flex to allow the chest to fall toward the wall. This maneuver stretches the scapula backward until the vertebral borders approach each other. Pectoral stretch can also be felt. After stretching slowly for 5 repetitions, the tempo is increased to create short bursts of stretching and pushing away from the wall. The body is allowed to fall toward the wall and then quickly is pushed back to the beginning position. These rapid pushups should be repeated 10 to 15 times.

Floor pushup (Fig. 24–2D): Floor pushups are done with the hands touching the floor and no farther apart than the width of the shoulders. The knees are allowed to touch the floor to reduce stress when pushup exercises are initiated. From 10 to 15 pushups are performed as tolerated. Some patients may be able to progress by doing the pushup from the toes without allowing the knees to touch the floor. Placement of the hands wider apart in relation to shoulder width adds further conditioning and is reserved for the rehabilitation of athletes.

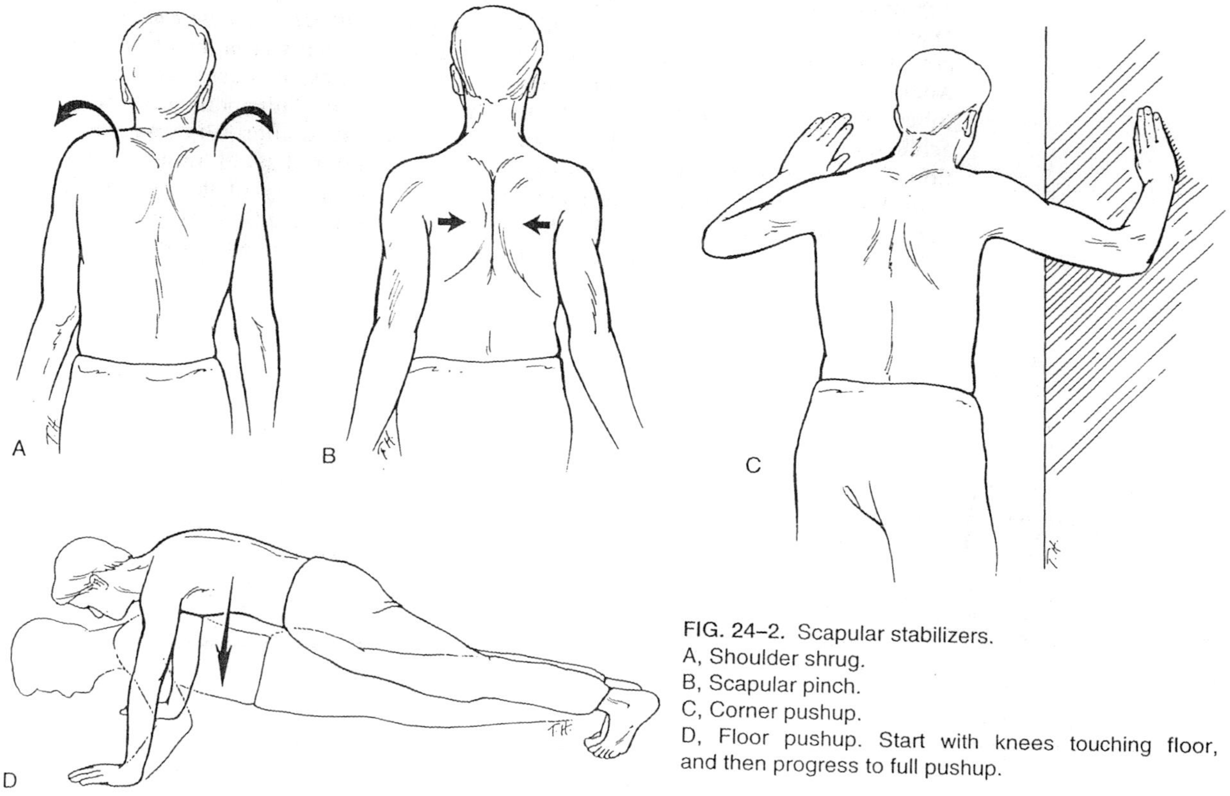

FIG. 24–2. Scapular stabilizers.
A, Shoulder shrug.
B, Scapular pinch.
C, Corner pushup.
D, Floor pushup. Start with knees touching floor, and then progress to full pushup.

E. Free weights and machines. Free weights are introduced when strengthening beyond the resistance afforded by elastic devices is desired. Beginning weights may vary from 3 to 5 pounds, depending on the patient's frame and muscular development.

External rotators (Fig. 24–3): External rotators are strengthened with the patient lying on the side. The elbow is bent to 90° with the arm resting against the body. The weight is repeatedly raised and lowered by slowly externally and internally rotating the shoulder. The patient then rolls onto the opposite side.

Internal rotators (Fig. 24–4): Internal rotators are exercised by internally rotating the shoulder while lying supine.

Prone position: The prone position is then assumed, and the arm hangs downward off the edge of the table with the hand holding the weight. From this position, the extended arm is alternately lifted forward and backward (Fig. 24–5A) and then is abducted through a range of 60° in each direction (Fig. 24–5B). We advise 15 repetitions. In time, the weight is increased gradually to 10 pounds. In every exercise involving weights, the number of repetitions is increased rather than overloading the joint with excessive weight. When weight is progressively increased at intervals, the number of repetitions should be reduced. This impingement protocol exercise is the first to allow forward flexion above shoulder height. If this exercise cannot be done without pain, forward flexion in the prone position should be eliminated until it can be done painlessly.

Seated position: Free weights may be introduced in the seated position, but only when they can be manipulated comfortably while prone. Starting with 3 to 5 pounds, the weight is then lifted through a 60° range in forward and backward extension, but only a 45° range in abduction. *Efforts to lift the arm in pure abduction are the most common cause of failure at this stage of impingement rehabilitation.* Abduction with the arm in internal or even neutral rotation causes the greater tuberosity to abut directly against the overlying acromion. Full abduction can be achieved only by combining this motion with external rotation. External rotation allows the greater tuberosity to clear the acromion and avoid impingement pain. For this reason, the forearm should be supinated as forward elevation with weight is progressed to shoulder level and beyond (Fig. 24–6). Holding the weight with the palm upward ensures external rotation during elevation.

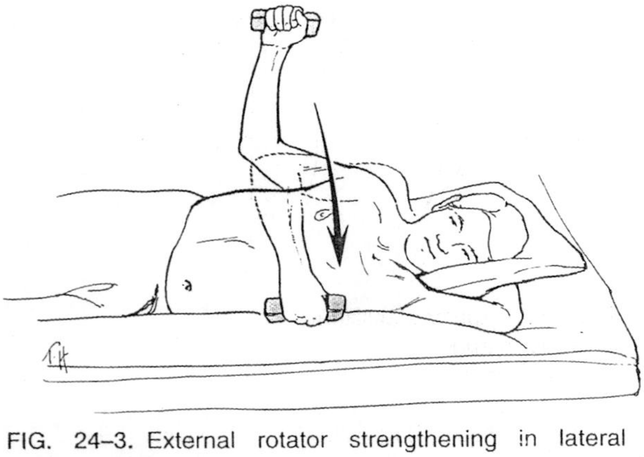

FIG. 24–3. External rotator strengthening in lateral recumbent position.

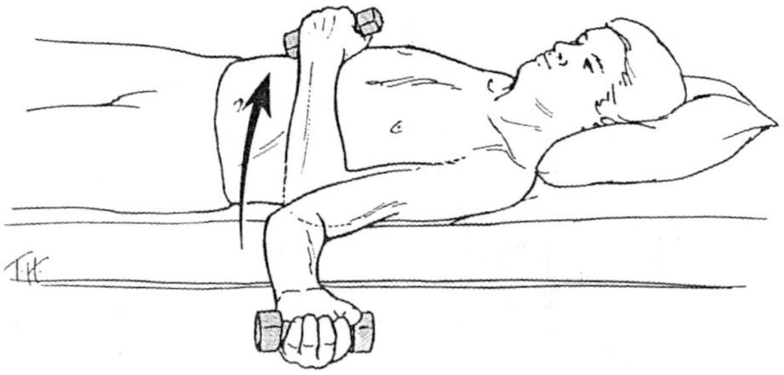

FIG. 24–4. Internal rotation strengthening while supine.

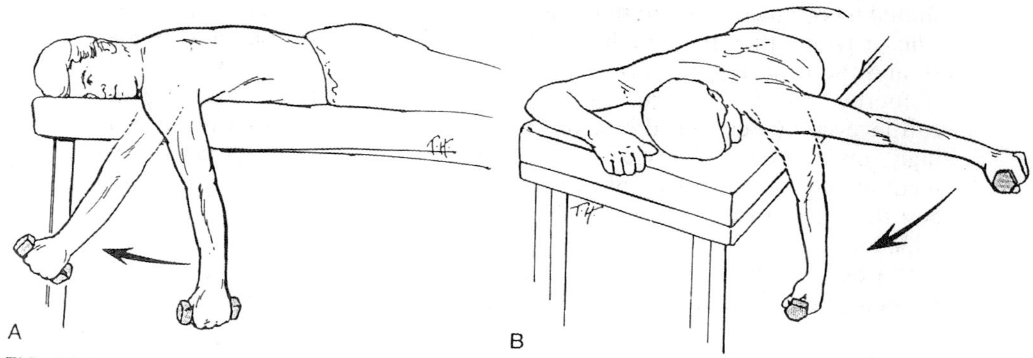

FIG. 24–5. Prone position.
A, Anterior-posterior deltoid strengthening while prone.
B, Lateral deltoid strengthening while prone.

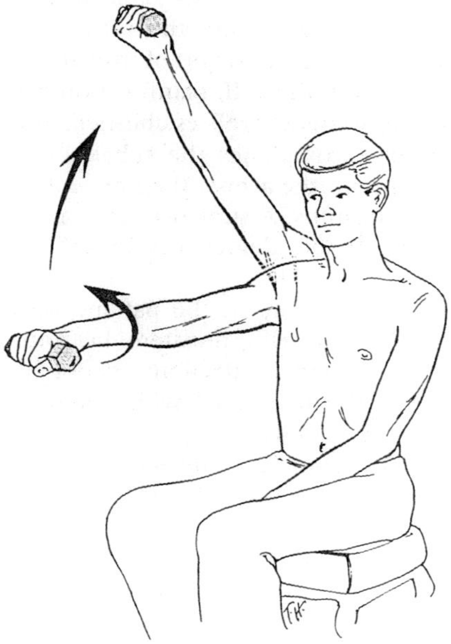

FIG. 24–6. Forward elevation is combined with external rotation to allow the greater tuberosity to clear the acromion and avoid impingement pin.

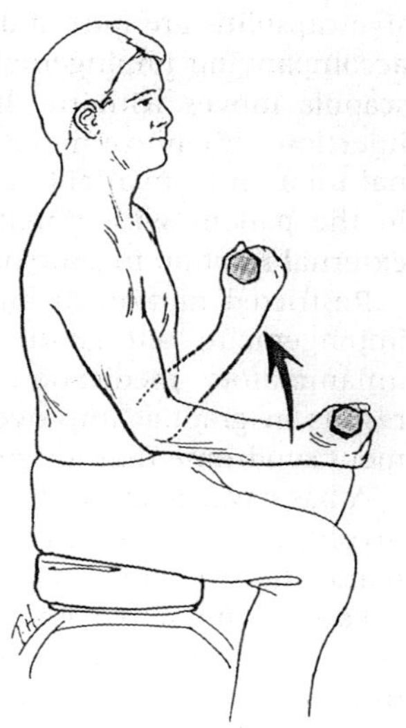

FIG. 24–7. Isolated curls.

Isolated curls: In the absence of bicipital tendinitis, isolated curls (flexion at elbow with arm at side) may be done early (Fig. 24–7), but extension of the curl into an overhead lift must be added cautiously. Bench presses are reasonably tolerated, because forward flexion does not actually extend to 90° unless the bench press is done on an incline. As stated earlier, frequent repetitions with lighter weights are preferable to overloading the shoulder with excessive weights.

F. Isotonic equipment. Stationary weight-training machinery can easily be adapted to the foregoing isotonic exercises. Preconditioning with free weights should be completed before undertaking more strenuous activities. The two specific activities that tend to be "widow-makers" for the rotator cuff are the behind-the-head military press with barbells or pull-down machinery and the "butterfly," to use the vernacular of the body-builder. Both exercises grind the cuff incessantly between the acromial arch and the humeral head. Not surprisingly, many body-builders eliminate these exercises voluntarily before seeking medical help. At the outset of treatment, the therapist or physician should suggest that these two exercises should not be resumed even after successful rehabilitation.

G. Isokinetic devices. Isokinetic devices are used for advanced conditioning of the elite athlete and are reviewed in Chapter 19.

STRETCHING EXERCISES

Some degree of restricted motion may accompany the chronic impingement syndrome. Forward flexion and internal rotation are commonly restricted as a result of pain and inactivity. An injection of local anesthetic into the subacromial space (impingement test, see Chap. 4) serves to differentiate the restriction caused by pain from that accompanying capsulitis. The early stages of true adhesive capsulitis are indeed difficult to differentiate from the stiff, painful shoulder accompanying impingement. When adhesive capsulitis is well established, the scapula moves with the humerus and no relief accompanies the subacromial injection. When examined in the supine position with the arm at the side, external rotation is invariably restricted in adhesive capsulitis. A similar examination in the patient with impingement permits a reasonable degree (25 to 45°) of external rotation in spite of local discomfort.

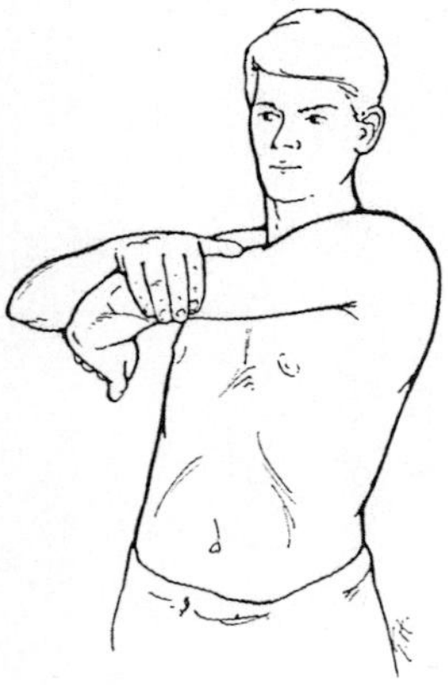

FIG. 24–8. Posterior capsule stretch.

Restricted motion in any range is difficult to overcome in the patient with impingement, but gentle stretching, in combination with nonsteroidal anti-inflammatory medication and one or two local steroid injections, generally results in gradual improvement much sooner in the individual with impingement syndrome than in the patient with adhesive capsulitis.

A basic warm-up stretch of the posterior cuff is accomplished by adducting the involved arm across the body, grasping it above the elbow with the opposite hand, and stretching to tolerance (Fig. 24–8).

Passive and active assisted stretching in both external and internal rotation is done in the subimpingement range. The patient uses a cane, a wand fashioned from a dowel, or a hand towel to assist in external rotation while supine with the elbow bent and the arm at the side (Fig. 24–9A). Internal rotation stretching may be done while standing. The restricted arm attempts to reach behind as far as possible. The opposite extremity grasps the arm at the wrist and attempts to stretch it farther. The wand or hand towel can be used in a similar fashion behind the back (Fig. 24–9B). The hand towel is particularly effective when stretching is performed during or immediately after a hot shower.

The most vigorous form of self-stretching to improve internal rotation is performed in the following fashion (Fig. 24–9C). The patient backs up to a desk or low chest of drawers with the arm held behind. The forearm is placed as flat as possible on the top of the desk or dresser. The knees are slowly bent while the trunk remains straight. A forceful internal rotation stretch is produced by this maneuver, and the patient is cautioned to proceed carefully. The stretch should be held for 10 seconds before releasing and repeating 5 times.

The doorjamb exercise affords an effective method of improving external rotation (Fig. 24–10). The patient stands before a doorway and elevates both arms to

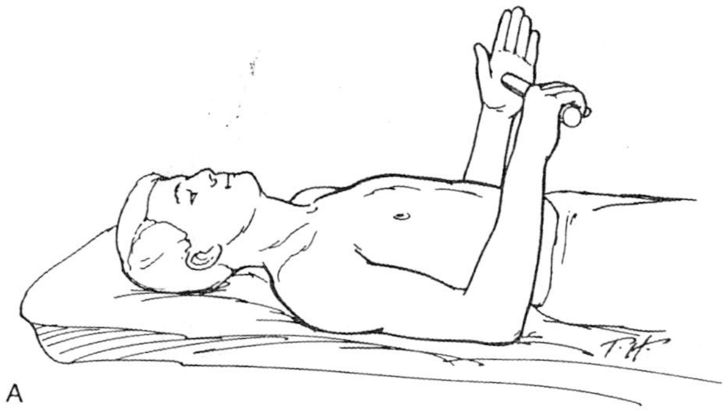

FIG. 24–9. A, External rotation contracture is stretched with arm at side and elbows bent to 90°. The opposite hand transmits force through a dowel.
B, Internal rotation stretch: A dowel is used behind the body to stretch for improvement in internal rotation contracture.
C, Greater internal rotation.

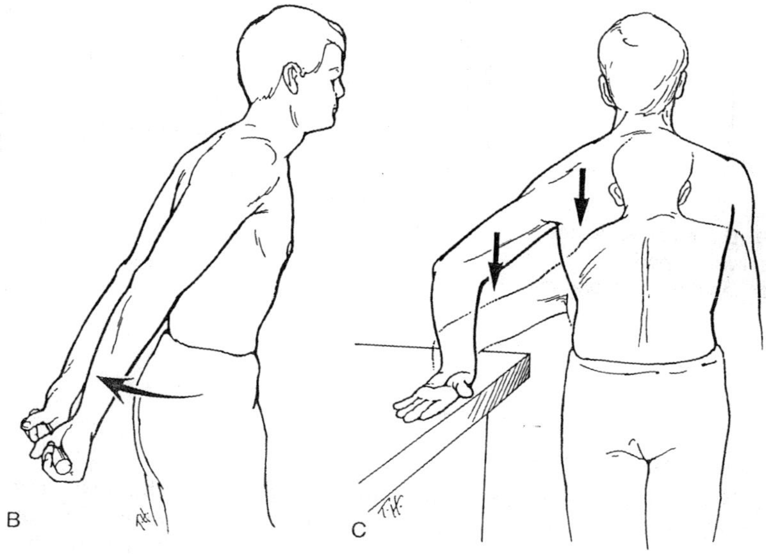

shoulder level with the elbows bent. The hands and forearms are rested, as best as possible, along the doorjamb on either side. The patient then leans forward to allow the weight of the body to pass through the doorway while the arms remain stationary. The leverage produced can be forceful, and the stretch should be performed cautiously.

POSTOPERATIVE REHABILITATION

Postoperative protocols accompany the descriptions of the various surgical procedures presented in the text. This section has been developed for the surgeon as well as the physical or occupational therapist and other health professionals concerned with shoulder rehabilitation. The basic principles and techniques required for rehabilitation are presented in detail.

PRINCIPLES OF SHOULDER REHABILITATION

Elimination of pain and restoration of function are the primary goals of rehabilitation. Three basic principles are involved.

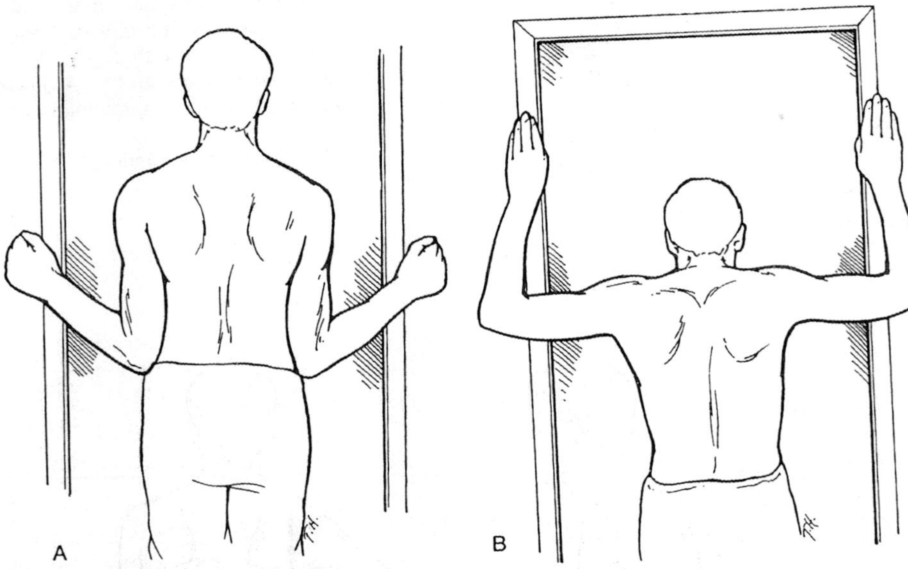

FIG. 24–10. Doorjamb stretches.
A, Elbows near the body.
B, Elevation increases as tolerated.

EARLY PASSIVE MOTION

The earliest possible mobilization that does not jeopardize the healing process or disrupt the stability of a reconstruction is desirable. Early passive motion is initiated to avoid the development of adhesions. The time to initiate passive motion is determined by the stress tolerance of the healing process. This variable requires the therapist to understand the technical aspects of any surgical reconstruction.

The tendinous insertion of a muscle that is detached for exposure and then resutured generally requires protection against active muscular contractions for 6 weeks. The same principle applies when the torn end of a rotator cuff tendon is reinserted into bone and held in place by transosseous sutures. Yet, in either instance, a secure reapproximation can tolerate gentle passive range of motion as early as 3 or 4 days postoperatively without endangering the end result. Arthroscopic subacromial decompression is performed without deltoid detachment. Although immediate active motion is allowed, some constraints are imposed until the denuded undersurface of the acromion has healed. Passive versus active motion must be defined in a consistent manner.

STRETCHING

Stretching is necessary to avoid or overcome adhesion formation as healing progresses. Initial stretching can be passive and quite gentle, whereas stretching exercises after healing are both passive and active and may involve significant force.

STRENGTHENING

Strengthening begins with simple isometrics. Early passive assisted exercises gradually become active assisted. When healing permits, the patient is allowed to lower and raise the shoulder against the resistance of gravity. Progressive resistance is added to restore strength. Improvement in strength may continue for as long as 2 years following shoulder surgery.

PHASES OF EXERCISE

The exercise program consists of three progressive phases, each of which has specific objectives.

Phase I: Passive exercises

1. To prevent early adhesion formation.
2. To promote relaxation and pain relief and to stretch the shoulder girdle musculature and begin isometric contractions of shoulder muscles.

Phase II: Active exercises

1. To strengthen shoulder muscles and continue to increase motion.
2. To promote increased range of motion and strengthening of shoulder muscles while controlling painful stimuli.

Phase III: Resistive exercises

1. To strengthen shoulder muscles further.
2. To eliminate remaining joint limitation.

SPECIFIC REHABILITATION PROTOCOLS

ARTHROSCOPIC SUBACROMIAL DECOMPRESSION (ARTHROSCOPIC ACROMIOPLASTY) WITHOUT FULL-THICKNESS ROTATOR CUFF TEAR

Arthroscopic acromioplasty is performed without detaching any portion of the deltoid insertion. For this reason, active motion may be resumed without the risk of deltoid detachment that accompanies the open procedure. A sling is not required postoperatively.

DAY 1 TO WEEKS

On the first postoperative day, the patient begins supine external rotation and then self-assisted forward elevation for 5 repetitions each. These movements are followed by pendulum exercises while standing (Fig. 24–11). The trunk should be flexed a full 90° so that it is horizontal to the floor. The purpose of these gentle range-of-motion exercises is to prevent adhesions from developing during the early postoperative period. They are performed every morning and evening for the first 3 weeks or longer if necessary to restore full motion.

3 WEEKS

After 3 weeks, the "ABC" strengthening exercises described earlier in this chapter are begun (see Fig. 24–1). These exercises are all performed in the sub-

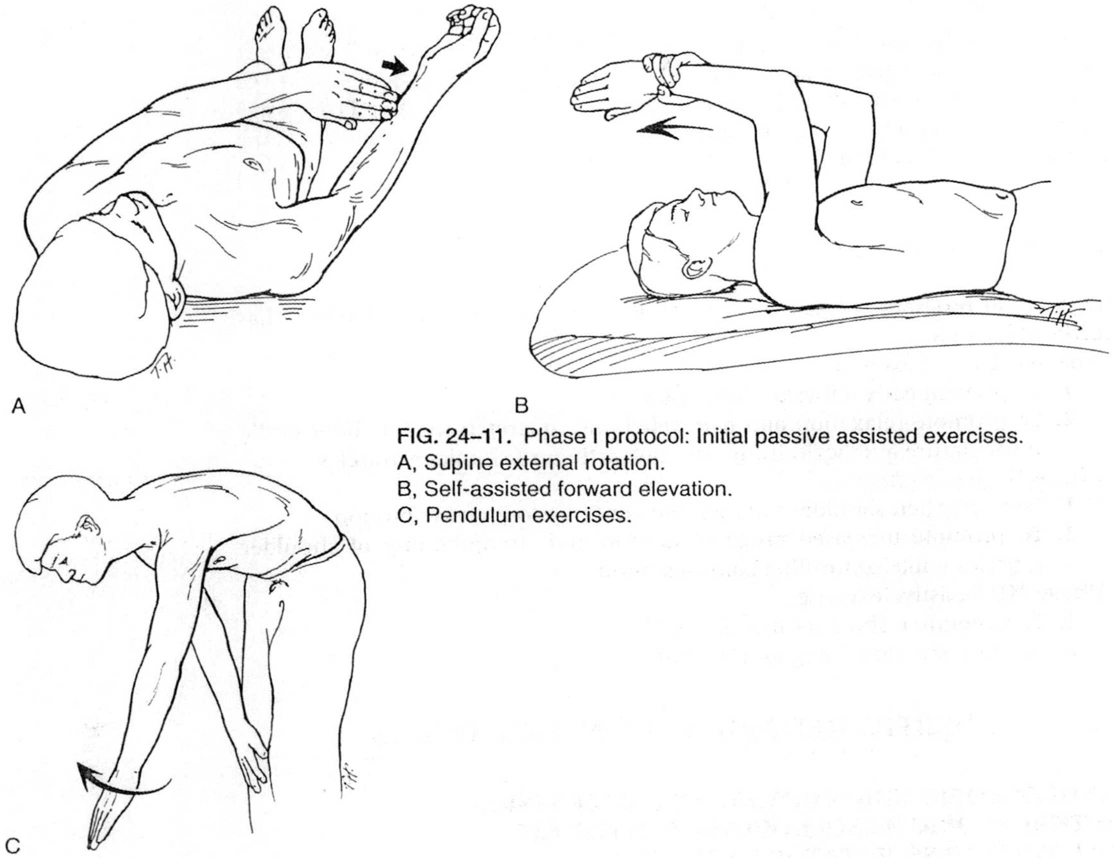

FIG. 24–11. Phase I protocol: Initial passive assisted exercises.
A, Supine external rotation.
B, Self-assisted forward elevation.
C, Pendulum exercises.

impingement range. Resistance and repetitions are increased as strength improves. If pain is provoked, the intensity of the exercises should be reduced.

6 WEEKS

After the sixth week, the phase III strengthening program is begun. Various progressively strenuous exercises are undertaken, depending on the individual's goal of rehabilitation. Exercise with free weights (3 to 5 pounds) begins in the prone position (see Fig. 24–5) and, after 1 or 2 weeks, progresses to the supine (see Figs. 24–3 and 24–4) and then to the seated position (see Figs. 24–6 and 24–7). Lifting should be done with the palms upward to ensure external rotation. The plane of the lift may range from forward flexion to the scapular plane, but lifts in pure abduction are avoided. Exercises designed to improve coordination and endurance also may be started gradually after the sixth week. A horizontal inertial exercise device has proved quite effective in restoring coordination (Fig. 24–12). The patient controls a designated amount of weight, which is propelled along a horizontal track in one direction and then the other. The control can be varied to simulate tennis or golf strokes (Fig. 24–13). Isotonic (Fig. 24–14) and isokinetic (Fig. 24–15) devices should be started at low resistance when introduced as early as 6 weeks. Sports-specific activity is allowed with restrictions at 6 weeks. Examples of such activity include ground strokes in ten-

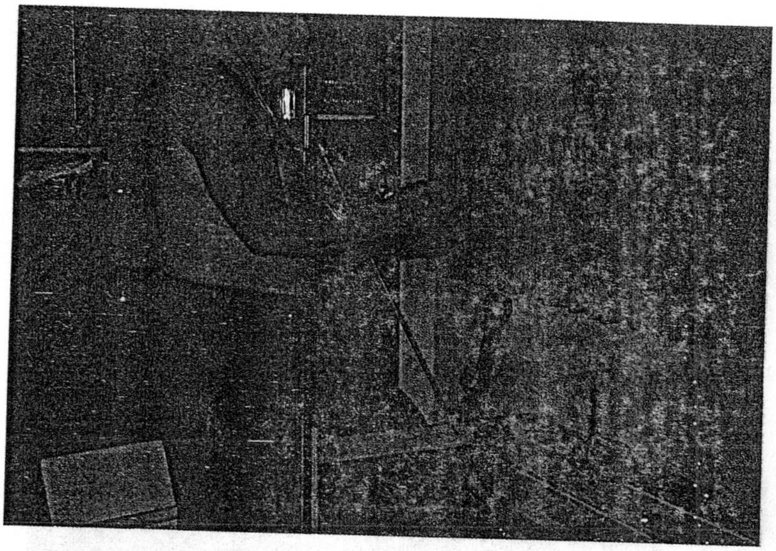

FIG. 24–12. Horizontal inertial exercise device.

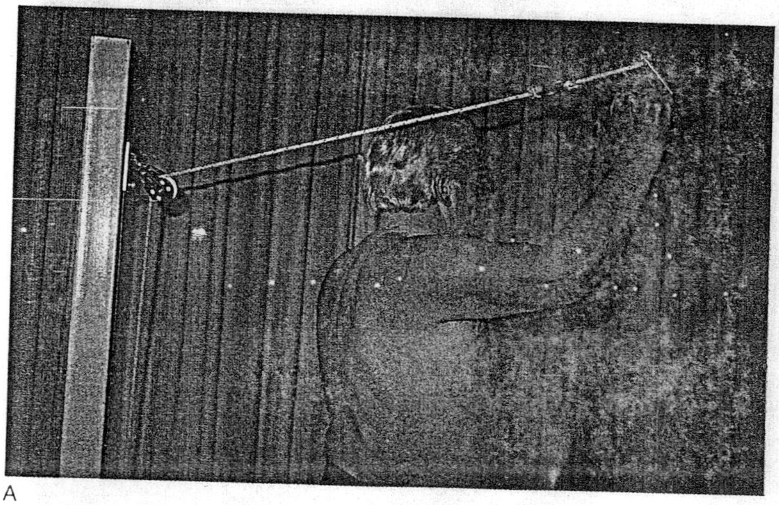

A

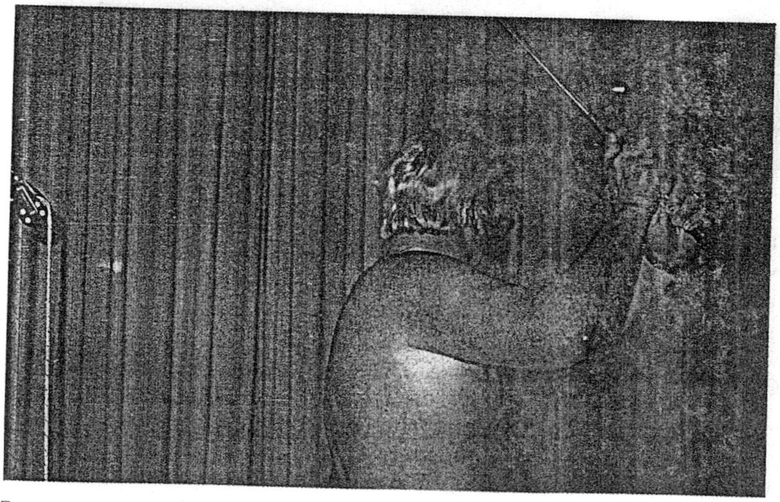

B

FIG. 24–13. Sports-specific exercise on inertial exerciser. A, Simulating backswing in golf.
B, Same patient holding golf club at top of backswing.

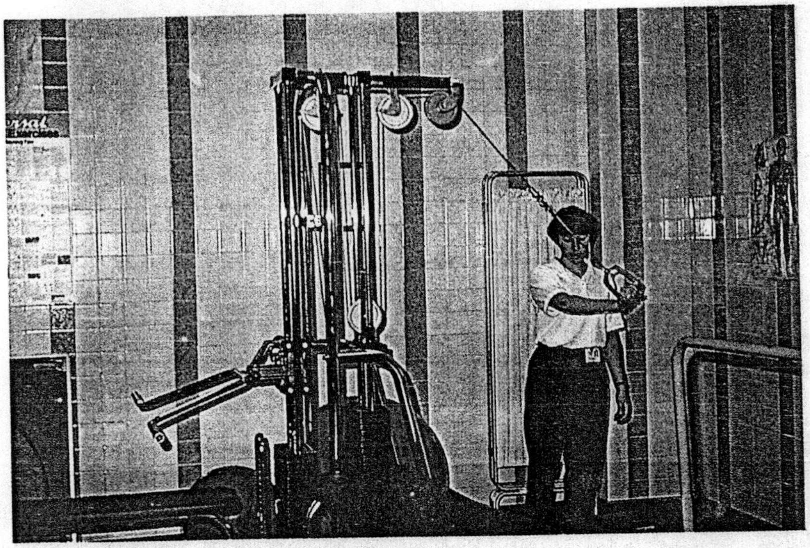

FIG. 24–14. Isotonic exercise device.

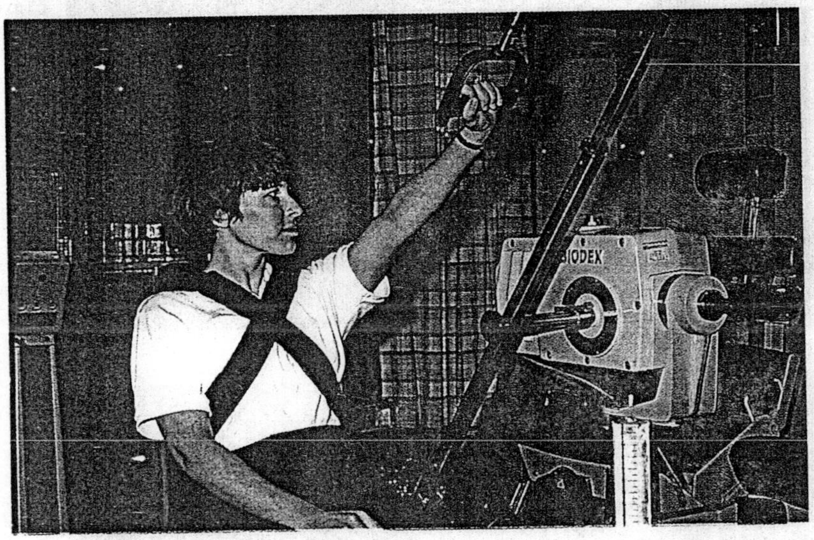

FIG. 24–15. Isokinetic exercise device.

nis or other racquet sports, chipping or pitching for the golfer, and underhand throwing for the ballplayer. Short overhead tosses may be started a few weeks later and then increased gradually.

3 MONTHS

Unrestricted sports activity or a return to strenuous overhead work is best delayed until after 3 months. The period from 6 weeks to 3 months is designed to gradually restore motion, strength, and endurance to the individual who performs overhead work or to the recreational athlete. The elite athlete must allow an even longer period (as long as 6 months) before attempting high performance at maximum exertion.

OPEN ACROMIOPLASTY WITHOUT FULL-THICKNESS ROTATOR CUFF TEAR

The open procedure either detaches the deltoid coronally from its insertion on the anterior acromion or otherwise peels away the deltoid by a midacromial sagittal incision that attempts to preserve the fibroperiosteal envelope that surrounds the anterior acromion (see Chap. 7). With either approach, the deltoid must be firmly reattached to the acromion following acromioplasty. Coronal detachments should be reconstructed with transosseous sutures through the decompressed acromion to ensure stability. In the sagittal dissection, the lateral portion of the fibroperiosteal sheath is often quite thin, and transosseous sutures are required to ensure strong closure.

The primary difference between rehabilitation following open and rehabilitation following arthroscopic acromioplasty is that a small portion of the anterior deltoid must be disrupted during the open procedure. The subsequent reconstruction of the deltoid insertion requires at least 5 or 6 weeks to pass before overhead elevation against the force of gravity can be accomplished without risk to the repair.

A sling is recommended for 3 to 6 weeks following open acromioplasty, depending on the extent of deltoid detachment and the security of the repair. The forearm and hand may be moved early to accomplish activities of daily living without actively raising the arm from the side. Failure of the deltoid reattachment is a serious complication, and the patient should be so advised to enlist maximum cooperation.

The day following open surgery, passive mobilization exercises to avoid stiffness are begun in external rotation, internal rotation, and forward flexion while supine (see Fig. 24–11). The exercise here is *passive only*, rather than the active assisted exercises that are permitted after arthroscopic acromioplasty (Fig. 24–16). Most patients can be taught to perform these passive exercises with the assistance of the sound arm.

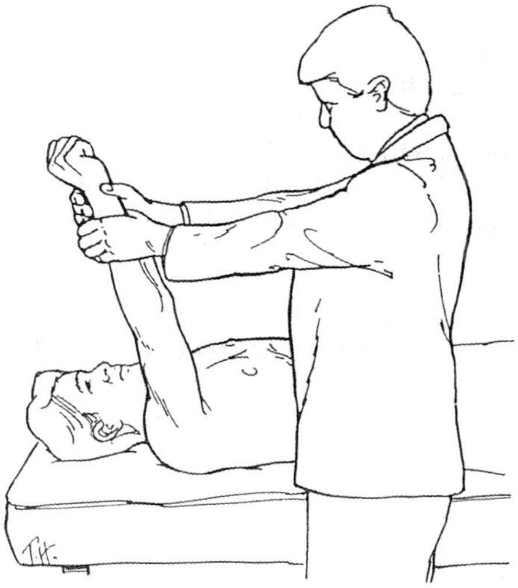

FIG. 24–16. Passive only forward elevation.

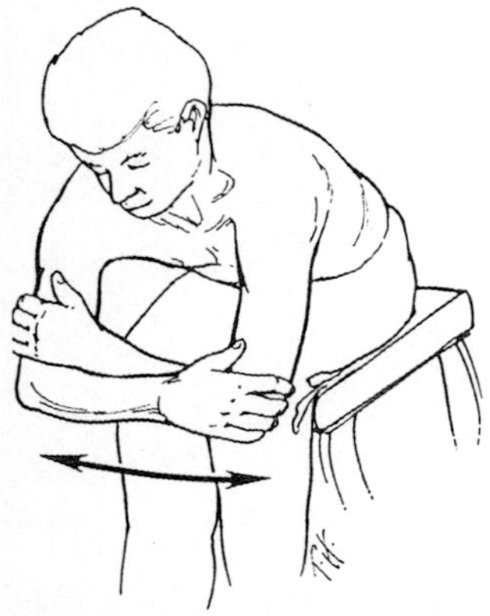

FIG. 24–17. Rock-a-bye exercises.

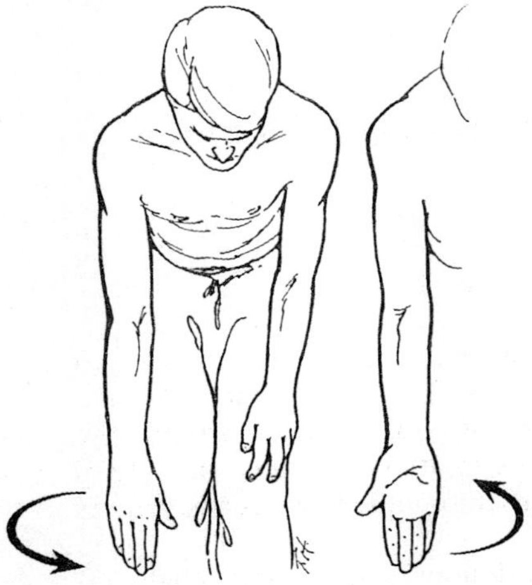

FIG. 24–18. Pendulum exercises: This exercise can be done combined with external rotation (supination) or internal rotation (pronation).

Rock-a-bye exercise is instructed on the first postoperative day (Fig. 24–17). The seated patient cradles the operated arm in the sling with the sound arm. While bending forward, the arms are allowed to fall away from the body until the elbows are beyond the knees. In this position, gentle circumduction is carried out.

The pendulum exercise replaces the rock-a-bye exercise within the first week (Fig. 24–18). The standing patient is instructed to bend forward until the trunk is parallel to the ground. The arm is allowed to fall away from the body until it hangs perpendicular to the body. A swaying motion of the body propels the relaxed shoulder into a series of pendulum-like motions. These motions may be side-to-side or in a circular pattern, first in one direction and then another. The forearm may be turned in both pronation and supination to achieve gentle internal and external rotation stretching. This exercise often relieves postoperative discomfort. The patient with a sound deltoid repair may perform the pendulum exercise 4 or 5 times daily.

Isometric strengthening in the subimpingement range may begin at 3 weeks, but the more strenuous "ABC" exercises (see Fig. 24–1) should not be attempted until 6 weeks have elapsed.

At 6 weeks, the phase II resisted exercises ("ABC") are begun in the subimpingement range. Phase II may be gradually progressed into phase III as tolerated. The rehabilitation protocol beyond this point is the same as that following arthroscopic acromioplasty without full-thickness rotator cuff tear.

OPEN REPAIR OF FULL-THICKNESS ROTATOR CUFF TEAR (INCLUDING OPEN ACROMIOPLASTY)

Prior to undergoing surgery for a torn rotator cuff, the patient is informed that the postoperative rehabilitation accounts for 50% of the result. The postoperative protocol is divided into 3 phases, modified from the principles advocated by Neer.

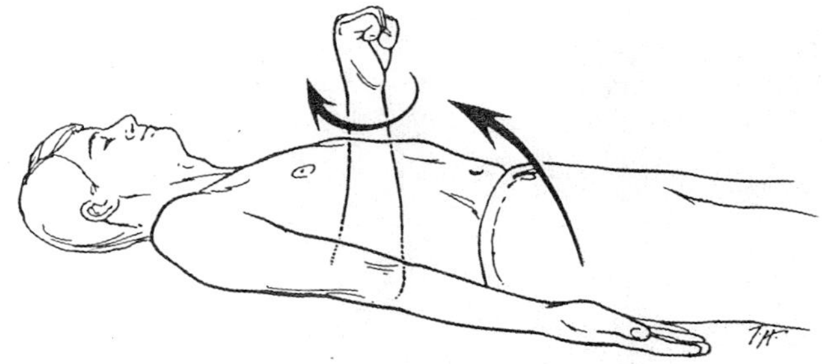

FIG. 24–19. Rotator cuff repair protocol: Phase I. While the patient is supine, elbow flexion and extension are permitted to improve circulation.

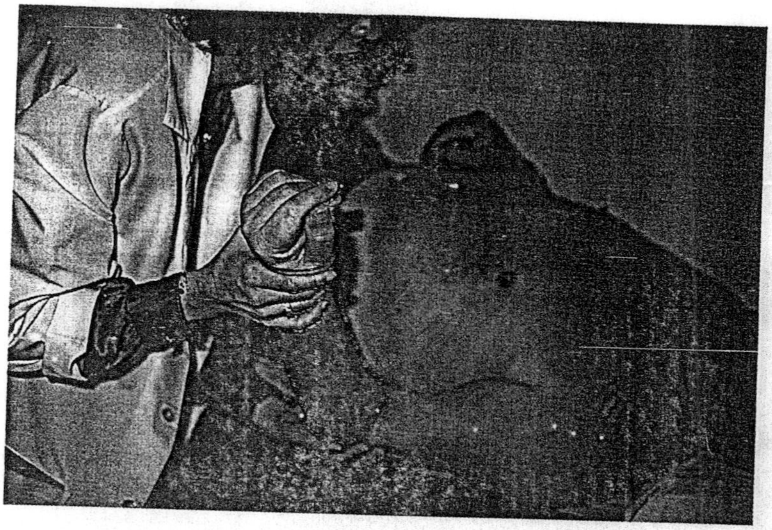

FIG. 24–20. Passive external rotation. Goal of 45° external rotation may require several days or longer to achieve.

PHASE I: PASSIVE EXERCISES

These exercises are designed primarily to prevent early adhesion formation without jeopardizing the repair. Approximately 6 weeks are required before a tendon-to-bony trough reconstruction can be strong enough to support the weight of the arm against gravity. For this reason, exercise is passive and limited to a range of motion imposed by the tension of the repair.

On the first postoperative day, with the patient resting supine in bed, the sling is released to allow the elbow to extend and flex while the arm remains at the side (Fig. 24–19). The fist is also clenched repeatedly and released. The elbow then is bent to 90° and assisted into external rotation (Fig. 24–20). The goal of at least 45° of external rotation may take several days or longer to achieve. The early restoration of external rotation range is a key to cuff rehabilitation. Before the wound is closed, the surgeon should establish the range of motion allowed without stressing the repair. Both patient and therapist should be informed of this range.

Passive forward flexion is begun with the arm firmly supported and the palm directed upward to achieve some external rotation (Fig. 24–21). Relaxation is essential and is more difficult for some patients to achieve than for others. Exhaling slowly with the mouth open as the arm is elevated is helpful. Elevation

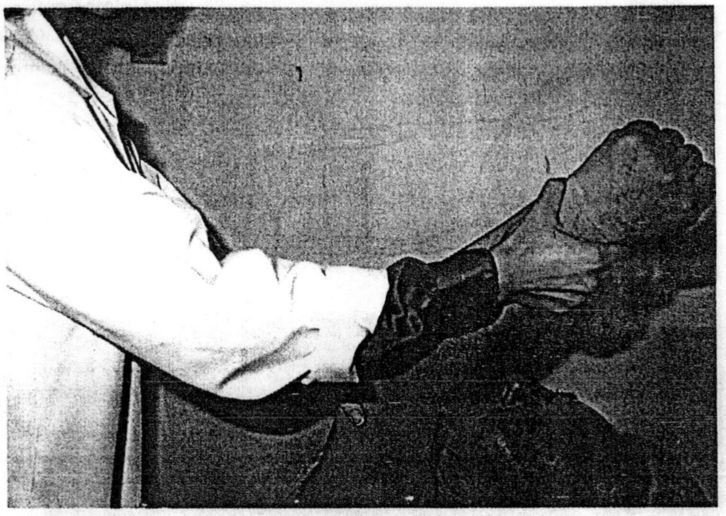

FIG. 24–21. Passive forward flexion.

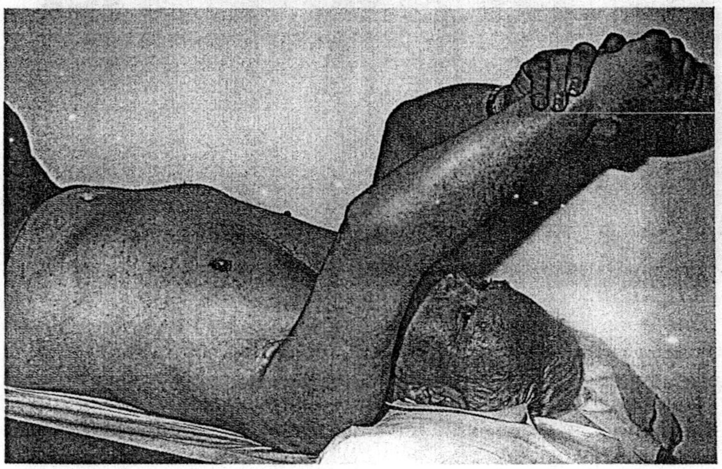

FIG. 24–22. Patient-assisted passive forward flexion.

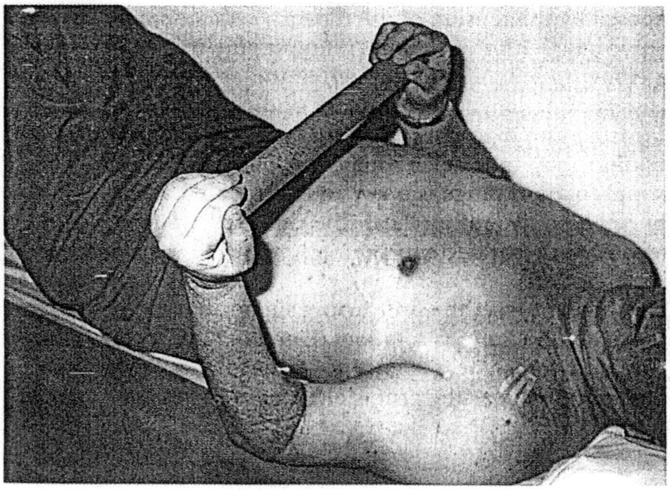

FIG. 24–23. Patient-assisted external rotation with dowel.

beyond 90° is seldom achieved in the first few days, but elevation should progress as rapidly as possible to a goal of 140° by the end of the first or second week.

The patient is also instructed in rock-a-bye exercises on the first day (Fig. 24–17). With the sling firmly supported by the sound arm, the patient bends forward until the elbows are beyond the knees. Nearly 90° of passive forward flexion can be achieved with this maneuver. The patient should be told that this position is comfortable for cleansing the axilla.

The surgeon should initiate these three passive exercises during the first and second day of hospitalization. The therapist then can continue the program. Because hospitalization may not be required beyond the third or fourth day, the phase I exercises are continued 2 to 3 times a week on an outpatient basis. Most patients learn to assist themselves in passive forward flexion (Fig. 24–22) and external rotation (Fig. 24–23) after 2 or 3 weeks. Once relaxation has been mastered, the sound arm can be used for support. Exercises are performed at home 2 times daily at this stage. The pendulum exercise (Fig. 24–24) may be substituted for the rock-a-bye exercise, and isometric contractures of the shoulder may begin at 3 weeks (Fig. 24–25). Efforts to improve scapular mobility are intensified at this time. Passive stretching should continue until a good range of passive motion is restored, hopefully by the sixth week.

PHASE II: ACTIVE EXERCISES

After the sixth week, active exercises are begun. Additional stretching may be required and may now be actively, as well as passively, assisted. Many patients tend to employ a shoulder shrug when attempting to lift the arm. This movement must be avoided as the cuff musculature is strengthened, because once established, the habit is difficult to overcome. Initial efforts to elevate the arm against gravity are best performed with the patient supine and the surgeon supervising (Fig. 24–26). The arm is elevated in the forward plane by the patient with the surgeon assisting. Once 90° of forward flexion is achieved, the patient takes over and holds the arm alone. Then the arm is lowered under the patient's control while the surgeon "spots" to ensure that a precipitous drop does not

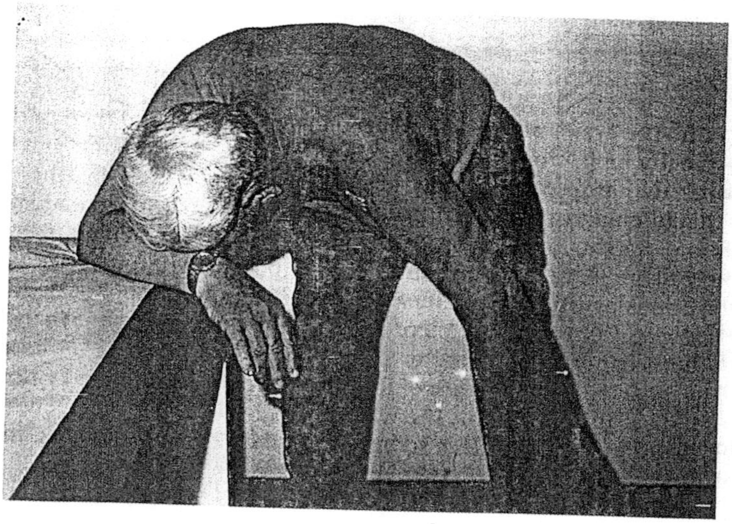

FIG. 24–24. Pendulum exercises.

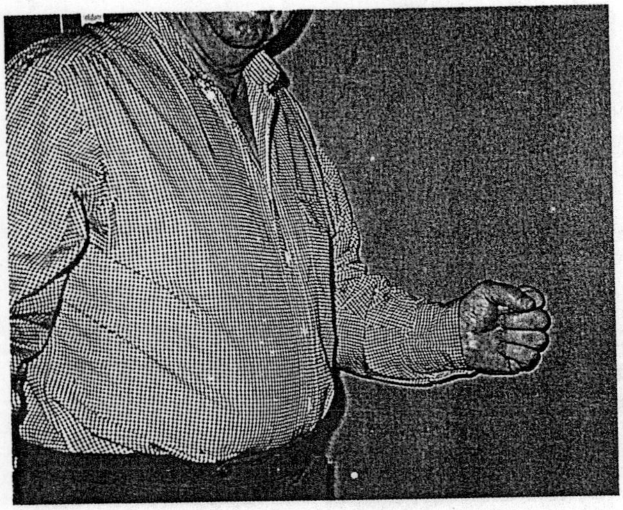

A

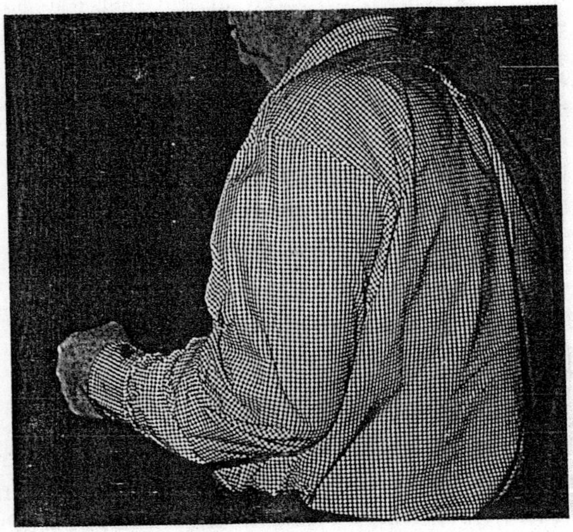

B

FIG. 24–25. Isometric exercises are begun in the third week.
A, Patient standing with back to wall presses elbow backward to strengthen posterior deltoid.
B, Patient faces the wall and pushes fist gently forward to tighten anterior deltoid.

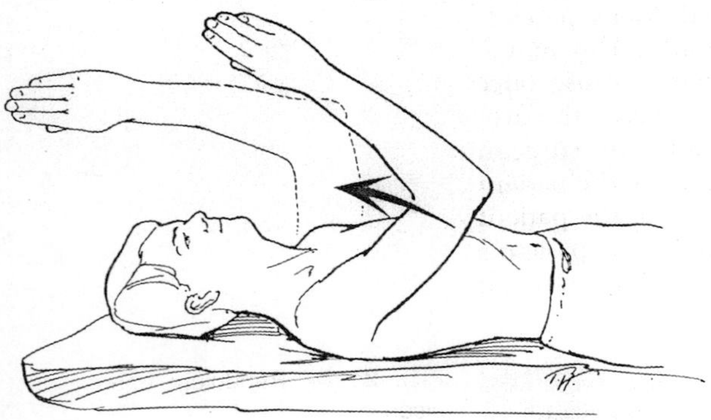

FIG. 24–26. Phase II: Active exercises. Initial active elevation is performed while patient is supine.

occur. The arm is allowed to go even lower than 90° and then to rise back to 90°. Strengthening proceeds in this position with much of the gravity eliminated, until the arm can be fully elevated from the side by the patient alone. Strengthening can proceed in the supine position with the addition of 1- to 3-pound weights. After 1 or 2 weeks of supine strengthening, the patient should be ready to elevate the arm in the seated position without a significant shrug.

Various assistive devices may be employed during phase II. A wand may be fashioned from a cane or piece of doweling 2 to 3 feet long. The wand is grasped by both hands while lying or seated and is brought into an overhead position (Fig. 24–27). The assistance of the sound arm is transmitted by the wand to raise and lower the other arm. The wand also adds a pressure element to the recovery of external rotation. The sound arm adds external rotation force while the patient is supine with elbows flexed to 90°.

Reciprocal overhead pulleys work in a similar fashion. The pulley may be hooked to an overhead support, such as an IV stand or the top of a door. The sound arm assists the healing arm in elevation (Fig. 24–28). The assistance is gradually diminished until the healing arm is doing most of the work.

Wall climbing can be combined with a more active phase II exercise (Fig. 24–29A). The patient faces the wall and climbs upward with the fingertips until the arm that was operated on is in maximum forward flexion. The hand is then moved away from the wall and held overhead. Even when the supraspinatus is quite weak, deltoid contraction and scapular migration to a position below the humeral head support the arm in this position. The patient turns 90° away from the wall and slowly lowers the arm (Fig. 24–29B). Because a full force of gravity develops as the arm is lowered, the sound arm should be ready to offer any required support.

PHASE III: RESISTIVE EXERCISES

Phase III resistive exercises are begun when the extremity can move synchronously against the force of gravity. This phase generally begins about 8 weeks postoperatively. Progressive resistance is added as the extremity strengthens. Light manual resistance is applied first (Fig. 24–30). Then elastic bands (Theraband) and surgical tubing are introduced. The resistance may be based on the opposite hand, as in the "ABC" exercises (see Fig. 24–1), or on a doorknob. Free weights are added as tolerated beginning with 1 to 3 pounds (see Figs. 24–5, 24–6, and 24–7). Exercises are designed to strengthen the anterior, middle, and posterior portions of the deltoid selectively, as well as the internal and external rotators and scapular stabilizers. Optimally, therapy continues 2 to 3 times weekly for the first 4 months. Rehabilitative methods, such as heat before treatment and ice afterward, are used to control discomfort that might occur.

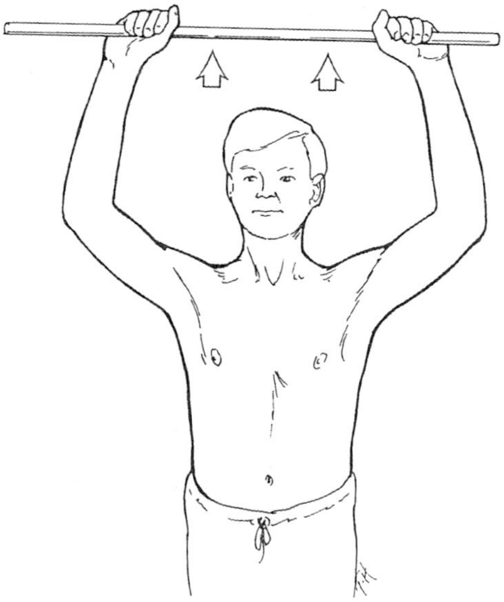

FIG. 24–27. Overhead elevation is assisted with a wand (dowel).

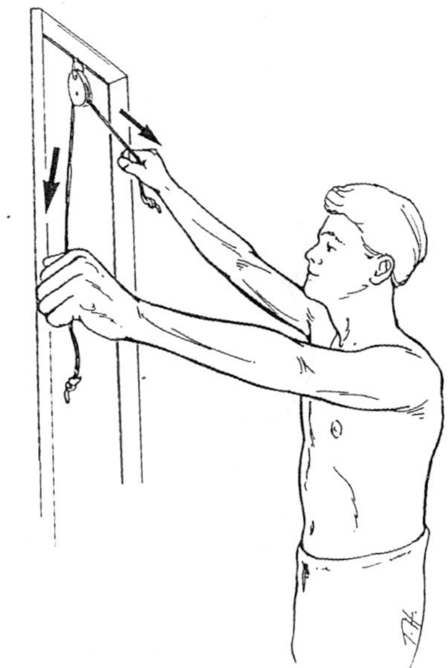

FIG. 24–28. Reciprocal overhead pulley exercise.

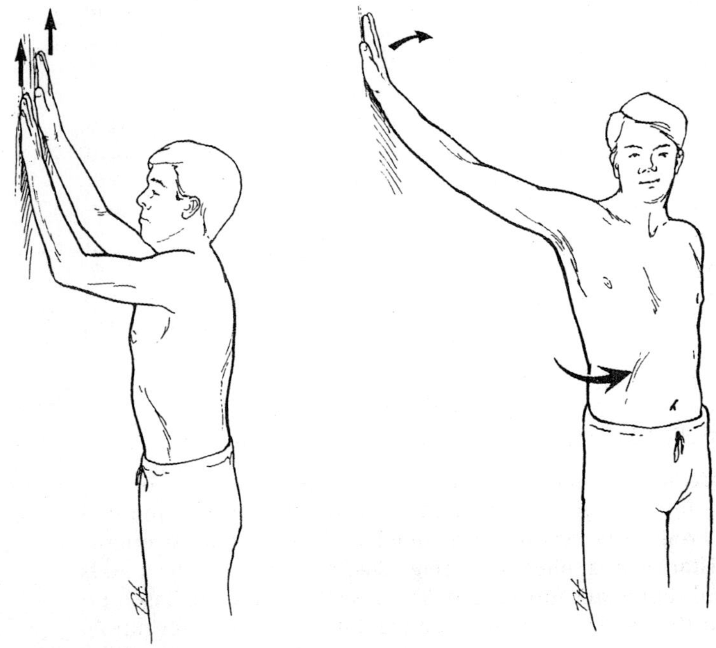

FIG. 24–29. Wall climbing.
A, Wall climbing combines active elevation with stretching.
B, After achieving good elevation, the hand is moved away from the wall. The patient then lowers the arm slowly against gravity.

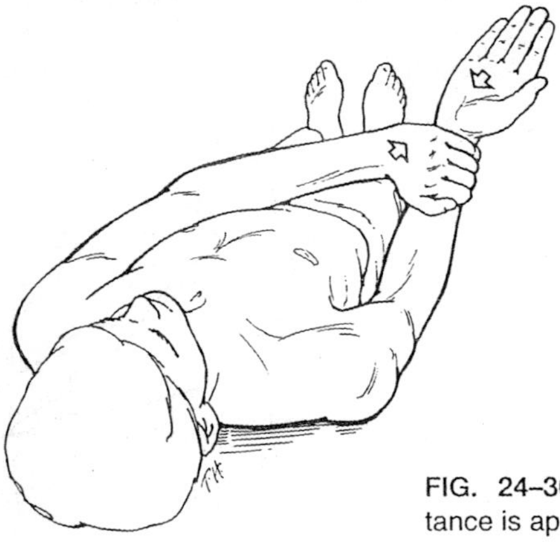

FIG. 24–30. Resistive exercises: Light manual resistance is applied by the left arm to the right arm.

The patient must conscientiously perform a home exercise program 4 to 6 times daily to supplement the therapy visits. After 4 months, the frequency of therapy visits is reduced in proportion to the patient's compliance and progress.

Active and active assisted stretching exercises should accompany phase III strengthening until full motion is restored. The doorjamb and internal rotation stretching exercises described earlier are quite valuable in this phase. Another doorway stretch is shown in Figure 24–31. In addition, a weight-bearing stretch to increase forward flexion is quite effective. The patient begins this exercise in the kneeling position and bears weight on both hands. The arms are gradually stretched forward as the body sinks into a prone position to eventually achieve full forward extension (Fig. 24–32).

The ultimate goal of cuff rehabilitation varies from a return to painless activities of daily living in an elderly patient to the achievement of preinjury form in an elite athlete. Athletes in general require additional therapy to restore coordination and endurance. Isotonic (both eccentric and concentric) and isokinetic exercises may continue under the supervision of a trainer after healing is secure. A golfer or recreational tennis player may begin play at 6 months, but throwers and weight-lifters are advised to wait at least 1 year before resuming strenuous competition. Following successful repair and rehabilitation of a full-thickness rotator cuff tear, strength generally continues to improve for at least 1 year. Follow-up examination after 2 years suggests that further improvement in strength occurs during the second year.

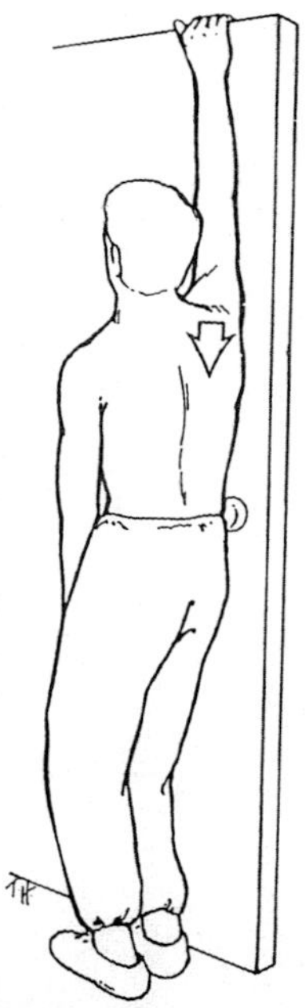

FIG. 24–31. Phase III stretching: Patient holds the top of the door and flexes knees to use body weight to stretch residual contracture.

ARTHROSCOPIC SUBACROMIAL DECOMPRESSION AND MINI-OPEN REPAIR OF FULL-THICKNESS ROTATOR CUFF TEARS

The rehabilitation protocol in these instances is similar but somewhat less demanding than that following open repair. Patients recover passive range of motion sooner and with less morbidity when the acromioplasty and repair are accomplished without deltoid detachment. When the tear is small enough to require only two sutures, or when an elliptic excision of a partial tear is reconstructed with side-to-side closure, phase II may begin at as early as 4 weeks.

DEBRIDEMENT AND DECOMPRESSION OF MASSIVE IRREPARABLE TEARS

Degenerative rotator cuff disease may progress to the point that reconstruction is virtually impossible. Rockwood has performed *open* acromioplasty and debridement of the irreparable cuff in a group of patients with such disease and reported satisfactory results.[38] Our experience with arthroscopic decompression and debridement has been similar to that of Rockwood in selected patients with irreparable cuff disease.

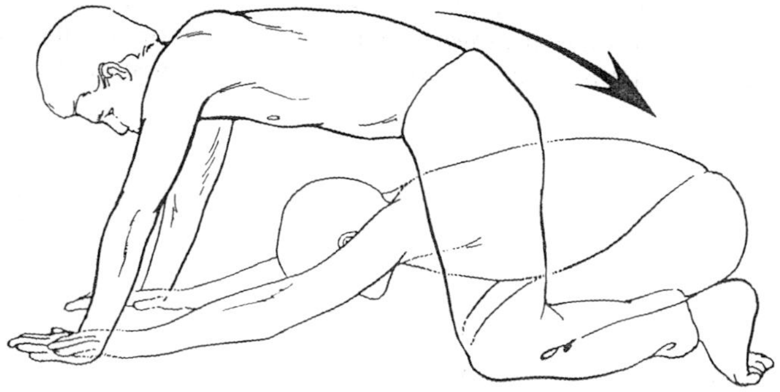

FIG. 24–32. Weight-bearing stretch: Patient rests on hands in kneeling position and then curls backward to use body weight for stretching.

When the procedure is performed *arthroscopically*, postoperative rehabilitation is similar to that following arthroscopic subacromial decompression without cuff tear. Active and active assisted motion should be started the day following surgery because the deltoid has not been disturbed. Rehabilitation following open debridement and decompression must be passively assisted until healing of the deltoid permits active elevation.

The goal after open and arthroscopic surgery is to strengthen the deltoid and scapular muscles so that functional elevation can occur in the absence of the supraspinatus and most of the infraspinatus. The "ABC" exercises with rubber tubing are started in the subimpingement range as soon as tolerated. The proprioceptive neuromuscular facilitation (PNF) pattern of obliquely abducting and elevating the arm while supine is particularly helpful in rehabilitating these patients. The hand is placed across the body in front of the contralateral hip. The arm is then lifted upward and outward to arrive overhead and moderately abducted in the plane of the scapula. Weights of 1 to 3 pounds are added gradually. This exercise is then progressed from the supine to the standing position. As pain from the acromioplasty subsides, efforts to strengthen the deltoid are maximized. Once the humeral head migrates upward into the coracoacromial arch, this pseudoarticulation captures the head and allows a strong deltoid to elevate the arm. Substitution patterns develop in these patients. If the biceps tendon is intact and hypertrophied, the patient may flex the elbow and roll into external rotation before elevation is accomplished. Others may achieve the overhead position by inclining the trunk forward slightly and then swinging the arm forward. The deltoid captures this momentum and completes the elevation. In our experience, 6 months to 1 year are required for functional elevation to develop in these patients for whom goals are limited. Few patients will be able to lift more than 3 to 5 pounds; however, pain relief has been gratifying.

ARTHROSCOPIC DEBRIDEMENT AND DECOMPRESSION OF REPARABLE FULL-THICKNESS ROTATOR CUFF TEARS

When reparable full-thickness rotator cuff tears are selected for arthroscopic debridement and decompression (based on age, activity, handedness, and size of tear), the rehabilitation is comparable to that following arthroscopic subacromial decompression without rotator cuff tear. Patients with rotator cuff tears take longer than patients without rotator cuff tears to achieve reasonable pain relief (as long as 3 months). Because the best results of treatment for full-thickness rotator cuff tears follow open repair rather than arthroscopic subacromial decompression and debridement, we routinely advise patients that the arthroscopic treatment is a compromise. Weakness persists or possibly increases, and the joint likely becomes painful if strenuous activity is resumed.

NONOPERATIVE AND POSTOPERATIVE REHABILITATION OF SHOULDER INSTABILITY

25

NONOPERATIVE REHABILITATION

The therapeutic exercises designed to overcome joint laxity are quite specific. An intense, prolonged rehabilitation effort is required to achieve a successful nonsurgical result, particularly in the athlete involved in throwing or racquet sports. Many individuals with congenital joint laxity also benefit from appropriate strengthening exercises. An exercise program designed to treat traumatic rupture of the capsulolabral mechanism (Bankart defect) usually fails. Reconstruction of the defect is required to restore unrestricted activity.

Stability depends mainly on two factors—ligamentous integrity and muscular control. The *capsular ligaments* are the primary static restraints of the shoulder and may be overstretched by throwing, racquet sports, weight training, swimming, or other strenuous activities. The *muscles* that control the shoulder form a secondary or dynamic restraint. Shoulder musculature may be divided into two groups—proximal humeral stabilizers and scapular stabilizers.

The proximal humerus is stabilized by the cuff musculature, the deltoid, pectoralis, and latissimus muscles. The scapular stabilizers (often overlooked in the rehabilitation program) include the rhomboids, levator scapulae, and serratus, as well as the trapezius and pectoralis minor. Because nonsurgical measures cannot alter an overstretched capsule, rehabilitation is directed toward the muscular stabilizers. When capsular contracture in one direction is a factor in displacing the humeral head in the opposite direction, this tightness must be overcome by stretching. Regardless of the direction of instability, all the muscles must be selectively strengthened to achieve dynamic stability. Strengthening should begin with isometric exercises and proceed to isotonic and finally isokinetic activities to achieve maximum results.

THERAPEUTIC EXERCISES

PROXIMAL HUMERAL STABILIZERS

The initial emphasis is placed on rotator cuff and deltoid strengthening. When impingement is associated with instability, the exercises should begin in the subimpingement range with the "ABC" elastic tubing exercises described in

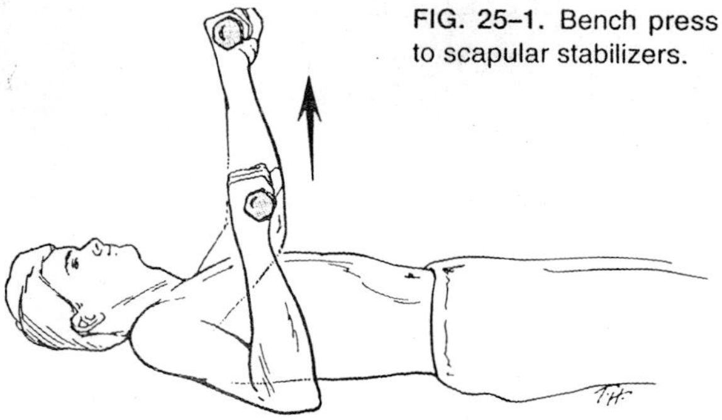

FIG. 25–1. Bench press with dumbbells to add strength to scapular stabilizers.

Chapter 24 (see Fig. 24–1). Free weights (3 to 5 pounds) then are used, first in the lateral recumbent position and then in the prone and seated positions as described (see Figs. 24–3 through 24–7). Supraspinatus strengthening is most effective when done in the scapular plane. The thumb should be pointing downward at the start and gradually rotated to point upward as full elevation with weight is achieved (see Fig. 24–6).

SCAPULAR STABILIZERS

Beyond their involvement in the preceding exercises, the scapular stabilizers require isolated strengthening. The shoulder shrug and scapular pinch exercises are used as warm-ups (see Fig. 24–2A and B). Corner pushups and floor pushups are added as strength improves (see Fig. 24–2C and D). The elbow should not pass posterior to the line of the body during a pushup to avoid overstretching of the anterior capsule.

The bench press with dumbbells adds strength to the scapular stabilizers (Fig. 25–1). The overhead military press, which allows the bar to pass behind the head, should be avoided. This exercise stretches the anterior capsule unduly.

POSTOPERATIVE REHABILITATION

Rehabilitation following surgical reconstruction of the unstable shoulder varies with the direction of instability and the method of stabilization. This section supplements the rehabilitation protocols outlined in Chapter 24 for specific surgical techniques.

ANTERIOR INSTABILITY

Anterior instability is invariably accompanied either by stretched, incompetent capsular ligaments, which allow chronic subluxation, or by a traumatic disruption of the capsulolabral attachment (Bankart lesion), which permits recurrent dislocation. A capacious capsule with intact labral attachment is tightened with some type of capsular reefing. This adjustment may be made adjacent to the glenoid, within the midportion of the capsule, or at the humeral insertion. In most circumstances, a superior shift of medial and inferior capsule is performed to balance the joint. When the capsulolabral mechanism is detached, the defect must be repaired to restore normal anatomic structure. When the capsule is both detached and redundant, some reefing is required, but in any instance, the capsule is sutured, stapled, tacked, or screwed back to the bony rim of the glenoid (see Chaps. 13 and 14).

Open surgical repair is routinely performed through the deltopectoral groove without disturbing the attachment of these contiguous muscles. The subscapularis is either detached near its tendinous insertion or split horizontally. On occasion, the conjoined tendon insertion must be loosened to allow additional exposure.

Postoperative mobilization must not unduly stress the healing of capsule to capsule, capsule to bone, or detached subscapularis tendon to its insertion, depending on the procedure.

2–3 DAYS

The goal of rehabilitation is to restore as much mobility as possible without sacrificing stability. The swath is removed on the second or third day to permit rock-a-bye exercises and then is replaced.

1 WEEK

Gentle passive mobilization exercises within the limits of the repair may be initiated after the first week. Most patients are quite protective of an open repair at this time, but generally permit forward flexion while supine to 90° with the arm internally rotated and to 30° of external rotation with the arm at the side.

2 WEEKS

After 2 weeks, resistance exercises are begun. These exercises include shoulder shrug, scapular pinch, and deltoid isometrics in anterior, posterior, and lateral directions (Fig. 25–2). The protective swath is eliminated after 2 weeks, and passive stretching continues to tolerance.

3 WEEKS

Cooperative patients may begin to gradually reduce the wearing time of the sling at 3 weeks following Bankart-type repairs, but protection with the sling is extended for as long as 6 weeks when a capsular reefing has been performed. The interval between the third and sixth weeks permits healing to mature while gentle mobilization and isometric conditioning continues.

6 WEEKS

Isotonic strengthening and active assisted range of motion strengthening begin in earnest after 6 weeks (phase II). Isolated scapular mobilization is emphasized. Healing by this time may have produced considerable anteroinferior capsular contracture. Stretching may have to continue progressively for 4 to 6 months to regain synchronous motion.

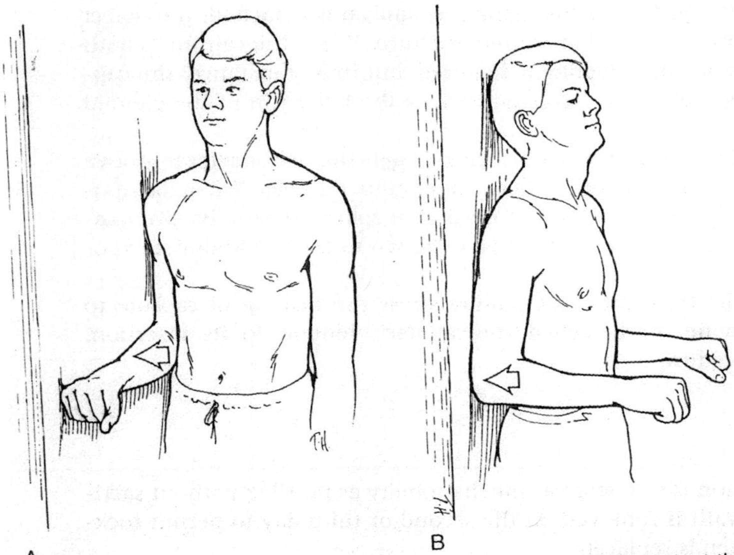

FIG. 25–2. A, Isometric deltoid exercise: Pressure is exerted against the wall to strengthen lateral deltoid.
B, Pressure is exerted posteriorly for isometric strengthening of the posterior deltoid. The direction is then reversed to strengthen the anterior deltoid.

The goal of active external rotation beyond 45 to 50° should not be exceeded, except when required for elite athletic endeavors. In this special category, the anterior capsular or labral reconstruction allows at least 45° external rotation at the end of the operation, and the patient is immobilized in an abduction splint in a position of approximately 40° abduction, 40° forward flexion, and 40° external rotation. In these patients, the splint is removed after 2 weeks, and rehabilitation progresses as described.

8 WEEKS

The phase III resistive exercises, including pushups, are started at this time. Active stretching should continue until full range of motion is restored (with care taken to avoid overstretching into external rotation). Isokinetics may be started now.

12 WEEKS

By 3 months post surgery, the patient should be capable of performing strengthening and stretching exercises in a home program with little more than occasional supervision from a therapist. Recreational sports activity can be resumed gradually between the third and sixth months, after which unrestricted activity is permitted. The elite athlete must continue to train under supervision to regain motion and endurance specific to a selected sport for as long as 1 year before resuming competition.

POSTERIOR INSTABILITY

Surgical techniques designed to overcome posterior instability include capsular reconstruction, bone block, and osteotomy to alter glenoid version.

Capsular reefing techniques, such as the posterior capsular shift or reverse Bankart procedure, require immobilization in neutral or slight external rotation. A "gunslinger" brace or spica cast is generally required. In these instances, the immobilization is carried out for 6 to 8 weeks to ensure adequate healing. The recurrence rate following posterior reconstructions is much higher than that following anterior stabilizations. Consequently, a more conservative approach is taken during the period of immobilization. Once the immobilization is removed, shoulder rehabilitation proceeds along the pattern described for rehabilitation following anterior instability repair.

The *bone block* and *osteotomy* techniques require at least 6 weeks of protection to allow for bone healing. The rehabilitation may then proceed as described previously.

MULTIDIRECTIONAL INSTABILITY

Multidirectional instability is now commonly appreciated as a clinical entity. Multidirectional instability may produce abnormal translation in a variety of directions: anterior and inferior, posterior and inferior, or a combination of anterior, posterior, and inferior.

Patients with the latter combination pattern of instability are apt to exhibit a degree of generalized ligamentous laxity approaching that characteristic of Ehlers-Danlos syndrome. Restoring stability in this subgroup of patients is challenging, and prolonged immobilization is required. A gunslinger brace or spica cast in the neutral position is required for a minimum of 8 weeks. Stretching exercises are used sparingly to achieve a maximum range of motion required for activities of daily living. Strengthening begins following immobilization, but resumption of strenuous activities should be delayed for as long as 1 year in patients with global instability.

The more common combination of *anteroinferior* or *posteroinferior* multidirectional instability requires a less rigid protocol. The direction of major instability usually dictates whether the operation is done through an anterior or a posterior approach. Our rehabilitation protocol dictates that patients who have had an anterior capsular shift are immobilized in a gunslinger brace set in 10° of internal rotation for 6 weeks. Gentle passive mobilization is allowed after 2 or 3 weeks, but great care is taken to avoid stressing the repair by externally rotating or flexing too much. When the capsular shift has been performed posteriorly, the gunslinger brace is set in 10° of external rotation and maintained for 6 weeks following an initial repair. The brace is maintained for 8 weeks if a prior attempt to repair posterior instability in the patient has failed.

POST-ARTHROSCOPIC SHOULDER STABILIZATION

The arthroscopic techniques described in Chapter 13 are designed to reattach a capsulolabral detachment or to tighten, as well as to reattach a capacious capsule. The preponderance of these procedures is performed for anterior instability. Multidirectional instability is considered a relative contraindication at present.

The minimum period of sling-and-swath immobilization following arthroscopic repair is 3 weeks. Because arthroscopic stabilization is performed without extensive incision or muscle detachment, the post-surgical pain of arthroscopic repair is much diminished in comparison to the pain experienced after open stabilization procedures. The protective pain response is eliminated, and patients are cautioned against sling removal or premature resumption of activities that jeopardize the repair.

Although a given technique may allow sling immobilization to end at 3 weeks, an additional 3 weeks of restricted stretching is advised to protect the anterior capsule. Significant or prolonged contracture is less likely following arthroscopic stabilization unless superior shift of the capsule has been excessive. The concern following arthroscopic stabilization is rather with the higher recurrence rate of redislocation. This high rate suggests a failure of the fixation technique, a failure to incorporate adequate tissue into the repair, or possibly a failure of the patient to forego premature stressful activity that disrupts the repair before it has had time to mature.

Isometrics are begun after 3 weeks, but isotonic exercises are delayed a full 6 weeks. Stretching and strengthening then progress gradually along the same protocol as that described following open reconstruction.

CONCLUSION

Successful shoulder rehabilitation results from the combined efforts of the physician, therapist, and patient. Following surgical intervention, the therapist must be aware of the muscles that have been released and reattached during the surgery, as well as of the quality of the tissue that has been repaired, the type of fixation device(s) used, and the security of the repair. This information is essential during early mobilization. The patient also should understand this same information to achieve maximum compliance with the program. Handouts can be made from the illustrations of various exercises, but the patient should be personally instructed as to what exercises to do and how to perform them. Post-surgical rehabilitation is as important as the surgical procedure in restoring shoulder function.

REFERENCES—CHRONOLOGIC

1. Neer, C.S. II: Anterior acromioplasty for the chronic impingement syndrome in the shoulder. A preliminary report. J. Bone Joint Surg., *54A*:41, 1972.
2. Gerber, C., and Ganz, R.: Clinical assessment of instability of the shoulder. J. Bone Joint Surg., *66B*:551, 1984.
3. Ellman, H., Harris, E., and Kay, S.P.: Early degenerative joint disease simulating impingement. Arthroscopy, *8(4)*:482, 1992.
4. Neviaser, R.J., and Neviaser, T.J.: The frozen shoulder diagnosis and management. Clin. Orthop., *223*:59, 1987.
5. DePalma, A.F.: Surgery of the Shoulder. 2nd Ed. Philadelphia, J.B. Lippincott, 1973.
6. Moseley, H.F., and Overgaard, B.: The anterior capsular mechanism in recurrent anterior dislocation of the shoulder. J. Bone Joint Surg., *44B*:913, 1962.
7. Detrisac, D.A., and Johnson, L.L.: Arthroscopic Shoulder Anatomy. New Jersey, Slack, 1986.
8. Bowen, M.K., et al.: Role of the inferior glenohumeral ligament complex in limiting inferior translation of the glenohumeral joint. American Shoulder and Elbow Surgeons, Specialty Day, February 23, 1992.
9. Smith, J.G.: Pathological appearances of seven cases of injury of the shoulder joint with remarks. London Medical Gazette, *14*:280, 1834 (reported in Am. J. Med. Sci., *16*:219, 1834).
10. Codman, E.A.: Obscure lesions of the shoulder; rupture of the supraspinatus tendon. Boston Med. Surg. J., *196*:381, 1927.
11. Codman, E.A.: The Shoulder. Boston, Thomas Todd, 1934.
12. Wilson, P.D.: Complete rupture of the supraspinatus tendon. JAMA, *96*:433, 1931.
13. Bosworth, D.M.: An analysis of 28 consecutive cases of incapacitating shoulder lesions radically explored and repaired. J. Bone Joint Surg., *22*:392, 1940.
14. McLaughlin, H.L.: Lesions of the musculotendinous cuff of the shoulder. I. The exposure and treatment of tears with retraction. J. Bone Joint Surg., *26*:41, 1944.
15. McLaughlin, H.L., and Asherman, E.G.: Lesions of the musculotendinous cuff of the shoulder. IV. Some observations based upon the results of surgical repair. J. Bone Joint Surg., *33A*:76, 1951.
16. McLaughlin, H.L.: Rupture of the rotator cuff. J. Bone Joint Surg., *44A*:979, 1962.
17. Moseley, H.F.: Ruptures of the rotator cuff. Br. J. Surg., *38*:340, 1951.
18. Debeyre, J., Patte, D., and Elmelik, E.: Repair of ruptures of the rotator cuff of the shoulder, with a note on advancement of the supraspinatus muscle. J. Bone Joint Surg., *47B(1)*:36, 1965.
19. Patte, D., Debeyre, J., and Goutallier, D.: Rotator cuff repair by muscle advancement. *In* Shoulder Surgery. Edited by I. Bayley and L. Kessel. Great Britain, Springer-Verlag, 1982.
20. Heikel, H.V.A.: Rupture of the rotator cuff of the shoulder: experiences of surgical treatment. Acta Orthop. Scand., *39*:477, 1968.
21. Godsil, R.D., Jr., and Linscheid, R.L.: Intratendinous defects of the rotator cuff. Clin. Orthop., *69*:181, 1970.
22. Neviaser, J.S.: Ruptures of the rotator cuff of the shoulder. New concepts in the diagnosis and operative treatment of chronic tears. Arch. Surg., *102*:483, 1971.
23. Wolfgang, G.L.: Surgical repair of tears of the rotator cuff of the shoulder. Factors influencing the results. J. Bone Joint Surg., *56A*:14, 1974.
24. Neviaser, J.S., Neviaser, R.J., and Neviaser, T.J.: The repair of chronic massive ruptures of the rotator cuff of the shoulder by use of a freeze-dried rotator cuff. J. Bone Joint Surg., *60A*:681, 1978.
25. Packer, N.P., Calvert, P.T., Bayley, J.I.L., and Kessel, L.: Operative treatment of chronic ruptures of the rotator cuff of the shoulder. J. Bone Joint Surg., *65B(2)*:171, 1983.
26. Post, M., Silver, R. and Singh, M.: Rotator cuff tear. Diagnosis and treatment. Clin. Orthop., *173*:78, 1983.
27. Hawkins, R.J., Misamore, G.W., and Hobeika, P.E.: Surgery for full-thickness rotator cuff tears. J. Bone Joint Surg., *67A*:1349, 1985.
28. Ellman, H., Hanker, G., and Bayer, M.: Repair of the rotator cuff. End-result study of factors influencing reconstruction. J. Bone Joint Surg., *68A*:1136, 1986.
29. Cofield, R.H.: Subscapular muscle transposition for repair of chronic rotator cuff tears. Surg. Gynecol. Obstet., *154*:677, 1982.
30. Neviaser, R.J., and Neviaser, T.J.: Transfer of subscapularis and teres minor for massive defects of the rotator cuff. *In* Shoulder Surgery. Edited by I. Bayley and L. Kessel. Berlin, Springer-Verlag, 1982.
31. Neer, C.S. II: Shoulder Reconstruction. Philadelphia, W.B. Saunders, 1990.

32. Gerber, C.: Latissimus dorsi transfer for treatment of irreparable tears of the rotator cuff. Clin. Orthop., *275*:152, 1992.
33. Bigliani, L.U., et al.: Operative repair of massive rotator cuff tears: long-term results. Orthop. Trans., *14*:251, 1990.
34. Takagishi, N.: Conservative treatment of the ruptures of the rotator cuff. J. Jpn. Orthop. Assoc., *52*:781, 1978.
35. Brown, J.T.: Early assessment of supraspinatus tears, procaine infiltration as a guide to treatment. J. Bone Joint Surg., *31B(3)*:423, 1949.
36. Wolfgang, G.L.: Rupture of the musculotendinous cuff of the shoulder. Clin. Orthop., *134*:230, 1978.
37. Samilson, R.L.: Rotator cuff tears: management and end results of over 400 cases. J. Bone Joint Surg., *62B*:277, 1984.
38. Rockwood, C.A., and Burkhead, W.Z.: Management of patients with massive rotator cuff defects by acromioplasty and rotator cuff debridement. Orthop. Trans., *12*:190, 1988.
39. Ellman, H., and Kay, S.P.: Arthroscopic subacromial decompression for chronic impingement: 2- to 5-year results. J. Bone Joint Surg., *73B*:395, 1991.
40. Ellman, H., Kay, S.P., and Wirth, M.: Arthroscopic treatment of full-thickness rotator cuff tears: mid-term follow-up study. Arthroscopy (in press).
41. Esch, C., et al.: Arthroscopic subacromial decompression: results according to the degree of rotator cuff tear. Arthroscopy, *4(4)*:241, 1988.
42. Codman, E.A., and Akerson, I.D.: The pathology associated with rupture of the supraspinatus tendon. Ann. Surg., *93*:348, 1931.
43. Lohr, J.F., and Uhthoff, H.K.: The pathogenesis of degenerative rotator cuff tears. Orthop. Trans., *11*:237, 1987.
44. Fukuda, H., Mikasa, M., and Yamanaka, K.: Incomplete thickness rotator cuff tears diagnosed by subacromial bursography. Clin. Orthop., *223*:51, 1987.
45. Neer, C.S. II, Craig, E.V., and Fukuda, H.: Cuff tear arthropathy. Orthop. Trans., *5*:447, 1981.
46. McCarty, D.J., et al.: Milwaukee shoulder. Association of microspheroids containing hydroxyapatite crystals, active collagens and neutral protease with rotator cuff defects. J. Clin. Aspects Arthritis Rheum., *24*:464, 1981.
47. DePalma, A.F.: Surgery of the Shoulder. Philadelphia, J.B. Lippincott, 1950.
48. Lindblom, K.: On the pathogenesis of ruptures of the tendon aponeurosis of the shoulder joint. Acta Radiol., *20*:548, 1939.
49. Moseley, H.F., and Goldie, I.: The arterial pattern of the rotator cuff. J. Bone Joint Surg., *45B*:780, 1963.
50. Rothman, R.H. and Parke, W.W.: The vascular anatomy of the rotator cuff. Clin. Orthop. *41*:176, 1965.
51. MacNab, I., and Rathbun, J.B.: The microvascular pattern of the rotator cuff. J. Bone Joint Surg., *52B*:540, 1970.
52. Andrews, J.R., Broussard, T.S., and Carson, W.G.: Arthroscopy of the shoulder in the management of partial tears of the rotator cuff: a preliminary report. Arthroscopy, *1*:117, 1985.
53. Harryman, D.T. II, et al.: Repairs of the rotator cuff. Correlation of functional result with integrity of the cuff. J. Bone Joint Surg., *73A*:982, 1991.
54. Uhthoff, H.K., Sarkar, K., and Maynard, J.A.: Calcifying tendinitis: a new concept of its pathogenesis. Clin. Orthop., *118*:164, 1976.
55. Bigliani, L.U., Morrison, D.S., and April, E.W.: The morphology of the acromion and its relationship to rotator cuff tears. Orthop. Trans., *10*:228, 1986.
56. Neer, C.S. II and Poppen, N.K.: Supraspinatus outlet. Orthop. Trans., *11*:234, 1987.
57. Petersson, C.J., and Gentz, C.F.: Ruptures of the supraspinatus tendon. The significance of distally pointing acromioclavicular osteophytes. Clin. Orthop., *174*:143, 1983.
58. Ellman, H.: Diagnosis and treatment of incomplete rotator cuff tears. Clin. Orthop., *254*:64, 1990.
59. Matsen, F.A. III: Personal communication.
60. Neer, C.S. II: Impingement lesions. Clin. Orthop., *173*:70, 1983.
61. Hawkins, R.J., and Kennedy, J.C.: The impingement syndrome in athletes. Am. J. Sports Med., *8*:151, 1980.
62. Constant, C.R., and Murley, A.H.G.: A clinical method of functional assessment of the shoulder. Clin. Orthop., *214*:160, 1987.
63. Fukuda, H., Hamada, K., and Kobayashi, Y.: Push-up views for the massive rotator cuff tear—a new roentgenographic projection. Orthop. Trans., *13*:240, 1989.
64. Golding, F.C.: The shoulder—the forgotten joint. Br. J. Radiol., *35*:149, 1962.
65. Weiner, D.S., and MacNab, I.: Superior migration of the humeral head. A radiological aid in the diagnosis of tears of the rotator cuff. J. Bone Joint Surg., *52B(3)*:524, 1970.

66. Cotton, R.E., and Rideout, D.F.: Tears of the humeral rotator cuff. A radiological and pathological necropsy survey. J. Bone Joint Surg., *46B(2)*:314, 1964.
67. Rockwood, C.A., Jr., et al.: X-ray evaluation of shoulder problems. *In* The Shoulder. Edited by C.A. Rockwood, Jr., and F.A. Matsen III. Philadelphia, W.B. Saunders, 1990.
68. Neer, C.S. II: Displaced proximal humeral fractures. J. Bone Joint Surg., *52A*:1077, 1970.
69. Neer, C.S. II: Unfused acromial epiphysis in impingement and cuff tears. American Academy of Orthopedic Surgeons, Instructional Course, 1978.
70. Lindblom, K.: Arthrography and roentgenography in ruptures of the tendon of the shoulder joint. Acta Radiol., *20*:548, 1939.
71. Kerwein, G.A., Rosenburg, B., and Sneed, W.R.: Arthrographic studies of the shoulder joint. J. Bone Joint Surg., *39A*:1267, 1957.
72. Resnick, D.: Shoulder arthrography. Radiol. Clin. North Am., *19*:243, 1981.
73. Ghelman, B., and Goldman, A.B.: The double contrast shoulder arthrogram: evaluation of rotary cuff tears. Radiology, *124*:251, 1977.
74. Mink, J., Harris, E., and Rappaport, M.: Rotator cuff tear evaluation using double contrast shoulder arthrography. Radiology, *157*:621, 1985.
75. Resch, H., Kadletz, R., Beck, E., and Helweg, G.: Single and double-contrast CT scanning in the examination of recurrent shoulder dislocations. Unfallchirurg, *89*:441, 1982.
76. Middleton, W.D., et al.: Ultrasonography of the rotator cuff: technique and normal anatomy. J. Ultrasound Med., *3*:549, 1984.
77. Mack, L.A., Gannon, M.K., Kilcoyne, R.F., and Matsen, F.A. III: Sonographic evaluation of rotator cuff: accuracy in patient without prior surgery. Clin. Orthop., *234*:21, 1988.
78. Hodler, J., Fretz, C.J., Terrier, F., and Gerber, C.: Rotator cuff tears: correlation of sonographic and surgical findings. Radiology, *169*:791, 1988.
79. Seeger, L.L., et al.: MR imaging of the normal shoulder. Am. J. Radiol., *148*:83, 1987.
80. Kneeland, J.B., et al.: MR imaging of the shoulder: diagnosis of rotator cuff tears. Am. J. Radiol., *149(2)*:333, 1988.
81. Reiser, M., et al.: Role of magnetic resonance imaging in the diagnosis of shoulder joint injuries. Radiologe, *28(2)*:79, 1988.
82. Seeger, L.L., Gold, R.H., Bassett, L.W., and Ellman, H.: Shoulder impingement syndrome: MR findings in 53 shoulders. Am. J. Radiol., *150*:343, 1988.
83. Hawkins, R.J., and Kennedy, J.C.: Impingement syndrome in athletes. Am. J. Sports Med., *8*:151, 1980.
84. Post, M., and Cohen, J.: Impingement syndrome—a review of late Stage II and early Stage III lesions. Clin. Orthop., *207*:126, 1986.
85. Raggio, C.L., Warren, R.F., and Sculco, T.: Surgical treatment of impingement syndrome: four-year follow-up. Orthop. Trans., *9*:48, 1985.
86. McShane, R.B., Leinberry, C.F., and Fenlin, J.M.: Conservative open anterior acromioplasty. Clin. Orthop., *233*:137, 1987.
87. Thorling, J., et al.: Acromioplasty for impingement syndrome. Acta Orthop. Scand., *56*:147, 1985.
88. Ellman, H.: Arthroscopic subacromial decompression: a preliminary report. Orthop. Trans., *9*:49, 1985.
89. Paulos, L.E., Chamberlain, S., and Murray, S.: Arthroscopic subacromial decompression. Orthop. Trans., *10*:222, 1986.
90. Ellman, H.: Arthroscopic subacromial decompression: analysis of 1- to 3-year results. Arthroscopy, *3(3)*:173, 1987.
91. Mendoza, F.X., Nicholas, J.A., and Rubinstein, M.P.: Arthroscopic treatment of stage II subacromial impingement. Orthop. Trans., *12(3)*:732, 1988.
92. Gartsman, G.M.: Arthroscopic acromioplasty for lesions of the rotator cuff. J. Bone Joint Surg., *72A*:169, 1990.
93. Altchek, D.W., et al.: Arthroscopic acromioplasty: technique and results. J. Bone Joint Surg., *72A*:1198, 1990.
94. Paulos, L.E., and Franklin, J.L.: Arthroscopic shoulder decompression—development and application. A five-year experience. Am. J. Sports Med., *18*:235, 1990.
95. Ryu, R.K.N.: Arthroscopic subacromial decompression: a clinical review. Arthroscopy, *8(2)*:141, 1992.
96. Van Holsbeeck, E., et al.: Subacromial impingement: open versus arthroscopic decompression. Arthroscopy, *8(2)*:173, 1992.
97. Yamanaka, K., and Fukuda, H.: Pathological studies of the supraspinatus tendon with reference to incomplete thickness tears. Proc. 3rd International Conference on Surgery of the Shoulder, Fukuoka, Japan, October 1986.

98. Warren, F.W., et al.: Arthroscopic acromioplasty: a prospective analysis of 43 patients. Proc. Am. Acad. Orthop. Surg. 56th Annual Meeting, Las Vegas, February 1989.
99. Snyder, S.J., et al.: Partial-thickness rotator cuff tears: results of arthroscopic treatment. Arthroscopy, 7:1, 1991.
100. Neviaser, T.J. and Neviaser, R.J.: The diagnosis and treatment of incomplete rotator cuff tears. Orthop. Trans., *15*:239, 1989.
101. Bateman, J.E.: The Shoulder and Neck. Philadelphia, W.B. Saunders, 1972.
102. Kessel, L., and Watson, M.: The painful arc syndrome. Clinical classification as a guide to management. J. Bone Joint Surg., *59B(2)*:166, 1977.
103. Gerber, C., et al.: Latissimus dorsi transfer for the treatment of massive tears of the rotator cuff. Clin. Orthop., *232*:51, 1988.
104. Mikasa, M.: Trapezius transfer for global tear of the rotator cuff. *In* Surgery of the Shoulder. Edited by J.E. Bateman and R.P. Welsh. Philadelphia, B.C. Decker, 1984.
105. Augereau, B.: Reconstruction of massive rotator cuff rupture using a deltoid muscle flap. Orthopade, *20(5)*:315, 1991.
106. Burkhart, S.S.: Arthroscopic treatment of massive rotator cuff tears. Clinical results and biomechanical rationale. Clin. Orthop., *267*:45, 1991.
107. Ogilvie-Harris, D.J., and Wiley, A.M.: Arthroscopic surgery of the shoulder: a general appraisal. J. Bone Joint Surg., *68B*:201, 1986.
108. Franklin, J.L., Barrett, W.P., Jackins, S.E., and Matsen, F.A. III: Glenoid loosening and total shoulder arthroplasty. Association with rotator cuff deficiency. J. Arthroplasty, *3*:39, 1988.
109. Arntz, C.T., Matsen, F.A. III, and Jackins, S.: Surgical management of complex irreparable rotator cuff deficiency. J. Arthroplasty, *6*:363, 1991.
110. McLaughlin, H.L.: Lesions of the musculotendinous cuff of the shoulder: observations of the pathology, course and treatment of calcific deposits. Ann. Surg., *124*:354, 1946.
111. Uhthoff, H.K., Lohr, J., and Sarkar, K.: The pathogenesis of rotator cuff tears. *In* The Shoulder. Edited by N. Takagishi. Tokyo, Professional Postgraduate Services, 1987.
112. DePalma, A.F., and Kruper, J.F.: Long-term study of shoulder joint afflicted with and treated for calcified tendinitis. Clin. Orthop., *20*:61, 1961.
113. Pinals, R.F., and Short, C.L.: Calcific periarthritis involving multiple sites. Arthritis Rheum., *9*:566, 1966.
114. McKendry, R.J.R., Uhthoff, H.K., Sarkar, K., and Hyslop, T.S.: Calcifying tendinitis of the shoulder: prognostic value of clinical, histologic, and radiologic features in 57 surgically treated cases. J. Rheumatol., *9*:75, 1982.
115. Ellman, H. and Kay, S.P.: Arthroscopic treatment of calcific tendinitis. Orthop. Trans., *13(2)*:240, 1989.
116. Ark, J.W., Flock, T.S., Flatow, E.L., and Bigliani, L.U.: Arthroscopic treatment of calcific tendinitis of the shoulder. Arthroscopy, *8(2)*:183, 1992.
117. Ellman, H., et al.: Role of arthroscopy in the treatment of calcifying tendinitis: the American experience. Presented at the Vth International Conference on Surgery of the Shoulder, Paris, July 1992.
118. Lippmann, R.K.: Frozen shoulder, periarthritis, bicipital tenosynovitis. Arch. Surg., *47*:283, 1943.
119. Crenshaw, A.H., and Kilgore, W.E.: Surgical treatment of bicipital tenosynovitis. J. Bone Joint Surg., *48A*:1496, 1966.
120. Post, M.: The Shoulder. Surgical and Nonsurgical Management. Philadelphia, Lea & Febiger, 1988.
121. Meyer, A.W.: Spontaneous dislocation and disruption of tendon of long head of biceps brachii: 59 instances. Arch. Surg., *17*:493, 1928.
122. Hitchcock, H.H., and Bechtol, C.O.: Painful shoulder. Observations on role of the tendon of the long head of the biceps brachii in its causation. J. Bone Joint Surg., *30A*:363, 1948.
123. Neer, C.S. II, Flatow, E.L., and Lech, O.: Tears of the rotator cuff: long-term results of anterior acromioplasty and repair. Presented at the Fourth Open Meeting of the American Shoulder and Elbow Surgeons, Atlanta, February 1988.
124. Bowen, M.K., and Warren, R.H.: Ligamentous control of shoulder stability based on selective cutting and static translation experiments. Clin. Sports Med., *10*:757, 1991.
125. Morgan, C.D., Rames, R., and Snyder, S.: Arthroscopic Assessment of Anatomic Variations of the Glenohumeral ligaments associated with Recurrent Anterior Shoulder Instability. Presented at The American Shoulder and Elbow Surgeons Meeting, Washington, D.C., 1992.
126. Baker, C.L., Uribe, J.W., and Whitman, C.: Arthroscopic evaluation of acute initial anterior shoulder dislocations. Am. J. Sports Med., *18(1)*:25, 1990.
127. Bankart, A.S.B.: Recurrent or habitual dislocation of the shoulder joint. Br. Med. J., *2*:1132, 1923.

128. Turkel, S.J., et al.: Stabilizing mechanisms preventing anterior dislocation of the glenohumeral joint. J. Bone Joint Surg., *63A*:1208, 1981.
129. Rodosky, M.W., et al.: The role of the biceps-superior glenoid labrum complex in anterior stability of the shoulder. Pittsburgh Orthop. J., *1*:57, 1990.
130. Glousman, R.E., et al.: Dynamic electromyographic analysis of the throwing shoulder with glenohumeral instability. J. Bone Joint Surg., *70A*:220, 1988.
131. Jobe, F.W., Giangarra, C.E., Kivtne, R.S., and Glousman, R.E.: Anterior capsulolabral reconstruction of the shoulder in athletes in overhand sports. Am. J. Sports Med., *19*:428, 1991.
132. Tibone, J.E., Jobe, F.W., and Kerlan, R.F.: Shoulder impingement syndrome in athletes treated by anterior acromioplasty. Clin. Orthop., *188*:134, 1985.
133. Rockwood, C.A., and Matsen, F.A.: The Shoulder. Philadelphia, W.B. Saunders, 1990.
134. Harryman, D.T., et al.: Translation of the humeral head on the glenoid with passive glenohumeral motion. J. Bone Joint Surg., *72A*:1334, 1990.
135. Neviaser, R.J., Neviaser, T.J., and Neviaser, J.S.: Concurrent rupture of the rotator cuff and anterior dislocation of the shoulder in the older patient. J. Bone Joint Surg., *70A*:1308, 1988.
136. Aronen, J.G., and Regan, K.: Decreasing the incidence of recurrence of first time anterior shoulder dislocations with rehabilitation. Am. J. Sports Med., *12*:283, 1984.
137. Calandra, J.J., Baker, C.L. and Uribe, J.: The incidence of Hill-Sachs' lesions in initial anterior shoulder dislocations. Arthroscopy, *5(4)*:254, 1989.
138. Hovelius, L.: Anterior dislocation of the shoulder in teenagers and young adults. J. Bone Joint Surg., *64*:254, 1982.
139. Simonet, W.T., and Cofield, R.H.: Prognosis in anterior shoulder dislocation. Am. J. Sports Med., *12(1)*:19, 1984.
140. Tijmes, J., Loyd, H.M., and Tullos, H.S.: Arthrography in acute shoulder dislocations. South. Med. J., *72*:564, 1979.
141. Wheeler, J.H., et al.: Arthroscopic versus nonoperative treatment of acute shoulder dislocations in young athletes. Arthroscopy, *5(3)*:213, 1989.
142. Hovelius, L., et al.: Recurrences after initial dislocation of the shoulder. J. Bone Joint Surg., *65*:343, 1983.
143. Warner, J.P., and Warren, R.F.: Arthroscopic Bankart repair using a cannulated, absorbable fixation device. Operative Techniques in Orthopedics, *1(2)*:192, 1991.
144. Altchek, D.W., Ortiz, G., Warren, R.F., and Wickiewicz, T.L.: Arthroscopic labral debridement—a three-year follow-up study. Orthop. Trans., *14(2)*: Summer 1990.
145. Glasgow, S.G., Bruce, R.A., Ysacobucci, G.N., and Torg, J.S.: Arthroscopic resection of glenoid labral tears in the athlete: a report of 29 cases. Arthroscopy, *8(1)*:48, 1992.
146. McGlynn, F.J., and Caspari, R.B.: Arthroscopic findings in the subluxing shoulder. Clin. Orthop., *183*:173, 1984.
147. Gross, R.M.: Arthroscopic shoulder capsulorrhaphy: does it work? Am. J. Sports Med., *17(4)*:495, 1989.
148. Morgan, C.D., and Bodenstab, A.B.: Arthroscopic Bankart suture repair: technique and early results. Arthroscopy, *3(2)*:111, 1987.
149. Caspari, R.B.: Arthroscopic reconstruction for anterior shoulder instability. Techniques in Orthopedics, *3*:59, 1988.
150. Maki, N.J.: Arthroscopic stabilization for recurrent shoulder instability. *In* Surgery of the Shoulder. Edited by Post, M., Morrey, B.F., and Hawkins, R.J. St. Louis, Mosby Yearbook, 1990.
151. Bartlett, E.C.: Evolution and use of pin and sleeve technique in suture anchor placement. Am. J. Arthroscopy, *5(1)*:21, 1991.
152. Hawkins, R.B.: Arthroscopic stapling repair for shoulder instability: a retrospective study of 50 cases. Arthroscopy, *5(2)*:122, 1989.
153. Johnson, L.L.: Shoulder arthroscopy. *In* Arthroscopic Surgery Principles & Practice. Edited by E.A. Klein, K.H. Falk, and T. O'Brien. St. Louis, CV Mosby, 1986.
154. Matthews, L.S., et al.: Arthroscopic staple capsulorrhaphy for recurrent anterior shoulder instability. Arthroscopy, *4(2)*:106, 1988.
155. Reider, B., and Inglis, A.E.: The Bankart procedure modified by the use of Prolene pull-out sutures. J. Bone Joint Surg., *64A(4)*:628, 1982.
156. Grana, W.A., Buckley, P.D., and Yates, C.K.: Arthroscopic Bankart Suture Repair. Presented at the American Orthopedic Society for Sports Medicine, 1992 Specialty Day Meeting, Washington, D.C.
157. Wolin, P.M. Arthroscopic glenoid labrum suture repair. Orthop. Trans., *14(3)*:597, 1990.
158. Moran, M.C., and Warren, R.F.: Development of a synovial cyst after arthroscopy of the shoulder. J. Bone Joint Surg., *71A(1)*:127, 1989.

159. Bach, B.R.: Arthroscopic removal of painful Bristow hardware. Arthroscopy, *6(4)*:324, 1990.
160. Zuckerman, J.D., and Matsen, F.A.: Complications about the glenohumeral joint related to the use of screws and staples. J. Bone Joint Surg., *66A*:175, 1984.
161. Bigliani, L.U., et al.: Tensile properties of the inferior glenohumeral ligament. J. Orthop. Res., *10*:187, 1992.
162. Neer, C.S., and Foster, C.R.: Inferior capsular shift for involuntary inferior and multidirectional instability of the shoulder. J. Bone Joint Surg., *62A*:897, 1980.
163. Rowe, C.R., Patel, D., and Southmayd, W.W.: The Bankart procedure: a long-term end-result study. J. Bone Joint Surg., *60A(1)*:1, 1978.
164. Adolfsson, L., and Lysholm, J.: Arthroscopy and stability testing for anterior shoulder instability. Arthroscopy, *5(4)*:315, 1989.
165. Dolk, T., and Gremark, O.: Arthroscopy and stability testing of the shoulder joint. Arthroscopy, *2(1)*:35, 1986.
166. Henderson, W.D.: Arthroscopic stabilization of the anterior shoulder. Clin. Sports Med., *6(3)*:581, 1987.
167. Lane, J.G., Sachs, R.A., and Riehl, B.: Arthroscopic staple capsulorrhaphy: a long-term follow-up. Arthroscopy, *7(3)*:324, 1991.
168. Rose, D.J.: Arthroscopic suture capsulorrhaphy for anterior shoulder instability. Orthop. Trans., *14(3)*:597, 1990.
169. Wiley, A.M.: Arthroscopy for shoulder instability and a technique for arthroscopic repair. Arthroscopy, *4(1)*:25, 1988.
170. Yahiro, M.A., and Matthews, L.S.: Arthroscopic stabilization procedures for recurrent anterior shoulder instability. Orthop. Rev. *18(11)*:1161, 1989.
171. Darby, A.J.: Osteoarthritis. *In* Graduate Textbook of Clinical Orthopaedics. Edited by W. Harris and P.S.E. Wright. 1983.
172. Creuss, C.L.: Rheumatoid arthritis of the shoulder. Orthop. Clin. North Am., *11(2)*:333, 1980.
173. Steinbrocker, O., Traeger, C.H. and Batterman, R.C.: Therapeutic criteria for rheumatoid arthritis. JAMA, *140*:659, 1949.
174. Inglis, A.E., Ranawat, C.S. and Straub, L.R.: Synovectomy and debridement of the elbow in rheumatoid arthritis. J. Bone Joint Surg., *53A*:652, 1971.
175. Pappas, A.M., Goss, T.P., and Kleinman, P.K.: Symptomatic shoulder instability due to lesions of the glenoid labrum. Am. J. Sports Med., *11(5)*:279, 1983.
176. Calhoun, J., Cantrell, J., and Mader, J.: Septic Shoulders. Presented at The American Shoulder and Elbow Surgeons 4th Open Meeting, Atlanta, GA, 1988.
177. Gelberman, R.H., Menon, J., Austerlitz, M.S., and Weisman, M.H.: Pyogenic arthritis of the shoulder in adults. J. Bone Joint Surg., *62A*:550, 1980.
178. Leslie, B.M., Harris, J., and Driscoll, D.: Septic arthritis of the shoulder in adults. J. Bone Joint Surg., *71A*:1516, 1989.
179. Kohn, D.: The clinical relevance of glenoid labrum lesions. Arthroscopy, *3(4)*:223, 1987.
180. Altchek, D.W., Ortiz, G., Warren, R.F., and Wickiewicz, T.L.: Arthroscopic labral debridement—a three-year follow-up study. Orthop. Trans., *14(2)*, Summer 1990.
181. Glasgow, S.G., Bruce, R.A., Yacobucci, G.N., and Torg, J.S.: Arthroscopic resection of glenoid labral tears in the athlete: a report of 29 cases. Arthroscopy, *8(1)*:48, 1992.
182. McMaster, W.C.: Anterior glenoid labrum damage: a painful lesion in swimmers. Am. J. Sports Med., *14(5)*:383, 1986.
183. Snyder, S.J., et al.: SLAP lesions of the shoulder. Arthroscopy, *6(4)*:274, 1990.
184. Field, L.D., and Savoie, F.H.: Arthroscopic Suture Repair of Superior Labral Detachment Lesions of the Shoulder. Presented at AOSSM Specialty Day, 59th Annual Meeting of the American Academy of Orthopedic Surgeons, Washington, D.C., 1992.
185. Detrisac, D.A., and Johnson, L.L.: Arthroscopic Shoulder Anatomy. New Jersey, Slack, 1986.
186. Cooper, D.E., et al.: Anatomy, histology, and vascularity of the glenoid labrum. An anatomical study. J. Bone Joint Surg., *74A*:46, 1992.
187. Rodosky, M.W., et al: The role of the biceps-superior glenoid labrum complex in anterior stability of the shoulder. Pittsburgh Orthop. J., *1*:57, 1990.
188. Rockwood, C.A., and Matsen, F.A.: The Shoulder. Philadelphia, W.B. Saunders, 1990.
189. Flatow, E.L., Cordasco, F.A., and Bigliani, L.U.: Arthroscopic resection of the outer end of the clavicle from a superior approach: a critical, quantitative, radiographic assessment of bone removal. Arthroscopy, *8(1)*:55, 1992.
190. Gartsman, G.M., et al.: Arthroscopic acromioclavicular joint resection. An anatomical study. Am. J. Sports Med., *19*:2, 1991.
191. Whipple, T.L.: Arthroscopic Treatment of Acromioclavicular Joint Arthritis. Presented at the Arthroscopy Association of North America, Boston, April, 1992.

192. Snyder, S.J., et al.: Arthroscopic Acromioclavicular Joint Debridement and Distal Clavicle Resection Utilizing the Claviculizer™. Presented at the American Academy of Orthopedic Surgeons, February, 1992.
193. Gartsman, G.M:: Arthroscopic resection of the acromioclavicular joint. Am. J. Sports Med., *21*:1993.
194. Bigliani, L.U., and Fischer, R.A.: Shoulder and elbow problems in the athlete. Curr Op in Ortho *1*:185, 1990.
195. Craig, E.V., and Hsu, K.C.: Shoulder problems in the weekend athlete. Orthop. Rev., *21(2)*:155, 1992.
196. Miniaci, A., and MacDonald, P.B.: Open surgical techniques in the athlete's shoulder. Clin. Sports Med., *10(4)*:929, 1991.
197. Neer, C.S., and Welsh, M.B.: The shoulder in sports. Orthop. Clin. North Am., *8(3)*:583, 1977.
198. Tibone, J.E., et al.: Surgical treatment of tears of the rotator cuff in athletes. J. Bone Joint Surg., *68A*:887, 1986.
199. Warren, R.F., and Marshall, J.L.: Athletic injuries of the shoulder. Surg. Rounds, 34, 1978.
200. Jobe, F.W., Perry, J., and Pink, M.: Electromyographic shoulder activity in men and women professional golfers. Am. J. Sports Med., *17(6)*:782, 1989.
201. Abrams, J.S.: Special shoulder problems in the throwing athlete: pathology, diagnosis, and nonoperative management. Clin. Sports Med., *10(4)*:839, 1991.
202. Hurley, J.A., and Anderson, T.E.: Shoulder arthroscopy: its role in evaluating shoulder disorders in the athlete. Am. J. Sports Med., *18(6)*:480, 1990.
203. Moynes, D.R., et al.: Electromyography and motion analysis of the upper extremity in sports. Phys. Ther., *66(12)*:1905, 1986.
204. Silliman, J.F., and Hawkins, R.J.: Current concepts and recent advances in the athlete's shoulder. Clin. Sports Med., *10(4)*:693, 1991.
205. Townsend, H., et al.: Electromyographic analysis of the glenohumeral muscles during a baseball rehabilitation program. Am. J. Sports Med., *19(3)*:264, 1991.
206. Lehman, R.C.: Shoulder pain in the elite weight lifter. Orthop. Trans., *14(3)*:685, 1990.
207. Neviaser, T.J.: Weight lifting. Risks and injuries to the shoulder. Arthros Update, *10(3)*:615, 1991.
208. Cook, F.F., and Tibone, J.E.: The Mumford procedure in athletes—an objective analysis of function. Am. J. Sports Med., *16(2)*:97, 1988.
209. Ferretti, A., Cerullo, G., and Russo, G.: Suprascapular neuropathy in volleyball players. J. Bone Joint Surg., *69A(2)*:260, 1987.
210. Kennedy, J.C., Hawkins, R., and Krissoff, W.B.: Orthopaedic manifestations of swimming. Am. J. Sports Med., *6(6)*:309, 1978.
211. Nuber, G.W., et al.: Fine wire electromyography analysis of muscles of the shoulder during swimming. Am. J. Sports Med., *14*:7, 1986.
212. Pink, M., et al.: The normal shoulder during freestyle swimming. An electromyographic and cinematographic analysis of twelve muscles. Am. J. Sports Med., *19(6)*:569, 1991.
213. Richardson, A.R., Jobe, F.W., and Collins, H.R.: The shoulder in competitive swimming. Am. J. Sports Med., *8*:159, 1980.
214. Scovazzo, M.L., et al.: The painful shoulder during freestyle swimming. Am. J. Sports Med., *19(6)*:577, 1991.
215. Weaver, J.K.: Skiing-related injuries to the shoulder. Clin. Orthop., *216*:24, 1987.
216. Priest, J.D.: The shoulder of the tennis player. Clin. Sports Med., *7(2)*:387, 1988.
217. Ryu, R.K., et al.: An electromyographic analysis of shoulder function in tennis players. Am. J. Sports Med., *16(5)*:481, 1988.
218. Bigliani, L.U., et al.: Inferior capsular shift procedure for anterior-inferior shoulder instability in athletes. Orthop. Trans., *13(3)*560, 1989.
219. Bigliani, L.U., Kimmel, J., McCann, P.D., and Wolfe, I.: Repair of rotator cuff tears in tennis players. Am. J. Sports Med., *20(2)*:112, 1992.
220. Whiting, W.C., Gregor, R.J., and Finerman, G.A.: Kinematic analysis of human upper extremity movements in boxing. Am. J. Sports Med., *16(2)*:130, 1988.
221. Fukuda, H., and Neer, C.: Recurrent posterior subluxation and dislocation of the shoulder in two archers. Orthopedics, *11(1)*:171, 1988.
222. Mann, D.L., and Littke, N.: Shoulder injuries in archery. Can. J. Sport Sci., *14(2)*:85, 1989.
223. Andrews, J.R., Kupferman, S.P., and Dillman, C.J.: Labral tears in throwing and racquet sports. Clin. Sports Med., *10(4)*:901, 1991.
224. Scarpinato, D.F., Bramhall, J.P., and Andrews, J.R.: Arthroscopic management of the throwing athlete's shoulder: indications, techniques, and results. Clin. Sports Med., *10(4)*:913, 1991.
225. Engelberg, A.L.: Guides to the Evaluation of Permanent Impairment. Chicago, American Medical Association, 1988.

226. Bigliani, L.U., Flatow, E., and DeLiz, E.: Complications of shoulder arthroscopy. Orthop. Rev., *20(9)*:743, 1991.
227. Bigliani L.U.: Complications of shoulder arthroscopy. *In* Management of Complications in Orthopaedics. Edited by O.H. Sherman and J. Minkoff. Baltimore, Williams & Wilkins, 1990.
228. Caspari, R.B.: Complications of shoulder arthroscopy. *In* Complications in Arthroscopy. Edited by N.F. Sprague, New York, Raven Press, 1989.
229. Curtis, A.S., Del Pizzo, W., Snyder, S.J., and Karzel, R.P.: Complications of Shoulder Arthroscopy. Presented at The American Orthopedic Society for Sports Medicine, 1992 Specialty Day Meeting, February 23, 1992.
230. Olson, E., and Fu, F.: Complication and pitfalls in shoulder arthroscopic operative techniques. Orthopedics, *1(3)*:253, 1991.
231. Rockwood, C.A.: Shoulder arthroscopy. Editorial. J. Bone Joint Surg., *12*:731, 1988.
232. Small, N.C.: Complications in arthroscopic surgery performed by experienced arthroscopists. Arthroscopy, *4*:215, 1988.
233. Ellman, H.: Arthroscopic subacromial decompression: analysis of one to three year results. Arthroscopy, *3(3)*:173, 1987.
234. Gartsman, G.M.: Arthroscopic acromioplasty for lesions of the rotator cuff. J. Bone Joint Surg., *72A*:169, 1990.
235. Paulos, L.E., and Franklin, J.L.: Arthroscopic shoulder decompression—development and application. A five year experience. Am. J. Sports Med., *18(3)*:235, 1990.
236. Burkhart, S.S.: Deep venous thrombosis after shoulder arthroscopy. Arthroscopy, *6(1)*:61, 1990.
237. Pitman, M.I., et al.: The use of somatosensory evoked potentials for detection of neuropraxia during shoulder arthroscopy. Arthroscopy, *4(4)*:250, 1988.
238. Klein, A., et al.: Measurement of brachial plexus strain in arthroscopy of the shoulder. Arthroscopy, *3(1)*:45, 1987.
239. Mullins, R.C., Drez, D., and Cooper, J.: Hypoglossal nerve palsy after arthroscopy of the shoulder and open operation with the patient in the beach-chair position. J. Bone Joint Surg., *74A*:137, 1992.
240. Bigliani L.U., Dalsey, R.M., McCann, P.D., and April, E.W.: An anatomical study of the suprascapular nerve. Arthroscopy, *6*:301, 1990.
241. Bryan, W.J., Schauder, K., and Tullos, H.S.: The axillary nerve and its relationship to common sports medicine shoulder problems. Am. J. Sports Med., *14*:113, 1986.
242. Burkhead, W.Z., Scheinberg, R.R., and Boc, G.: Surgical anatomy of the axillary nerve. J. Shoulder Elbow Surg., *1(1)*:31, 1992.
243. Flatow, E.L., Bigliani, L.U., and April, E.W.: An anatomical study of the coracoid muscles. Clin. Orthop., *244*:166, 1989.
244. Caspari, R.B., and Thal, R.: A technique for arthroscopic subacromial decompression. Arthroscopy, *8(1)*:23, 1992.
245. Sampson, T.G., Nisbet, J.K., and Glick, J.M.: Precision acromioplasty in arthroscopic subacromial decompression of the shoulder. Arthroscopy, *7(3)*:301, 1991.
245a. Fulkerson, J.P., and Winters, T.F.: Articular cartilage response to arthroscopic surgery: a review of current knowledge. Arthroscopy, *2(3)*:184, 1986.
246. Morrison, D.S., and Schaefer, R.K.: Relationship between subacromial space pressure, blood pressure and visual clarity during arthroscopic subacromial decompression. Orthop. Trans., *14*:564, 1990.
247. Hawkins, R.B.: Arthroscopic stapling repair for shoulder instability: a retrospective study of 50 cases. Arthroscopy, *5(2)*:122, 1989.
248. O'Driscoll, S.W., Evans, D.C., and Scarborough, O.N.: Long term results of the staple capsulorrhaphy: twenty years experience in the Toronto teaching hospitals. Orthop. Trans., *12*:674, 1988.
249. Norwood, L., and Fowler, L.: Rotator cuff tears. A shoulder arthroscopy complication. Am. J. Sports Med., *17(6)*:837, 1989.
250. Burkhart, S.: Arthroscopic treatment of massive rotator cuff tears. Clinical results and biomechanical rationale. Clin. Orthop., *267*:45, 1991.
251. Montgomery, T.J., Savoie, F.H., and Yerger, B.: A Comparison of Arthroscopic Debridement with Open Surgical Repair for Full Thickness Tears of the Rotator Cuff. Presented at the 8th Open Meeting, American Shoulder and Elbow Surgeons, Washington, D.C., February 1992.
252. D'Angelo, G., and Ogilvie-Harris, D.J.: Septic arthritis following arthroscopy, with cost/benefit analysis of antibiotic prophylaxis. Arthroscopy, *4(1)*:10, 1988.
253. Sherman, O.H., et al.: Arthroscopy—"no problem surgery." An analysis of complications in two thousand six hundred and forty cases. J. Bone Joint Surg., *68A*:256, 1986.
254. Small, N.C.: Complications in arthroscopy: the knees and other joints. Committee on complications of the Arthroscopy Association of North America. Arthroscopy, *2*:253, 1986.

255. Ogilvie-Harris, D.J., and Boynton, E.: Arthroscopic acromioplasty extravasation of fluid into the deltoid muscle. Arthroscopy, *6(1)*:52, 1990.
256. Reagan, B.F., et al.: Irrigating solutions for arthroscopy. J. Bone Joint Surg., *65A*:629, 1983.
257. Burkhart, S.S., Barnett, C.R., and Snyder, S.S.: Transient postoperative blindness as a possible effect of glycine toxicity. Arthroscopy, *6(2)*:112, 1990.
258. Marshall, G.J., et al.: Synovisol as an irrigant for electrosurgery of joints. Arthroscopy, *4(3)*:187, 1988.
259. Fly, W.R., et al.: Arthroscopic subacromial decompression in athletes less than 40 years old. Orthop. Trans., *14*:250, 1990.
260. Gartsman, G.M., Blair, M.E., Jr., Noble, P.C., Bennett, J.B., and Tullos, H.S.: Arthroscopic Subacromial Decompression. An Anatomical Study. Am. J. Sports Med., *16*:48, 1988.

REFERENCES-ALPHABETICAL

Abrams, J.S.: Special shoulder problems in the throwing athlete: pathology, diagnosis, and nonoperative management. Clin. Sports Med., *10(4)*:839, 1991.

Adolfsson, L., and Lysholm, J.: Arthroscopy and stability testing for anterior shoulder instability. Arthroscopy, *5(4)*:315, 1989.

Altchek, D.W., et al.: Arthroscopic acromioplasty: technique and results. J. Bone Joint Surg., *72A*:1198, 1990.

Altchek, D.W., Ortiz, G., Warren, R.F., and Wickiewicz, T.L.: Arthroscopic labral debridement—a three-year follow-up study. Orthop. Trans., *14(2)*, Summer 1990.

Andrews, J.R., Broussard, T.S., and Carson, W.G.: Arthroscopy of the shoulder in the management of partial tears of the rotator cuff: a preliminary report. Arthroscopy, *1*:117, 1985.

Andrews, J.R., Kupferman, S.P., and Dillman, C.J.: Labral tears in throwing and racquet sports. Clin. Sports Med., *10(4)*:901, 1991.

Ark, J.W., Flock, T.S., Flatow, E.L., and Bigliani, L.U.: Arthroscopic treatment of calcific tendinitis of the shoulder. Arthroscopy, *8(2)*:183, 1992.

Arntz, C.T., Matsen, F.A. III, and Jackins, S.: Surgical management of complex irreparable rotator cuff deficiency. J. Arthroplasty, *6*:363, 1991.

Aronen, J.G., and Regan, K.: Decreasing the incidence of recurrence of first time anterior shoulder dislocations with rehabilitation. Am. J. Sports Med., *12*:283, 1984.

Augereau, B.: Reconstruction of massive rotator cuff rupture using a deltoid muscle flap. Orthopade, *20(5)*:315, 1991.

Bach, B.R.: Arthroscopic removal of painful Bristow hardware. Arthroscopy, *6(4)*:324, 1990.

Baker, C.L., Uribe, J.W., and Whitman, C.: Arthroscopic evaluation of acute initial anterior shoulder dislocations. Am. J. Sports Med., *18(1)*:25, 1990.

Bankart, A.S.B.: Recurrent or habitual dislocation of the shoulder joint. Br. Med. J., *2*:1132, 1923.

Bartlett, E.C.: Evolution and use of pin and sleeve technique in suture anchor placement. Am. J. Arthroscopy, *5(1)*:21, 1991.

Bateman, J.E.: The Shoulder and Neck. Philadelphia, W.B. Saunders, 1972.

Bigliani, L.U.: Complications of shoulder arthroscopy. *In* Management of Complications in Orthopaedics. Edited by O.H. Sherman and J. Minkoff. Baltimore, Williams & Wilkins, 1990.

Bigliani, L.U., and Fischer, R.A.: Shoulder and elbow problems in the athlete. Curr Op in Ortho *1*:185, 1990.

Bigliani, L.U., Dalsey, R.M., McCann, P.D., and April, E.W.: An anatomical study of the suprascapular nerve. Arthroscopy, *6*:301, 1990.

Bigliani, L.U., et al.: Tensile properties of the inferior glenohumeral ligament. J. Orthop. Res., *10*:187, 1992.

Bigliani, L.U., et al.: Operative repair of massive rotator cuff tears: long-term results. Orthop. Trans., *14*:251, 1990.

Bigliani, L.U., et al.: Inferior capsular shift procedure for anterior-inferior shoulder instability in athletes. Orthop. Trans. *13(3)*:560, 1989.

Bigliani, L.U., Flatow, E., and DeLiz, E.: Complications of shoulder arthroscopy. Orthop. Rev., *20(9)*:743, 1991.

Bigliani, L.U., Kimmel, J., McCann, P.D., and Wolfe, I.: Repair of rotator cuff tears in tennis players. Am. J. Sports Med., *20(2)*:112, 1992.

Bigliani, L.U., Morrison, D.S., and April, E.W.: The morphology of the acromion and its relationship to rotator cuff tears. Orthop. Trans., *10*:228, 1986.

Bosworth, D.M.: An analysis of 28 consecutive cases of incapacitating shoulder lesions radically explored and repaired. J. Bone Joint Surg., *22*:392, 1940.

Bowen, M.K., and Warren, R.H.: Ligamentous control of shoulder stability based on selective cutting and static translation experiments. Clin. Sports Med., *10*:757, 1991.

Bowen, M.K., et al.: Role of the inferior glenohumeral ligament complex in limiting inferior translation of the glenohumeral joint. American Shoulder and Elbow Surgeons, Specialty Day, February 23, 1992.

Brown, J.T.: Early assessment of supraspinatus tears, procaine infiltration as a guide to treatment. J. Bone Joint Surg., *31B(3)*:423, 1949.

Bryan, W.J., Schauder, K., and Tullos, H.S.: The axillary nerve and its relationship to common sports medicine shoulder problems. Am. J. Sports Med., *14*:113, 1986.

Burkhart, S.S., Arthroscopic treatment of massive rotator cuff tears. Clinical results and biomechanical rationale. Clin. Orthop., *267*:45, 1991.

Burkhart, S.S.: Deep venous thrombosis after shoulder arthroscopy. Arthroscopy, *6(1)*:61, 1990.

Burkhart, S.S., Barnett, C.R., and Snyder, S.S.: Transient postoperative blindness as a possible effect of glycine toxicity. Arthroscopy, *6(2)*:112, 1990.

Burkhead, W.Z., Scheinberg, R.R., and Boc, G.: Surgical anatomy of the axillary nerve. J. Shoulder Elbow Surg., *1(1)*:31, 1992.

Calandra, J.J., Baker, C.L., and Uribe, J.: The incidence of Hill-Sachs' lesions in initial anterior shoulder dislocations. Arthroscopy, *5(4)*:254, 1989.

Calhoun, J., Cantrell, J., and Mader, J.: Septic Shoulders. Presented at The American Shoulder and Elbow Surgeons 4th Open Meeting, Atlanta, GA, 1988.

Caspari, R.B.: Complications of shoulder arthroscopy. *In* Complications in Arthroscopy. Edited by N.F. Sprague, New York, Raven Press, 1989.

Caspari, R.B.: Arthroscopic reconstruction for anterior shoulder instability. Techniques in Orthopedics, *3*:59, 1988.

Caspari, R.B., and Thal, R.: A technique for arthroscopic subacromial decompression. Arthroscopy, *8(1)*:23, 1992.

Codman, E.A.: The Shoulder. Boston, Thomas Todd, 1934.

Codman, E.A.: Obscure lesions of the shoulder: rupture of the supraspinatus tendon. Boston Med. Surg. J., *196*:381, 1927.

Codman, E.A., and Akerson, I.D.: The pathology associated with rupture of the supraspinatus tendon. Ann. Surg., *93*:348, 1931.

Cofield, R.H.: Subscapular muscle transposition for repair of chronic rotator cuff tears. Surg. Gynecol. Obstet., *154*:677, 1982.

Constant, C.R., and Murley, A.H.G.: A clinical method of functional assessment of the shoulder. Clin. Orthop., *214*:160, 1987.

Cook, F.F., and Tibone, J.E.: The Mumford procedure in athletes—an objective analysis of function. Am. J. Sports Med., *16(2)*:97, 1988.

Cooper, D.E., et al.: Anatomy, histology and vascularity of the glenoid labrum. An anatomical study. J. Bone Joint Surg., *74A*:46, 1992.

Cotton, R.E., and Rideout, D.F.: Tears of the humeral rotator cuff. A radiological and pathological necropsy survey. J. Bone Joint Surg., *46B(2)*:314, 1964.

Craig, E.V., and Hsu, K.C.: Shoulder problems in the weekend athlete. Orthop. Rev., *21(2)*:155, 1992.

Crenshaw, A.H., and Kilgore, W.E.: Surgical treatment of bicipital tenosynovitis. J. Bone Joint Surg., *48A*:1496, 1966.

Creuss, C.L.: Rheumatoid arthritis of the shoulder. Orthop. Clin. North Am., *11(2)*:333, 1980.

Curtis, A.S., Del Pizzo, W., Snyder, S.J., and Karzel, R.P.: Complications of Shoulder Arthroscopy. Presented at The American Orthopedic Society for Sports Medicine, 1992 Specialty Day Meeting, February 23, 1992.

D'Angelo, G., and Ogilvie-Harris, D.J.: Septic arthritis following arthroscopy, with cost/benefit analysis of antibiotic prophylaxis. Arthroscopy, *4(1)*:10, 1988.

Darby, A.J.: Osteoarthritis. *In* Graduate Textbook of Clinical Orthopaedics. Edited by W. Harris and P.S.E. Wright. 1983.

Debeyre, J., Patte, D., and Elmelik, E.: Repair of ruptures of the rotator cuff of the shoulder, with a note on advancement of the supraspinatus muscle. J. Bone Joint Surg., *47B(1)*:36, 1965.

DePalma, A.F.: Surgery of the Shoulder. 2nd Ed. Philadelphia, J.B. Lippincott, 1973.

DePalma, A.F.: Surgery of the Shoulder. Philadelphia, J.B. Lippincott, 1950.

DePalma, A.F., and Kruper, J.F.: Long-term study of shoulder joint afflicted with and treated for calcified tendinitis. Clin. Orthop., *20*:61, 1961.

Detrisac, D.A., and Johnson, L.L.: Arthroscopic Shoulder Anatomy. New Jersey, Slack, 1986.

Dolk, T., and Gremark, O.: Arthroscopy and stability testing of the shoulder joint. Arthroscopy, *2(1)*:35, 1986.

Ellman, H.: Diagnosis and treatment of incomplete rotator cuff tears. Clin. Orthop., *254*:64, 1990.

Ellman, H.: Arthroscopic subacromial decompression: analysis of one to three year results. Arthroscopy, *3(3)*:173, 1987.

Ellman, H.: Arthroscopic subacromial decompression: a preliminary report. Orthop. Trans., *9*:49, 1985.

Ellman, H., and Kay, S.P.: Arthroscopic subacromial decompression for chronic impingement: 2- to 5-year results. J. Bone Joint Surg., *73B*:395, 1991.

Ellman, H., and Kay, S.P.: Arthroscopic treatment of calcific tendinitis. Orthop. Trans., *13(2)*:240, 1989.

Ellman, H., et al.: Role of arthroscopy in the treatment of calcifying tendinitis: the American experience. Presented at the Vth International Conference on Surgery of the Shoulder, Paris, July 1992.

Ellman, H., Hanker, G., and Bayer, M.: Repair of the rotator cuff. End-result study of factors influencing reconstruction. J. Bone Joint Surg., *68A*:1136, 1986.

Ellman, H., Harris, E., and Kay, S.P.: Early degenerative joint disease simulating impingement. Arthroscopy, *8(4)*:482, 1992.

Ellman, H., Kay, S.P., and Wirth, M.: Arthroscopic treatment of full-thickness rotator cuff tears: mid-term follow-up study. Arthroscopy (in press).

Engelberg, A.L.: Guides to the Evaluation of Permanent Impairment. Chicago, American Medical Association, 1988.

Esch, C., et al.: Arthroscopic subacromial decompression: results according to the degree of rotator cuff tear. Arthroscopy, *4(4)*:241, 1988.

Ferretti, A., Cerullo, G., and Russo, G.: Suprascapular neuropathy in volleyball players. J. Bone Joint Surg., *69A(2)*:260, 1987.

Field, L.D., and Savoie, F.H.: Arthroscopic Suture Repair of Superior Labral Detachment Lesions of the Shoulder. Presented at AOSSM Specialty Day, 59th Annual Meeting of the American Academy of Orthopedic Surgeons, Washington, D.C., 1992.

Flatow, E.L., Bigliani, L.U., and April, E.W.: An anatomical study of the coracoid muscles. Clin. Orthop., *244*:166, 1989.

Flatow, E.L., Cordasco, F.A., and Bigliani, L.U.: Arthroscopic resection of the outer end of the clavicle from a superior approach: a critical quantitative, radiographic assessment of bone removal. Athroscopy, *8(1)*:55, 1992.

Fly, W.R., et al.: Arthroscopic subacromial decompression in athletes less than 40 years old. Orthop. Trans., *14*:250, 1990.

Franklin, J.L., Barrett, W.P., Jackins, S.E., and Matsen, F.A. III: Glenoid loosening and total shoulder arthroplasty. Association with rotator cuff deficiency. J. Arthroplasty, *3*:39, 1988.

Fukuda, H., and Neer, C.: Recurrent posterior subluxation and dislocation of the shoulder in two archers. Orthopedics, *11(1)*:171, 1988.

Fukuda, H., Hamada, K., and Kobayashi, Y.: Push-up views for the massive rotator cuff tear—a new roentgenographic projection. Orthop. Trans., *13*:240, 1989.

Fukuda, H., Mikasa, M., and Yamanaka, K.: Incomplete thickness rotator cuff tears diagnosed by subacromial bursography. Clin. Orthop., *223*:51, 1987.

Fulkerson, J.P., and Winters, T.F.: Articular cartilage response to arthroscopic surgery: a review of current knowledge. Arthroscopy, *2(3)*:184, 1986.

Gartsman, G.M.: Arthroscopic resection of the acromioclavicular joint. Am. J. Sports Med., 21:1993.

Gartsman, G.M.: Arthroscopic acromioplasty for lesions of the rotator cuff. J. Bone Joint Surg., *72A*:169, 1990.

Gartsman, G.M., et al.: Arthroscopic acromioclavicular joint resection. An anatomical study. Am. J. Sports Med., *19*:2, 1991.

Gartsman, G.M., Blair, M.E., Noble, P.C., Bennett, J.B., and Tullos, H.S.: Arthroscopic Subacromial Decompression. An Anatomical Study. Am. J. Sports Med., *16*:48, 1988.

Gelberman, R.H., Menon, J., Austerlitz, M.S., and Weisman, M.H.: Pyogenic arthritis of the shoulder in adults. J. Bone Joint Surg., *62A*:550, 1980.

Gerber, C.: Latissimus dorsi transfer for treatment of irreparable tears of the rotator cuff. Clin. Orthop., *275*:152, 1992.

Gerber, C., and Ganz, R.: Clinical assessment of instability of the shoulder. J. Bone Joint Surg., *66B*:551, 1984.

Gerber, C., et al.: Latissimus dorsi transfer for the treatment of massive tears of the rotator cuff. Clin. Orthop., *232*:51, 1988.

Ghelman, B., and Goldman, A.B.: The double contrast shoulder arthrogram: evaluation of rotary cuff tears. Radiology, *124*:251, 1977.

Glasgow, S.G., Bruce, R.A., Ysacobucci, G.N., and Torg, J.S.: Arthroscopic resection of glenoid labral tears in the athlete: a report of 29 cases. Arthroscopy, *8(1)*:48, 1992.

Glousman, R.E., et al.: Dynamic electromyographic analysis of the throwing shoulder with glenohumeral instability. J. Bone Joint Surg., *70A*:220, 1988.

Godsil, R.D., Jr., and Linscheid, R.L.: Intratendinous defects of the rotator cuff. Clin. Orthop., *69*:181, 1970.

Golding, F.C.: The shoulder—the forgotten joint. Br. J. Radiol., *35*:149, 1962.

Grana, W.A., Buckley, P.D., and Yates, C.K.: Arthroscopic Bankart Suture Repair. Presented at the American Orthopedic Society for Sports Medicine, 1992 Specialty Day Meeting, Washington, D.C.

Gross, R.M.: Arthroscopic shoulder capsulorrhaphy: does it work? Am. J. Sports Med., *17(4)*:495, 1989.

Harryman, D.T. II, et al.: Repairs of the rotator cuff. Correlation of functional result with integrity of the cuff. J. Bone Joint Surg., *73A*:982, 1991.

Harryman, D.T., et al.: Translation of the humeral head on the glenoid with passive glenohumeral motion. J. Bone Joint Surg., *72A*:1334, 1990.

Hawkins, R.B.: Arthroscopic stapling repair for shoulder instability: a retrospective study of 50 cases. Arthroscopy, *5(2)*:122, 1989.

Hawkins, R.J., and Kennedy, J.C.: The impingement syndrome in athletes. Am. J. Sports Med., *8*:151, 1980.

Hawkins, R.J., Misamore, G.W., and Hobeika, P.E.: Surgery for full-thickness rotator cuff tears. J. Bone Joint Surg., *67A*:1349, 1985.

Heikel, H.V.A.: Rupture of the rotator cuff of the shoulder: experiences of surgical treatment. Acta Orthop. Scand., *39*:477, 1968.

Henderson, W.D.: Arthroscopic stabilization of the anterior shoulder. Clin. Sports Med., *6(3)*:581, 1987.

Hitchcock, H.H., and Bechtol, C.O.: Painful shoulder. Observations on role of the tendon of the long head of the biceps brachii in its causation. J. Bone Joint Surg., *30A*:363, 1948.

Hodler, J., Fretz, C.J., Terrier, F., and Gerber, C.: Rotator cuff tears: correlation of sonographic and surgical findings. Radiology, *169*:791, 1988.

Hovelius, L., et al.: Recurrences after initial dislocation of the shoulder. J. Bone Joint Surg., *65*:343, 1983.

Hovelius, L.: Anterior dislocation of the shoulder in teenagers and young adults. J. Bone Joint Surg., *64*:254, 1982.

Hurley, J.A., and Anderson, T.E.: Shoulder arthroscopy: its role in evaluating shoulder disorders in the athlete. Am. J. Sports Med., *18(6)*:480, 1990.

Inglis, A.E., Ranawat, C.S., and Straub, L.R.: Synovectomy and debridement of the elbow in rheumatoid arthritis. J. Bone Joint Surg., *53A*:652, 1971.

Jobe, F.W., Giangarra, C.E., Kivtna, R.S., and Glousman, R.E.: Anterior capsulolabral reconstruction of the shoulder in athletes in overhand sports. Am. J. Sports Med., *19*:428, 1991.

Jobe, F.W., Perry, J., and Pink, M.: Electromyographic shoulder activity in men and women professional golfers. Am. J. Sports Med., *17(6)*:782, 1989.

Johnson, L.L.: Shoulder arthroscopy. *In* Arthroscopic Surgery Principles & Practice. Edited by E.A. Klein, K.H. Falk, and T. O'Brien. St. Louis, CV Mosby, 1986.

Kennedy, J.C., Hawkins, R., and Krissoff, W.B.: Orthopaedic manifestations of swimming. Am. J. Sports Med., *6(6)*:309, 1978.

Kerwein, G.A., Rosenburg, B., and Sneed, W.R.: Arthrographic studies of the shoulder joint. J. Bone Joint Surg., *39A*:1267, 1957.

Kessel, L., and Watson, M.: The painful arc syndrome. Clinical classification as a guide to management. J. Bone Joint Surg., *59B(2)*:166, 1977.

Klein, A., et al.: Measurement of brachial plexus strain in arthroscopy of the shoulder. Arthroscopy, *3(1)*:45, 1987.

Kneeland, J.B., et al.: MR imaging of the shoulder: diagnosis of rotator cuff tears. Am. J. Radiol., *149(2)*:333, 1988.

Kohn, D.: The clinical relevance of glenoid labrum lesions. Arthroscopy, *3(4)*:223, 1987.

Lane, J.G., Sachs, R.A., and Riehl, B.: Arthroscopic staple capsulorrhaphy: a long-term follow-up. Arthroscopy, *7(3)*:324, 1991.

Lehman, R.C.: Shoulder pain in the elite weight lifter. Orthop. Trans., *14(3)*:685, 1990.

Leslie, B.M., Harris, J., and Driscoll, D.: Septic arthritis of the shoulder in adults. J. Bone Joint Surg., *71A*:1516, 1989.

Lindblom, K.: Arthrography and roentgenography in ruptures of the tendon of the shoulder joint. Acta Radiol., *20*:548, 1939.

Lindblom, K.: On the pathogenesis of ruptures of the tendon aponeurosis of the shoulder joint. Acta Radiol., *20*:548, 1939.

Lippmann, R.K.: Frozen shoulder, periarthritis, bicipital tenosynovitis. Arch. Surg., *47*:283, 1943.

Lohr, J.F., and Uhthoff, H.K.: The pathogenesis of degenerative rotator cuff tears. Orthop. Trans., *11*:237, 1987.

Mack, L.A., Gannon, M.K., Kilcoyne, R.F., and Matsen, F.A. III: Sonographic evaluation of rotator cuff: accuracy in patient without prior surgery. Clin. Orthop., *234*:21, 1988.

MacNab, I., and Rathbun, J.B.: The microvascular pattern of the rotator cuff. J. Bone Joint Surg., *52B*:540, 1970.

Maki, N.J.: Arthroscopic stabilization for recurrent shoulder instability. *In* Surgery of the Shoulder. Edited by Post, M., Morrey, B.F., and Hawkins, R.J. St. Louis, Mosby Yearbook, 1990.

Mann, D.L., and Littke, N.: Shoulder injuries in archery. Can. J. Sport Sci., *14(2)*:85, 1989.

Marshall, G.J., et al.: Synovisol as an irrigant for electrosurgery of joints. Arthroscopy, *4(3)*:187, 1988.

Matsen, F.A. III: Personal communication.

Matthews, L.S., et al.: Arthroscopic staple capsulorrhaphy for recurrent anterior shoulder instability. Arthroscopy, *4(2)*:106, 1988.

McCarty, D.J., et al.: Milwaukee shoulder. Association of microspheroids containing hydroxyapatite crystals, active collagens and neutral protease with rotator cuff defects. J. Clin. Aspects Arthritis Rheum., *24*:464, 1981.

McGlynn, F.J., and Caspari, R.B.: Arthroscopic findings in the subluxing shoulder. Clin. Orthop., *183*:173, 1984.

McKendry, R.J.R., Uhthoff, H.K., Sarkar, K., and Hyslop, T.S.: Calcifying tendinitis of the shoulder: prognostic value of clinical, histologic, and radiologic features in 57 surgically treated cases. J. Rheumatol., *9*:75, 1982.

McLaughlin, H.L.: Lesions of the musculotendinous cuff of the shoulder: observations of the pathology, course and treatment of calcific deposits. Ann. Surg., *124*:354, 1946.

McLaughlin, H.L.: Lesions of the musculotendinous cuff of the shoulder. I. The exposure and treatment of tears with retraction. J. Bone Joint Surg., *26*:41, 1944.

McLaughlin, H.L.: Rupture of the rotator cuff. J. Bone Joint Surg., *44A*:979, 1962.

McLaughlin, H.L., and Asherman, E.G.: Lesions of the musculotendinous cuff of the shoulder. IV. Some observations based upon the results of surgical repair. J. Bone Joint Surg., *33A*:76, 1951.

McMaster, W.C.: Anterior glenoid labrum damage: a painful lesion in swimmers. Am. J. Sports Med., *14(5)*:383, 1986.

McShane, R.B., Leinberry, C.F., and Fenlin, J.M.: Conservative open anterior acromioplasty. Clin. Orthop., *233*:137, 1987.

Mendoza, F.X., Nicholas, J.A., and Rubinstein, M.P.: Arthroscopic treatment of stage II subacromial impingement. Orthop. Trans., *12(3)*:732, 1988.

Meyer, A.W.: Spontaneous dislocation and disruption of tendon of long head of biceps brachii: 59 instances. Arch. Surg., *17*:493, 1928.

Middleton, W.D., et al.: Ultrasonography of the rotator cuff: technique and normal anatomy. J. Ultrasound Med., *3*:549, 1984.

Mikasa, M.: Trapezius transfer for global tear of the rotator cuff. *In* Surgery of the Shoulder. Edited by J.E. Bateman and R.P. Welsh. Philadelphia, B.C. Decker, 1984.

Miniaci, A., and MacDonald, P.B.: Open surgical techniques in the athlete's shoulder. Clin. Sports Med., *10(4)*:929, 1991.

Mink, J., Harris, E., and Rappaport, M.: Rotator cuff tear evaluation using double contrast shoulder arthrography. Radiology, *157*:621, 1985.

Montgomery, T.J., Savoie, F.H., and Yerger, B.: A Comparison of Arthroscopic Debridement with Open Surgical Repair for Full Thickness Tears of the Rotator Cuff. Presented at the 8th Open Meeting, American Shoulder and Elbow Surgeons, Washington, D.C., February 1992.

Moran, M.C., and Warren, R.F.: Development of a synovial cyst after arthroscopy of the shoulder. J. Bone Joint Surg., *71A(1)*:127, 1989.

Morgan, C.D., and Bodenstab, A.B.: Arthroscopic Bankart suture repair: technique and early results. Arthroscopy, *3(2)*:111, 1987.

Morgan, C.D., Rames, R., and Snyder, S.: Arthroscopic Assessment of Anatomic Variations of the Glenohumeral Ligaments Associated with Recurrent Anterior Shoulder Instability. Presented at The American Shoulder and Elbow Surgeons Meeting, Washington, D.C., 1992.

Morrison, D.S., and Schaefer, R.K.: Relationship between subacromial space pressure, blood pressure and visual clarity during arthroscopic subacromial decompression. Orthop. Trans., *14*:564, 1990.

Moseley, H.F.: Ruptures of the rotator cuff. Br. J. Surg., *38*:340, 1951.

Moseley, H.F., and Goldie, I.: The arterial pattern of the rotator cuff. J. Bone Joint Surg., *45B*:780, 1963.

Moseley, H.F., and Overgaard, B.: The anterior capsular mechanism in recurrent anterior dislocation of the shoulder. J. Bone Joint Surg., *44B*:913, 1962.

Moynes, D.R., et al.: Electromyography and motion analysis of the upper extremity in sports. Phys. Ther., *66(12)*:1905, 1986.

Mullins, R.C., Drez, D., and Cooper, J.: Hypoglossal nerve palsy after arthroscopy of the shoulder and open operation with the patient in the beach-chair position. J. Bone Joint Surg., *74A*:137, 1992.

Neer, C.S. II: Shoulder Reconstruction. Philadelphia, W.B. Saunders, 1990.

Neer, C.S. II: Impingement lesions. Clin. Orthop., *173*:70, 1983.

Neer, C.S. II: Unfused acromial epiphysis in impingement and cuff tears. American Academy of Orthopedic Surgeons, Instructional Course, 1978.

Neer, C.S. II: Anterior acromioplasty for the chronic impingement syndrome in the shoulder. A preliminary report. J. Bone Joint Surg., *54A*:41, 1972.

Neer, C.S. II: Displaced proximal humeral fractures. J. Bone Joint Surg., *52A*:1077, 1970.

Neer, C.S., and Foster, C.R.: Inferior capsular shift for involuntary inferior and multidirectional instability of the shoulder. J. Bone Joint Surg., *62A*:897, 1980.

Neer, C.S. II, and Poppen, N.K.: Supraspinatus outlet. Orthop. Trans., *11*:234, 1987.

Neer, C.S., and Welsh, M.B.: The shoulder in sports. Orthop. Clin. North Am., *8(3)*:583, 1977.

Neer, C.S. II, Craig, E.V., and Fukuda, H.: Cuff tear arthropathy. Orthop. Trans., *5*:447, 1981.

Neer, C.S. II, Flatow, E.L., and Lech, O.: Tears of the rotator cuff: long-term results of anterior acromioplasty and repair. Presented at the Fourth Open Meeting of the American Shoulder and Elbow Surgeons, Atlanta, February 1988.

Neviaser, J.S.: Ruptures of the rotator cuff of the shoulder. New concepts in the diagnosis and operative treatment of chronic tears. Arch. Surg., *102*:483, 1971.

Neviaser, J.S., Neviaser, R.J., and Neviaser, T.J.: The repair of chronic massive ruptures of the rotator cuff of the shoulder by use of a freeze-dried rotator cuff. J. Bone Joint Surg., *60A*:681, 1978.

Neviaser, R.J., and Neviaser, T.J.: The frozen shoulder diagnosis and management. Clin. Orthop., *223*:59, 1987.

Neviaser, R.J., and Neviaser, T.J.: Transfer of subscapularis and teres minor for massive defects of the rotator cuff. *In* Shoulder Surgery. Edited by I. Bayley and L. Kessel. Berlin, Springer-Verlag, 1982.

Neviaser, R.J., Neviaser, T.J., and Neviaser, J.S.: Concurrent rupture of the rotator cuff and anterior dislocation of the shoulder in the older patient. J. Bone Joint Surg., *70A*:1308, 1988.

Neviaser, T.J.: Weight lifting. Risks and injuries to the shoulder. Arthros Update, *10(3)*:615, 1991.

Neviaser, T.J., and Neviaser, R.J.: The diagnosis and treatment of incomplete rotator cuff tears. Orthop. Trans., *15*:239, 1989.

Norwood, L., and Fowler, L.: Rotator cuff tears. A shoulder arthroscopy complication. Am. J. Sports Med., *17(6)*:837, 1989.

Nuber, G.W., et al.: Fine wire electromyography analysis of muscles of the shoulder during swimming. Am. J. Sports Med., *14*:7, 1986.

O'Driscoll, S.W., Evans, D.C., and Scarborough, O.N.: Long term results of the staple capsulorrhaphy: twenty years experience in the Toronto teaching hospitals. Orthop. Trans., *12*:674, 1988.

Ogilvie-Harris, D.J., and Boynton, E.: Arthroscopic acromioplasty extravasation of fluid into the deltoid muscle. Arthroscopy, *6(1)*:52, 1990.

Ogilvie-Harris, D.J., and Wiley, A.M.: Arthroscopic surgery of the shoulder: a general appraisal. J. Bone Joint Surg., *68B*:201, 1986.

Olson, E., and Fu, F.: Complication and pitfalls in shoulder arthroscopic operative techniques. Orthopedics, *1(3)*:253, 1991.

Packer, N.P., Calvert, P.T., Bayley, J.I.L., and Kessel, L.: Operative treatment of chronic ruptures of the rotator cuff of the shoulder. J. Bone Joint Surg., *65B(2)*:171, 1983.

Pappas, A.M., Goss, T.P., and Kleinman, P.K.: Symptomatic shoulder instability due to lesions of the glenoid labrum. Am. J. Sports Med., *11(5)*:279, 1983.

Patte, D., Debeyre, J., and Goutallier, D.: Rotator cuff repair by muscle advancement. *In* Shoulder Surgery. Edited by I. Bayley and L. Kessel. Great Britain, Springer-Verlag, 1982.

Paulos, L.E., and Franklin, J.L.: Arthroscopic shoulder decompression—development and application. A five year experience. Am. J. Sports Med., *18(3)*:235, 1990.

Paulos, L.E., Chamberlain, S., and Murray, S.: Arthroscopic subacromial decompression. Orthop. Trans., *10*:222, 1986.

Petersson, C.J., and Gentz, C.F.: Ruptures of the supraspinatus tendon. The significance of distally pointing acromioclavicular osteophytes. Clin. Orthop., *174*:143, 1983.

Pinals, R.F., and Short, C.L.: Calcific periarthritis involving multiple sites. Arthritis Rheum., *9*:566, 1966.

Pink, M., et al.: The normal shoulder during freestyle swimming. An electromyographic and cinematographic analysis of twelve muscles. Am. J. Sports Med., *19(6)*:569, 1991.

Pitman, M.I., et al.: The use of somatosensory evoked potentials for detection of neuropraxia during shoulder arthroscopy. Arthroscopy, *4(4)*:250, 1988.

Post, M.: The Shoulder. Surgical and Nonsurgical Management. Philadelphia, Lea & Febiger, 1988.

Post, M., and Cohen, J.: Impingement syndrome—a review of late State II and early Stage III lesions. Clin. Orthop., *207*:126, 1986.

Post, M., Silver, R., and Singh, M.: Rotator cuff tear. Diagnosis and treatment. Clin. Orthop., *173*:78, 1983.

Priest, J.D.: The shoulder of the tennis player. Clin. Sports Med., *7(2)*:387, 1988.

Raggio, C.L., Warren, R.F., and Sculco, T.: Surgical treatment of impingement syndrome: four-year follow-up. Orthop. Trans., *9*:48, 1985.

Reagan, B.F., et al.: Irrigating solutions for arthroscopy. J. Bone Joint Surg., *65A*:629, 1983.

Reider, B., and Inglis, A.E.: The Bankart procedure modified by the use of Prolene pull-out sutures. J. Bone Joint Surg., *64A(4)*:628, 1982.

Reiser, M., et al.: Role of magnetic resonance imaging in the diagnosis of shoulder joint injuries. Radiologe, *28(2)*:79, 1988.

Resch, H., Kadletz, R., Beck, E., and Helweg, G.: Single and double-contrast CT scanning in the examination of recurrent shoulder dislocations. Unfallchirurg, *89*:441, 1982.

Resnick, D.: Shoulder arthrography. Radiol. Clin. North Am., *19*:243, 1981.

Richardson, A.R., Jobe, F.W., and Collins, H.R.: The shoulder in competitive swimming. Am. J. Sports Med., *8*:159, 1980.

Rockwood, C.A.: Shoulder arthroscopy. Editorial. J. Bone Joint Surg., *12*:731, 1988.

Rockwood, C.A., and Burkhead, W.Z.: Management of patients with massive rotator cuff defects by acromioplasty and rotator cuff debridement. Orthop. Trans., *12*:190, 1988.

Rockwood, C.A., and Matsen, F.A.: The Shoulder. Philadelphia, W.B. Saunders, 1990.

Rockwood, C.A., Jr., et al.: X-ray evaluation of shoulder problems. *In* The Shoulder. Edited by C.A. Rockwood, Jr., and F.A. Matsen III. Philadelphia, W.B. Saunders, 1990.

Rodosky, M.W., et al.: The role of the biceps-superior glenoid labrum complex in anterior stability of the shoulder. Pittsburgh Orthop. J., *1*:57, 1990.

Rose, D.J.: Arthroscopic suture capsulorrhaphy for anterior shoulder instability. Orthop. Trans., *14(3)*:597, 1990.

Rothman, R.H., and Parke, W.W.: The vascular anatomy of the rotator cuff. Clin. Orthop., *41*:176, 1965.

Rowe, C.R., Patel, D., and Southmayd, W.W.: The Bankart procedure: a long-term end-result study. J. Bone Joint Surg., *60A(1)*:1, 1978.

Ryu, R.K.N.: Arthroscopic subacromial decompression: a clinical review. Arthroscopy, *8(2)*:141, 1992.

Ryu, R.K., et al.: An electromyographic analysis of shoulder function in tennis players. Am. J. Sports Med., *16(5)*:481, 1988.

Samilson, R.L.: Rotator cuff tears: management and end results of over 400 cases. J. Bone Joint Surg., *62B*:277, 1984.

Sampson, T.G., Nisbet, J.K., and Glick, J.M.: Precision acromioplasty in arthroscopic subacromial decompression of the shoulder. Arthroscopy, *7(3)*:301, 1991.

Scarpinato, D.F., Bramhall, J.P., and Andrews, J.R.: Arthroscopic management of the throwing athlete's shoulder: indications, techniques, and results. Clin. Sports Med., *10(4)*:913, 1991.

Scovazzo, M.L., et al.: The painful shoulder during freestyle swimming. Am. J. Sports Med., *19(6)*:577, 1991.

Seeger, L.L., et al.: MR imaging of the normal shoulder. Am. J. Radiol., *148*:83, 1987.

Seeger, L.L., Gold, R.H., Bassett, L.W., and Ellman, H.: Shoulder impingement syndrome: MR findings in 53 shoulders. Am. J. Radiol., *150*:343, 1988.

Sherman, O.H., et al.: Arthroscopy—"no problem surgery." An analysis of complications in two thousand six hundred and forty cases. J. Bone Joint Surg., *68A*:256, 1986.

Silliman, J.F., and Hawkins, R.J.: Current concepts and recent advances in the athlete's shoulder. Clin. Sports Med., *10(4)*:693, 1991.

Simonet, W.T., and Cofield, R.H.: Prognosis in anterior shoulder dislocation. Am. J. Sports Med., *12(1)*:19, 1984.

Small, N.C.: Complications in arthroscopic surgery performed by experienced arthroscopists. Arthroscopy, *4*:215, 1988.

Small, N.C.: Complications in arthroscopy: the knees and other joints. Committee on complications of the Arthroscopy Association of North America. Arthroscopy, *2*:253, 1986.

Smith, J.G.: Pathological appearances of seven cases of injury of the shoulder joint with remarks. London Medical Gazette, *14*:280, 1834 (reported in Am. J. Med. Sci., *16*:219, 1834).

Snyder, S.J., et al.: Arthroscopic Acromioclavicular Joint Debridement and Distal Clavicle Resection Utilizing the Claviculizer™. Presented at the American Academy of Orthopedic Surgeons, February, 1992.

Snyder, S.J., et al.: Partial-thickness rotator cuff tears: results of arthroscopic treatment. Arthroscopy, *7*:1, 1991.

Snyder, S.J., et al.: SLAP lesions of the shoulder. Arthroscopy, *6(4)*:274, 1990.

Steinbrocker, O., Traeger, C.H., and Batterman, R.C.: Therapeutic criteria for rheumatoid arthritis. JAMA, *140*:659, 1949.

Takagishi, N.: Conservative treatment of the ruptures of the rotator cuff. J. Jpn. Orthop. Assoc., *52*:781, 1978.

Thorling, J., et al.: Acromioplasty for impingement syndrome. Acta Orthop. Scand., *56*:147, 1985.

Tibone, J.E., et al.: Surgical treatment of tears of the rotator cuff in athletes. J. Bone Joint Surg., *68A*:887, 1986.

Tibone, J.E., Jobe, F.W., and Kerlan, R.F.: Shoulder impingement syndrome in athletes treated by anterior acromioplasty. Clin. Orthop., *188*:134, 1985.

Tijmes, J., Loyd, H.M., and Tullos, H.S.: Arthrography in acute shoulder dislocations. South. Med. J., *72*:564, 1979.

Townsend, H., et al.: Electromyographic analysis of the glenohumeral muscles during a baseball rehabilitation program. Am. J. Sports Med., *19(3)*:264, 1991.

Turkel, S.J., et al.: Stabilizing mechanisms preventing anterior dislocation of the glenohumeral joint. J. Bone Joint Surg., *63A*:1208, 1981.

Uhthoff, H.K., Lohr, J., and Sarkar, K.: The pathogenesis of rotator cuff tears. *In* The Shoulder. Edited by N. Takagishi. Tokyo, Professional Postgraduate Services, 1987.

Uhthoff, H.K., Sarkar, K., and Maynard, J.A.: Calcifying tendinitis: a new concept of its pathogenesis. Clin. Orthop., *118*:164, 1976.

Van Holsbeeck, E., et al.: Subacromial impingement: open versus arthroscopic decompression. Arthroscopy, *8(2)*:173, 1992.

Warner, J.P., and Warren, R.F.: Arthroscopic Bankart repair using a cannulated, absorbable fixation device. Operative Techniques in Orthopedics, *1(2)*:192, 1991.

Warren, R.F., and Marshall, J.L.: Athletic injuries of the shoulder. Surg. Rounds, 34, 1978.

Warren, F.W., et al.: Arthroscopic acromioplasty: a prospective analysis of 43 patients. Proc. Am. Acad. Orthop. Surg. 56th Annual Meeting, Las Vegas, February 1989.

Weaver, J.K.: Skiing-related injuries to the shoulder. Clin. Orthop., *216*:24, 1987.

Weiner, D.S., and MacNab, I.: Superior migration of the humeral head. A radiological aid in the diagnosis of tears of the rotator cuff. J. Bone Joint Surg., *52B(3)*:524, 1970.

Wheeler, J.H., et al.: Arthroscopic versus nonoperative treatment of acute shoulder dislocations in young athletes. Arthroscopy, *5(3)*:213, 1989.

Whipple, T.L.: Arthroscopic Treatment of Acromioclavicular Joint Arthritis. Presented at the Arthroscopy Association of North America, Boston, April, 1992.

Whiting, W.C., Gregor, R.J., and Finerman, G.A.: Kinematic analysis of human upper extremity movements in boxing. Am. J. Sports Med., *16(2)*:130, 1988.

Wiley, A.M.: Arthroscopy for shoulder instability and a technique for arthroscopic repair. Arthroscopy, *4(1)*:25, 1988.

Wilson, P.D.: Complete rupture of the supraspinatus tendon. JAMA, *96*:433, 1931.

Wolfgang, G.L.: Rupture of the musculotendinous cuff of the shoulder. Clin. Orthop., *134*:230, 1978.

Wolfgang, G.L.: Surgical repair of tears of the rotator cuff of the shoulder. Factors influencing the results. J. Bone Joint Surg., *56A*:14, 1974.

Wolin, P.M.: Arthroscopic glenoid labrum suture repair. Orthop. Trans., *14(3)*:597, 1990.

Yahiro, M.A., and Matthews, L.S.: Arthroscopic stabilization procedure for recurrent anterior shoulder instability. Orthop. Rev., *18(11)*:1161, 1989.

Yamanaka, K., and Fukuda, H.: Pathological studies of the supraspinatus tendon with reference to incomplete thickness tears. Proc. 3rd International Conference on Surgery of the Shoulder, Fukuoka, Japan, October 1986.

Zuckerman, J.D., and Matsen, F.A.: Complications about the glenohumeral joint related to the use of screws and staples. J. Bone Joint Surg., *66A*:175, 1984.

INDEX

Note: Page numbers in *italics* indicate figures; t indicates tables.